Covid-19 and Dentistry: Oral Health Impacts, Management and Future Preparedness

Covid-19 and Dentistry: Oral Health Impacts, Management and Future Preparedness

Editor: Alicia Dexter

hayle medical

New York

Hayle Medical,
750 Third Avenue, 9th Floor,
New York, NY 10017, USA

Visit us on the World Wide Web at:
www.haylemedical.com

ISBN 978-1-64647-557-5 (Hardback)

Cataloging-in-Publication Data

Covid-19 and dentistry : oral health impacts, management and future preparedness / edited by Alicia Dexter.
p. cm.
Includes bibliographical references and index.
ISBN 978-1-64647-557-5
1. Dentistry. 2. COVID-19 (Disease)--Complications. 3. Mouth--Care and hygiene.
4. Mouth--Diseases. 5. Mouth--Diseases--Treatment. I. Dexter, Alicia.

RK51.5 .C68 2023
617.6--dc23

Contents

Preface

In my initial years as a student, I used to run to the library at every possible instance to grab a book and learn something new. Books were my primary source of knowledge and I would not have come such a long way without all that I learnt from them. Thus, when I was approached to edit this book; I became understandably nostalgic. It was an absolute honor to be considered worthy of guiding the current generation as well as those to come. I put all my knowledge and hard work into making this book most beneficial for its readers.

Coronavirus disease (COVID-19) refers to a type of contagious respiratory disease caused through the SARS-CoV-2 virus. The virus is transmitted from an infected person to a healthy person through droplets released while sneezing, coughing and speaking. The practice of dentistry has been seriously impacted by the COVID-19 outbreak, majorly due to the generation of large amounts of droplets and aerosols combined with the patient's blood or saliva during dental procedures. Dental professionals are at a high risk since SARS-CoV-2 has been found in the saliva of infected people. There is a high risk of cross infection between patients and dental health care personnel (DHCP) because of the characteristics of dental environments. Thus, it is likely to trigger changes in the delivery of dental care in the future, such as changes in layout and workflow of dental clinics. This book provides comprehensive insights on the impact of Covid-19 on dentistry. It is appropriate for students seeking detailed information on oral health impacts, management and future preparedness regarding this virus in the field of dentistry. Those in search of information to further their knowledge will be greatly assisted by this book.

I wish to thank my publisher for supporting me at every step. I would also like to thank all the authors who have contributed their researches in this book. I hope this book will be a valuable contribution to the progress of the field.

Editor

1

The Dental Team: An Additional Resource for Delivering Vaccinations

Stefan Serban[1,2], Zhain Mustufvi[1], Jing Kang[1], Sally Eapen Simon[2], Siobhan Grant[2] and Gail Douglas[1]*

[1] *School of Dentistry, University of Leeds, Leeds, United Kingdom,* [2] *Public Health England, North East and Yorkshire Regional Office, Leeds, United Kingdom*

Keywords: COVID-19, coronavirus, dentistry, dental team, vaccinations, influenza, flu, immunisation

***Correspondence:**
Stefan Serban
s.t.serban@leeds.ac.uk

INTRODUCTION

Influenza is regarded by the World Health Organization (WHO) as a "serious global health threat" and is responsible for a significant number of deaths worldwide (1, 2). Influenza vaccines are usually delivered in primary care physician practices as well as in pharmacy settings. Dental practices are generally not seen as routine providers of influenza vaccines, although certain countries have been recently starting to develop frameworks to facilitate this (3, 4). Potential workforce capacity gaps, expansion of the eligible cohorts, requirement to drive improvements in uptake, and to reduce inequalities support the rationale for members of the dental team to join the vaccinator workforce. We propose a few potential models, some of which are currently being piloted in certain areas of the United Kingdom, and suggest that the members of the dental team might be ideally placed to contribute to national immunization programs.

The coronavirus pandemic has had a devastating effect on people's lives, pushing the limits of healthcare systems and placing enormous economic and political pressures on governments. As with other pandemics throughout history it has also highlighted the vulnerabilities of our society and forced us to reflect on our values and priorities, compelling us to develop new ways of delivering care, adapted to the new realities of the world around us (5). Face to face consultations became the exceptions and remote consultations the new norm (6). Thousands of clinical and non-clinical staff have been redeployed from their usual workplace into new settings to support the pandemic response (7).

In several countries around the world, the multi-skilled dental workforce has demonstrated that dentistry is ready to support the national health systems response in a time of emergency (8, 9). Members of the dental team were redeployed based on their set of competencies into various roles including medical history taking, phlebotomy, cannulation, suturing, and others (10). A properly trained and indemnified dental workforce would be ideally placed to support the delivery of the flu vaccination program for the next season (11). In 2009, during the H1N1 (swine flu) pandemic a precedent has been established when certain US states commissioned dentists to administer flu vaccines in order to increase capacity for delivery and meet the increased demand in a short time frame (12, 13).

DELIVERY MODELS

The delivery models for seasonal flu vaccinations and for school vaccination programs vary between different healthcare systems around the globe. The next section presents some of the models that are currently being explored in the UK. These could be adapted for different healthcare settings based on the existing structures and processes developed nationally (14). The members of the dental team could support the delivery of the seasonal influenza vaccine, as well as other immunization programs such as the childhood vaccination program and potentially the large-scale delivery of COVID-19 vaccines, should a safe and effective vaccine become available in the future.

Flu Vaccinations

Every year, the arrival of autumn means also the beginning of the flu season. Seasonal influenza has been a constant challenge for healthcare systems across the world and it is estimated to be responsible for nearly 400,000 deaths every year world-wide (2).

The uptake of influenza vaccines varies between different countries. The most accurate and comparable data is on vaccination rates for people over the age of 65. These rates present large variations from 10.2% in Estonia to 85.1% in South Korea (15). This year, national health systems are facing the risk of a dual threat created by seasonal influenza and the potential resurgence of COVID-19, which could have devastating effects especially in the high-risk groups. Certain governments have recognized this threat and established a set of preventative measures. For example, the UK Government has decided to expand the eligibility criteria for influenza vaccinations to include additional groups in the national immunization schemes. These additional groups consist of all people over the age of 50, people who are shielding from COVID-19 and their households, as well as secondary school children in England. This represents an estimated total of 30 million people, which represent an increase of 5 million people compared to the previous year (16, 17). This broadening of the eligibility criteria would lead to operational and logistical challenges for delivery in a timely manner. Expanding the workforce capacity to include the members of the dental team could attenuate some of these challenges.

The following models might serve as potential avenues that could be explored by policy makers in different countries.

Provision of Additional Personnel for Local Delivery Programs

Additional health protection measures have been imposed by COVID-19, such as dental surgery fallow time after an aerosol generating procedure and increased decontamination demands (18, 19). As a result, some dental teams may be utilizing less personnel and therefore these staff members could join existing immunization teams to deliver vaccinations in various settings such as schools, primary care, and specially allocated community settings. This would increase the available workforce capacity to deliver vaccinations in a short time frame. This is an important advantage as to maximize protection for the entire flu season, it would be essential to cover as many eligible people as possible as soon as the vaccines become available in the first few months of the season (20, 21). The most cost-effective solution would be to utilize dental nurses or hygienists/therapist to support this model however we believe that the option to administer vaccinations should be available to all members of the dental team as long as they are properly trained, competent, and indemnified.

Use of Premises

Dental surgeries represent a large network of clinical settings that are known and easily accessible to the public. Evidence suggests that certain cohorts of patients visit the dental surgery more frequently than their general physician (22). Larger dental surgeries are likely to have capacity in terms of surgery or floor space that could be used temporarily by immunization teams. Dental practices are also well-equipped to deal with rare but serious adverse reactions.

One-Stop Shop

Patients could choose to receive their influenza vaccine at the same time as their dental appointment. This model would support the principle of reduction of the number of contacts between patients and healthcare settings and reduce the risks associated with multiple journeys, especially in more rural areas where traveling longer distances is often required. It could be done both opportunistically as well as in a targeted manner for specific cohorts. This approach has already been successfully implemented in certain states in the US (13).

Childhood Immunization Programs

Besides helping the delivery of influenza vaccines, members of the dental team could be deployed to support the catch-up initiatives for childhood immunization programs. In several countries around the world, the COVID-19 pandemic has led to school closures for a significant amount of time and this has created a backlog in terms of delivering immunization programs for school aged children with the increased risk of community outbreaks (23).

COVID-19 Vaccinations

It is believed that a COVID-19 vaccine would be the best way to speed up the economic recovery and protect public health from the damage caused by the pandemic. The race to develop a safe and effective coronavirus vaccine has demonstrated the need for innovative thinking and collaboration between researchers from different scientific disciplines (24). The success or failure of any large-scale immunization program depends on the uptake of the vaccines by the majority of the population and it will raise significant logistic challenges (25, 26). If the above-mentioned models for flu vaccination could be piloted and evaluated, the lessons learned from these initiatives could inform the planning and delivery of a large-scale COVID-19 mass immunization program, with a vaccinator workforce which included dental team members.

DISCUSSION

Any of the above models would need to take into consideration certain factors such as:

- Approval from the regulatory bodies of dental care providers and professional indemnity providers;
- Approval from national regulatory agencies for medicines;
- Information governance and access to clinical data including patients' full medical history and robust intra-operability between data systems across dental and medical systems;
- Clear funding mechanism.

Research into the effectiveness, safety and cost-effectiveness of these interventions should be encouraged in order to inform future evidence-based decisions. Any service evaluation should also include a qualitative component for capturing the experiences of the new dental vaccinators as well the views of the existing vaccinating teams and patients.

It has become clear that the coronavirus pandemic highlighted the stark inequalities in our society. It was marked by a strong socioeconomic gradient, affecting disproportionately the most vulnerable groups. Public health measures such as prevention and health promotion are the among the key interventions to reduce the impact of inequalities (27, 28). Dental leaders have long been advocating the idea of "putting the mouth back in the body" (29, 30). There is a short window of opportunity, before the beginning of the flu season, to explore the untapped resource of the dental workforce in supporting the delivery of an enhanced immunization program. There is no better time to consider innovative solutions aimed to challenge the traditional boundaries between the different parts of the healthcare system (31). This is a crucial time to reconsider the segregated models of the past and move toward more integration of resources to support the uptake of one of the largest flu vaccination programs to date (32). Seasonal influenza has the potential to place additional strains on the health and social care systems which were already hard-hit by the coronavirus pandemic. This is the time to design preventative measures to mitigate the dual threat caused by influenza and COVID-19 and to think holistically about the resources available in the healthcare system. Engaging the dental team for delivering influenza vaccinations could further strengthen the collaboration between medicine and dentistry and is likely to set an important precedent to meet the demands of future public health crisis.

AUTHOR CONTRIBUTIONS

SS prepared the first draft of the manuscript. All the other co-authors contributed with comments and approved the final version.

REFERENCES

1. The World Health Organization. *Global Influenza Strategy 2019-2030*. (2019). Available online at: https://www.who.int/influenza/Global_Influenza_Strategy_2019_2030_Summary_English.pdf?ua=1 (accessed September, 2020).
2. Paget J, Spreeuwenberg P, Charu V, Taylor RJ, Iuliano AD, Bresee J, et al. Global mortality associated with seasonal influenza epidemics: New burden estimates and predictors from the GLaMOR Project. *J Glob Health*. (2019) 9:020421. doi: 10.7189/jogh.09.020421
3. Oregon State Legislature. *Relating to Vaccines Administered by Dentists; and Declaring an Emergency*. (2019). Available online at: https://olis.leg.state.or.us/liz/2019R1/Measures/Overview/HB2220. (accessed September, 2020).
4. The Scottish Government. *Memorandum to NHS: PCA(D)(2020)12*. (2020). Available online at: https://www.sehd.scot.nhs.uk/pca/PCA2020(D)12.pdf (accessed September, 2020).
5. Snowden FM. *Epidemics and Society: From the Black Death to the Present*. New Haven, CT; London: Yale University Press (2019).
6. Greenhalgh T, Wherton J, Shaw S, Morrison C. Video consultations for covid-19. *BMJ*. (2020) 368:m998. doi: 10.1136/bmj.m998
7. Adams JG, Walls RM. Supporting the health care workforce during the COVID-19 global epidemic. *JAMA*. (2020) 323:1439–40. doi: 10.1001/jama.2020.3972
8. Hurley S. Why re-invent the wheel if you've run out of road? *Br Dent J*. (2020) 228:755–6. doi: 10.1038/s41415-020-1646-z
9. Yang Y, Zhou Y, Liu X, Tan J. Health services provision of 48 public tertiary dental hospitals during the COVID-19 epidemic in China. *Clin Oral Investig*. (2020) 24:1861–4. doi: 10.1007/s00784-020-03267-8
10. Johnston L, Archer N, Martin K. Swapping drills for dressings: redeployment of dentists to community nursing. *Br J Community Nurs*. (2020) 25:266–70. doi: 10.12968/bjcn.2020.25.6.266
11. NHS. *Redeploying the Clinical Dental Workforce to Support the NHS Clinical Delivery Plan for COVID-19*. (2020). Available online at: https://www.england.nhs.uk/coronavirus/wp-content/uploads/sites/52/2020/04/C0301-Permissions-Redeploying-our-people-clinical-dental-workforce-v2.pdf (accessed July, 2020).
12. The Boston Globe. *State Takes Extra Steps to Battle Flu in Fall*. (2009). Available online at: http://archive.boston.com/news/health/articles/2009/08/13/state_asks_volunteers_to_aid_flu_vaccinations/ (accessed July, 2020).
13. Simon L, editor. *How Will Dentistry Respond to the Coronavirus Disease 2019 (COVID-19) Pandemic?*. JAMA Health Forum. American Medical Association (2020).
14. Serban S, Eapen-Simon S, Grant S. Dental team immunisation. *Br Dent J*. (2020) 229:209. doi: 10.1038/s41415-020-2071-z
15. The Organisation for Economic Co-operation and Development (OECD). *Influenza Vaccination Rates*. (2018). Available online at: https://data.oecd.org/healthcare/influenza-vaccination-rates.htm#indicator-chart (accessed September, 2020).
16. UK Government Press Office. *Most Comprehensive Flu Programme in UK History will be Rolled out This Winter*. (2020). Available online at: https://www.gov.uk/government/news/most-comprehensive-flu-programme-in-uk-history-will-be-rolled-out-this-winter (Accessed July, 2020).
17. UK Government Press Office. *25 Million to be Offered Free NHS Flu Jab This Winter*. (2019). Available online at: https://www.gov.uk/government/news/25-million-to-be-offered-free-nhs-flu-jab-this-winter (accessed September, 2020).
18. Meng L, Hua F, Bian Z. Coronavirus disease 2019 (COVID-19): emerging and future challenges for dental and oral medicine. *J Dent Res*. (2020) 99:481–7. doi: 10.1177/0022034520914246
19. Cochrane Oral Health Group. *Recommendations for the Re-opening of Dental Services: A Rapid Review of International Sources*. (2020). Available online at: https://oralhealth.cochrane.org/news/recommendations-re-opening-dental-services-rapid-review-international-sources (accessed September, 2020).
20. National Institute for Health and Care Excellence. *Flu Vaccination: Increasing Uptake*. (2018). Available online at: https://www.nice.org.uk/guidance/ng103/resources/flu-vaccination-increasing-uptake-pdf-66141536272837 (accessed September, 2020).
21. Dexter LJ, Teare MD, Dexter M, Siriwardena AN, Read RC. Strategies to increase influenza vaccination rates: outcomes of a nationwide cross-sectional survey of UK general practice. *BMJ Open*. (2012) 2:e000851. doi: 10.1136/bmjopen-2011-000851
22. Yonel Z, Sharma P, Yahyouche A, Jalal Z, Dietrich T, Chapple IL. Patients' attendance patterns to different healthcare settings and perceptions of stakeholders regarding screening for chronic, non-communicable diseases in high street dental practices and community pharmacy: a cross-sectional study. *BMJ Open*. (2018) 8:e024503. doi: 10.1136/bmjopen-2018-024503
23. Joint Committee on Vaccination and Immunisation. *Statement on the Delivery of the HPV Vaccine*. (2020). Available online at: https://www.gov.uk/government/publications/delivery-of-the-hpv-vaccine-and-impact-of-school-closures-statement-from-the-jcvi/joint-committee-on-vaccination-and-immunisation-statement-on-the-delivery-of-the-hpv-vaccine (accessed July, 2020).
24. Michie S, West R. Behavioural, environmental, social, and systems interventions against covid-19. *BMJ*. (2020) 370:m2982. doi: 10.1136/bmj.m2982

25. Constable C, Caplan A. Comparison of the implementation of human papillomavirus and hepatitis B vaccination programs in the United States: implications for future vaccines. *Vaccine.* (2020) 38:954–62. doi: 10.1016/j.vaccine.2019.11.073
26. Wigle J, Coast E, Watson-Jones D. Human papillomavirus (HPV) vaccine implementation in low and middle-income countries (LMICs): health system experiences and prospects. *Vaccine.* (2013) 31:3811–7. doi: 10.1016/j.vaccine.2013.06.016
27. Van Lancker W, Parolin Z. COVID-19, school closures, and child poverty: a social crisis in the making. *Lancet Public Health.* (2020) 5:e243–e4. doi: 10.1016/S2468-2667(20)30084-0
28. UK Government. *Prevention is Better than cuRe - Matt Hancock's Speech to the International Association of National Public Health Institutes.* (2018). Available online at: https://www.gov.uk/government/speeches/prevention-is-better-than-cure-matt-hancocks-speech-to-ianphi (accessed July, 2020).
29. Hurley S. Enhanced role for oral health in imminent NHS long-term plan. *BDJ.* (2018) 225:689. doi: 10.1038/sj.bdj.2018.943
30. Donoff B, McDonough JE, Riedy CA. Integrating oral and general health care. *N Engl J Med.* (2014) 371:2247–9. doi: 10.1056/NEJMp1410824
31. Lamster IB, Myers-Wright N. Oral health care in the future: expansion of the scope of dental practice to improve health. *J Dent Educ.* (2017) 81:eS83–eS90. doi: 10.21815/JDE.017.038
32. Watt RG, Serban S. Multimorbidity: a challenge and opportunity for the dental profession. *Br Dent J.* (2020) 229:282–6. doi: 10.1038/s41415-020-2056-y

2

The Impact of the COVID-19 Epidemic on Orthodontic Patients in China: An Analysis of Posts on Weibo

Feiyang Guo [1†], Bojun Tang [1†], Danchen Qin [1†], Tingting Zhao [1], Yu-xiong Su [2], Colman McGrath [3], Fang Hua [4,5] and Hong He [1*]*

[1] Department of Orthodontics, Hubei-MOST KLOS & KLOBM, School & Hospital of Stomatology, Wuhan University, Wuhan, China, [2] Discipline of Oral and Maxillofacial Surgery, Faculty of Dentistry, The University of Hong Kong, Hong Kong, China, [3] Applied Oral Sciences & Community Dental Care, Faculty of Dentistry, The University of Hong Kong, Hong Kong, China, [4] Center for Evidence-Based Stomatology, Hubei-MOST KLOS & KLOBM, School & Hospital of Stomatology, Wuhan University, Wuhan, China, [5] Division of Dentistry, School of Medical Sciences, Faculty of Biology, Medicine and Health, University of Manchester, Manchester Academic Health Science Centre, Manchester, United Kingdom

Correspondence:
Fang Hua
huafang@whu.edu.cn
Hong He
drhehong@whu.edu.cn

† These authors have contributed equally to this work

Background: During the COVID-19 pandemic, many dental care services including orthodontic practice were suspended. Orthodontic patients turned to social media platforms to communicate, share experiences, and look for solutions. Our study aimed to investigate the attitudes and perspectives of orthodontic patients during the COVID-19 epidemic in China by analyzing orthodontics-related posts on Sina Weibo (a Chinese counterpart of Twitter).

Materials and Methods: Potentially eligible posts on Sina Weibo platform were collected between December 30, 2019, and April 18, 2020. Posts related to both orthodontics and COVID-19 were included and then coded and classified into specific appliances and themes. Geographic and temporal distributions of the included posts were analyzed. In addition, time-lagged cross correlation was performed to explore the association between the number of daily posts and daily new COVID-19 cases/deaths in China. Chi-square tests were employed to compare the differences between fixed appliances and aligners in *problems/difficulties* and *feelings* during the epidemic.

Results: Of the 28,911 posts identified, 4,484 were included in the analysis. The most frequently mentioned themes were *appointments* ($n = 2,621$, 58.5%), *negative feelings* ($n = 2,189$, 48.8%), and *problems/difficulties* ($n = 1,155$, 25.8%). A majority of posts were tweeted in regions with high levels of economic development and population density in eastern China and from February to March. The number of daily posts had a significantly positive correlation with daily new COVID-19 cases/deaths in China ($P < 0.05$). Compared with clear aligners, patients with fixed appliances reported more *problems/difficulties* ($P < 0.001$) and *negative feelings* ($P < 0.001$), but fewer *positive feelings* ($P < 0.001$).

Conclusions: The analysis of Weibo posts provided a timely understanding of the impact of COVID-19 on orthodontic patients. Delayed appointments were their greatest concern, and negative feelings and untreated orthodontic problems increased during the suspension of dental care services. However, patients with clear aligners reported fewer negative feelings and problems than those with fixed appliances. The findings highlighted the need to consider both treatment- and psychology-related issues of orthodontic patients and how to handle them appropriately during the epidemic.

Keywords: COVID-19, orthodontics, social media, dental care, online health

INTRODUCTION

The coronavirus disease 2019 (COVID-19) caused by severe acute respiratory syndrome coronavirus 2 (SARS-CoV-2) has spread rapidly throughout the world and triggered a global pandemic after being discovered in Wuhan, China, in December 2019 (1). The coronavirus showed high contagiousness and rapid spread, and as of June 9, 2020, the World Health Organization (WHO) reported 7,039,918 confirmed COVID-19 cases and 404,396 deaths (2).

The characteristics of dental practices, such as close face-to-face communication, droplet- and aerosol-generating procedures, and contaminated surfaces, expose dental patients and practitioners to high levels of pathogenic microorganisms and high risks of cross infection (3, 4). In addition, standard precautions are insufficient to protect practitioners and patients from the infection of COVID-19, which brings great challenges to dental services in this period (3). Therefore, most epidemic-attacked regions in China enforced strict regulations to dental health services in late January 2020, which only permitted emergent dental services (4). After 2 months of effective anti-epidemic efforts, China moved into a mitigation stage in April (5), and dental facilities began to gradually resume routine services under strict protective measures.

Scheduled orthodontic appointments and most orthodontic problems were deemed nonemergent; thus, most orthodontic departments and clinics were suspended during the epidemic (6). During the time of orthodontic practice suspension and home quarantine, many orthodontists and patients were at home and communicated by smartphones or online telemedicine services (4, 7). Given the failure to attend regular appointments, orthodontic problems such as loosening of brackets and archwires could not be treated timely in this long period of dental service suspension (6), which had a considerable impact on the lives and treatments of orthodontic patients. Therefore, being aware of patients' mental and physical conditions was necessary for orthodontists to give appropriate suggestions to patients during the epidemic and to prioritize the needs of patients after dental service reopening.

Social media have shown unique advantages in the dissemination of information, and the activities on social media platforms have increased sharply in the special period of transportation restriction and home quarantine (8). As a Chinese counterpart of Twitter, Sina Weibo is a popular social media platform that allows users to share their experiences, opinions, and perspectives, as well as to follow and communicate with others (9). The large scale of users, huge volume of information, and availability of free and immediate access have made it possible for researchers to investigate the public perception of public health events such as MERS-CoV and H7N9 through Sina Weibo (10). In addition, Weibo, regarded as an ideal tool to search large-scale, comprehensive information in a short time, was widely adopted in research related to impact of COVID-19 on public opinions, dental service, and psychology (11–13).

Previous studies have indicated that the COVID-19 epidemic had a negative impact on the public (14, 15). However, to our knowledge, its impact on orthodontic patients has not been explored, and Weibo has not been applied in the orthodontic field before. Therefore, this study aimed to investigate attitudes and perspectives of orthodontic patients during the COVID-19 epidemic, by analyzing the geographic location, time, and content of orthodontic-related posts on Weibo during the COVID-19 epidemic in China.

MATERIALS AND METHODS

Ethics

This study was approved by the Ethics Committee of School & Hospital of Stomatology, Wuhan University (no. 2020-B46). As the study utilized open information on the Internet, personal privacy and clinical data of the research subjects were not involved. Therefore, an exemption for informed consent was granted (11).

Data Collection

Potentially eligible posts were searched and collected retrospectively by two authors (F.G. and B.T.) from the Sina Weibo platform between December 30, 2019, and April 18, 2020. We used 9 keywords regarding COVID-19 and 10 keywords about orthodontics (**Table 1**), which were searched in

TABLE 1 | Keywords for searching the posts (translated from Chinese).

COVID-19-related keywords	Orthodontic-related keywords
Pneumonia	Orthodontics
Novel coronavirus	Correction
Virus	Orthodontic treatment
Epidemic	Invisalign®[a]
Anti-epidemic	Angelalign®[b]
Epidemic prevention	Braces
Battle against the epidemic	Brackets
COVID-19	Archwires
NCP (novel coronavirus pneumonia)	Oral myofunction
	Sleep disordered breathing

[a] *Align Technology, Santa Clara, CA, USA.*
[b] *EA Medical Instruments, Shanghai, China.*

TABLE 2 | Main themes and specific appliances for coding with definition and example.

Category[a]	Definition	Example
Main theme[b]		
Problems/difficulties	Problems related to orthodontic treatment	"…epidemic… The rubber bands have been used up. And the wire deformed when I just ate the braised chicken."
Appointments	Able/unable to attend orthodontic appointments	"…I haven't made an appointment of my appliances for 3 months because of the epidemic…."
Negative feelings	Obvious emotional words and/or emoticons expressing negative feelings	"If it wasn't for the epidemic, I would have started orthodontic treatment! I'm mad!!!"
Positive feelings	Obvious emotional words and/or emoticons expressing positive feelings	"…because of this epidemic…Finally I got the new aligners and my treatment will soon come to an end. I can see the dawn of victory!"
Contact with dentists	Able/unable to contact the dentist during the epidemic	"…clinics provided the online follow-up consultation warm-heartedly and professionally, and send new aligners and rubber bands…"
Consultation	Orthodontic consultation with netizens for advice	"I can't see the dentist during the epidemic and found my teeth becoming a little bit irregular. I want to ask what's wrong with my teeth ?"
Orthodontic plans	Plans for orthodontic treatment after the epidemic	"I'm not afraid of tooth extraction, I just want to put on braces after pneumonia"
Others	Other COVID-19- and orthodontic-related posts could not be classified into the above-mentioned themes, e.g., routine records	"Today is my 496th day of wearing Invisalign®. During the epidemic, I persisted in wearing aligners and now I'm wearing the 49th maxillary and 57th mandibular aligner."
Specific appliances[c]		
Fixed appliances	Posts with key words indicating fixed appliances, for example, brackets or archwires	"My brackets are lost! Pain! Please let the epidemic end soon!"
Clear aligners	Posts with key words indicating clear aligners, for example, Invisalign® or Angelalign®	"…This is the 11th week to wear Invisalign®…"
Retainers	Posts with key words indicating retainers	"…My retainer on the table was thrown by others…I can't get another pair during the epidemic"

[a] *A post could be classified into both main theme and specific appliances.*
[b] *A post was classified into more than one main theme if containing miscellaneous information.*
[c] *Only posts that contained key indicating words and could be identified as a specific type of appliances were coded.*

combinations (i.e., one COVID-19 keyword combined with one orthodontic keyword). A Python-based platform Gooseeker was employed to collect all the Weibo posts and extract data from each post, including Weibo number, Weibo username, full-text content, posting date, and location tag (optional when posting). In addition to the location tag, we also extracted geographic location information from full-text posts.

After the collection of posts, duplicate posts were initially removed by Microsoft Excel (2019), and then the remaining posts were screened by two authors (F.G. and D.Q.) to identify eligible posts. As decided *a priori*, only Weibo posts pertaining to both COVID-19 and the users' own orthodontic experience were included. Posts not related to COVID-19 (e.g., other types of pneumonia or other viral infections), irrelevant to orthodontic experience (e.g., prosthodontic treatment or other dental experience), posted by dental professionals, containing advertisements, or having a geographic location outside of China were excluded.

Coding Procedure

The included posts were read iteratively to familiarize two authors (F.G. and D.Q.) with the contents before coding. Inductive and deductive manual coding approaches were used (16). Initial primary coding categories for type of appliances and post contents were developed based on our study objective and previous research (17–19). Each category had several main themes (**Table 2**). A pilot coding on a subset of posts (10% randomly selected posts) was then conducted independently and in duplicate by two authors (F.G. and D.Q.) using the predetermined codes. Posts that could not be categorized with the initial codes were given a new code. Any disagreement was resolved via discussion with two experts (F.H. and H.H.). After coding, data were examined to identify potential subcategories within each primary category.

Prior to the formal coding procedure, 60 randomly selected posts were coded by two authors (F.G. and D.Q.) independently and in duplicate to achieve an agreement on the understanding of themes and subthemes. Thereafter, all posts were coded and sorted into primary categories and/or subcategories by the same two authors. If new codes emerged during this procedure, the temporary coding categories would be revised accordingly. All disagreements in classification and naming of themes and subthemes were resolved by discussion with two experts (F.H. and H.H.).

Data Analysis

Descriptive statistics were performed to summarize the characteristics of the included posts. For geographic distribution analysis, the number of posts with location was compared with the cumulative number of COVID-19 cases in each region of China. Epidemiological data were retrieved from the

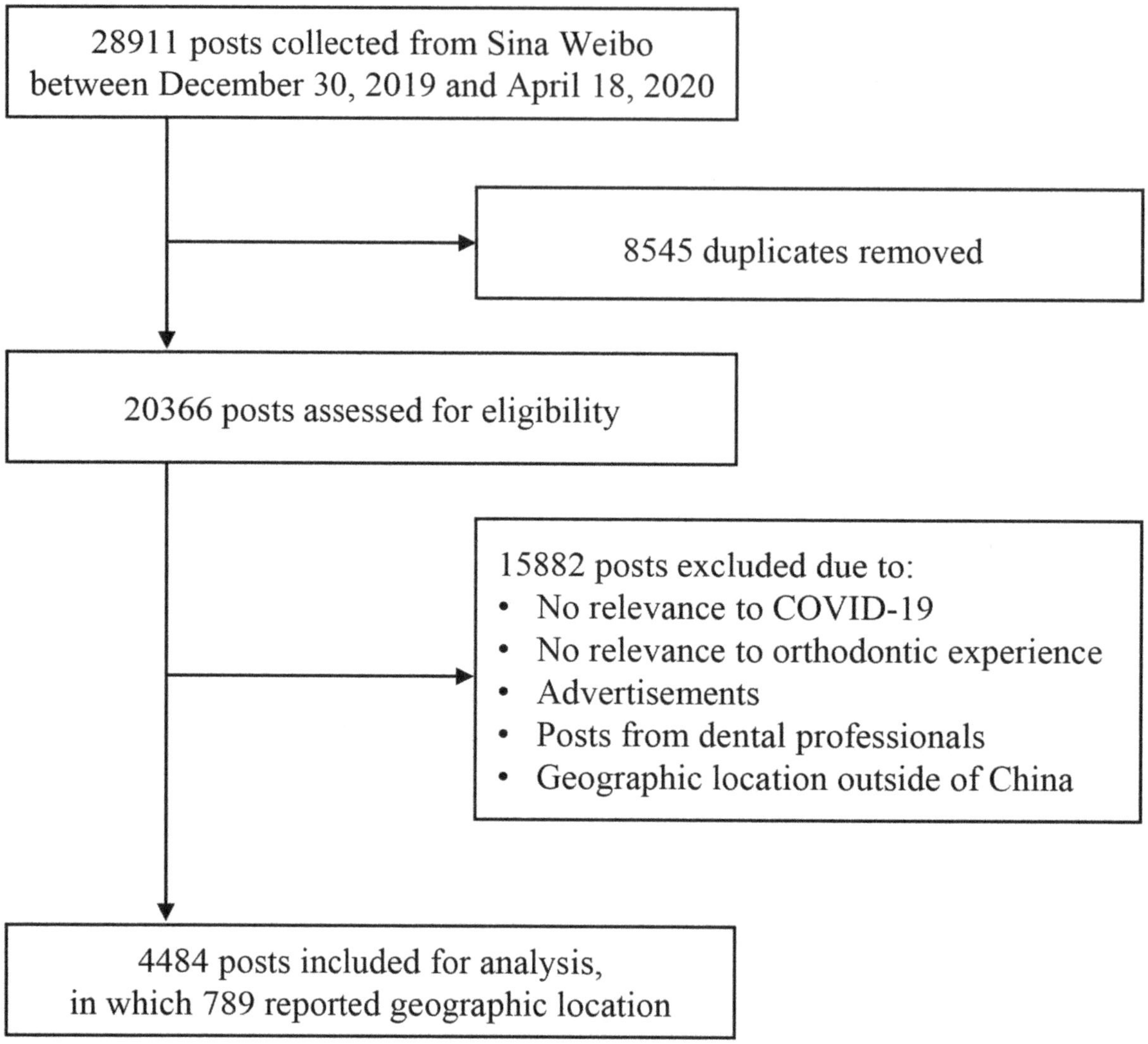

FIGURE 1 | Flow chart of posts selection.

official website of the Chinese Center for Disease Control and Prevention (CCDC) (5).

Temporal distribution analysis was performed to (1) present the change of number of posts and confirmed new COVID-19 cases/deaths each day in China; (2) display the daily number of posts related to orthodontic problems; (3) compare the daily number of posts of *positive feelings* with that of *negative feelings*; and (4) analyze the number of posts each day related to ability (able or unable) to attend an appointment during the epidemic. Time-lagged cross correlation (TLCC) was used to investigate the association between daily number of posts and daily confirmed new COVID-19 cases/deaths in China.

Chi-square tests were employed to compare the differences between fixed appliances and aligners in *problems* and *positive* and *negative feelings*. IBM SPSS Statistics 23.0 was used for statistical analysis, and a two-tailed $P < 0.05$ was considered significant.

RESULTS

Inclusion and Basic Characteristics of Posts

A total of 28,911 Weibo posts were collected, of which 4,484 were finally included in the analysis (**Figure 1**). Although we identified 305 posts regarding oral myofunction or sleep disordered breathing, none of these posts were concerning orthodontics. Among 4,484 included posts, 1,835 could be identified and coded as a specific type of appliances, in which 786 (42.8%) were related to fixed appliances, 985 (53.7%) clear aligners, and 64 (3.5%) retainers (**Table 3**).

Geographic Distribution of Posts

Among the 4,484 included posts, only 789 (17.6%) reported geographic information. The results of geographic distribution analysis are presented in **Figure 2**. In western China with

TABLE 3 | Number of posts for specific appliances (n = 1,835)[a].

Appliances	Number	Percentage (%)
Fixed appliances	786	42.8%
Clear aligners	985	53.7%
Retainers	64	3.5%
Total	1,835	100%

[a]*Among 4,484 included posts, 1,835 could be identified as a specific type of appliances and were coded.*

<100 COVID-19 cases confirmed, posts were less frequently distributed. More than half of the posts containing location information were posted from eastern China, where four provinces (Guangdong, Beijing, Shanghai, and Shandong) had the most posts (>60). However, <40 posts were from Hubei, the original epicenter and worst-affected province of COVID-19 in China.

Frequency of Main Themes and Subthemes

Figure 3 illustrates the percentage of posts in each main theme. The most frequently mentioned themes were *appointments* (n = 2,621, 58.5%), *negative feelings* (n = 2,189, 48.8%), *problems/difficulties* (n = 1,155, 25.8%), and *positive feelings* (n = 750, 16.7%). *Negative feelings* were reported 3 times more frequently than *positive feelings*. Only a few posts mentioned *contact with dentists* (n = 196, 4.4%) and *consultation* (n = 146, 3.3%).

The frequency and distribution of subthemes within each main theme are shown in **Table 4**. Among the 1,155 posts related to *problems/difficulties*, the most commonly listed issue was "loose brackets or archwires" (n = 479, 41.5%), followed by "shortage of subsequent aligners" (n = 268, 23.2%) and "poking archwires or ligatures" (n = 175, 15.2%). In terms of 2,126 Weibo posts regarding *appointments*, three-quarters were regarding "unable to attend an appointment" (n = 1,875, 71.5%). However, only a relatively small proportion of posts mentioned being "able to attend an appointment" (n = 747, 28.5%). In accordance with the *appointments* and *problems/difficulties*, 2,189 posts expressed feelings in a negative tone, in which most of them were related to treatment delay (n = 1,933, 88.3%), followed by "complaint about pain from orthodontic appliances" (n = 132, 6.0%).

In 750 posts related to *positive feelings*, one-third were concerning clear aligners, including "pleased to get new aligners during the epidemic" (n = 149, 19.9%) and "convenience/comfort of clear aligners" (n = 115, 15.3%). "Excellent dental care service," with key words such as "warm-hearted" and "careful," was mentioned 10 times more commonly than "poor dental care service" (217 vs. 20). Other reasons for positive feelings were "looking forward to ending orthodontic treatment" (n = 135, 18.0%) and "pleased to attend an appointment" (n = 131, 17.5%). Moreover, according to 196 posts with respect to *contact with dentists*, most patients could contact their dentists (n = 180, 91.8%) and make online consultation or face-to-face appointments with them, whereas a few lost contacts with their dentists (n = 16, 8.2%).

Temporal Distribution of Weibo Posts and Specific Themes

The temporal distribution of Weibo posts is presented in **Figure 4A**. No posts were identified before January 21. Then the number of posts began to increase from late January to early February, which was in accordance with the trend of daily new COVID-19 cases/deaths. The number of posts maintained a steady high level for 2 months, about 60 to 80 posts per day. In late March, the number of posts started to decline gradually.

The trend of posts related to *problems/difficulties* during this period (**Figure 4B**) was consistent with that of total posts. The number of posts related to orthodontic problems reached a plateau between mid-February and mid-March and then gradually declined. *Positive and negative feelings* showed opposite trends during the epidemic (**Figure 4C**). Posts related to *negative feelings* increased sharply in late January and early February and decreased gradually in late March, while those regarding *positive feelings* rocketed in late February. Similar trends were seen in *appointments* (**Figure 4D**), in which posts related to "unable to attend an appointment" increased quickly in late January and decreased in late March and those regarding "able to attend an appointment" started to increase gradually in early March.

As **Table 5** shows, the total number of daily posts was significantly correlated with the daily new cases ($r = 0.323$) and deaths ($r = 0.555$) in lag (−2) ($P < 0.05$), which suggested that the increase in the number of posts happened 2 days before that of new cases or deaths. *Negative feelings* also rose 2 days before the increase of deaths ($r = 0.287$, $P < 0.05$) but were not significantly associated with daily new cases. In addition, the number of posts regarding positive feelings showed a significant negative correlation with daily new cases ($r = -0.331$) and deaths ($r = -0.272$) in lag (5), which indicated that *positive feelings* increased 5 days after the decline of daily new cases or deaths.

Comparison Between Fixed Appliances and Clear Aligners

As shown in **Table 6**, 75.4% of the posts regarding fixed appliances reported problems arising during the epidemic and only 35.4% of those regarding clear aligners. The difference in *problems/difficulties* between the two appliances was significant ($P < 0.001$). For positive feelings, 44.9% of aligners expressed *positive feelings*, which were significantly more than that of fixed appliances (8.8%, $P < 0.001$). On the contrary, the difference between two appliances in *negative feelings* was significant ($P <$ 0.001), as more fixed appliances (70.9%) were related to *negative feelings* compared with clear aligners (28.9%). Moreover, posts of fixed appliances expressed more *negative feelings* than *positive feelings*, while clear aligners were in the opposite situation.

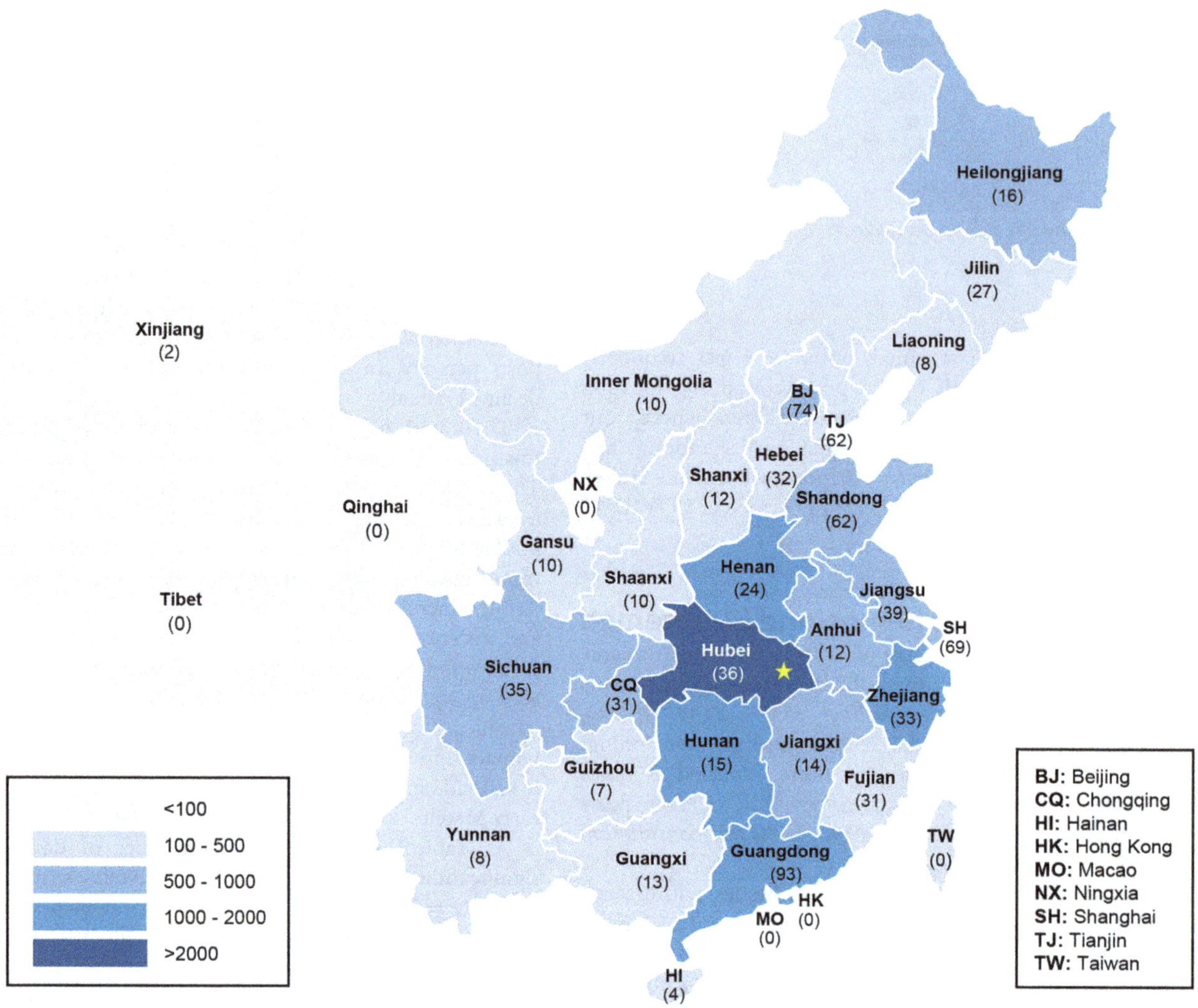

FIGURE 2 | Geographic distribution of Weibo posts and total cases of COVID-19 in China ($n = 789$). The number of posts in each region is presented in parentheses. The gradient of colors displays the cumulative number of confirmed COVID-19 cases (by June 3). The yellow star marks the location of Wuhan.

DISCUSSION

Orthodontic Services and the COVID-19 Pandemic

The outbreak of COVID-19 has brought about considerable changes to people's daily life. To control and prevent the spread of COVID-19, in late January, Chinese authorities imposed traffic restriction and appealed to the public to take a series of actions, including self-isolation and quarantine, social distancing, and mask-wearing in public places (20). The outbreak of disease and changes in life are reported to have a psychological impact on the public, such as panic, anxiety, and depression (21, 22).

For orthodontic patients, except for the above-mentioned situations, orthodontics-related problems were also their main concerns. Relevant governments in most regions in China set regulations on dental care services during the epidemic, and all elective dental treatments were suspended including orthodontic practice (4, 23). As a result of the regulation of dental practice as well as travel restriction, orthodontic patients could not attend an appointment on a routine basis, leaving problems untreated and with consequences for a prolonged duration of treatment.

About 1 month after the outbreak of COVID-19, as the epidemic was controlled in most provinces, the regulations began to relax and dental care services gradually resumed in these regions. To investigate the attitudes and perspectives of orthodontic patients during the COVID-19 epidemic, we have adopted a new data search platform, social media Weibo. The application of Weibo in orthodontic research can fit well with the COVID-19 epidemic, due to its advantages in studying population-level health behaviors, social opinions, and public responses to health issues in a timely and dynamic way. Therefore, 4,484 included posts in Sina Weibo were collected between December 30, 2019, and April 18, 2020, about 1 month

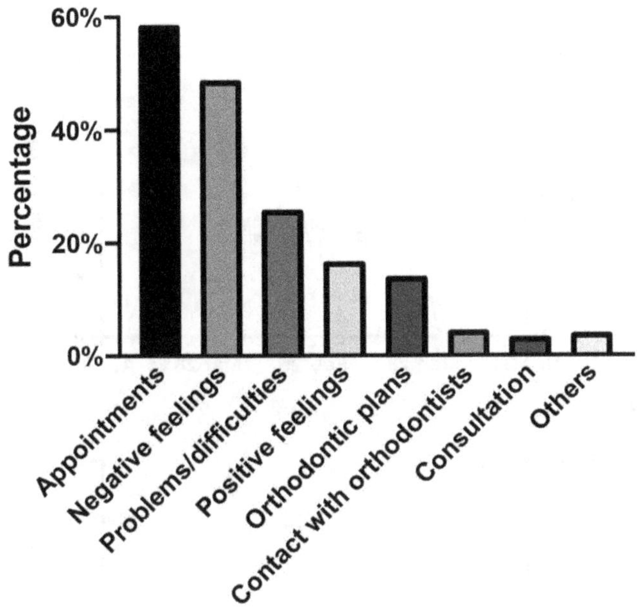

FIGURE 3 | Percentage of posts in each main theme (n = 4,484).

TABLE 4 | Frequency and distribution of subthemes within each main theme (n = 4,484).

Main theme	Total	Subtheme	*N* (%)
Problems/difficulties[a]	1,155	Loose brackets or archwires	479 (41.5%)
		Shortage of subsequent aligners	268 (23.2%)
		Poking archwires or ligatures	175 (15.2%)
		Broken appliances	72 (6.2%)
		Loss of aligners/retainers	55 (4.8%)
		Insufficient rubber bands	34 (2.9%)
		Aligners worn irregularly	32 (2.8%)
		Failed attachments	29 (2.5%)
		Loose temporary anchorage devices	23 (2.0%)
		Unfit aligners	13 (1.1%)
		Others	54 (4.7%)
Appointments	2,621	Unable to attend an appointment	1,875 (71.5%)
		Able to attend an appointment	746 (28.5%)
Negative feelings[a]	2,189	Negative feelings toward treatment delay	1,933 (88.3%)
		Complaint about pain from orthodontic appliances	132 (6.0%)
		Concerns about orthodontic visits during the epidemic	110 (5.0%)
		Fear of the COVID-19 epidemic	23 (1.1%)
		Poor dental care services	20 (0.9%)
		Others	54 (2.5%)
Positive feelings[a]	750	Excellent dental care service	217 (28.9%)
		Pleased to get new aligners during the epidemic	149 (19.9%)
		Looking forward to ending orthodontic treatment	135 (18.0%)
		Pleased to attend an appointment	131 (17.5%)
		Convenience/comfort of clear aligners	115 (15.3%)
		Others	126 (16.8%)
Contact with dentists	196	Able to contact dentists	180 (91.8%)
		Losing contact with dentists	16 (8.2%)

[a]A post was classified into more than one subtheme if containing miscellaneous information.

before the outbreak and after the relief of COVID-19, to provide insights into the changes in the influence of COVID-19 on orthodontic patients during the period of the progression and remission of the epidemic.

Distribution of Weibo Posts

In this study, posts were mainly from eastern regions that generally had a high level of economic development and population density in China. Three province-level regions including Guangdong, Beijing, and Shanghai posted 2 to 3 times more posts than did Hubei, the most virus-hit province. A previous study focusing on the Weibo posts with COVID-19-related oral health information showed a similar geographic distribution (12). Guangdong, Beijing, and Shanghai are the most economically developed and densely populated areas in China, and more people used Weibo to express their opinions during the epidemic (11). In addition, since orthodontic treatment is relatively expensive and not covered under health insurance in China, more people in these regions with better economic condition receive orthodontic treatment; economically developed regions also have more dental hospitals and clinics and therefore have more orthodontic patients (23). As people were more sensitive to epidemic and social events in these areas with a large population, convenient transportation, and high network penetration, negative feelings caused by epidemic were more likely to emerge (11, 14). Thereby, attention should be paid to the psychological management of orthodontic patients from developed regions.

The trend of Weibo posting was associated with the pattern of reports of daily new cases and death cases of COVID-19, which can be divided into three main stages: rising, stable, and falling. This trend was similar to a previous study on H7N9-related posts on Weibo (24). After the official confirmation of human-to-human transmission of COVID-19 on January 20 and the steep rise in the number of newly confirmed cases, the number of daily posts increased substantially from late January to early February. Then the number of posts reached a plateau and lasted until mid-March, about half a month after the initial control of the epidemic. During this period, most dental practices were suspended as well as orthodontic treatment, and orthodontic patients could only consult via online services (4). As the daily new COVID-19 cases decreased to a relatively low level and dental services began to resume in less-affected regions, the number of posts gradually declined.

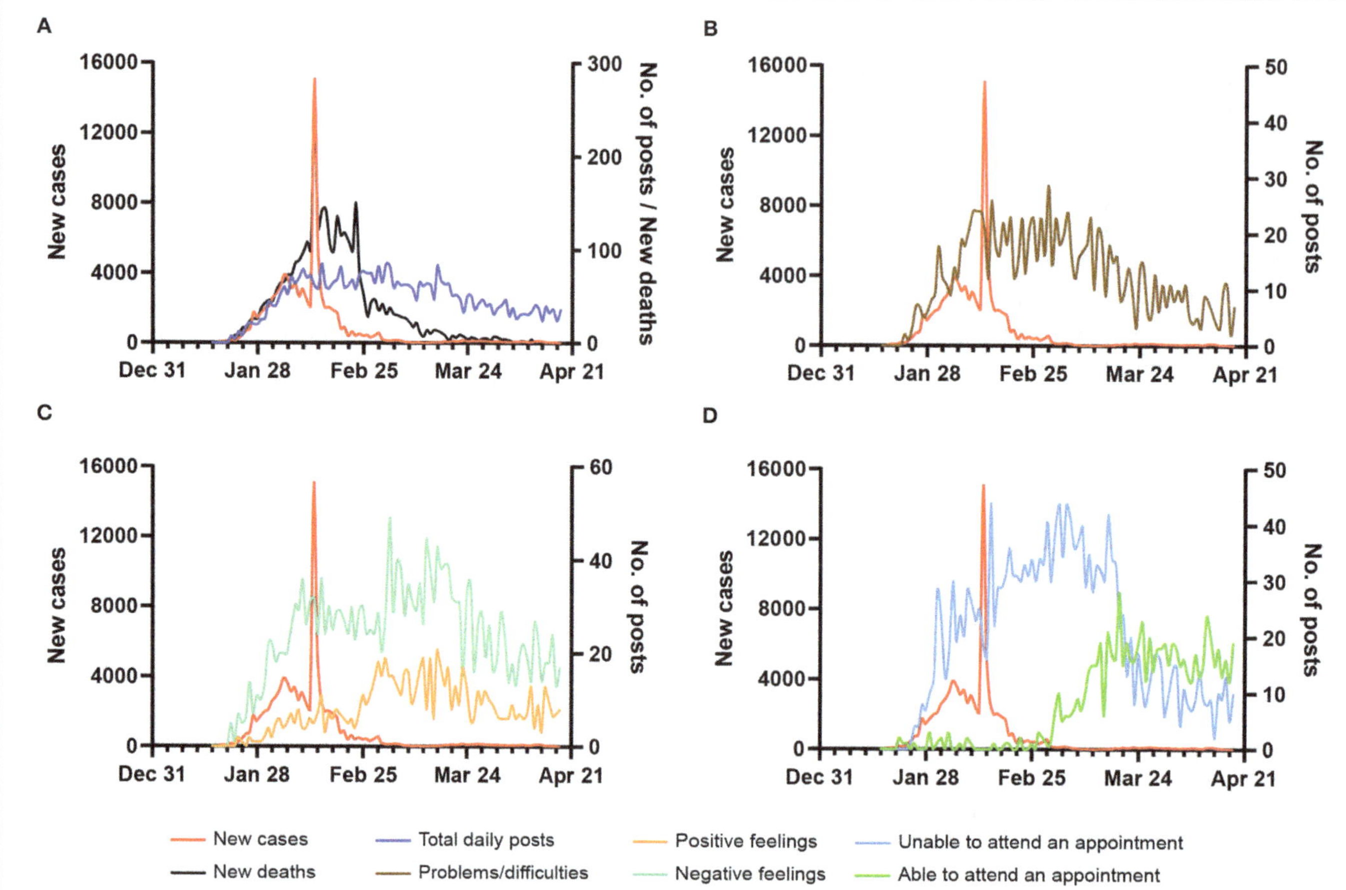

FIGURE 4 | Number of Weibo posts and daily new COVID-19 cases/deaths in China. Total number of posts **(A)**, and number of posts related to problems **(B)**, positive and negative feelings **(C)** and if able to attend an appointment **(D)** are compared with daily new cases/deaths.

TABLE 5 | Time-lag correlation coefficients between the number of posts and daily new confirmed COVID-19 cases or daily new deaths (n = 4,484)[a].

Lag	−5	−4	−3	−2	−1	0	1	2	3	4	5
Daily new cases											
Total number of posts	**0.297**	**0.265**	**0.249**	**0.323**[b]	**0.229**	0.201	0.196	0.149	0.141	0.073	−0.004
Positive feelings	−0.183	−0.174	**−0.238**	−0.141	−0.182	**−0.231**	**−0.241**	**−0.290**	**−0.320**	**−0.275**	**−0.331**[b]
Negative feelings	0.099	0.120	0.074	0.138	0.050	0.079	0.050	−0.019	0.011	−0.052	−0.100
Daily new deaths											
Total number of posts	**0.517**	**0.533**	**0.517**	**0.555**[b]	**0.517**	**0.502**	**0.499**	**0.440**	**0.421**	**0.393**	**0.322**
Positive feelings	−0.013	−0.028	−0.097	−0.063	−0.106	−0.148	−0.157	−0.203	**−0.237**	**−0.228**	**−0.272**[b]
Negative feelings	**0.225**	**0.263**	**0.228**	**0.287**[b]	**0.244**	**0.260**	**0.238**	0.175	0.182	0.130	0.086

[a] *Values in bold are statistically significant (<0.05).*

[b] *The largest correlation between the number of posts and daily new confirmed COVID-19 cases or daily new deaths among different time lags.*

As aforementioned, time of each fluctuation of the number of posts was related to the date of major events, especially regulations about dental practice. Likewise, during the "hepatitis B vaccine crisis," the trend of public reactions on Weibo was also influenced by the number of deaths and the suspension of relevant vaccine (25). In addition, we found a moderate positive correlation between the number of posts and negative feelings and that of new cases or deaths 2 days before and a negative association between positive feelings and number of new cases and deaths 5 days after. Our findings suggest that the popularity of Weibo topics related to COVID-19 and orthodontics was associated with the severity of the COVID-19 epidemic (11), and the implementation of public health interventions could have an impact on patients' reaction to their treatment and feelings in outbreaks of diseases (25).

The Content of Weibo Posts

In our study, the most frequent reasons for tweeting were delayed appointments and expression of negative feelings. Negative feelings were mainly toward treatment delay including worries about missing appointments, annoyance arising from orthodontic problems, and extension of the duration. A recent study has suggested that the COVID-19 epidemic impacted orthodontic appointments and provoked patients' anxiety, and the biggest concern of over half of the patients was also the delay of treatment (26).

Due to the suspension of orthodontic practices during the epidemic, lots of orthodontic problems remained untreated. A previous study showed that the need for orthodontic treatment ranked second in all dental problem-related Weibo posts during the epidemic (12). In our study, a quarter of posts mentioned orthodontic problems, in which loose brackets and archwires were the most common problems. However, some orthodontic procedures that are aerosol generating were still restricted in high-risk regions after the resumption of orthodontic practice. Therefore, to reduce nosocomial infection, orthodontists should give priority to deal with the patients whose treatment would not have aerosol generated after work resumption and avoid appointments with patients whose treatment was restricted (27).

Telemedicine, the approach of online consultation and remote management of patients, developed rapidly and was widely applied during the COVID-19 epidemic (6, 7). However, in this study, a few patients stated that they were unable to contact their dentists, which compromised patients' confidence in treatment (28, 29). Thus, orthodontists should provide patients with correct contact information in case of any emergent situation. In addition, due to the high risk of infection in dental settings, patients may hesitate to attend an appointment after work resumption (26). Therefore, online consultation may still serve as the main communication method at the beginning of work resumption and is also useful in patient triage in this busy time (30).

In summary, our study on the distribution and content of Weibo posts provided an updated understanding of the attitudes and perspectives of orthodontic patients during the COVID-19 epidemic. With accessible resources to acquire timely and large-scale information (13), the social media platform Weibo was recommended to be used by orthodontists to better understand the physical and psychological conditions of orthodontic patients as well as their needs (31). Given the suspension of routine dental practices, more patients with orthodontic problems would seek support and relevant information about treatment through the Internet. However, this online information remains to be doubtful and might be incorrect or unfounded (18). Previous research has indicated that Weibo was more efficient in disseminating information than conventional ways (24). Therefore, orthodontics can use Weibo to spread professional knowledge regarding the management of orthodontic emergencies, such as the use of orthodontic wax for poking archwires for patients, especially for those who lost contact with their orthodontists. Moreover, our findings can provide data based on which patient management during and after the epidemic can be optimized (29). Since adolescents who are a susceptible population of COVID-19 comprise the majority of orthodontic patients and asymptomatic COVID-19 infection may exist after the epidemic, strict infection control measures are necessary for orthodontists (30). Except for the management mentioned above (including restriction on aerosol-generated practices, online consultation, and strict precautions), it is also recommended to schedule patient appointments carefully and reduce the number of patients to avoid crowds gathering/waiting in the consultation area of dental hospitals and clinics.

TABLE 6 | Frequency and distribution in different themes between fixed appliances and aligners ($n = 1,771$).

Themes	Fixed appliances ($n = 786$)	Aligners ($n = 985$)	*P*
Problems/difficulties	593 (75.4%)	349 (35.4%)	<0.001
Positive feelings	69 (8.8%)	442 (44.9%)	<0.001
Negative feelings	557 (70.9%)	285 (28.9%)	<0.001

Differences Between Fixed Appliances and Clear Aligners

In the present study, clear aligners showed many advantages over fixed appliances during this epidemic; problems with clear aligners were significantly less than those with fixed appliances. Many patients chose fixed appliances due to lower cost and shorter treatment duration (32); however, they experienced high incidence of bracket detachment and poking archwires, which could not be treated timely during the epidemic (27). In contrast, the main concerns of aligners were shortage of aligners and aligner breakage, which were easier to manage during the lockdown period. Patients were required to extend the wearing time of each available aligner and to wear it carefully to avoid breakage, and after work resumption, they could get the remaining aligners on delivery without the need for an appointment (29). As for feelings, there was a significant difference in positive and negative feelings between fixed appliances and aligners, and patients with fixed appliances were more inclined to get anxious. Previous studies also suggested that aligners had less impact on patients' daily life, and patients felt more satisfaction and less discomfort compared to patients with conventional fixed appliances (33, 34). It seems that patients with clear aligners were easier to manage than those with fixed appliances during the COVID-19 epidemic; therefore, more attention should be paid to the management of patients with fixed appliances.

Limitations

The present study has some limitations. First, the inclusion of Weibo users alone may not reflect the overall situation in the whole population. However, samples from social media should be representative of adolescents, which predominate the orthodontic patients (18). Although there are other popular social media platforms such as WeChat in China, Weibo is the largest one with ample public opinions and accessible information. In addition, Weibo is the most often used platform for discussing breaking news and events, with 550 million monthly active users in the first quarter of 2020 (35). Second, the present study was based only on the Chinese population, which may not reflect populations from other countries. Further research is needed to study the situation in other countries and regions, which may identify cross-cultural differences. Third, data quality issues and privacy issues are frequently mentioned in social media research (36). Since Weibo users can choose to share posts with the public or specific people and only open public data can be searched, some information was inevitably unavailable. However, such selection bias is common in health care-related research using social media (19, 37). So far, there have been no commonly accepted guidelines or consensus about the ethics of user privacy and data use on social media-based studies. In this study, we only collected public information and strictly avoided direct quotations and presentation of any personal information (38).

CONCLUSIONS

The analysis of Weibo posts provided a timely understanding of the impact of COVID-19 on orthodontic patients. Delayed appointments were their greatest concern, and negative feelings and untreated orthodontic problems increased during the suspension of dental care services. However, patients with clear aligners reported fewer negative feelings and problems than those with fixed appliances. The findings highlighted the need to consider both treatment and psychological issues of orthodontic patients and how to handle them appropriately during the epidemic.

AUTHOR CONTRIBUTIONS

FH: study conception. FG, BT, DQ, TZ, FH, and HH: study design. FG, BT, DQ, FH, and HH: data collection. FG, DQ, and FH: data analysis. TZ, Y-xS, CM, and HH: data interpretation. FG, BT, and DQ: manuscript drafting. TZ, Y-xS, CM, FH, and HH: critical revision of the manuscript. All authors: approval of the final version.

ACKNOWLEDGMENTS

The authors would like to thank Dr. Kun He from the School of Cyber Science and Engineering, Wuhan University for technical assistance.

REFERENCES

1. Zhu N, Zhang D, Wang W, Li X, Yang B, Song J, et al. A novel coronavirus from patients with pneumonia in China, 2019. *N Engl J Med.* (2020) 382:727–33. doi: 10.1056/NEJMoa2001017
2. World Health Organization. *Coronavirus disease 2019 (COVID-19): situation report-141.* (2020). Available online at: https://www.who.int/docs/default-source/coronaviruse/situation-reports/20200609-covid-19-sitrep-141.pdf?sfvrsn=72fa1b16_2 (accessed June 10, 2020).
3. Peng X, Xu X, Li Y, Cheng L, Zhou X, Ren B. Transmission routes of 2019-nCoV and controls in dental practice. *Int J Oral Sci.* (2020) 12:9. doi: 10.1038/s41368-020-0075-9
4. Meng L, Hua F, Bian Z. Coronavirus disease 2019 (COVID-19): emerging and future challenges for dental and oral medicine. *J Dent Res.* (2020) 99:481–7. doi: 10.1177/0022034520914246
5. Chinese Center for Disease Control and Prevention. *Distribution of New Coronavirus Pneumonia.* (2020). Available online at: http://2019ncov.chinacdc.cn/2019-nCoV/ (accessed May 12, 2020)
6. Suri S, Vandersluis YR, Kochhar AS, Bhasin R, Abdallah MN. Clinical orthodontic management during the COVID-19 pandemic. *Angle Orthod.* (2020) 90:473–84. doi: 10.2319/033120-236.1
7. Machado RA, de Souza NL, Oliveira RM, Martelli Júnior H, Bonan PRF. Social media and telemedicine for oral diagnosis and counselling in the COVID-19 era. *Oral Oncol.* (2020) 105:104685. doi: 10.1016/j.oraloncology.2020.104685
8. China Internet Network Information Center. *The 45th China statistical report on internet development.* (2020). Available online at: http://www.cnnic.net.cn/hlwfzyj/hlwxzbg/hlwtjbg/202004/P020200428596599037028.pdf (accessed May 25, 2020).
9. Li J, Xu Q, Cuomo R, Purushothaman V, Mackey T. Data mining and content analysis of the chinese social media platform weibo during the early COVID-19 outbreak: retrospective observational infoveillance study. *JMIR Public Health Surveill.* (2020) 6:e18700. doi: 10.2196/18700
10. Fung IC, Fu KW, Ying Y, Schaible B, Hao Y, Chan CH, et al. Chinese social media reaction to the MERS-CoV and avian influenza A(H7N9) outbreaks. *Infect Dis Poverty.* (2013) 2:31. doi: 10.1186/2049-9957-2-31
11. Han X, Wang J, Zhang M, Wang X. Using social media to mine and analyze public opinion related to COVID-19 in China. *Int j environ res public health.* (2020) 17:2788. doi: 10.3390/ijerph17082788
12. Tao Z, Chu G, McGrath C, Hua F, Leung YY, Yang W, et al. Nature and diffusion of COVID-19-related oral health information on chinese social media: an analysis of tweets on weibo. *J Med Internet Res.* (2020) 22:e19981. doi: 10.2196/19981
13. Li S, Wang Y, Xue J, Zhao N, Zhu T. The impact of COVID-19 epidemic declaration on psychological consequences: a study on active weibo users. *Int j environ res public health.* (2020) 17:2032. doi: 10.3390/ijerph17062032
14. Liu N, Zhang F, Wei C, Jia Y, Shang Z, Sun L, et al. Prevalence and predictors of PTSS during COVID-19 outbreak in China hardest-hit areas: gender differences matter. *Psychiatry Res.* (2020) 287:112921. doi: 10.1016/j.psychres.2020.112921
15. Zhang Y, Ma ZF. Impact of the COVID-19 pandemic on mental health and quality of life among local residents in Liaoning Province, China: a cross-sectional study. *Int j environ res public health.* (2020) 17:2381. doi: 10.3390/ijerph17072381
16. Chan A, Antoun JS, Morgaine KC, Farella M. Accounts of bullying on twitter in relation to dentofacial features and orthodontic treatment. *J Oral Rehabil.* (2017) 44:244–50. doi: 10.1111/joor.12487
17. Noll D, Mahon B, Shroff B, Carrico C, Lindauer SJ. Twitter analysis of the orthodontic patient experience with braces vs invisalign. *Angle Orthod.* (2017) 87:377–83. doi: 10.2319/062816-508.1
18. Rachel Henzell M, Margaret Knight A, Morgaine KC, Antoun JS, Farella M. A qualitative analysis of orthodontic-related posts on twitter. *Angle Orthod.* (2014) 84:203–7. doi: 10.2319/051013-355.1
19. Al-Moghrabi D, Johal A, Fleming PS. What are people tweeting about orthodontic retention? A cross-sectional content analysis. *Am J Orthod Dentofacial Orthop.* (2017) 152:516–22. doi: 10.1016/j.ajodo.2017.04.021
20. Pan A, Liu L, Wang C, Guo H, Hao X, Wang Q, et al. Association of public health interventions with the epidemiology of the COVID-19 outbreak in Wuhan, China. *JAMA.* (2020) 323:1–9. doi: 10.1001/jama.2020.6130
21. Bao Y, Sun Y, Meng S, Shi J, Lu L. 2019-nCoV epidemic: address mental health care to empower society. *Lancet.* (2020) 395:e37–8. doi: 10.1016/s0140-6736(20)30309-3
22. Rubin GJ, Wessely S. The psychological effects of quarantining a city. *BMJ.* (2020) 368:m313. doi: 10.1136/bmj.m313
23. Yang Y, Zhou Y, Liu X, Tan J. Health services provision of 48 public tertiary dental hospitals during the COVID-19 epidemic in China. *Clin oral invest.* (2020) 24:1861–4. doi: 10.1007/s00784-020-03267-8
24. Zhang EX, Yang Y, Di Shang R, Simons JJ, Quek BK, Yin XF, et al. Leveraging social networking sites for disease surveillance and public sensing: the case of the 2013 avian influenza A(H7N9) outbreak in China. *West Pac surveill response j.* (2015) 6:66–72. doi: 10.5365/wpsar.2015.6.1.013
25. Chen B, Zhang JM, Jiang Z, Shao J, Jiang T, Wang Z, et al. Media and public reactions toward vaccination during the 'hepatitis b vaccine crisis' in China. *Vaccine.* (2015) 33:1780–5. doi: 10.1016/j.vaccine.2015.02.046

26. Cotrin PP, Peloso RM, Oliveira RC, Oliveira RCG, Pini NIP, Valarelli FP, et al. Impact of coronavirus pandemic in appointments and anxiety/concerns of patients regarding orthodontic treatment. *Orthod Craniofac Res.* (2020) 23:455–61. doi: 10.1111/ocr.12395
27. Saltaji H, Sharaf K. COVID-19 and orthodontics—a call for action. *Am J Orthod Dentofacial Orthop.* (2020) 158:12–3. doi: 10.1016/j.ajodo.2020.04.006
28. Stephens R, Ryan FS, Cunningham SJ. Information-seeking behavior of adolescent orthodontic patients. *Am J Orthod Dentofacial Orthop.* (2013) 143:303–9. doi: 10.1016/j.ajodo.2012.10.018
29. Caprioglio A, Pizzetti GB, Zecca PA, Fastuca R, Maino G, Nanda R. Management of orthodontic emergencies during 2019-NCOV. *Prog Orthod.* (2020) 21:10. doi: 10.1186/s40510-020-00310-y
30. Turkistani KA. Precautions and recommendations for orthodontic settings during the COVID-19 outbreak: a review. *Am J Orthod Dentofacial Orthop.* (2020) 158:175–81. doi: 10.1016/j.ajodo.2020.04.016
31. Papadimitriou A, Kakali L, Pazera P, Doulis I, Kloukos D. Social media and orthodontic treatment from the patient's perspective: a systematic review. *Eur j orthod.* (2019) 42:23—41. doi: 10.1093/ejo/cjz029
32. Pithon MM, Baião FCS, Sant Anna L, Paranhos LR, Cople Maia L. Assessment of the effectiveness of invisible aligners compared with conventional appliance in aesthetic and functional orthodontic treatment: a systematic review. *J invest clin dent.* (2019) 10:e12455. doi: 10.1111/jicd.12455
33. White DW, Julien KC, Jacob H, Campbell PM, Buschang PH. Discomfort associated with invisalign and traditional brackets: a randomized, prospective trial. *Angle Orthod.* (2017) 87:801–8. doi: 10.2319/091416-687.1
34. Azaripour A, Weusmann J, Mahmoodi B, Peppas D, Gerhold-Ay A, Van Noorden CJF, et al. Braces versus invisalign®: gingival parameters and patients' satisfaction during treatment: a cross-sectional study. *BMC Oral Health.* (2015) 15:69. doi: 10.1186/s12903-015-0060-4
35. China Internet Watch. *Statistics: Weibo monthly active users (MAU) & DAU.* (2020). Available online at: https://www.chinainternetwatch.com/statistics/weibo-mau/ (accessed October 12, 2020).
36. Krasnova H, Günther O, Spiekermann S, Koroleva K. Privacy concerns and identity in online social networks. *Identity Inform Soc.* (2009) 2:39–63. doi: 10.1007/s12394-009-0019-1
37. Huber J, Woods T, Fushi A, Duong MT, Eidelman AS, Zalal AR, et al. Social media research strategy to understand clinician and public perception of health care messages. *JDR clin translational res.* (2020) 5:71–81. doi: 10.1177/2380084419849439
38. Moreno MA, Goniu N, Moreno PS, Diekema D. Ethics of social media research: common concerns and practical considerations. *Cyberpsychol Behav Social Networking.* (2013) 16:708–13. doi: 10.1089/cyber.2012.0334

3

Systemic Management of Pandemic Risks in Dental Practice: A Consolidated Framework for COVID-19 Control in Dentistry

Habib Benzian[1,2*†], *Eugenio Beltrán-Aguilar*[1†] *and Richard Niederman*[3†]

[1] *Department Epidemiology and Health Promotion, World Health Organization Collaborating Center Quality Improvement and Evidence-Based Dentistry, College of Dentistry, New York University, New York, NY, United States,* [2] *Global Health Center, Geneva Graduate Institute for Policy Studies, Geneva, Switzerland,* [3] *Department Epidemiology and Health Promotion, College of Dentistry, New York University, New York, NY, United States*

***Correspondence:**
Habib Benzian
habib.benzian@nyu.edu

†ORCID:
Habib Benzian
orcid.org/0000-0003-3692-4849
Eugenio Beltrán-Aguilar
orcid.org/0000-0003-2202-0507
Richard Niederman
orcid.org/0000-0001-6674-1774

Dental teams and their workplaces are among the most exposed to airborne and bloodborne infectious agents, and therefore at the forefront of pandemic-related changes to how dental care is organized and provided to patients. The increasing complexity of guidelines makes is challenging for clinicians to navigate the multitude of COVID-19 guidelines issued by different agencies. A comparative analysis of guidance issued for managing COVID-19 in dental settings leading U.S. agencies was conducted, including documents of the Occupational Safety and Health Administration (OSHA), an agency of the U.S. Secretary of Labor, and of the U.S. Centers for Disease Prevention and Control (CDC), an agency of the U.S. Secretary of Health and Human Services. Details of infection control and other risk mitigation measures were reviewed for consistency, overlaps and similarities, then clustered according to thematic areas covering all domains of managing a dental healthcare setting. The analysis revealed five distinct areas of pandemic control, comprising (1) planning and protocols, (2) patient screening, (3) preparation of facilities, (4) PPE and infection control, and (5) procedures and aerosol control; thereby covering systematically all aspects requiring adaptation in a pandemic context. The "Pandemic-5 Framework for COVID-19 Control in Dentistry" provides an opportunity to simplify comprehensive decision-making from a clinical practitioner perspective. The framework supports a comprehensive systems-driven approach by using dental clinics as a setting to integrate pandemic clinical responses with the implementation of appropriate infection control protocols. Traditionally these two aspects are addressed independently from each other in separate concepts.

Keywords: infection control, workplace safety and health, hierarchy of risk control, airborne transmission of pathogens, dental procedure, systems thinking, dentistry, practice management dental

SAFETY OF DENTAL CARE UNDER COVID-19

The COVID-19 pandemic has pushed safety precautions and infection control to the limelight, forcing the entire healthcare sector to review protocols and practices to ensure continued safety of care for patients and healthcare workers in an evolving context. Recognizing, understanding and managing the risks of emerging, previously unknown infections, while continuing to provide care, are complex processes. They require a systematic and systemic adaptation of multiple interlinked aspects, such as population protection and risk containment measures, healthcare service practices including infection control; and workplace health and safety for providers and patients, including surveillance of workplace-related adverse events (1–8).

Dental teams and their clinical work places are among the most affected by exposure to airborne and bloodborne infectious agents and therefore at the forefront of pandemic-related changes how dental care is organized and provided to patients (9–12). Early reports from China highlighted the risks of droplet and aerosol transmission in dental care, which led to service limitations or shut-downs in many countries worldwide, following governmental restrictions (13–15). Subsequently, numerous national recommendations for dental services have been rapidly developed, detailing adaptations of practice management, use of personal protective equipment (PPE) and other aspects of clinical dental care (15–17). In the U.S., like in many other countries, different agencies and organizations with different scopes of work are guiding infection control, workplace health and safety, and other related matters. In addition, federal and state regulations may be requiring pandemic changes to oral healthcare services.

For dental teams managing a clinical dental workplace it becomes increasingly complex to navigate this patchwork of COVID-19 guidelines issued by different agencies, also because they address different aspects of pandemic response and often reflect the organizational remit of the issuing organization. This puts a high burden on individual practitioners and practice owners. Clinicians are expected to keep themselves updated with the latest information so that they can take responsible managerial and clinical decisions to provide the safest possible healthcare environment.

This paper presents a new and consolidated framework for managing the COVID-19 pandemic risks in dental settings using five distinct areas of control. By combining approaches of different and overlapping guideline concepts of two leading U.S. public health agencies, the framework aims at simplifying decision-making and adaptations in the dental setting to mitigate the risks of COVID-19 transmission.

CURRENT FRAMEWORKS ADDRESSING OCCUPATIONAL RISKS AND INFECTION CONTROL IN DENTAL SETTINGS

In the U.S., two agencies provide public health and workplace guidance to address COVID-19: The Occupational Safety and Health Administration (OSHA), an agency of the U.S. Secretary of Labor, and the U.S. Centers for Disease Prevention and Control (CDC), an agency of the U.S. Secretary of Health and Human Services. Both have developed recommendations throughout the course of the pandemic with repeated updates accounting for the constantly evolving context. In developing these recommendations, both organizations built on their existing frameworks for risks to occupational health and infection control in healthcare and dentistry.

OSHA's "Hierarchy of Controls" addresses workplace health and safety, including healthcare settings. The concept identifies four areas of intervention with decreasing efficiency of protection for staff: Risk elimination, engineering controls, administrative practices and PPE (18). This approach has been used to issue guidance on preparing workplaces for COVID-19, as well as develop specific recommendations for "Dentistry Workers and Employers" (19, 20). OSHA places dental health care providers in the "very high" or "high" risk category because of their exposure to aerosols during dental care. For aspects of PPE and specific infection control the guidance refers to the relevant CDC recommendations.

In 2016, the CDC defined "basic expectations for safe care" in dental settings (21). The set of standard precautions comprises hand hygiene, PPE, respiratory etiquette, safe injection practice, storage and handling of instruments, and the disinfection of instruments and practice environment. In addition, a set of transmission-based precautions cover the identification of infectious patients, contact precautions, droplet and aerosol precautions. These fundamental principles are taking a clinical service provision perspective, thereby complementing OSHA's health and safety approach. The CDC's COVID-19-related recommendations for dental settings build on these standard and transmission-based precautions, but also incorporate elements of engineering controls from OSHA's framework and reference additional guidance from the American Dental Association (22, 23).

In addition, U.S. state agencies, the American Dental Association, and several dental professional associations provided further guidance, which may or may not be aligned with the advice of OSHA or the CDC. The multitude of guideline-generating agencies places dentists and their teams in a dilemma where they need to actively search for, obtain, read and compare several sources of practice recommendations. They need to appraise the quality of information provided and the relevance for their own context in order to make appropriate decisions in the best interest of patient, staff and the wider public's safety. In the current highly dynamic pandemic context this is a challenging task.

A comparative analysis of the CDC and OSHA guidance was undertaken in order to identify areas of overlap and complementarity. Clustering of thematic areas of infection control and measures for health and safety at the workplace resulted in a consolidated framework comprising five areas of intervention. **Figure 1** shows the areas of intervention of CDC's and OSHA's guidance and their respective links to the proposed new framework with five areas of control.

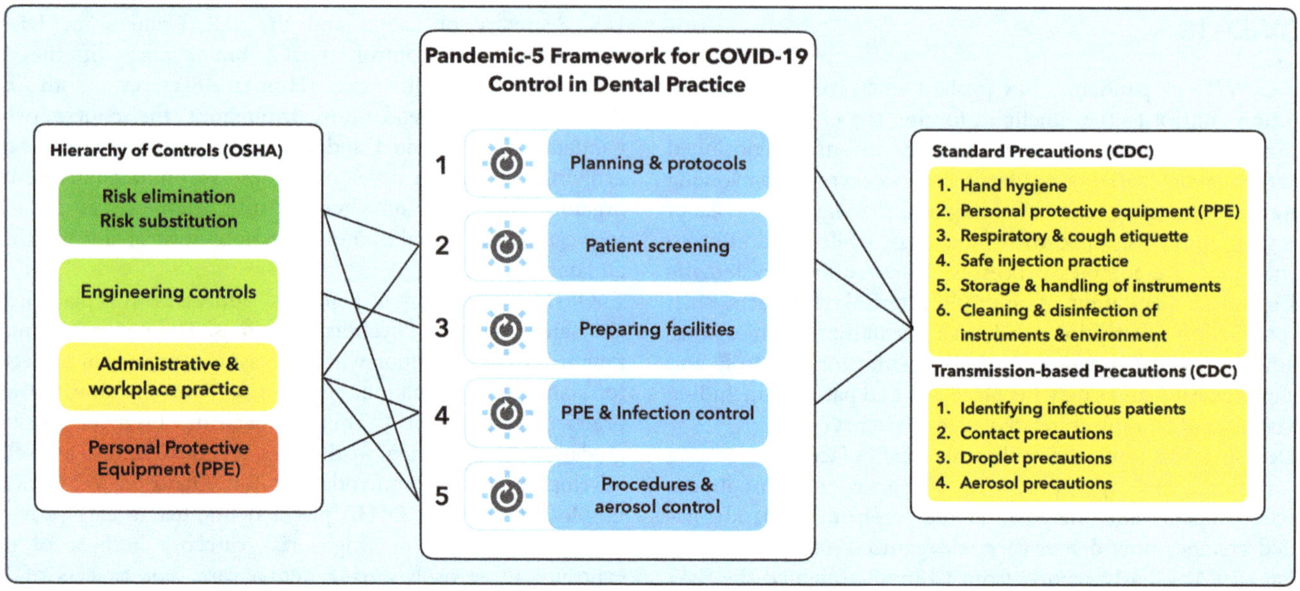

FIGURE 1 | Pandemic-5 framework for COVID-19 control in dental practice.

A SYSTEMS-THINKING APPROACH TO MANAGING RISKS OF COVID-19

Systems-thinking is increasingly applied to public health (24), hospital infections and infectious disease control (25, 26). Using the dental workplace as a system to analyze challenges and solutions in several interconnected and pandemic-related domains allows for a more holistic and comprehensive adaptation and response to COVID-19 in the dental practice.

The "Pandemic-5 Framework for COVID-19 Control in Dental Practice" synthesizes the elements of OSHA's "Hierarchy of Controls" and CDC's "Standard and Transmission-based Precautions" into a new, consolidated and simplified model (**Figure 1**).

The framework is inspired by the model for health system reform developed by Roberts et al. (27), which uses the metaphor of "control knobs" to describe core areas of intervention or change in a complex health system setting. The Pandemic-5 Framework uses the control-knob principle to systematically identify the five areas of possible interventions to manage and control the risk of COVID-19 in dental settings. The five areas and selected control interventions for each area comprise:

1. Planning and protocols
   Pandemic preparedness and response require planning and anticipation, risk assessments, thinking through different scenarios, and putting control and mitigation measures in place. Preparedness also includes communication and participation of the entire dental team and communication with patients. Staff training, rehearsing of protocols and monitoring compliance should be planned and formalized as well. Some aspects of planning and documentation may even be required as part of legal and licensing regulations. Ideally, all control measures are covered by a written plan including protocols, checklists and practical control measures.
2. Patient screening
   This area of control relates to simple assessments of the patient's health status and oral health care need. The objective is to limit or select who has access to the clinical setting. Pre-screening *via* phone or online using questionnaires and/or software are used to determine whether the patient is currently ill, has any particular risks of being infected, or is at part of a high-risk group for infection. Tele-consultations may already address the patient's problem. Through this screening process, patients with urgent problems may receive palliative care while being scheduled treatment at the dental clinic, where additional COVID-19 screening may be performed prior to providing care. Depending on the pandemic situation and infection risks, patient visits for elective procedures may be either post-poned or performed (17).
3. Preparing facilities
   The preparation of facilities comprises a range of measures to ensure physical distancing in waiting and reception areas, signage and patient flow, separation of operatories, ventilation and air filtration, enabling regular hand hygiene for patient and staff through additional disinfection dispensers. Depending on official guidance and context, additional measures to reduce aerosols and surface contamination may be taken such as spacing waiting rooms, opening windows, negative pressure rooms, or touchless doors and faucets. The area of engineering controls from OHSA's "Guidance for workplace health and safety" provides further details.

4. PPE and infection control
   Personal protective equipment is a key aspect for dental teams working in close proximity to the patient's face. A range of measures, including different types and protective levels of face masks, face shields, disposable gowns, head caps, gloves, eye protection or goggles are available and should be selected depending on the nature and length of patient contact, as well as the type of procedure performed. All of the CDC's "Standard and Transmission-based Precautions" for infection control remain in place, and additional measures for surface decontamination and operatory cleaning between patients may be recommended.
5. Procedures and aerosol control
   With the remaining uncertainty around the risk of aerosol transmission of SARS-CoV-2, dental procedures must be selected and delivered carefully. Clinicians have the choice between aerosol-generating procedures involving water-air cooled rotary instruments, ultrasonic scalers and other technology for which maximum suction methods and rubber dam should be used as much as possible. Alternatively, procedure with minimal or no aerosol potential may be chosen, such as the approach of the Safe, Aerosol-free, Emergent (SAFE) Dentistry concept (28). New measures of aerosol control might be considered such as innovative suction technology, once their efficiency and evidence have been demonstrated.

The description of possible activities and risk mitigation measures under each control area is merely illustrative and not meant to be comprehensive, nor is the aim to provide specific guidance on actual measures that need to be taken in a specific setting or situation. Organizations and professional associations are encouraged to structure their guidance according to the five areas of control, thereby making it easier for clinicians to systematically follow and implement. Dental teams may also use the framework to review available information from different sources and to collate them to the five control areas, which simplifies staying updated and taking informed decisions about increasing, maintaining or loosening control measures.

Whatever the choices in the five control areas are, it is important to keep three fundamental principles in mind: consider every patient to be potentially infectious, focus on precautions to prevent droplet/aerosol transmission, and use the best possible PPE for protection of patients and staff (5). In contrast to OSHA's hierarchy of controls, all five control areas are equally important and need to be considered in order to provide the best possible occupational safety and infection control. The combination of measures in all five areas provides best possible safety and protection.

THE CONTINUUM OF UNCERTAINTY AND RISK UNDER COVID-19

Knowing the characteristics of a new infectious agent and its transmission mode, infectivity, disease patterns and many other aspects are part of the foundational determinants for an effective pandemic response, including appropriate infection control measures (29). Only when these aspects are known, the risks of certain events and outcomes can be fully assessed. This empirical analysis of observations, epidemiological surveillance, laboratory and virologic insights is highly complex and dynamic. It resembles a giant puzzle where over time different pieces are coming together toward a more complete picture. Less than a year after the first identification a lot is already known about SARS-Cov-2 and the clinical features of COVID-19 infections. Even though uncertainty is decreasing, and knowledge is increasing on a daily basis, reaching full understanding of the pandemic will take more time. Uncertainties about fundamental properties of the disease and the resulting risks will remain and impact on clinical decisions.

The role of airborne transmission *via* droplets and aerosols is one of the major areas of uncertainty for dentistry, since many of the frequently-used interventions are classified as aerosol-generating procedures (30, 31). Consequently, the current situation limits managerial control in dental settings and leaves a probability for failure (**Figure 2**). So far there have been no reports of major SARS-CoV-2 transmission events in dental settings, but several factors are limiting knowledge and reporting of such incidents; it is likely that more details will emerge over time (5, 32).

Understanding the dynamic nature of the situation, where progress toward full certainty and knowledge of risks may not be a linear process; and where new unexpected challenges may appear at any time, is important when deciding on adapting control and risk management in dental services to the COVID-19 pandemic. Ideally, such measures would need to be equally dynamic and adaptive in order to provide effective protection.

SCENARIO PLANNING USING THE PANDEMIC-5 FRAMEWORK FOR COVID-19 CONTROL IN DENTISTRY

Systems thinking opens the door to a number of analysis and modeling approaches that help understand the relationships and interlinkages between different elements of the system (24). Scenario planning is among the tools that link problem-driven analysis with goal-oriented solutions (33). The principle of a "control knob" to step up or decrease precautions allows for flexible adaptation in the COVID-19 or other novel infectious agent contexts. External factors beyond control of the dental team, such as the level of community spread, availability of PPE or availability of a vaccine, are determining the adaptive measures within the control framework. The overall goal of the adaptations is to maintain and provide safe care for patients and clinicians, without the risk of infection or disease transmission.

SHIFTING RESPONSIBILITY FOR PANDEMIC CONTROL AND RESPONSE REQUIRES HIGH COMPLIANCE

When the first peak of the pandemic subsided, governments or states were allowing the gradual re-opening of dental

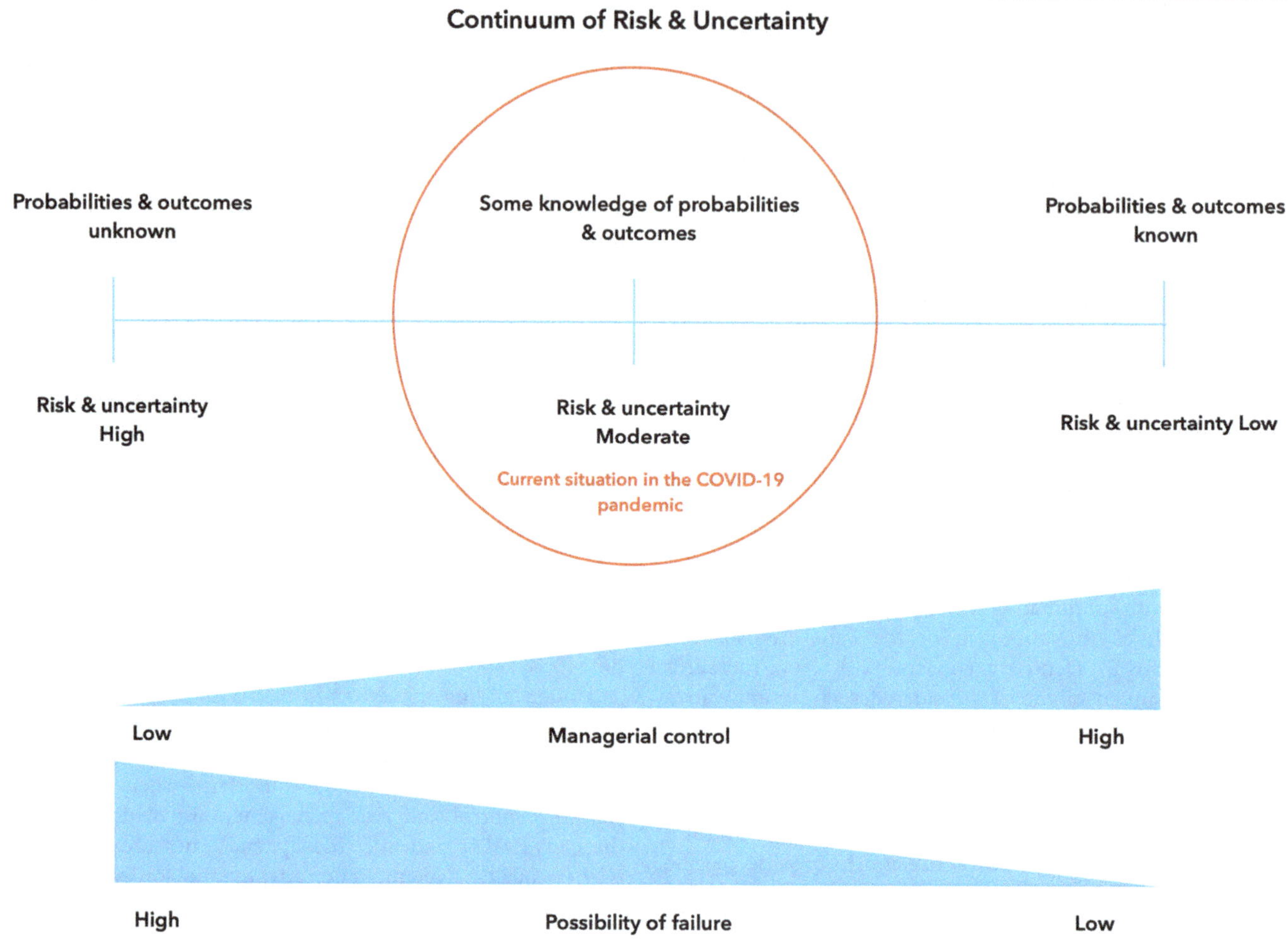

FIGURE 2 | Continuum of risk, uncertainty and managerial control.

services. This process implied shifting aspects of population-wide containment measures to clinic-level measures. By implication, individual practitioners and dental teams had to make the required clinical COVID-19 control decisions based on the most current guidance and their best professional judgment. This is a crucial step in devolving elements of the COVID-19 (or any future airborne infectious disease) preparedness and response, and one which requires confidence that appropriate measures will be uniformly followed.

However, dental teams express concerns over a multitude of uncertainties. These uncertainties include the understanding of community transmission, shortages of PPE, and safety of care without full PPE (34). On the other hand, previous studies show that dentists frequently tend to downplay risks and display a degree of over-confidence with their infection control measures, which may contribute to potentially lower compliance with new recommendations (35, 36). Others may even consider external guidance as an intrusion of their professional autonomy (37–39).

The Pandemic-5 Framework for COVID-19 Control in Dentistry provides an opportunity to simplify and systematize decisions from a clinical setting and practitioner perspective. The framework supports a comprehensive systems-driven approach by using dental clinics as a setting to integrate pandemic clinical responses with the implementation of appropriate infection control protocols. Traditionally these two aspects are addressed independently from each other in separate concepts.

The proposed framework shifts the locus of control back to the clinical setting and the provider's decision realm. Decisions are made based on rational assessments of uncertainty and risk, taking into account external uncontrollable factors. A clinician who feels in control, has decision autonomy and confidence, is more likely to adapt to change and to comply responsibly with service recommendations (40). The knowledge of the five control areas and options to fine-tune the pandemic response empowers and facilitates active management of the pandemic risk.

The concept also facilitates system adaptations in resource-poor settings where governmental or robust epidemiological guidance may not be available. Validation of the concept of the five pandemic control areas, using other international guidelines is encouraged and should not be too complex. Other areas of healthcare are facing similar challenges related to aerosols and proximity to patients, such as anesthesiology, maxillo-facial or ear-nose-throat surgery. Future research may show to what extent the Pandemic-5 Model might also be applicable to these clinical disciplines.

AUTHOR CONTRIBUTIONS

All authors contributed equally to conceptualizing, drafting, and finalizing the manuscript.

REFERENCES

1. Pan Y, Liu H, Chu C, Li X, Liu S, Lu S. Transmission routes of SARS-CoV-2 and protective measures in dental clinics during the COVID-19 pandemic. *Am J Dent.* (2020) 33:129–34.
2. Hamedani S, Farshidfar N, Ziaei A, Pakravan H. The dilemma of COVID-19 in dental practice concerning the role of saliva in transmission: a brief review of current evidence. *Eur Oral Res.* (2020) 54:92–100. doi: 10.26650/eor.20200050
3. Sommerstein R, Swissnoso, Fux CA, Vuichard-Gysin D, Abbas M, Marschall J, et al. Risk of SARS-CoV-2 transmission by aerosols, the rational use of masks, and protection of healthcare workers from COVID-19. *Antimicrob Resist Infect Control.* (2020) 9. doi: 10.1186/s13756-020-00763-0
4. Gallagher JE, Johnson I, Verbeek JH, Clarkson JE, Innes N. Relevance and paucity of evidence: a dental perspective on personal protective equipment during the COVID-19 pandemic. *Br Dental J.* (2020) 229:121–4. doi: 10.1038/s41415-020-1843-9
5. Beltrán-Aguilar E, Benzian H, Niederman R. Rational perspectives on risk and certainty for dentistry during the COVID-19 pandemic. *Am J Infect Control.* (2021) 49:131–3. doi: 10.1590/SciELOPreprints.537
6. Volgenant CMC, Persoon IF, Ruijter RAG, Soet JJH. Infection control in dental health care during and after the SARS-CoV-2 outbreak. *Oral Dis.* (2020). doi: 10.1111/odi.13408. [Epub ahead of print].
7. Casamassimo PS. Safety in dental care: where is our surveillance imperative. *J Am Dent Assoc.* (2020) 151:381. doi: 10.1016/j.adaj.2020.02.019
8. Organization for Safety, Asepsis and Prevention (OSAP), DentaQuest Partnership for Oral Health Advancement (DQP). *Best Practices for Infection Control in Dental Clinics During the COVID-19 Pandemic.* Atlanta, Boston: OSAP/DQP (2020).
9. Samaranayake LP, Peiris M. Severe acute respiratory syndrome and dentistry: a retrospective view. *J Am Dent Assoc.* (2004) 135:1292–302. doi: 10.14219/jada.archive.2004.0405
10. Bali Z, Bali RK, Nagrath S. Prion diseases: risks, characteristics, and infection control considerations in dentistry. *J Investig Clin Dent.* (2011) 2:236–40. doi: 10.1111/j.2041-1626.2011.00080.x
11. Scully C, Samaranayake LP. Emerging and changing viral diseases in the new millennium. *Oral Dis.* (2016) 22:171–9. doi: 10.1111/odi.12356
12. Gamio L. *The Workers Who Face the Highest Coronavirus Risk.* New York, NY: New York Times (2020).
13. Peng X, Xu X, Li Y, Cheng L, Zhou X, Ren B. Transmission routes of 2019-nCoV and controls in dental practice. *Int J Oral Sci.* (2020) 12:9. doi: 10.1038/s41368-020-0075-9
14. Meng L, Hua F, Bian Z. Coronavirus disease 2019 (COVID-19): emerging and future challenges for dental and oral medicine. *J Dent Res.* (2020) 99:481–7. doi: 10.1177/0022034520914246
15. COVID-19 Dental Services Evidence Review (CoDER) Working Group. *Recommendations for the Re-Opening of Dental Services: A Rapid Review of International Sources (Version 1.3).* Available online at: https://oralhealth.cochrane.org/sites/oralhealth.cochrane.org/files/public/uploads/covid19_dental_reopening_rapid_review_07052020.pdf (accessed May 13, 2020).
16. Jamal M, Shah M, Almarzooqi SH, Aber H, Khawaja S, El Abed R, et al. Overview of trans-national recommendations for COVID-19 transmission Control in dental care settings. *Oral Dis.* (2020). doi: 10.1111/odi.13431. [Epub ahead of print].
17. World Health Organization (WHO). *Consideration for the Provision of Essential Oral Health Services in the Context of COVID-19.* Interim guidance. Available online at: https://www.who.int/publications/i/item/who-2019-nCoV-oral-health-2020.1 (accessed August 3, 2020).
18. Occupational Safety and Health Administration (OSHA). *Recommended Pratices for Safety and Health Programs* (OSHA3885) (2016) Available online at: https://www.osha.gov/Publications/OSHA3885.pdf (accessed December 20, 2020).
19. Occupational Safety and Health Administration (OSHA), Department of Labor. *Guidance on Preparing Workplaces for COVID-19 (OSHA 3990-02 2020).* Available online at: www.osha.gov/Publications/OSHA3990.pdf (accessed December 20, 2020).
20. Occupational Safety and Health Administration (OSHA). *COVID-19 Control and Prevention—Dentistry Workers and Employers.* (2020). Available online at: https://www.osha.gov/SLTC/covid-19/dentistry.html (accessed December 20, 2020).
21. Centers for Disease Control and Prevention (CDC). *Summary of Infection Prevention Practices in Dental Settings: Basic Expectations for Safe Care.* Atlanta: CDC, US Dept of Health and Human Services (2016).
22. Centers for Disease Control and Prevention (CDC). *Guidance for Dental Settings: Interim Infection Prevention and Control Guidance for Dental Settings During the COVID-19 Response.* (2020). Available online at: https://www.cdc.gov/coronavirus/2019-ncov/hcp/dental-settings.html (May 19, 2020).
23. American Dental Association (ADA). *What Constitutes a Dental Emergency?* (2020). Available online at: https://success.ada.org/~/media/CPS/Files/Open%20Files/ADA_COVID19_Dental_Emergency_DDS.pdf?utm_source=adaorg&utm_medium=covid-resources-lp&utm_content=cv-pm-emerg-def&utm_campaign=covid-19 (March 27, 2020).
24. Peters DH. The application of systems thinking in health: why use systems thinking. *Health Res Policy Syst.* (2014) 12:51. doi: 10.1186/1478-4505-12-51
25. Chuang S, Howley PP, Lin SH. Implementing systems thinking for infection prevention: The cessation of repeated scabies outbreaks in a respiratory care ward. *Am J Infect Control.* (2015) 43:499–505. doi: 10.1016/j.ajic.2015.02.002
26. Xia S, Zhou XN, Liu J. Systems thinking in combating infectious diseases. *Infect Dis Poverty.* (2017) 6:144. doi: 10.1186/s40249-017-0339-6
27. Roberts MJ, Hsiao W, Berman P, Reich M. *Getting Health Reform Right. Anniversary Edition: A Guide to Improving Performance and Equity.* New York, NY: Oxford University Press (2019). p. 360.
28. Benzian H, Niederman R. A dental response to the COVID-19 pandemic—safer aerosol-free emergency (SAFER) dentistry. *Front Med.* (2020) 7:520. doi: 10.3389/fmed.2020.00520
29. Bizzoca ME, Campisi G, Muzio LL. Covid-19 pandemic: What changes for dentists and oral medicine experts? A narrative review and novel approaches to infection containment. *Int J Environ Res Public Health.* (2020) 17:3793. doi: 10.3390/ijerph17113793
30. Harrel SK, Molinari J. Aerosols and splatter in dentistry: a brief review of the literature and infection control implications. *J Am Dent Assoc.* (2004) 135:429–37. doi: 10.14219/jada.archive.2004.0207
31. Zemouri C, de Soet H, Crielaard W, Laheij A. A scoping review on bio-aerosols in healthcare and the dental environment. *PLoS ONE.* (2017) 12:e0178007. doi: 10.1371/journal.pone.0178007
32. Estrich CG, Mikkelsen M, Morrissey R, Geisinger ML, Ioannidou E, Vujicic M, et al. Estimating COVID-19 prevalence and infection control practices among US dentists. *J Am Dental Assoc.* (2020) 151:815–24. doi: 10.1016/j.adaj.2020.09.005
33. Schoemaker P. Multiple scenario development: Its conceptual and behavioral foundation. *Strat Manag J.* (1993) 14:193–213. doi: 10.1002/smj.4250140304
34. Janes C. *Amid Coronavirus Concerns, Dentists Face a Fraught Road to Reopening.* The Washington Post (2020). Available online at: https://www.washingtonpost.com/health/amid-coronavirus-concerns-dentists-face-a-fraught-road-to-reopening/2020/05/28/187f5e30-9909-11ea-ac72-3841fcc9b35f_story.html (May 29, 2020).
35. Chambers DW. The role of dentists in dentistry. *J Dent Educ.* (2001) 65:1430–40. doi: 10.1002/j.0022-0337.2001.65.12.tb03502.x
36. Oosthuysen J, Potgieter E, Blignaut E. Compliance with infection control recommendations in South African dental practices: a review of

studies published between 1990 and 2007. *Int Dent J.* (2010) 60:181–9. doi: 10.1922/IDJ_2371Oosthuysen09
37. Franzén C. State governance versus dentists' autonomy—the case of Swedish dental care. *Acta Odontol Scand.* (2018) 76:125–9. doi: 10.1080/00016357.2017.1390151
38. Soares de Morais Freitas C. Conflicts in the practice of dentistry: the autonomy in question. *Interface Comunicação.* (2007) 11. doi: 10.1590/S1414-32832007000100004
39. van der Sanden WJ, Mettes DG, Plasschaert AJ, van't Hof MA, Grol RP, Verdonschot EH. Clinical practice guidelines in dentistry: opinions of dental practitioners on their contribution to the quality of dental care. *Qual Saf Health Care.* (2003) 12:107–111. doi: 10.1136/qhc.12.2.107
40. Chen J, Wang L. Locus of control and the three components of commitment to change. *Pers Individ Diff.* (2007) 42:503–12. doi: 10.1016/j.paid.2006.07.025

4

Optimizing Safe Dental Practice During the COVID-19 Pandemic: Recommendations Based on a Guide Developed for Dental Practices in China

Li Li†, Mianyan Zeng†, Xiao Chen, Shuman Cai, Cuixia Xu, Wei Xia, Lijun Jiang, Xiaoyan Zou, Pei Chen and Mingdeng Rong**

Department of Periodontology and Oral Implantology, Stomatological Hospital, Southern Medical University, Guangzhou, China

***Correspondence:**
Pei Chen
cpei3057@126.com
Mingdeng Rong
rmdeng@smu.edu.cn

† These authors share first authorship

The current global coronavirus disease 2019 (COVID-19) outbreak is still exerting severe global implications, and its development in various regions is complex and variable. The high risk of cross-infection poses a great challenge to the dental practice environment; it is therefore urgent to develop a set of pandemic prevention measures to ensure dental practice safety during the COVID-19 outbreak. Therefore, we combined the epidemiological characteristics of severe acute respiratory syndrome coronavirus 2 (SARS-CoV-2), public emergency measures for COVID-19, characteristics of dental practice, and relevant literature reports to develop a set of dynamic practice measures for dental practices in high-, medium-, and low-risk areas affected by COVID-19. This will help dental practices to achieve standard prevention and ensure their safe and smooth operation during the pandemic. It is hoped that these measures will provide a reference basis for dental hospitals and dental clinics in their care and pandemic prevention work.

Keywords: COVID-19, SARS-CoV-2, infection control, dental clinics, public health, prevention, disinfection

INTRODUCTION

From the beginning of 2019 to March 25, 2021, the cumulative number of confirmed cases of coronavirus disease 2019 (COVID-19) in the world is more than 125,700,000 and causing more than 2,756,000 deaths, which shows that COVID-19 is still spreading around the world. COVID-19 vaccines have been developed currently. However, due to the emergence of a variety of mutated strains of severe acute respiratory syndrome coronavirus 2 (SARS-CoV-2) (1), coupled with the uncertainty of vaccine efficacy, the pandemic is still severe and undoubtedly poses a huge threat and harm to the health of people worldwide. It also presents a great challenge to dental practices, which are characterized by a great demand for consultation and emergency treatment, as well as an environment that has a high level of spattering (2). This is greatly increasing the risk of cross-infection in the dental clinical practice process. Thus, how can dental staff establish effective protection to ensure safe and smooth dental practice implementation?

Studies have shown that the main routes of transmission of SARS-CoV-2 are respiratory droplets and contact transmission, with an additional possibility of air and aerosol transmission (prolonged, closed, high concentrations). Furthermore, SARS-CoV-2 can be isolated from stool, urine, and conjunctival secretions. Thus, attention should also be paid to contact or aerosol transmission caused by its contamination of the environment (3–6). It is well-known that instruments and operations commonly used in dentistry are prone to generate large amounts of droplets and aerosols, and dental care personnel are therefore at risk of inhaling large amounts of aerosols. SARS-CoV-2 can persist in aerosols for up to 3 h (7). Due to the direct contact operation on the dental cavity, the dental mucosa is considered a potential high-risk route for SARS-CoV-2 infection (8). Moreover, the complex structure of the turbine handpiece, saliva ejector, and dental chair drainage pipe that are not easily cleaned and disinfected and the use of sharp instruments during practice makes dental care personnel prone to occupational exposure (9). This may cause an increase in cross-infection among dentists, nurses, and patients and could become a difficult point for prevention and control during the COVID-19 pandemic. To truly and comprehensively identify studies on the prevention and control of the pandemic in dental practice, the authors used keywords such as "COVID-19," "SARS-CoV-2," "COVID-19 dental," "dental," and "infection control" on the PubMed and China National Knowledge Infrastructure (CNKI) websites. It was hoped that the literature would provide insights into the measures and experiences of dental practices in other countries during the COVID-19 pandemic (10–16). Among them, Italy, Latin America, and Poland recommend that patients should undergo pretesting and triage, as well as reinforce personal protective equipment (PPE) usage and hand hygiene. A mouthwash that is effective against COVID-19, disinfection and sterilization, rubber dams in dental practice should also be used. Singapore suggested a "Proposed color-coded framework for dental practice during the COVID-19 pandemic" (17). However, the measures described in these articles are still not detailed or specific enough and lack dynamic guidelines for pandemic prevention.

Therefore, there is an urgent need to develop scientific and comprehensive dynamic guidelines applicable to the dental clinic and dental hospital practice. This should be based on the characteristics and policies related to the COVID-19 pandemic in different periods and regions. It would help control infection sources in time, cut off the transmission pathways, protect the safety of the three parties involved (namely, doctors, nurses, and patients), and ensure the safe and smooth operationalization of dental practice work. Therefore, based on the development of the COVID-19 pandemic and the dental clinical practice, we summarized the practice measures implemented by Chinese dental clinics during the COVID-19 pandemic. The effectiveness of these dynamic measures has been confirmed because no dentists have been infected with COVID-19, except for a few dentists in Wuhan, who were reported to be infected with COVID-19 at the beginning of the outbreak, so we hope that these measures can guide domestic and foreign dental hospitals and dental clinics for smooth and safe practice during the COVID-19 pandemic. The specific practice measures are as follows.

BE GUIDED BY THE COVID-19 PREVENTION POLICIES AND MEASURES ISSUED BY NATIONAL AND REGIONAL HEALTH AUTHORITIES

China issued eight editions of the Diagnosis and Treatment Protocol for COVID-19 from January 15, 2020, to August 19, 2020 (18). These were issued in conjunction with daily updates for areas at high, medium, and low risk of an outbreak, making important dynamic guidelines for people to recognize and implement effective measures against the COVID-19 outbreak. As of March 1, 2021, 48 online learning sessions on infection control during hospital outbreaks have been held (19). Meanwhile, Guangdong Province issued daily dynamic guidelines for hospital outbreak prevention and control according to the pandemic changes. All regional dental hospitals and dental clinics have adjusted their systems and measures for conducting the dental practice promptly according to the policies and measures issued by the state and local provinces and municipalities.

INTRODUCTION OF "HEALTH CODES" AND COMMUNICATION BIG DATA TRIP CARDS FOR RAPID IDENTIFICATION OF PATIENT RISK LEVELS

The "health code" is filled in by the individual using information such as the identity card number, location information, health status, exposure history, and travel and residence history. The platform reviews the information and grants the applicant a QR code in red, yellow, or green. Holders of red and yellow codes are subject to a 14- and 7-day intensive or home quarantine, respectively, while holders of green codes are allowed normal passage. This system dynamically assesses and regrants codes according to the risk level of the pandemic.

The Communication Big Data Trip Card is a software developed by the China Academy of Information and Communication Technology, in conjunction with three basic telecommunication companies, allowing mobile phone users to check information on all the cities and regions they visited in the past 14 days (20, 21).

These two "electronic bodies" can help dental institutions quickly identify the risk level of patients, reduce triage time, achieve the purpose of less exposure for people, and more proper government supervision, making a significant contribution to China in the control of pandemics (22).

However, there will be no digital identity for those who buy smartphones unconditionally or have behavioral and cognitive limitations. The operation of the health code considers the plight of ""people without codes" in advance, and coresidents can help people without codes apply for health codes. These can be saved or even printed and have a validity period of 14 days (23). Nonetheless, it is still difficult to implement these digital technologies in countries where smartphones and the Internet are not widely available.

Because of the large amount of personal data collected to apply for electronic identity, there is the possibility of privacy breaches, as some privacy advocates still refuse to apply for electronic identity. For now, without electronic identity, their daily travel will be impacted. In this regard, several recent studies have discussed the future of electronic identity after the pandemic (24–26). A number of issues have been highlighted, such as whether to upgrade, improve, or delete the electronic identity after the pandemic, whether the private information can be completely deleted, and whether it could be used by criminals. These are issues that China needs to resolve in the near future. The author believes that to prevent unauthorized access to such data that could be used for criminal activity, it is necessary to develop new privacy software and establish more ideal confidentiality systems and laws.

DENTAL INSTITUTIONS SHOULD IMPROVE ALL PANDEMIC PREVENTION WORK AND POLICIES BEFORE STARTING A DENTAL PRACTICE

Establish a COVID-19 Pandemic Prevention and Control Team to Strengthen Supervision and Guidance Work and Strive to Promote and Improve the Level of Nosocomial Infection Control

Through networking, train whole staff in all protocols, including the receiving process and in the use of protective equipment. All personnel must be trained and qualified before taking up their duties, and it is particularly important to strengthen training on infection control for the dental support staff; even if they are not involved in direct patient care, they are often in contact with the patients' environment, leading to the possibility of contact transmission at any time (27, 28).

Implement Whole-Staff Health Confirmation Before Starting a Dental Practice

Hospital staff returning from low-risk areas will be required to return to work with a green code for health and with no abnormalities in their communication big data trip. Hospital staff returning from medium- and high-risk areas need to be isolated at home or centrally for 14 days and test negative for viral nucleic acid before returning to work. Daily temperature checks are required for all commuting to and from work, and no gatherings are allowed to avoid cluster infections. Regular nucleic acid testing for hospital staff should be carried out after starting dental practice to rule out nosocomial infections.

Implementation of Online Booking and Dental Care Consultation Services

Online appointments should be implemented in separate time slots to control the number of people attending each time slot, and only one patient should be booked per hour to avoid crowding. Fill in the epidemiological questionnaire form during online appointments to initially screen high-risk individuals. Online appointment numbers should be limited to patients with acute conditions such as severe dental pain, pericoronitis, post-operative osteitis, dry socket or abscess, cellulitis, tooth fracture or dislocation, and certain emergency restorative procedures (29). Furthermore, non-urgent patients should be encouraged to postpone their visits. Simultaneously, an "Internet + telephone" consultation service should be developed to actively provide health assessment, consultation guidance, psychological guidance, and other services. Additionally, detailed epidemiological history should be collected to correctly guide patients to the dental clinic in an orderly manner to reduce the risk of infection (30).

Development of Contingency Plans for COVID-19 Outbreaks in Dental Specialties

Since dental clinics are generally not designated clinics for treating COVID-19 patients, when four categories of people (confirmed cases, suspected cases, patients with febrile symptoms, and close contacts) are screened out, they need to be transferred to the designated COVID-19 clinics for further treatment (**Figure 1**). A separate isolation room should be set up at the location nearest to the dental practice facility's exit for temporary housing of patients pending transfer. The transfer route should be delineated to achieve the shortest outdoor distance and least contact with people (31), with daily access closed and only passable when the emergency plan is activated. Simultaneously, each department should set up a separate, well-ventilated, and disinfected single room as an isolation clinic and an isolation surgery room in the operating room, which is not open daily and is used only for the emergency treatment of these four categories of people. Because it is difficult to accurately predict the changes and development of the pandemic, it is important to reflect on the emergency management ability of hospitals to respond well to these changes (32).

Dental patients with fever or severe respiratory symptoms but no abnormalities in green health code or communication big data trip cards should be immediately notified to the department and the person in charge of COVID-19 infection control. Under secondary protection (see **Table 1** for details), the receiver should lead the patient to the isolation room through a special emergency channel. The hospital's COVID-19 infection control staff should bring the patient to the fever clinic for consultation. After the nucleic acid test and computed tomography (CT) examination are found to be unremarkable, and a specialist rules out the COVID-19 infection, the patient can visit the dental clinic. After that patient leaves, the area through which he or she passes should be fully disinfected. The receiving staff should be isolated at home or centrally while awaiting the patient's screening results. If the results are unremarkable, the receiving staff can go to work normally; if the results are abnormal, they need to be observed in centralized isolation for 14 days. A negative nucleic acid test should be received before they can return to work.

If a dental patient is found to be in close contact of a suspected or confirmed COVID-19 case, the department and the person

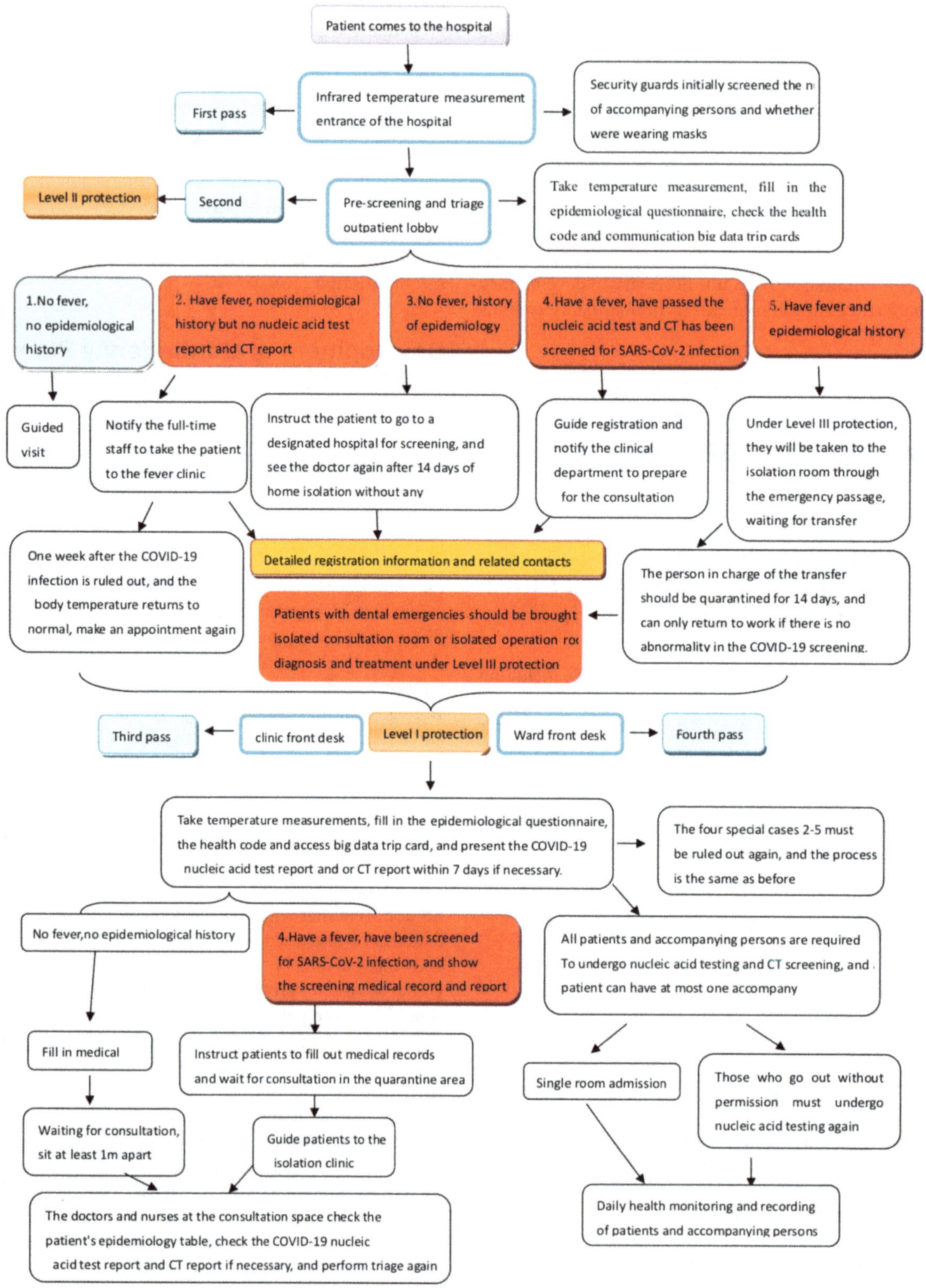

FIGURE 1 | Pre-screening and triage process in dental institutions during the coronavirus disease 2019 (COVID-19) pandemic.

in charge of COVID-19 infection control should be notified immediately, and the local Centers for Disease Control and Prevention (CDC) should be notified as well. The receiver should bring the patient to the isolation room *via* the emergency lane under Level III protection. Furthermore, the patient will wait to be brought by the CDC personnel to the designated COVID-19 treatment facility for treatment. In the event of an emergency requiring immediate treatment or surgery for the four above categories of people or patients with unknown epidemiologic history, the patients should be placed in an isolation consultation or isolation surgery room for consultation or surgery under Level III protection (33), with proper isolation and disinfection measures and timely screening for SARS-CoV-2 infection after treatment (34, 35). If the vital signs are stable, the patient should be promptly transferred to a designated treatment facility for the subsequent consultation and treatment of COVID-19. The personnel involved in the practice need to be isolated at home or centrally for 14 days and must test negative for nucleic acid before returning to work.

However, the emergency passage can only be temporarily developed according to the current building structure, and there is no special emergency passage. When transferring the four categories of people, it is difficult to completely avoid crowds. It is only possible to arrange personnel to evacuate the crowd in time to ensure the transfer route's safety as far as possible when a similar situation occurs. Therefore, in the future, the buildings of dental hospitals or dental institutions should set up special emergency passages for the timely and safe evacuation of special groups of people in response to similar public health emergencies.

SYSTEM FOR STARTING THE PRACTICE OF DENTAL INSTITUTIONS DURING A PANDEMIC

Implementation of a Three-Level Pre-screening and Triage System for Dentistry

Guarding should be implemented at the four entrances of the dental institution: the entrance of the main gate of the dental hospital or dental clinic, the entrance of the outpatient lobby on the first floor, the entrance of the front desk of the clinic, and the entrance of the ward Three-level pre-screening and triage should also be implemented for the outpatient clinic: the first level at the outpatient lobby, the second level at the front desk of the clinic, and the third level at the dental chair (36). The staff at the outpatient hall is under Level II protection. The staff at the front desk of the clinic is under Level I protection. The staff at the dental chair is under Level II protection (see **Table 1**, **Figure 2** for details). Different levels of protection for different positions should also be implemented, at least three epidemiological history inquiries and temperature measurements for all patients should also be conducted, and the nucleic acid test reports and CT reports should also be checked when necessary. Each level in the three-level pre-screening and triage is indispensable.

TABLE 1 | Requirements and scope of application of three levels of wearable protective.

Protection level	Wearing requirements	Scope of application
Level I	Disposable work caps, overalls, medical-surgical masks	The front desk of all outpatient departments and wards
Level II	Disposable work caps, overalls, medical-surgical masks or medical protective masks, goggles or protective face shields, disposable isolation suits, disposable latex gloves	Pre-screening triage staff in the primary outpatient lobby Tertiary clinic operators; exposure to patients with severe fever or respiratory symptoms but without unusual epidemiological history Cleaning personnel
Level III	Disposable work caps, overalls, medical-surgical masks or medical protective masks, goggles or protective face shields, protective clothing, disposable latex gloves, waterproof boot covers	Exposure to suspected or confirmed COVID-19 cases

The pre-screening and triage site should be marked, relatively self-contained, well-ventilated, and equipped with rapid hand disinfectant, surface disinfectant, PPE, and temperature detection devices. The pre-screening and triage counters and items should be disinfected every 2 h and whenever contamination is encountered.

Differentiation of Dental Practice Items by Risk Level

The high-, medium-, and low-risk areas released daily by the state are divided according to the zoning and classification criteria, which are refined to community-based units. The risk level of the pandemic is dynamically adjusted and announced on time. The pandemic is handled according to the principles of "early, small, strict, and practical" (37). The specific classification principles are (**Table 2**): ① High-risk areas are defined as areas with more than 50 new cases of COVID-19, with a cluster outbreak within the last 14 days; ② Medium-risk areas are defined as areas with new confirmed cases of COVID-19 within 14 days, but with the total number of confirmed cases of COVID-19 not exceeding 50 cases, or areas with the total number of confirmed cases of COVID-19 exceeding 50 cases, but with no cluster outbreak within 14 days; ③ Low-risk areas are defined as areas with no confirmed cases of COVID-19 or no new cases of COVID-19 for 14 days.

This shows that the classification of the pandemic's risk level in each region is dynamic and constantly changing. Dynamic adjustments should be made in practice items, and dental chair arrangements according to the national and regional pandemic changes and the different risk levels of COVID-19 in different regions. Studies have shown that the bacterial load is five times higher after simultaneous dental treatment in multiple chairs, while this difference is reduced to two times higher with single chairs (38). Therefore, it is important to rationalize practice items and chair settings during a pandemic to achieve four-handed dentistry to reduce infection and occupational exposure risk.

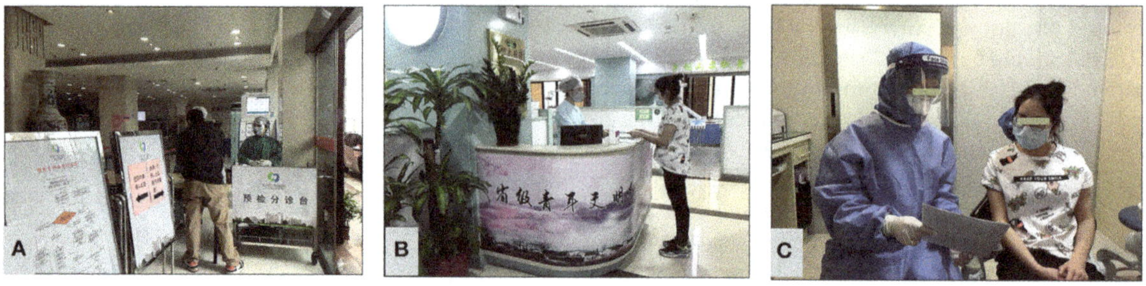

FIGURE 2 | Three-level pre-screening and triage. **(A)** Level 1 lobby triage. **(B)** Level 2 clinic front desk triage. **(C)** Level 3 consultation space triage.

Furthermore, dental chairs should be set up in well-ventilated consultation rooms with air sterilization equipment (3, 38). The measures for performing dental practice during periods of different risk levels are as follows:

High-Risk Areas

In such areas, dental clinics are completely closed, while dental hospitals, depending on their scale, retain 4–6 medical staff and one guide per day for dental emergencies and on-site consultations. A dedicated infection control specialist is also established to supervise and guide medical staff in infection control and achieve standard prevention. Patients attending the clinic must hold a green code and communication big data without abnormality. Furthermore, they must present the results of a nucleic acid test taken within 7 days and CT reports within 7 days only if necessary. Medical practice should be conducted in a separate room with good ventilation and sterilization equipment, and only one dental chair can be used in a large multi-chair room. The practice items are mainly for dental emergencies, and slow handpieces can be used for emergencies. The orthodontics department can receive return visits and suspend spattering operations, but the inpatient department of maxillofacial surgery must postpone elective surgery and only accept patients with dental emergencies requiring inpatient treatment. Patients are admitted in a single room, and only one person is allowed to accompany each patient. Patients and accompanying persons need to undergo nucleic acid detection and CT screening before being admitted to the hospital, and they can only be admitted if there is no abnormality. During hospitalization, the patient and accompanying staff should be monitored for body temperature and respiratory symptoms every day. They should not go out without permission. Nucleic acid testing and CT screening must be repeated after going out.

Medium-Risk Areas

At this time, some dental outpatient consultations can be gradually resumed, and the number of the medical staff at work can be increased appropriately according to the number of patients. Except for periodontal treatment, dental implants, and dental preparations, which are highly spattering procedures, the rest of the procedures can be resumed gradually. Dental practices should be carried out in separate consultation rooms. Furthermore, two consecutive dental chairs in a large multi-chair room cannot be used simultaneously. Seats at an interval of one chair should be used. Attending patients should present their green code and communication big data without abnormalities. Furthermore, a COVID-19 nucleic acid test report and/or CT report taken within the last 7 days should be presented if necessary. During the medium-risk period, principles for admitting patients to the ward remain the same as those during the high-risk period.

Low-Risk Areas

Daily dental outpatient practice will resume at this time. For highly spattering operations such as tooth extraction (except for deciduous teeth), periodontal treatment, and dental implants, patients will be required to hold a green code and communication big data without abnormalities, as well as present a 7-day COVID-19 nucleic acid test report and, if necessary, a 7-day CT report. Conversely, other procedures do not require a nucleic acid test report. All chairs can be used normally (except dental isolation chairs). The ward may add elective procedures as appropriate, and single-room admission should be adopted as far as possible. For multi-bed wards, patients should be placed one bed apart, windows should be opened regularly for ventilation in the ward, and the patients' and accompanying persons' temperature should be monitored. Moreover, respiratory symptoms should be observed daily during hospitalization. Nucleic acid testing and CT screening are still required before the hospitalization of patients and accompanying persons.

DEVELOPMENT OF A SYSTEM FOR THE MANAGEMENT OF PATIENTS AND ACCOMPANYING PERSONS IN DENTAL FACILITIES

Investigating the Epidemiological History

During the pandemic, each patient and the accompanying person must fill out the COVID-19 Epidemiological Questionnaire (39). The health code and communication big data trip cards should be reviewed, and the hospital should keep the questionnaire. The questionnaire's content should be dynamically adapted to the epidemiological characteristics of COVID-19, taking into account the daily release of areas at high risk of the pandemic.

TABLE 2 | Hierarchical differential guidelines for dental institutions to start practice.

	High-risk areas	Medium-risk areas	Low-risk areas
Consultation settings	Separate consultation rooms are open, and only one consultation space is available in large multi-place rooms	A separate consultation room starts a dental practice, with multiple consecutive consultations with one consultation space interval.	Resumption of daily consultation schedule
Dental practice items allowed	The entire hospital should be closed for routine outpatient care, and a 24-h emergency clinic should be set up, with a focus on emergencies and the use of low-speed turbines if necessary	Suspend high spattering operations; remaining items can be phased in, using low-speed turbine handpieces if necessary	Resumption of daily starting dental practice program
Patient sources	Emergency	A small number of online or telephone appointment numbers and emergency numbers in different time slots	The appropriate number of online or telephone appointments and emergency numbers in different time slots
Patient visit requirements	Need to have nucleic acid test report within 7 days and CT report if necessary	Present nucleic acid test report and CT report within 7 days if necessary	Nucleic acid test report within 7 days for high spattering operations and CT report if necessary
No anomalies in health code green code or communication big data	Need	Need	Need
Disinfection of objects surfaces	Terminal disinfection four times a day, disinfection of the dental chair after each consultation, and terminal disinfection of dental chairs after splattering operations	Terminal disinfection four times a day, disinfection of the dental chair after each consultation, and terminal disinfection of dental chairs after each splattering operation	Twice-daily Terminal disinfection, disinfection of the dental chair after each consultation, and terminal disinfection of dental chairs after each splattering operation
Floor and wall disinfection	Avoid dry sweeping, disinfect four times a day, disinfect wall height 2–2.5 m, disinfect anytime there is contamination	Avoid dry sweeping, disinfect twice a day, disinfect walls at the height of 2–2.5 m, disinfect whenever there is contamination	Avoid dry sweeping, disinfect twice a day, disinfect walls at the height of 2–2.5 m, disinfect whenever there is contamination
Surface disinfectants	1,000 mg/L chlorinated disinfectant solution can be used; see "8.1 Surface disinfectants" for other details	A disinfectant solution containing 500–1,000 mg/L chlorine can be used; see "8.1 Surface disinfectants" for other details	500 mg/L chlorinated disinfectant can be used; see "8.1 Surface disinfectants" for other details
Elevators	Elevator keys and cabs are disinfected every 2 h, and whenever there is contamination	Elevator keys and cabs are disinfected every 2 h, and whenever there is contamination	Elevator keys and cabs are disinfected every 2 h, and whenever there is contamination
Elevator disinfectants	500 mg/L chlorinated disinfectant or 75% alcohol	Same as high-risk areas	Same as high-risk areas
Toilet	Disinfect four times a day and whenever there is contamination	Disinfect four times a day and whenever there is contamination	Disinfect twice daily and whenever there is contamination
Toilet disinfectants	1,000 mg/L chlorinated disinfectant	Same as high-risk areas	500 mg/L chlorinated disinfectant
Air	Use the air disinfector throughout the practice, and use the UV lamp for 30–60 min when no one is around, and open the windows twice a day for more than 30 min each time	Same as high-risk areas	Same as high-risk areas
Air disinfectants	See "8.2.1 Air disinfectants" for details	Same as high-risk areas	Same as high-risk areas

For example, at the beginning of the pandemic, Wuhan was the center of the outbreak, so the location for investigating the epidemiological history was Wuhan. Any visits to Wuhan or contact with people who visited Wuhan within 14 days were ruled out (40), body temperature were tested, and respiratory symptoms were ruled out. On April 26, 2020, the COVID-19 patients in Wuhan were cleared, so Wuhan was no longer included in the epidemiological survey questionnaire.

Provide COVID-19 Nucleic Acid Report and/or CT Findings as Necessary

Rapid sequencing of the SARS-CoV-2 genome has led to the development of real-time multiplex reverse transcription-polymerase chain reaction (RT-PCR) assays as the gold standard for detecting viral RNA and identifying patients with COVID-19 and asymptomatic carriers (41). Furthermore, it is currently the main type of test used to determine whether a patient is infected with SARS-CoV-2 in China. Patients with mild COVID-19 can have no pneumonia symptoms; therefore, CT results alone cannot be used as a criterion to rule out COVID-19 infection. However, nucleic acid testing can be affected by the disease's course, specimen collection, testing procedure, or testing reagents, among other factors. The test should be performed at a medical institution qualified for nucleic acid testing to improve the testing's positive rate. The specimens should be collected by professionals and sent for testing as soon as possible (3). The government qualifies nucleic acid testing institutions in China, and nucleic acid testing institution search, APPs, has been launched, through which the names and locations of testing institutions can be checked at any time.

Strengthen Patient Waiting Management in Dental Institutions

When patients visit dental institutions, they must all wear masks, and no accompanying persons can enter. In the case of the elderly, children, or patients with limited ability to act due to illness, one accompanying person may be allowed to enter and is required to wear a mask throughout. Patients should also be screened for green codes and communication big data to confirm lack of abnormalities before entering. A dedicated person should maintain order on the site, instructing patients to maintain a minimum distance of 1 m from each other (42), be seated one chair away from each other, maintain good cough etiquette, and avoid gathering of people.

INCREASE SELF-PROTECTION OF MEDICAL PERSONNEL IN DENTAL INSTITUTIONS

Selecting the Right Personal Protective Equipment

Since dental consultations are performed close to the patient, the operator's facepiece, eye mask, face mask, and operating arm are the areas closest to the patient and are the most contaminated (43). Thus, protection requirements should be at least Level II; Level III should be achieved when receiving the above four categories of people. Disposable protective equipment should be discarded after use and replaced when there is significant contamination with blood or body fluids. It is also necessary to avoid the overuse of PPE. Overlapping protective clothing is prone to breakage that is not easy to detect. It is more likely to be soaked with sweat during work, reducing the protective performance. Scientific and reasonable use of protective equipment can effectively reduce the risk of infection (44). The eye shields worn during operation often fog up, resulting in unclear vision, and are prone to occupational exposure. The anti-fogging method for the endoscope lens in the operating room can be borrowed; that is, iodophor can be evenly applied to the inner side of the eyepiece. The ionic iodine becomes molecular iodine, which plays an oxidizing role and forms a protective film that can last for 4–5 h against fogging.

Before the outbreak, dental practices generally used Level I protection with protective face shields or eye shields for highly spattering operations. The outbreak was so rapid that the vast majority of dental practices had inadequate protection measures in place. There was a shortage of protective materials, resulting in inadequate protective equipment for medical staff. If disposable gowns are not available, they can be temporarily replaced by cloth surgical gowns, which can be changed once every 4 h and washed and disinfected centrally. This can also have a protective effect (**Figure 2A**). In the case of sufficient materials, it is strongly recommended to use disposable isolation gowns, surgical masks, or medical protective masks. However, neither isolation nor surgical clothing can effectively protect the neck of medical staff, posing a risk of infection. Moreover, the use of disposable protective clothing is seldom applied during diagnosis and treatment in the Stomatology Department due to the high cost and shortage of materials. Therefore, the disposable shawl cap was quickly developed. This can be used with isolation or surgical clothing to strengthen the protective measures of medical personnel (**Figure 2C**), and standard prevention could be achieved insofar as high-risk environments are involved.

Strengthening Hand Hygiene

Many studies have shown the critical role of healthcare workers' (HCWs) hands in transmitting microorganisms in the healthcare setting and ultimately to patients (45). Handwashing can therefore slow the spread of the virus (46). Nonetheless, before the outbreak, hand hygiene compliance was poor among HCWs (47–49). Studies have shown that hand sanitizer dispensers and gloves are the most contaminated PPE (50). Therefore, it is very important to improve compliance to and accuracy of hand hygiene. WHO also issues an annual global call to action to health workers through its SAVE LIVES: Clean Your Hands campaign, held annually in the month of May. This campaign aims to educate health workers and patients on the importance of effective handwashing, which has become more urgent with the COVID-19 pandemic.

Use the seven-step handwashing technique and master the five moments requiring handwashing: two before and three after, two before: before contact with the patient and before aseptic operation; three after: after contact with the patient, after contact with the patient's surroundings and related objects, and after exposure to body fluids. When handwashing is not available, adequate rapid hand sanitizer should be deployed in the best configuration within the medical staff's reach, which will reduce unnecessary walking of medical staff and make it easier to improve hand hygiene implementation.

With the improvements in hand hygiene implementation rate, the frequency of handwashing and hand disinfection has greatly increased, consequently followed by an increase in the incidence of hand eczema (51–53). Several studies have reported that oral medical staff have a high incidence of hand eczema owing to different factors of moisture-related operations such as frequent handwashing, increased irritation from hand disinfectants, and the long-term use of rubber gloves (54–57). Because hand eczema involves macules, papules, vesicles, edema, scaling, hyperkeratosis, fissures, etc. (58), skin damage increases the susceptibility of acquiring contact infection. Moreover, wearing gloves can aggravate the symptoms of hand eczema; therefore, people with hand eczema who have been treated with the corresponding drug treatments should still daub emollients, temporarily rest after work, and reduce hand stimulation to avoid aggravation (59, 60).

Proper Donning and Doffing of Protective Equipment Are More Important

Wearing proper PPE can help medical staff reduce the risk of infection, but incorrectly donning and doffing PPE can expose medical staff to hazardous conditions that make them highly susceptible to infection. Multiple publications during the outbreak reported proper PPE donning and doffing (61–64), with hand hygiene implementation throughout the process of proper PPE donning and doffing. Since gloves are the most heavily contaminated protective equipment, both the Glove-in-Glove Technique and Bird Beak Technique methods of glove removal can be used (65) to reduce the chance of hand contamination. Proper donning and doffing of PPE are necessary to reduce the chances of infection effectively.

STRENGTHEN INFECTION CONTROL AND PREVENTION IN THE DENTAL CLINIC ENVIRONMENT

Sterilization of Object Surfaces and the Environment in the Dental Clinic

Studies have shown that coronaviruses can survive from 2 h to 9 days on surfaces of various materials such as plastic, metal, or glass (66, 67). Furthermore, self-service printers, desks/keyboards, desktops, door handles, medical equipment, utilities, and walls and floors are the most contaminated areas in the clinic (50), especially those that are subject to high-frequency use, such as elevator buttons and bathrooms. Therefore, the dental clinic should be kept clean and tidy, desktop items should be kept in cabinets as much as possible, and object surfaces should be properly disinfected to reduce environmental contamination.

Object surface disinfectant: ① use 75% alcohol to wipe object surfaces two times and allow action for 3 min (spray disinfection is prohibited); ② use a chlorine-containing disinfectant at a concentration of 500–1,000 mg/L to wipe or soak for 30 min; ③ use quaternary ammonium salt disinfectant at a concentration of 1,000–2,000 mg/L to spray or wipe; ④ use 0.1–0.2% peroxyacetic acid or 3% hydrogen peroxide to spray or soak for disinfection for an action time of 30 min. In cases of obvious pollution, water-absorbent materials containing 10,000 mg/L chlorine disinfectant can be used to wrap the pollutants and can be cleaned for disinfection again (68).

Measures to Reduce Aerosols in the Dental Clinic

Air Purification

(1) The fresh air system should be turned on in the dental clinic while ensuring the cleanliness of the fresh air system air intake and its surroundings; when there is no fresh air system, the doors or windows should be opened to enhance air circulation (69). An outbreak of COVID-19 was reported in an air-conditioned restaurant in Guangzhou, China, due to poor air circulation without a fresh air system and ventilation windows (70). Ventilating the clinic by opening windows to inject fresh outdoor air directly into the clinic is one of the quickest and most effective methods to reduce the amount of aerosols in the air inside the clinic (38).

(2) Air disinfection machines with human–machine co-presence may be used and kept running at all times during operation. These can also be used in an unoccupied environment with UV lamp irradiation for at least 30–60 min. If the temperature is lower than 20°C or higher than 40°C and indoor humidity is >60%, the irradiation time needs to be extended, while the power of the UV lamp should be tested regularly and the UV lamp should be cleaned 1–2 times a week. Every day after the end of the consultation, 0.2% peroxyacetic acid or 3% hydrogen peroxide can be sprayed using the aerosol spray method, with the dosage calculated as 20–30 ml/m^3 (1 g/m^3), and ventilation after 60 min of disinfection action. A total of 15% peroxyacetic acid can also be used for heating fumigation, with the dosage calculated as 7 ml/m^3 and ventilation after 1–2 h of fumigation action (68).

Patients Should Properly Gargle Before Dental Consultation

Several studies have confirmed that preoperative patient gargling reduces room air bacteria caused by dental procedures. Furthermore, during the COVID-19 pandemic, pre-consultation gargling should be performed with 1.5–3% hydrogen peroxide or 0.5–1.5% povidone-iodine for at least 30 s (71–73). Simultaneously, the patient should be instructed to gently spit into the gargling cup, use a strong aspiration device to aspirate the liquid from the gargling cup, and to try not to use or reduce the mouthwash basin's use to reduce droplet and aerosol production. SARS-CoV-2 has also been shown to be insensitive to chlorhexidine and Hibitane, so gargling with these solutions is not recommended (3, 74). However, recent studies have shown that in SARS-CoV-2-positive subjects, gargling with 1% hydrogen peroxide does not reduce oral viral load (75). However, the sample size in this experiment was small, and only RT-PCR was used as the detection method; thus, the statistical power of the results remains questionable. The author hopes that more studies can be conducted to assess the relationship between the use of mouthwash and SARS-CoV-2 to identify the type, method, and concentration of mouthwash that can reduce or even inactivate SARS-CoV-2 instantly, so that it can be applied in oral diagnosis and treatment to reduce the risk of infection.

Use Four-Handed and Six-Handed Operation for Oral Treatment, Prevention, and Control

According to several literature reports, the use of four-handed and six-handed operations in oral diagnosis and treatment can effectively improve work efficiency, reduce the work intensity of oral medical staff, and concomitantly achieve better standard prevention (76–81). Therefore, during the pandemic period, four-handed operations are a necessity for oral diagnosis and treatment (82, 83). Six-handed operations, if available, are better, as they can improve work efficiency and effectiveness, shorten the working time, reduce the time of medical personnel's exposure to aerosol pollution, and reduce the risk of infection. However, some institutions believe that the implementation of four-handed and six-handed operations requires more human resources, and the operation cost will be greatly increased. Therefore, currently, many oral hospitals and dental clinics involved in daily oral treatment operations do not apply four-handed or six-handed operation. The author's unit has practiced four-handed operations for many years; during this pandemic, we realized the superiority of four-handed operation in the prevention and control of the pandemic in dental institutions, and we believe that the effective implementation of four-handed operations will increase the economic benefits of oral institutions and patient comfort.

Application of Powerful Aspiration Devices

To effectively reduce splatter contamination from dental operations, the literature emphasizes and recommends using strong aspiration devices. Studies have shown that the use of strong aspiration devices could reduce droplet splatter area by 93%. A strong aspiration group reduced aerosol particles by ~90% compared to a weak aspiration group (84); thus, they should be used in conjunction with strong and weak aspiration in clinical operations. An extra-dental vacuum aspirator (EOVA) can be used, if conditions permit, to reduce droplet and aerosol contamination. The use of EOVA has been mentioned in the literature as an effective method to reduce air pollution in dental clinics. It is recommended for the treatment of patients with infectious diseases (85–88). EOVA devices were heavily promoted during the COVID-19 pandemic, but these devices were relatively expensive and not easily accessible across the board.

Use Anti-suction Turbo Dental Handpieces for Oral Treatment

In recent years, more attention has been directed toward the pollution of the dental treatment table water system. The pollution sources are mainly municipal water pollution and sudden stoppage of turbo dental handpieces, which causes patients' saliva and blood to flow through the turbo dental handpieces and into the lumen of the dental table water system (89, 90). The pollutants, after the back suction, will be ejected again the next time they are used, which can easily cause nosocomial infections (91). Although a variety of disinfectants have been used for the disinfection of dental treatment table water system in recent years (92, 93), it is possible to fundamentally solve the problem by using anti-suction turbo dental handpieces to prevent regurgitation. However, this will also increase the cost of oral institutions to a certain extent, and popularization and promotion may require time. Nevertheless, the authors believe that in the current pandemic period, effective prevention and control of each link are the first issues that oral doctors should consider. It is reported that 0.5 vol% H_2O_2 added to the water spray of dental handpieces drastically reduced the possibility of coronavirus spread during aerosol-generating dental procedures (94). Although these results still require confirmation, it may be a promising method to deal with water pollution in the future.

Use of Rubber Dams in Dental Practice

Studies have shown that using rubber dams during operations reduced colony counts by 82.7% (lamp-side sampling) and 83.9% (chest-side sampling) (95). Most studies have formed a broad consensus that rubber dams effectively reduced splatter transmission by 33% and reduced surface bacterial contamination by 80–99% during aerosol generation (96). Therefore, the use of rubber dams, where possible, can be effective in reducing aerosol formation during clinical operations.

DENTAL PANORAMIC RADIOGRAPHY AND CONE BEAM COMPUTED TOMOGRAPHY ARE RECOMMENDED FOR ORAL RADIOGRAPHY DURING THE PANDEMIC

Intraoral radiography, dental panoramic radiography, and cone beam computed tomography (CBCT) are commonly used imaging techniques in the Department of Stomatology. As mentioned earlier, SARS-CoV-2 can be present in saliva and aerosols (97–99). Since intraoral radiography easily induces nausea and cough, there is a high risk of transmission. Concomitantly, since it is necessary to put the sensor into the patient's mouth, there is also a risk of cross-infection. Dental panoramic radiography and cone beam computed tomography are, therefore, recommended during the pandemic (100, 101). However, some dental clinics are less equipped and only have intraoral radiography. The sensors can be covered with a disposable plastic film. After the film is soaked with 1,000 mg/L chlorine-containing disinfectant for 30 min, it is discarded into a medical waste bag (102), and the sensor is disinfected with 75% alcohol.

Radiologists should also conduct secondary protection. Patients should use povidone-iodine or hydrogen peroxide gargle for at least 30 s before undergoing oral radiology examination. After each patient's examination, 75% alcohol or 500 mg/L chlorine-containing disinfectant should be used to disinfect the examination room and equipment (103, 104).

STERILIZATION OF DENTAL CHAIRS BEFORE AND AFTER PRACTICE

Disinfection of Dental Chairs Before Starting Dental Practice

Routinely turn on the dental chair water line rinse for 2–5 min before starting practice to drain the residual fluid in the pipe from the previous day's consultation; this can reduce the bacterial content in the pipe by one third (**Table 2**). For dental chairs with a pipe disinfection function, the pipe should be disinfected before the consultation. Conversely, for dental chairs without pipe disinfection function, the water pipe can be flushed and disinfected before starting dental practice with 500 mg/L of chlorine-containing disinfection solution, 3% hydrogen peroxide, and 5% silver peroxide ion, and the air pipe of the dental chair should be flushed for 20–30 s (105, 106). Several studies have demonstrated that daily pre-consultation rinsing can flush out plankton deposited in the pipeline the night before and reduce the number of bacteria in the pipeline.

Disinfection of Dental Chairs Should Be Carried Out After Each Spraying Operation

During patient visits, the stain-proof film can be used to avoid stains in the frequently touched areas. At the end of each consultation, remove the stain-proof film, disinfect the dental chair's surface, and flush the pipes. A chlorine solution at 500–1,000 mg/L can be used for terminal disinfection of the dental chair after each splattering operation. The higher the concentration of chlorine-containing disinfectant, the more effective the disinfection, but the more corrosive it is to the pipes; therefore, this is an emergency practice measure under the COVID-19 pandemic.

Terminal Disinfection

During the pandemic period, terminal disinfection using 500–1,000 mg/L of chlorine disinfectant is performed 2–4 times a day. Disinfection of the dental chair pipe should also be performed simultaneously. For dental chairs without the pipeline disinfection function, the same disinfection method for the dental chair pipe before starting practice should be carried out. After rinsing, the power should be turned off and the pipe should be left for 30 min and rinsed with clean water. The pipe disinfectant's concentration should then be tested to prevent the disinfectant from corroding the dental chair pipe.

DENTAL APPLIANCE HANDLING

According to the Regulation for Disinfection and Sterilization Technique of Dental Instruments (WS 506–2016), the hazard degree of oral instruments can be divided into three groups: critical dental instruments, semi-critical dental instruments, and non-critical dental instruments. According to these requirements, it is important to choose the appropriate disinfection and storage methods (107). Among them, semi-critical and non-critical oral instruments only need to be cleaned and preserved after disinfection. However, during the pandemic period, oral instruments should be sterilized using high temperature and high-pressure steam and stored separately (except instruments with low temperature resistance) (108). Only one person should conduct sterilization or disinfection to avoid cross-infection. Separating semi-critical and non-critical dental instruments after packaging sterilization greatly increases the operating costs of oral medical institutions, especially of smaller dental clinics. This will cause them to not sterilize their equipment, and the equipment will be sent to other oral medical institutions for sterilization. Such scenarios not only increase the operation cost but also increase the workload. However, only by doing an adequate job of infection control in every detail of oral diagnosis and treatment operation can we avoid cross-infection and protect the safety of doctors, nurses, and patients.

After use, dental instruments are placed separately and recycled promptly, depending on the instrument material, function, and disposal method (107). A disinfection-cleaning-disinfection process can be used to treat dental instruments during an outbreak. It is advisable to pre-treat dental instruments at the chairside, decontaminated by wiping with 75% alcohol. It has been shown that the contamination rate of instruments decreases substantially after chairside pre-cleaning, while the cleaning time can be shortened, and the damage rate of instruments can be reduced (109). After chairside pre-treatment, instruments can be placed in 75% alcohol for 30–60 min, or in a chlorine-containing disinfectant solution at 1,000–2,000 mg/L for 30 min, before being soaked in a 1:150 multi-enzyme solution and sealed. Instruments that cannot be soaked (e.g., high-speed turbine handpieces or scaling machine handles) are stored dry and sealed after surface pre-treatment and promptly recycled to the supply room for centralized cleaning and disinfection. Dental instruments used by the four categories of people should be sealed after immediate chairside disinfection and stored wet or dry in a special sealed box, recovered by the supply room specialist, and sent to the supply room for disinfection *via* a special channel. The supply room should make contingency plans for instruments after use by the four categories of people before starting a dental practice. Designated personnel should be appointed to clean and disinfect them, which should reach Level 3 protection, and separate cleaning rooms should be set up. Disinfection equipment should be marked with clear and conspicuous labels to distinguish them from other instruments to avoid cross-infection.

MEDICAL WASTE MANAGEMENT FOR DENTAL PRACTICE

Medical waste, a hazardous by-product, carries the risk of infection. During outbreaks of major infectious diseases, improper collection, storage, transportation, or disposal of medical waste will cause ecological pollution and increase the risk of disease transmission (110).

The dress code for cleaning personnel performing waste collection during an outbreak includes long-sleeved overalls, disposable hat, disposable surgical mask, disposable isolation gown, waterproof latex gloves, waterproof boots, and face shield. Recovery of items after use for the four categories of people should be under Level III protection.

A storage room for isolation items should be designated to recover items after use for the above four categories of people, and the special bags and sharps boxes for medical waste should be carefully checked to ensure that they are not damaged or leaking. Double-layered bags should be used for medical waste, with a gooseneck knot closure, to seal them in layers. Each bag and sharps box should be tied or affixed with a Chinese label, and the label content should include medical waste generation unit, generation department, generation date, and category. The items should be marked as having been used for the four categories of people to enhance the warning effect. Before leaving the contaminated area, these items should be disinfected by spraying the bag's surface with 1,000 mg/L chlorine disinfectant (pay attention to spraying evenly) or adding a medical layer waste bag on the outside prior to transportation to the government-designated COVID-19 patient medical waste disposal facility. At the end of the transport, the transportation tool should be disinfected with 1,000 mg/L chlorine-containing disinfectant solution (111).

COVID-19 VACCINATION

China has been developing and producing the COVID-19 vaccine and has gradually started vaccinating key populations (e.g., medical personnel, frozen food industry, and logistics) with the COVID-19 vaccine since the end of December 2020, with rollout gradually being extended to all citizens. As of 24:00, February 9, 2021, 40.52 million doses of vaccination have been administered nationwide. The authors received COVID-19 vaccination on February 4 and March 4, 2021, respectively, without adverse reactions. However, recently, a new study showed that SARS-CoV-2 had evolved into more than 800 different subtypes or branches since the outbreak at the end of 2019 (112), with some strains not even detectable by nucleic acid tests. Admittedly, the protection rate of the COVID-19 vaccine currently in use is difficult to determine. This is a major challenge for future pandemic prevention and control; therefore, pandemic prevention and control cannot be slackened.

LIMITATIONS

These measures also have limitations. For example, a health code, a three-level pre-testing triage, three-level protection, and four-handed operation are easier to implement in countries with abundant medical resources. According to the literature, many countries are experiencing shortages of supplies during the pandemic. Because of poor detection capabilities and insufficient knowledge of infection prevention and control (IPC) protocols (113–118), it is difficult to implement these measures. But during the pandemic, we must strive to achieve standard prevention and to avoid cross-infection. The authors recommend the following measures in response to these situations.

- Set up an IPC team to develop an IPC policy and emergency plan, considering the available resources, to guide medical staff and patients to protect themselves during the pandemic. Strengthen IPC knowledge by training, including that in handwashing, PPE use, etc. (119).
- In case of insufficient medical staff, the number and frequency of patient visits should be reduced to decrease the pressure on medical staff. Also, reassign the medical staff posted in the pre-testing and triage positions when all oral diagnoses and treatments cannot be guaranteed with four-handed operations, which should be performed for as many high-spray procedures as possible, to reduce aerosol pollution.
- When there is no air disinfection equipment, the operation should be conducted in a well-ventilated consulting room.
- Manual instruments should be used as much as possible to reduce aerosol pollution (120). During periodontal treatment, manual scaling can be used instead of ultrasonic cleaning; use slow dental handpieces instead of high-speed handpieces when the use of handpieces is necessary.
- Frequent handwashing should be performed in situations where hand sanitizers are in short supply.
- When a mask is not obviously contaminated or damaged, it should be disinfected with vaporous hydrogen peroxide, ultraviolet germicidal irradiation, and moist heat (121, 122). However, this method is only to be used when masks are in short supply.
- Cloth isolation gowns or surgical gowns can be used instead of disposable gowns. Although either cloth or surgical gowns can be used, they exhibit higher bacterial detection rates than do disposable gowns (123); however, one should change the cloth or surgical gown every 4 h and have centralized cleaning and disinfection facilities available. These gowns can be used in an emergency in case of a shortage of disposable gowns, but they have a high permeability (124), and should be replaced when there is obvious contamination.
- In the case of shortage of disposable protective face shields, one shield can be used repeatedly, but it must be strictly disinfected and stored in a clean area. The commonly used disinfection methods are as follows: After wiping and disinfecting with 75% alcohol, irradiate under ultraviolet light for 1 h (125); soak in 1% sodium hypochlorite solution for at least 10 min; soak in 2% glutaraldehyde for 10 min, rinse with normal saline, and then air-dry; and ethylene oxide (ETO) sterilization (126). Without a disposable protective face shield, a simple protective face shield can be made using a transparent, flexible plastic film and rope (127).

CONCLUSION

Although the global COVID-19 pandemic is still ongoing, dental care for patients with dental diseases cannot be stopped. We should learn from experience and actively implement pre-screening and triage to control the infection source, taking into account the pandemic trend and the above dynamic measures on dental practice under the pandemic. According to the etiological and epidemiological characteristics of the COVID-19 virus, and to its pathogenic and epidemiological characteristics, the key to infection control is the reasonable, correct, and effective use of disinfectants. Simultaneously, we should adequately implement infection control and prevention and cut off transmission routes. Additionally, we should achieve standard prevention, protect susceptible people, protect doctors and patients in both directions, and avoid cross-infection to ensure safe and smooth dental practice.

AUTHOR CONTRIBUTIONS

LL was responsible for the study concepts and design, and literature research. MZ was responsible for the clinical studies and experimental studies. XC was responsible for the data acquisition and analysis. SC was responsible for the statistical analysis. CX was responsible for the manuscript preparation. WX was responsible for the manuscript editing. LJ was responsible for the study design. XZ was responsible for the experimental studies.

PC was responsible for the guarantor of integrity of the entire study, definition of intellectual content, and manuscript review. MR was responsible for the guarantor of integrity of the entire study and manuscript review. All authors read and approved the final manuscript.

ACKNOWLEDGMENTS

The authors would like to thank the team from the Department of Periodontology and Oral Implantology, Stomatological Hospital, Southern Medical University.

REFERENCES

1. Benvenuto D, Benedetti F, Demir AB, Ciccozzi M, Zella D. Analysis of three mutations in Italian strains of SARS-CoV-2: implications for pathogenesis. *Chemotherapy*. (2021). doi: 10.1159/000515342. [Epub ahead of print].
2. Harrel SK, Molinari J. Aerosols and splatter in dentistry: a brief review of the literature and infection control implications. *J Am Dent Assoc.* (2004) 135:429–37. doi: 10.14219/jada.archive.2004.0207
3. Diagnosis and treatment protocol for COVID-19 (trial Edition 8). Available online at: http://www.nhc.gov.cn/cms-search/downFiles/a449a3e2e2c94d9a856d5faea2ff0f94.pdf
4. Mukhra R, Krishan K, Kanchan T. Possible modes of transmission of Novel coronavirus SARS-CoV-2: a review. *Acta Biomed.* (2020) 91:e2020036. doi: 10.23750/abm.v91i3.10039
5. Transmission of SARS-CoV-2: implications for infection prevention precautions. Available online at: https://www.who.int/news-room/commentaries/detail/transmission-of-sars-cov-2-implications-for-infection-prevention-precautions
6. Wang W, Xu Y, Gao R, Lu R, Han K, Wu G, et al. Detection of SARS-CoV-2 in different types of clinical specimens. *JAMA.* (2020) 323:1843–4. doi: 10.1001/jama.2020.3786
7. Van Doremalen N, Bushmaker T, Morris DH, Holbrook MG, Gamble A, Williamson BN, et al. Aerosol and surface stability of SARS-CoV-2 as compared with SARS-CoV-1. *N Engl J Med.* (2020) 382:1564–7. doi: 10.1056/NEJMc2004973
8. Xu H, Zhong L, Deng J, Peng J, Dan H, Zeng X, et al. High expression of ACE2 receptor of 2019-nCoV on the epithelial cells of oral mucosa. *Int J Oral Sci.* (2020) 12:8. doi: 10.1038/s41368-020-0074-x
9. Chen WP, Huang SH. Preventive measures of environmental infection propagation in department of stomatology. *Chin J Pract Stomatol.* (2015) 8:56–60. Available online at: https://kns.cnki.net/kcms/detail/detail.aspx?FileName=ZSKQ201501018&DbName=CJFQ2015
10. Izzetti R, Nisi M, Gabriele M, Graziani F. COVID-19 transmission in dental practice: brief review of preventive measures in Italy. *J Dent Res.* (2020) 99:1030–8. doi: 10.1177/0022034520920580
11. Mayta-Tovalino F, Diaz-Soriano A, Munive-Degregori A, Pérez-Vargas F, Luza S, Bocanegra R, et al. Proposal for a provisional protocol for the care and identification of dental transmission routes of COVID-19 in Latin America: a literature review. *J Clin Exp Dent.* (2020) 12:e979–90. doi: 10.4317/jced.57762
12. Shamsoddin E, DeTora LM, Tovani-Palone MR, Bierer BE. Dental care in times of the COVID-19 pandemic: a review. *Med Sci (Basel).* (2021) 9:13. doi: 10.3390/medsci9010013
13. Amato A, Caggiano M, Amato M, Moccia G, Capunzo M, De Caro F. Infection control in dental practice during the COVID-19 pandemic. *Int J Environ Res Public Health.* (2020) 17:4769. doi: 10.3390/ijerph17134769
14. Tysiac-Miśta M, Dziedzic A. The attitudes and professional approaches of dental practitioners during the COVID-19 outbreak in Poland: a cross-sectional survey. *Int J Environ Res Public Health.* (2020) 17:4703. doi: 10.3390/ijerph17134703
15. Pereira LJ, Murata RM, Pardi V, Mattos FF. Streamlining the dental care during COVID-19 pandemic: updated clinical recommendations and infection control management framework. *Braz Oral Res.* (2021) 35:e046. doi: 10.1590/1807-3107bor-2021.vol35.0046
16. Villani FA, Aiuto R, Paglia L, Re D. COVID-19 and dentistry: prevention in dental practice, a literature review. *Int J Environ Res Public Health.* (2020) 17:4609. doi: 10.3390/ijerph17124609
17. Tay JRH, Ng E, Ong MMA, Sim C, Tan K, Seneviratne CJ. A risk-based approach to the COVID-19 pandemic: the experience in National Dental Centre Singapore. *Front Med (Lausanne).* (2020) 7:562728. doi: 10.3389/fmed.2020.562728
18. National Health Commission of the people's Republic of China. Available online at: http://zs.kaipuyun.cn/s?searchWord=%25E6%2596%25B0%25E5%259E%258B%25E5%2586%25A0%25E7%258A%25B6%25E7%2597%2585%25E6%25AF%2592%25E8%2582%25BA%25E7%2582%258E%25E8%25AF%258A%25E7%2596%2597%25E6%2596%25B9%25E6%25A1%2588&column=%25E5%2585%25A8%25E9%2583%25A8&wordPlace=0&orderBy=0&startTime=&endTime=&pageSize=10&pageNum=0&timeStamp=0&siteCode=bm24000006&sonSiteCode=&checkHandle=1&searchSource=1&strFileType=&govWorkBean=%257B%257D&sonSiteCode=&areaSearchFlag=0&secondSearchWords=&topical=&docName=&label=&countKey=0&uc=0&left_right_index=0
19. Health Commission of Guangdong Province. Available online at: http://wsjkw.gd.gov.cn/zwgk_gsgg/content/post_3230777.html
20. Cha YF. Health code: automated rating and utilization of individual epidemic risk. *Zhejiang J.* (2020) 03:28–35. doi: 10.16235/j.cnki.33-1005/c.2020.03.005
21. Wu J. From health code to data-body: bio-politics in a digitalized era. *J Nantong Univ (Soc Sci Ed).* (2021) 37:8–15. doi: 10.3969/j.issn.1673-2359.2021.01.002
22. Shi C, Ma L. *Collaborative Governance, Technological Innovation and Smart Epidemic Prevention: a Case Study based on "Health Codes"*. Vol. 04 (2020). p. 107–16. doi: 10.13903/j.cnki.cn51-1575/d.20200421.001
23. Wang L. *'Remainder Life': Ethical Reflections on Health Code in the Fight Against COVID-19.* Vol. 21 (2021). p. 27–32. doi: 10.16112/j.cnki.53-1160/c.2021.01.004
24. Wu GJ. Health QR code, digital person, and the remainder-life — — Technopolitical and biopolitical reflection. *Explor Free Views.* (2020) 09:115–22 + 159. Available online at: https://kns.cnki.net/kcms/detail/detail.aspx?FileName=TSZM202009025&DbName=DKFX2020
25. Yao JY. *Whether the health code can be upgraded to "universal code": after the epidemic, whether the health code information is destroyed or retained "financial magazine"*. WeChat official account (2020). Available online at: https://mp.weixin.qq.com/s/QLC5n5sVQX6PS6YVt9_Jyw
26. Hu Y. After the outbreak, what is the future of health code. *Xinhua Daily* (2020).
27. Li XX, Su ZW, Yin W. Current situation of hospital infection management of hospital logistics staffs and cleaners. *Mod Prev Med.* (2006) 06:117–8. doi: 10.3969/J.ISSN.1003-8507.2006.06.047
28. Wang Y. Standardize the training of hospital infection knowledge for cleaners to prevent hospital infection. *Cap Med.* (2014) 21:9. doi: 10.3969/j.issn.1005-8257.2014.16.006
29. American Dental Association what constitutes a dental emergency? Available online at: https://success.ada.org/~/media/CPS/Files/Open%20Files/ADA_COVID19_Dental_Emergency_DDS.pdf
30. Notice on further consolidation of achievements and improvement of COVID-19 prevention and treatment capability in medical institutions. Available online at: http://www.nhc.gov.cn/xcs/zhengcwj/202004/9ceeac520d944e1a94301d06d1e9dcce.shtml
31. Notice of the general Office of the National Health commission on strengthening the management of fever outpatient service in key hospitals in key areas and the prevention and control of infections in medical institutions; (2020). Available online at: http://www.nhc.gov.cn/yzygj/s7659/202002/485aac6af5d54788a05b3bcea5a22e34.shtml
32. Notice on further improving the current COVID-19 epidemic prevention and control (2020). Available online at: http://www.gov.cn/xinwen/2020-06/11/content_5518727.htm
33. Lee Y, Zhang LY. The interpretation of Consensus on emergency surgery and infection prevention and control for severe trauma patients with 2019 novel corona virus pneumonia. *Med J Chin Peoples Liberation Army.* (2020) 45:113–7. doi: 10.11855/j.issn.0577-7402.2020.02.02
34. Ma J, Lu JB, Guo J, Liu ZE, Yong Q, Li X, et al. Protection standards for stomatological hospitals during the epidemic period of COVID-19(X III):

procedure management of dental and maxillofacial surgery ward. *J Pract Stomatol.* (2020) 36:207–11. doi: 10.3969/j.issn.1001-3733.2020.02.014
35. Chinese Ministry of Health. Technique standard for isolation in hospitals. *Chin J Nosocomiol.* (2009) 19:1612–6. Available online at: https://kns.cnki.net/kcms/detail/detail.aspx?FileName=SCSD000005873386&DbName=SCSD
36. Lu WH. Triage of preview and triage ensure the safety of medical treatment. *Health News* (2020).
37. Prevention and control plan for COVID-19. 7th ed. Available from: http://www.nhc.gov.cn/cms-search/downFiles/f9ea38ce2c2d4352bf61ab0feada439f.pdf.
38. An N, Yue L, Zhao B. Droplets and aerosols in dental clinics and prevention and control measures of infection. *Zhonghua Kou Qiang Yi Xue Za Zhi.* (2020) 55:223–8. doi: 10.3760/cma.j.cn112144-20200221-00081
39. Cai GJ, Suo JJ, Liu YX, Zhang SB. Preliminary study on experience in epidemiological survey of COVID-19 epidemic. *Chin J Nosocomiology.* (2020) 30:1147–51. Available online at: http://kns.cnki.net/kcms/detail/detail.aspx?FileName=ZHYY202008008&DbName=DKFX2020
40. Lauer SA, Grantz KH, Bi Q, Jones FK, Zheng Q, Meredith HR, et al. The incubation period of coronavirus Disease (2019). (COVID-19) from publicly reported confirmed cases: estimation and application. *Ann Intern Med.* (2020) 172:577–82. doi: 10.7326/M20-0504
41. Green DA, Zucker J, Westblade LF, Whittier S, Rennert H, Velu P, et al. Clinical performance of SARS-CoV-2 molecular tests. *J Clin Microbiol.* (2020) 58:e00995–20. doi: 10.1128/JCM.00995-20
42. Chu DK, Akl EA, Duda S, Solo K, Yaacoub S, Schünemann HJ. COVID-19 Systematic Urgent Review Group Effort (SURGE) study authors. Physical distancing, face masks, and eye protection to prevent person-to-person transmission of SARS-CoV-2 and COVID-19: a systematic review and meta-analysis. *Lancet.* (2020) 395:1973–87. doi: 10.1016/j.jvs.2020.07.040
43. Innes N, Johnson IG, Al-Yaseen W, Harris R, Jones R, Kc S, et al. A systematic review of droplet and aerosol generation in dentistry. *J Dent.* (2021) 105:103556. doi: 10.1016/j.jdent.2020.103556
44. Wu YH, Cao Y, Gao Y, Rongmeng J, Jiqiu K, Jun Z, et al. Research on documentary standards for safety and protection of medical staff during Corona Virus Disease 2019 epidemic and current status. *Chin J Nosocomiol.* (2020) 30:1161–6. Available online at: https://kns.cnki.net/kcms/detail/detail.aspx?FileName=ZHYY202008011&DbName=DKFX2020
45. Allegranzi B, Pittet D. Role of hand hygiene in healthcare-associated infection prevention. *J Hosp Infect.* (2009) 73:305–15. doi: 10.1016/j.jhin.2009.04.019
46. Ma QX, Shan H, Zhang HL, Li GM, Yang RM, Chen JM. Potential utilities of mask-wearing and instant hand hygiene for fighting SARS-CoV-2. *J Med Virol.* (2020) 92:1567–71. doi: 10.1002/jmv.25805
47. Mathai E, Allegranzi B, Kilpatrick C, Pittet D. Prevention and control of health care-associated infections through improved hand hygiene. *Indian J Med Microbiol.* (2010) 28:100–6. doi: 10.4103/0255-0857.62483
48. Awoke N, Geda B, Arba A, Tekalign T, Paulos K. Nurses practice of hand hygiene in Hiwot Fana specialized University Hospital, Harari regional state, Eastern Ethiopia: observational study. *Nurs Res Pract.* (2018) 2018:2654947. doi: 10.1155/2018/2654947
49. Saitoh A, Sato K, Magara Y, Osaki K, Narita K, Shioiri K, et al. Improving hand hygiene adherence in healthcare workers before patient contact: a multimodal intervention in four tertiary care hospitals in Japan. *J Hosp Med.* (2020) 15:262–7. doi: 10.12788/jhm.3446
50. Ye G, Lin H, Chen S, Wang S, Zeng Z, Wang W, et al. Environmental contamination of SARS-CoV-2 in healthcare premises. *J Infect.* (2020) 81:e1–5. doi: 10.1016/j.jinf.2020.04.034
51. Guertler A, Moellhoff N, Schenck TL, Hagen CS, Kendziora B, Giunta RE, et al. Onset of occupational hand eczema among healthcare workers during the SARS-CoV-2 pandemic: comparing a single surgical site with a COVID-19 intensive care unit. *Contact Dermatitis.* (2020) 83:108–14. doi: 10.1111/cod.13618
52. Erdem Y, Altunay IK, Aksu Çerman A, Inal S, Ugurer E, Sivaz O, et al. The risk of hand eczema in healthcare workers during the COVID-19 pandemic: do we need specific attention or prevention strategies? *Contact Dermatitis.* (2020) 83:422–3. doi: 10.1111/cod.13632
53. Singh M, Pawar M, Bothra A, Choudhary N. Overzealous hand hygiene during the COVID 19 pandemic causing an increased incidence of hand eczema among general population. *J Am Acad Dermatol.* (2020) 83:e37–41. doi: 10.1016/j.jaad.2020.04.047
54. Pradhan S, Kroumpouzos G, Goldust M. Hand eczema due to frequent hand washing in combat with COVID-19. *J Cosmet Dermatol.* (2020) 19:2474–5. doi: 10.1111/jocd.13639
55. Kvam MS, Alfonso JH, Berents TL, Randem BG, Stylianou E. Work-related hand eczema [published correction appears in. Tidsskr Nor Laegeforen (2019) 139(3):10.4045/tidsskr.18.0213. Published 2019 Feb 5;139(4):]. Arbeidsrelatert håndeksem [published correction appears in Tidsskr Nor Laegeforen.;Feb 08. Tidsskr Nor Laegeforen.:2019]. doi: 10.4045/tidsskr.18.0213
56. Minamoto K, Watanabe T, Diepgen TL. Self-reported hand eczema among dental workers in Japan - a cross-sectional study. *Contact Dermatitis.* (2016) 75:230–9. doi: 10.1111/cod.12656
57. Meding B, Wrangsjö K, Hosseiny S, Andersson E, Hagberg S, Torén K, et al. Occupational skin exposure and hand eczema among dental technicians-need for improved prevention. *Scand J Work Environ Health.* (2006) 32:219–24. doi: 10.5271/sjweh.1002
58. Agner T, Elsner P. Hand eczema: epidemiology, prognosis and prevention. *J Eur Acad Dermatol Venereol.* (2020) 34(Suppl. 1):4–12. doi: 10.1111/jdv.16061
59. Silvestre Salvador JF, Heras Mendaza F, Hervella Garcés M, Palacios-Martínez D, Sánchez Camacho R, Senan Sanz R, et al. Guidelines for the diagnosis, treatment, and prevention of hand eczema. *Actas Dermo Sifiliogr.* (2020) 111:26–40. doi: 10.1016/j.ad.2019.04.005
60. Blicharz L, Czuwara J, Samochocki Z, Goldust M, Chrostowska S, Olszewska M, et al. Hand eczema-A growing dermatological concern during the COVID-19 pandemic and possible treatments. *Dermatol Ther.* (2020) 33:e13545. doi: 10.1111/dth.13545
61. Guidance for wearing and removing personal protective equipment in healthcare settings for the care of patients with suspected or confirmed COVID-19. Available online at: https://www.ecdc.europa.eu/sites/default/files/documents/COVID-19-guidance-wearing-and-removing-personal-protective-equipment-healthcare-settings-updated.pdf
62. McCarthy R, Gino B, d'Entremont P, Barari A, Renouf TS. The importance of personal protective equipment design and donning and doffing technique in mitigating infectious disease spread: a technical report. *Cureus.* (2020) 12:e12084. doi: 10.7759/cureus.12084
63. Mahmood SU, Crimbly F, Khan S, Choudry E, Mehwish S. Strategies for rational use of personal protective equipment (PPE) among healthcare providers during the COVID-19 crisis. *Cureus.* (2020) 12:e8248. doi: 10.7759/cureus.8248
64. Personal Protective Equipment Use in Health Care. (2020). Available online at: http://www.health.govt.nz/our-work/diseases-and-conditions/covid-19-novel-coronavirus/covid-19-novel-coronavirus-information-specific-audiences/covid-19-advice-workers-including-personal-protective-equipment/personal-protective-equipment-use-health-careHauora., M.o.H.M., Personal protective equipment use in health care.2020
65. Two Techniques to Safely Remove Contaminated nitrile Gloves. Available online at: https://communityattire.com/two-techniques-to-safely-remove-contaminated-nitrile-gloves/
66. Carraturo F, Del Giudice C, Morelli M, Cerullo V, Libralato G, Galdiero E, et al. Persistence of SARS-CoV-2 in the environment and COVID-19 transmission risk from environmental matrices and surfaces. *Environ Pollut.* (2020) 265:115010. doi: 10.1016/j.envpol.2020.115010
67. Derraik JGB, Anderson WA, Connelly EA, Anderson YC. Rapid review of SARS-CoV-1 and SARS-CoV-2 viability, susceptibility to treatment, and the disinfection and reuse of PPE, particularly filtering facepiece respirators. *Int J Environ Res Public Health.* (2020) 17:6117. doi: 10.3390/ijerph17176117
68. National Health Commission of the People's Republic of China. Regulation of disinfection technique in healthcare settings (WS/T 367-2012).[Z]; 2012-04-17. Available online at: http://www.nhc.gov.cn/wjw/s9496/201204/54510/files/2c7560199b9d42d7b4fce28eed1b7be0.PDF
69. Hygienic specifications for operation and management of air-conditioning ventilation systems in office buildings and public places during COVID-19 epidemic. Available online at: http://www.nhc.gov.cn/fzs/s7852d/202007/992a8d0b6c754e0db3df7458d604962e/files/53c4073f2f7d45538566792daf51745b.pdf

70. Lu J, Gu J, Li K, Xu C, Su W, Lai Z, et al. COVID-19 outbreak associated with air conditioning in restaurant, Guangzhou, China, (2020). *Emerg Infect Dis.* (2020) 26:1628–31. doi: 10.3201/eid2607.200764
71. Bidra AS, Pelletier JS, Westover JB, Frank S, Brown SM, Tessema B. Comparison of *in vitro* inactivation of SARS CoV-2 with hydrogen peroxide and povidone-iodine oral antiseptic rinses. *J Prosthodont.* (2020) 29:599–603. doi: 10.1111/jopr.13220
72. Reis INR, do Amaral GCLS, Mendoza AAH, das Graças YT, Mendes-Correa MC, Romito GA, et al. Can preprocedural mouthrinses reduce SARS-CoV-2 load in dental aerosols? *Med Hypo.* (2021) 146:110436. doi: 10.1016/j.mehy.2020.110436
73. Anderson DE, Sivalingam V, Kang AEZ, Ananthanarayanan A, Arumugam H, Jenkins TM, et al. Povidone-iodine demonstrates rapid *in vitro* virucidal activity against SARS-CoV-2, the virus causing COVID-19 disease. *Infect Dis Ther.* (2020) 9:669–75. doi: 10.1007/s40121-020-00316-3
74. Peng X, Xu X, Li Y, Cheng L, Zhou X, Ren B. Transmission routes of 2019-nCoV and controls in dental practice. *Int J Oral Sci.* (2020) 12:9. doi: 10.1038/s41368-020-0075-9
75. Gottsauner MJ, Michaelides I, Schmidt B, Scholz KJ, Buchalla W, Widbiller M, et al. A prospective clinical pilot study on the effects of a hydrogen peroxide mouthrinse on the intraoral viral load of SARS-CoV-2. *Clin Oral Investig.* (2020) 24:3707–13. doi: 10.1007/s00784-020-03549-1
76. Qiao LH, Chen ML, Wu SM. Observation on the curative effect of four-handed operation matching method in the extraction of low-mandibular impacted wisdom teeth. *Nurs Pract Res.* (2021) 18:118–21. doi: 10.3969/j.issn.1672-9676.2021.01.033
77. Liu PL, Lu XP, Sa XJ. Application analysis of four-hand technique nursing in the preparation of tooth restoration. *Nurs Pract Res.* (2020) 17:112–4. doi: 10.3969/j.issn.1672-9676.2020.15.042
78. Xiong FY. Application of four-handed manipulation technique in hospital infection control of oral outpatient department. *J Med Theor Pract.* (2019) 32:1946–7. doi: 10.19381/j.issn.1001-7585.2019.12.080
79. Wang YF. Advantages of four-hand operation technology and its application value in oral nursing. *Electron J Gen Stomatol.* (2019) 6:9–10. doi: 10.16269/j.cnki.cn11-9337/r.2019.29.005
80. Chiang PC, Johnson R. An approach to improving the six-handed technique in oral rehabilitation. *J Am Dent Assoc.* (1978) 96:1020–4. doi: 10.14219/jada.archive.1978.0245
81. Feng RM, Zhou YZ, Lin LT. Effect of six-handed operation and nursing cooperation in stomatology department and its effect on prevention of cross infection. *Chin Gen Pract Nurs.* (2019) 17:1609–11. doi: 10.12104/j.issn.1674-4748.2019.13.029
82. Xu PY, Deng XY. Infection control and prevention in the dental clinic during coronavirus disease 2019 epidemic. *Chin J Nurs.* (2020) 55(Suppl. 1):614–5. Available online at: https://kns.cnki.net/kcms/detail/detail.aspx?FileName=ZHHL2020S1248&DbName=CJFQ2020
83. Huang XH, Liu B, Lee XN, Wang MY, Ma WS, Xu YB. Oral splashing treatment of four-hand operation and nursing cooperation during Covid-19 epidemic period. *Nurs Pract Res.* (2020) 17:17–9. Available online at: https://kns.cnki.net/kcms/detail/detail.aspx?FileName=HLSJ202007006&DbName=CJFQ2020
84. Harrel SK, Barnes JB, Rivera-Hidalgo F. Reduction of aerosols produced by ultrasonic scalers. *J Periodontol.* (1996) 67:28–32. doi: 10.1902/jop.1996.67.1.28
85. Zhou LW, Gao YB, Lin DX, Chen LX, Yang YF. Comparison of two different methods for air pollution control in dental scaling rooms. (2012) 18:32–3. doi: 10.3969/j.issn.1009-4393.2012.14.019
86. Suyama Y, Ozaki T, Takaku S, Fukuzawa Y, Mochizuki H, Ishii T, et al. Eliminating effects of an air purifier on infectants during dental procedure. *Bull Tokyo Dent Coll.* (1995) 36:27–31.
87. Noro A, Yanaka N, Takahashi K, Ishikawa T, Ogino J, Takahashi E, et al. A study on prevention of hospital infection control caused by tooth preparation dust in the dental clinic. Part 1. Preventive measures against environmental pollution in the dental clinic caused by microbial particles. *Bull Tokyo Dent Coll.* (1995) 36:201–6.
88. Shahdad S, Patel T, Hindocha A, Cagney N, Mueller JD, Seoudi N, et al. The efficacy of an extraoral scavenging device on reduction of splatter contamination during dental aerosol generating procedures: an exploratory study. *Br Dent J.* (2020). doi: 10.1038/s41415-020-2112-7. [Epub ahead of print].
89. Hu T, Zuo YL, Zhou XD. [Comparison of preventive effects of two kinds of dental handpieces on viral contamination at different rotating times]. *Hua Xi Kou Qiang Yi Xue Za Zhi.* (2004) 22:293–4.
90. Fu CL, Hu T, Zhou XD. Effect of antisuction designed handpiece on formation and contamination of biofilm in the waterlines of dental unit. *Chin J Nosocomiology.* (2004) 05:29–31. doi: 10.3321/j.issn:1005-4529.2004.05.008
91. Guo Q, Deng WZ, Huang RX,Luo JQ, Lee WN, Chen YW. Analysis of the effect of preventing the water pollution of the dental treatment table by using anti-suction turbo dental handpieces drastically. *Chin Youjiang Med J.* (2008) 05:575–6. doi: 10.3969/j.issn.1003-1383.2008.05.030
92. Pankhurst Caroline L, Crispian S, Lakshman S. Dental unit water lines and their disinfection and management: a review. *Dent Update.* (2017) 44:284–5:289–92. doi: 10.12968/denu.2017.44.4.284
93. Cheng L, Naibijiang N, Hasenbai A, Dong H, He H. Bacteriostatic effects of nanometer silver disinfectant on the biofilms in dental unit water lines. *J Dent Sci.* (2021) 16:327–32. doi: 10.1016/j.jds.2020.03.015
94. Ionescu AC, Brambilla E, Manzoli L, Orsini G, Gentili V, Rizzo R. Aerosols modification with H_2O_2 reduces airborne contamination by dental handpieces. *J Oral Microbiol.* (2021) 13:1881361. doi: 10.1080/20002297.2021.1881361
95. Qian HH. The efficacy of the rubber dam in reducing atmospheric bacterial contamination during dental treatment. *Chin J.* (2009) 44:821–2. doi: 10.3761/j.issn.0254-1769.2009.09.021
96. Bahador M, Alfirdous RA, Alquria TA, Griffin IL, Tordik PA, Martinho FC. Aerosols generated during endodontic treatment: a special concern during the coronavirus disease 2019 Pandemic. *J Endod.* (2021) 47:732–9. doi: 10.1016/j.joen.2021.01.009
97. Takeuchi Y, Furuchi M, Kamimoto A, Honda K, Matsumura H, Kobayashi R. Saliva-based PCR tests for SARS-CoV-2 detection. *J Oral Sci.* (2020) 62:350–1. doi: 10.2334/josnusd.20-0267
98. Batista AUD, Silva PLPD, Melo LA, Carreiro ADFP. Prosthodontic practice during the COVID-19 pandemic: prevention and implications. *Braz Oral Res.* (2021) 35:e049. doi: 10.1590/1807-3107bor-2021.vol35.0049
99. To KK, Tsang OT, Yip CC, Chan KH, Wu TC, Chan JM. Consistent detection of 2019 novel coronavirus in saliva. *Clin Infect Dis.* (2020) 71:841–3. doi: 10.1093/cid/ciaa149
100. MacDonald DS, Colosi DC, Mupparapu M, Kumar V, Shintaku WH, Ahmad M. Guidelines for oral and maxillofacial imaging: COVID-19 considerations. *Oral Surg Oral Med Oral Pathol Oral Radiol.* (2021) 131:99–110. doi: 10.1016/j.oooo.2020.10.017
101. Sushanth A, Srivastava KC, Shrivastava D, Hosni HA, Khan ZA, al-Johani K, et al. Recommendations, practices and infrastructural model for the dental radiology set-up in clinical and academic institutions in the COVID-19 Era. *Biology (Basel).* (2020) 9:334. doi: 10.3390/biology9100334
102. Su XH, Hu FY, Dong YJ. Emergency response to COVID-19 outbreak in general hospital stomatology department. *Chin J Nurs.* (2020) 55;Suppl 1:622–3.
103. Cral WG, Lima CAS, Queluz DP. COVID-19 and oral radiology. *Imaging Sci Dent.* (2020) 50:181–2. doi: 10.5624/isd.2020.50.2.181
104. Hamedani S, Farshidfar N. The practice of oral and maxillofacial radiology during COVID-19 outbreak. *Oral Radiol.* (2020) 36:400–3. doi: 10.1007/s11282-020-00465-8
105. Barbot V, Robert A, Rodier MH, Imbert C. Update on infectious risks associated with dental unit waterlines. *FEMS Immunol Med Microbiol.* (2012) 65:196–204. doi: 10.1111/j.1574-695X.2012.00971.x
106. Su J. Status and thinking of dental unit water lines management. *Chin J Pract Stomatol.* (2018) 11:713–7. doi: 10.19538/j.kq.2018.12.002
107. Regulation for disinfection and sterilisation technique of dental instruments WS 506-2016. *Chin J Infect Control.* (2017) 16:784–92. Available online at: https://kns.cnki.net/kcms/detail/detail.aspx?FileName=GRKZ201708024&DbName=CJFQ2017
108. Liu J, Sun J, Yue T, Lee YB, Liu HC. Thoughts on use, cleaning and disinfection management of oral medical devices during COVID-19 epidemic period. *Infect Dis Inf.* (2020) 33:378–82. Available online at: https://kns.cnki.net/kcms/detail/detail.aspx?FileName=CRBX202004024&DbName=CJFQ2020
109. Li XR, Hu LY, Zhang Y, Chen HF. The effects of cleaning dental appliances on cleaning performance. *Today Nurse.* (2013) 02:128–9.

Available online at: https://kns.cnki.net/kcms/detail/detail.aspx?FileName=DDHS201302080&DbName=CJFQ2013

110. Wei HL, Liang Y, Zhang Z, Jiao YY, Liu GL, Zheng Y, et al. Emergency management and disposal of medical waste in the COVID-19 epidemic. *Environ Monit China.* (2020) 36:8–13. doi: 10.19316/j.issn.1002-6002.2020.05.02
111. Novel management and technical guidelines for emergency disposal of medical waste in coronavirus (trial). Ministry of ecological and environment of the people's Republic of China; (2020). Available online at: http://www.mee.gov.cn/ywdt/hjywnews/202001/t20200129_761043.shtml
112. Feng YN, Chen ZX, Meng Y, Zhao X, Song Y, Wang J, et al. Global early transmission of SARS-COV-2 VOC 202012/01 and evolutionary characteristics of its spike protein. *Chin J Virol.* (2021) 37:267–73. doi: 10.13242/j.cnki.bingduxuebao.003866
113. Zawiah M, Al-Ashwal FY, Saeed RM, et al. Assessment of healthcare system capabilities and preparedness in yemen to confront the Novel Coronavirus (2019). (COVID-19) outbreak: a perspective of healthcare workers. *Front Public Health.* (2020) 8:419. doi: 10.3389/fpubh.2020.00419
114. Aronu CO, Ekwueme GO, Sol-Akubude VI, Okafor PN. Coronavirus (COVID-19) in Nigeria: Survival rate. *Sci Afr.* (2021) 11:e00689. doi: 10.1016/j.sciaf.2020.e00689
115. Ahmed J, Malik F, Bin Arif T, Majid Z, Chaudhary MA, Ahmad J, et al. Availability of Personal Protective Equipment (PPE) among US and Pakistani doctors in COVID-19 Pandemic. *Cureus.* (2020) 12:e8550. doi: 10.7759/cureus.8550
116. Saqlain M, Munir MM, Ahmed A, Tahir AH, Kamran S. Is Pakistan prepared to tackle the coronavirus epidemic?. *Drugs Ther Perspect.* (2020). doi: 10.1007/s40267-020-00721-1. [Epub ahead of print].
117. Ilesanmi OS, Afolabi AA, Akande A, Raji T, Mohammed A. Infection prevention and control during COVID-19 pandemic: realities from health care workers in a north central state in Nigeria. *Epidemiol Infect.* (2021) 149:e15. doi: 10.1017/S0950268821000017
118. Al-Ashwal FY, Kubas M, Zawiah M, et al. Healthcare workers' knowledge, preparedness, counselling practices, and perceived barriers to confront COVID-19: A cross-sectional study from a war-torn country, Yemen. *PLoS ONE.* (2020) 15:e0243962. doi: 10.1371/journal.pone.0243962
119. Pethani AS, Allana RR, Hussain M. Emerging challenges and threats for dental health care sector attributable to COVID-19: tale of a developing country. *Asia Pac J Public Health.* (2020) 32:278–80. doi: 10.1177/1010539520932708
120. Blignaut E, Nemutandani S, Samaranayake L. Strategic implementation of dental infection control in resource-poor jurisdictions during COVID-19 pandemic: a perspective from South Africa. *Acta Odontol Scand.* (2020) 78:614–7. doi: 10.1080/00016357.2020.1804073
121. CDC. Decontamination and Reuse of Filtering Facepiece Respirators (2020). Available online at: https://www.cdc.gov/coronavirus/2019-ncov/hcp/ppe-strategy/decontamination-reuse-respirators.html (accessed April 8, 2020).
122. Lore MB, Heimbuch BK, Brown TL, Wander JD, Hinrichs SH. Effectiveness of three decontamination treatments against influenza virus applied to filtering facepiece respirators. *Annals Occupational Hygiene.* (2012) 56:92–101. doi: 10.1093/annhyg/mer054
123. Ward WG Sr, Cooper JM, Lippert D, Kablawi RO, Neiberg RH, Sherertz RJ. Glove and gown effects on intraoperative bacterial contamination. *Ann Surg.* (2014) 259:591–7. doi: 10.1097/SLA.0b013e3182a6f2d9
124. Lankester BJ, Bartlett GE, Garneti N, Blom AW, Bowker KE, Bannister GC. Direct measurement of bacterial penetration through surgical gowns: a new method. *J Hosp Infect.* (2002) 50:281–5. doi: 10.1053/jhin.2001.1154
125. Xu XL, Cui L, Ye YS, Liu X, Liu B. Self-made simple protective face shield to prevent and control COVID-19. *J Nurs.* (2020) 27:58–9. doi: 10.16460/j.issn1008-9969.2020.12.00
126. Khan MM, Parab SR. Safety guidelines for sterility of face shields during COVID 19 pandemic. *Indian J Otolaryngol Head Neck Surg.* (2020) 73:1–2. doi: 10.1007/s12070-020-01865-2
127. Ademola-Popoola D, Lloyd F. How to make a protective face shield or visor. *Community Eye Health.* (2020) 33:34–5.

5

An Online Cross-Sectional Survey on Oral Healthcare Among School-Age Children During COVID-19 Epidemic in Wuhan, China

Zhen Li, Yuhong Li, Chang Liu, Han Jiang, Chenzheng Zhang and Minquan Du**

The State Key Laboratory Breeding Base of Basic Science of Stomatology (Hubei-MOST) & Key Laboratory of Oral Biomedicine Ministry of Education, School and Hospital of Stomatology, Wuhan University, Wuhan, China

***Correspondence:**
Chenzheng Zhang
zhangchenzheng@foxmail.com
Minquan Du
duminquan@whu.edu.cn

Background: Since the outbreak of Coronavirus disease 2019 (COVID-19), the government of China adopted many measures which changed people's lifestyle including oral health-related lifestyle to control the transmission. The aim of this study was to investigate oral health status, oral healthcare behaviors, and parental attitudes toward oral healthcare among school-age children in Wuhan during the COVID-19 outbreak and what the status would be when the outbreak is under control.

Methods: This study was an online cross-sectional survey facing elementary school students in Wuhan. The questionnaire was completed by children's parents or other family members. The information on demographic data, oral health status, oral healthcare behaviors, and parental attitudes toward oral healthcare was collected at the end of school closure. The chi-square test was used to test the association of different questionnaire items.

Results: A total of 18,383 subjects aged 6–13 years with complete data were included in this investigation, and 44.2% of them suffered pain or discomfort related to teeth and gums during the epidemic. While there might be an increasing need and concern of oral healthcare during the outbreak and even when the outbreak was controlled, the worry of infection made it difficult for people to meet their demands of dental attendance.

Conclusion: The risk of cross-infection during the treatment had a negative influence on parental attitudes toward dental attendance. Effective measures should be taken to meet people's demands of dental attendance.

Keywords: Wuhan, school-age children, oral health, epidemic, COVID-19

INTRODUCTION

Coronavirus disease 2019 (COVID-19) is a respiratory disease caused by a novel coronavirus named severe acute respiratory syndrome coronavirus 2 (SARS-CoV-2). The World Health Organization (WHO) officially recognized the outbreaks as a public health emergency of international concern on January 30, 2020 (1). As of June 8, 2020, a total of 6,931,000 confirmed cases and 400,857 deaths has been recognized in the whole world (2). This is a great challenge not only for China, but also for the world.

Oral disease is a major public health problem which affects children worldwide (3). Moreover, it would impact children's eating, speaking, emotional well-being, and general health when it happened to children (4). It is widely accepted that lifestyles are closely associated with oral disease (5), and great changes have happened on children's daily life since the outbreak of COVID-19.

Currently, the transmission of COVID-19 is regarded as starting with an animal-to-human transmission, followed by human-to-human spread. The modes of its interpersonal transmission include respiratory droplets, contact transmission, and aerosol routes. In addition, some asymptomatic spread cases were also reported (6). Considering these transmission characteristics of COVID-19, dentistry practices have a high risk of infection such as the frequent production of aerosols, constant presence of saliva, and the unavoidable touch of mouth, nose, and eyes (7). As a result, general non-emergency dental treatment was suspended and only emergency dental services were provided across China since January 2020 (8). Besides the limitation of dental attendance, many other measures, including lockdown for the whole Hubei province, quarantining infected and suspected people, restricting access to public spaces, and issuing a home quarantine order to all the residents, were adopted by the government of China to control the transmission efficiently. During this special domiciliary time, people have spent most of their time staying at home. For citizens in Wuhan, only online shopping provided by local supermarkets and markets was available and a narrow range of goods could be bought. This epidemic also has an indirect impact on people's lifestyle through psychology. It was reported that over half of Chinese suffered moderate-to-severe psychological impact during the initial phase of the COVID-19 outbreak (9).

With all of these changes, we hypothesized that the oral health status, the oral healthcare behaviors, and the attitudes toward oral healthcare of school-age children may have also changed. Wuhan, as the city facing the severest epidemic condition across China (10), may face more challenges than other cities on oral healthcare.

The aim of this study was to investigate oral health status, oral healthcare behaviors, and parental attitudes toward oral healthcare among school-age children in Wuhan during the COVID-19 outbreak and what the status would be when the outbreak is under control, thereby providing guidance for the following preventive and therapeutic oral healthcare in Wuhan and other districts which are affected by the epidemic.

MATERIALS AND METHODS

Ethical Clearance

This questionnaire survey was undertaken by the Department of Preventive Dentistry, School & Hospital of Stomatology of Wuhan University. The questionnaire was anonymous to ensure privacy protection. Ethical approval (Approval no. HGGC-035) for the study was obtained from the Ethics Committee of the School & Hospital of Stomatology of Wuhan University, and informed consent was obtained from the guardian of each subject.

Study Participants

This survey faces to elementary school students in Wuhan. In view of their age, parents or other family members are allowed to fill in the questionnaire instead.

Data collection was conducted from May 1 to 7, 2020. An online data collection was conducted because of the home quarantine order. The questionnaire was published on Wenjuanxing, and it was set as "per IP address and WeChat account can only submit the questionnaire once" through the platform to prevent double entry from participants. Then, we posted the link and the quick response code of the questionnaire, on WeChat groups and moments, attaching with a brief introduction, and asked people for passing on to their friends and relatives.

Questionnaire Survey

The questionnaire consisted of four parts: (1) demographic data; (2) oral health status; (3) oral healthcare behaviors; and (4) attitudes toward oral healthcare during and after the epidemic situation.

Demographic data was collected on gender, age, and living region, including each district in Wuhan and the other regions in China.

To understand oral health status, we listed options including dental caries, bleeding while brushing teeth, loss of restorative material, tooth trauma, bad breath, oral ulcer, and other oral discomfort (an open-ended option) for people to multiply choose. In addition, we also afforded "I don't know" and "I don't have any discomfort" options. A self-assessment regarding oral health status was required in the end of the questionnaire.

In the aspect of oral healthcare behaviors, questions were designed covering several areas: (1) the choices about using oral healthcare products for the home; (2) the choices about using oral health services toward prevention; (3) meal times; (4) frequency of having confectionery; (5) frequency of having sweet drinks; (6) frequency of having sugared drinks like milk, yogurts, milk powders, tea, soybean milk, and coffees; and (7) frequency of toothbrushing.

Attitudes toward oral healthcare were measured by questions for during and after the epidemic situation, respectively, including the level of concern on oral health, the level of concern on access to treatment, the level of worry on being infected in the process of oral treatment, and the attitudes toward dental attendance.

In this questionnaire, "before the epidemic" means the period when there is no outbreak of epidemic (before January 23, 2020); "during the epidemic" means during Wuhan lockdown (from January 23, 2020, to April 8, 2020); and "after the epidemic" means the period that the epidemic is under control.

Statistical Analysis

Data analysis was performed using the SPSS (PC version 23.0) software with the level of statistical significance set at $P < 0.001$. Subjects with missing data were excluded from the analysis.

The Optimal Binning method was used to select the optimal cutoff point of age. The chi-square test was used to test the association of different questionnaire items. McNemar's test was taken into account to find out the different attitudes toward oral healthcare in different epidemic situations.

RESULTS

A total of 18,694 subjects took part in this investigation. Of these subjects, 159 children were excluded because their living region was out of Wuhan and 152 subjects were excluded because of their age. At last, 18,383 subjects (9,753 boys and 8,630 girls) between the ages of 6 and 13 years were included in this study. The age range of 9–10 is the cutoff point between younger and older school-age children in this study. The characteristics of the study group are shown in **Table 1**.

Table 2 presents children's oral health status during the epidemic. Almost half of the children (44.2%) suffered oral discomfort, and the younger group had a higher proportion than the older group (47.5 vs. 40.3%). Besides, more children aged 6–9 years had an increase in the severity of oral discomfort than the children aged 10–13 years during the epidemic (7.6 vs. 4.7%). No significant difference was found for gender in the items above. As for detailed experience of pain/discomfort the children suffered, the younger group had a higher rate of dental caries and loss of restorative material than the older group while more girls than boys suffered bleeding while brushing teeth.

Table 3 provides information on oral healthcare behaviors. As for the use of oral healthcare products for the home, the proportion of subjects who used electric toothbrush (33.1 vs. 30.2%), fluoride toothpaste (26.1 vs. 20.2%), mouth rinse (16.1 vs. 7.0%), and dental floss (8.8 vs. 8.0%) after the epidemic was higher than that during the epidemic. What is more, little difference was found for gender and significant difference was found for age in the use of oral healthcare products for the home. No matter the situation was during the epidemic or after the epidemic, the younger group had a higher rate of the usage of electric toothbrush and fluoride toothpaste while the older group had a higher rate of the usage of mouth rinse.

With regard to dental service utilization for preventive need, 28.3, 19.7, 10.1, and 8.7% of children took a routine check-up, pit and fissure sealant, fluoride varnish, and routine supragingival scaling before the epidemic, respectively. Moreover, the corresponding proportions were 55.1, 15.0, 10.2, and 18.6% when the epidemic was controlled. Children aged 6–9 years had a higher proportion of taking routine check-up (29.6 vs. 26.8%) and fluoride varnish (12.5 vs. 7.3%) than the older children and a lower proportion of taking pit and fissure sealant (18.6 vs. 21.0%) and routine supragingival scale (6.6 vs. 11.2%) before the epidemic. Besides, the parents of younger children had a higher willing of taking routine check-up (57.6 vs. 52.3%), fluoride varnish (13.0 vs. 7.0%), and pit and fissure sealant (17.8 vs. 11.8%) than the parents of older children and a lower

TABLE 1 | General characteristics of the study group.

	Male		Female		Total
	N	%	*N*	%	
Age (years)					
6	205	55.26%	166	44.74%	371
7	1,864	52.43%	1,691	47.57%	3,555
8	1,675	52.82%	1,496	47.18%	3,171
9	1,460	53.11%	1,289	46.89%	2,749
10	1,722	52.20%	1,577	47.80%	3,299
11	1,375	52.28%	1,255	47.72%	2,630
12	1,257	54.51%	1,049	45.49%	2,306
13	195	64.57%	107	35.43%	302
Total	9,753	53.05%	8,630	46.95%	18,383

TABLE 2 | Chi-square test for relationship of gender/age and oral health status during the epidemic.

	Gender					Age				*P*-value	Total	
	Male		Female		*P*-value	6–9 years		10–13 years				
	N	%	*N*	%		*N*	%	*N*	%		*N*	%
Experience of pain/discomfort related to teeth and gums					0.484					<0.001		
Yes	4,331	44.4%	3,788	43.9%		4,678	47.5%	3,441	40.3%		8,119	44.2%
No	5,422	55.6%	48,42	56.1%		5,168	52.5%	5,096	59.7%		10,264	55.8%
Severity of oral pain/discomfort compared with that before the epidemic					0.374					<0.001		
Increase	595	6.4%	505	6.1%		713	7.6%	387	4.7%		1,100	6.2%
No change	7,978	85.5%	7,130	86.2%		8,133	86.1%	6,975	85.4%		15,108	85.8%
Decrease	761	8.2%	636	7.7%		595	6.3%	802	9.8%		1,397	7.9%
Detailed experience of pain/discomfort related to teeth and gums												
Dental caries	1,511	35.8%	1,391	37.6%	0.246	1,888	41.1%	1,014	30.4%	<0.001	2,902	36.6%
Bad breath	1,173	27.8%	950	25.7%	0.031	1,109	24.2%	1,014	30.4%	0.194	2,123	26.8%
Oral ulcer	1,121	26.6%	916	24.7%	0.058	1,047	22.8%	990	29.7%	0.038	2,037	25.7%
Bleeding while brushing teeth	313	7.4%	397	10.7%	<0.001	358	7.8%	352	10.6%	0.087	710	9.0%
Loss of restorative material	256	6.1%	251	6.8%	0.241	351	7.6%	156	4.7%	<0.001	507	6.4%
Tooth trauma	35	0.8%	20	0.5%	0.115	29	0.6%	26	0.8%	0.901	55	0.7%

TABLE 3 | Chi-square test for relationship of age and oral healthcare behaviors during the epidemic.

	6–9 years		10–13 years		*P*-value	Total	
	N	%	*N*	%		*N*	%
Use of oral healthcare products for the home							
During the epidemic							
Manual toothbrush	7,197	73.5%	6,349	75.0%	0.050	13,546	74.2%
Electric toothbrush	3,144	32.1%	2,361	27.9%	<0.001	5,505	30.2%
Fluoride toothpaste	2,085	21.3%	1,598	18.9%	<0.001	3,683	20.2%
Mouth rinse	532	5.4%	755	8.9%	<0.001	1,287	7.0%
Dental floss	799	8.2%	663	7.8%	0.383	1,462	8.0%
After the epidemic							
Manual toothbrush	5,768	60.0%	5,316	63.9%	<0.001	11,084	61.8%
Electric toothbrush	3,407	35.4%	2,527	30.4%	<0.001	5,934	33.1%
toothpaste	2,643	27.5%	2,040	24.5%	<0.001	4,683	26.1%
Mouth rinse	1,422	14.8%	1,463	17.6%	<0.001	2,885	16.1%
Dental floss	857	8.9%	715	8.6%	0.427	1,572	8.8%
Use of oral health services toward prevention							
Before the epidemic							
Routine check-up	2,912	29.6%	2,287	26.8%	<0.001	5,199	28.3%
Pit and fissure sealant	1,829	18.6%	1,792	21.0%	<0.001	3,621	19.7%
Fluoride varnish	1,226	12.5%	625	7.3%	<0.001	1,851	10.1%
Routine supragingival scaling	648	6.6%	954	11.2%	<0.001	1,602	8.7%
After the epidemic							
Routine check-up	5,668	57.6%	4,466	52.3%	<0.001	10,134	55.1%
Pit and fissure sealant	1,751	17.8%	1,009	11.8%	<0.001	2,760	15.0%
Fluoride varnish	1,281	13.0%	597	7.0%	<0.001	1,878	10.2%
Routine supragingival scaling	1,566	15.9%	1,855	21.7%	<0.001	3,421	18.6%

willing of taking routine supragingival scale (15.9 vs. 21.7%) than the parents of older children after the epidemic. No dental service but routine check-up (26.4% for boys and 30.4% for girls before the epidemic; 54.0% for boys and 56.4% for girls after the epidemic) had a utilization difference for gender.

Table 4 shows the frequency of eating and toothbrushing. A percentage of 20.2% of children had a change of meal times. The proportion of children who had an increase in the frequency of confectionery, sweet drinks, and sugared drinks like milk, yogurts, milk powders, tea, soybean milk, and coffees was 18.4, 10.3, and 22.9%, respectively. With 7.4% of children who had an increase in the frequency of toothbrushing, only 62.3% of children brushed their teeth more than twice a day during the epidemic. The proportion of girls who had a stable meal time (81.3 vs. 78.4%) and who brush their teeth more than twice a day (65.3 vs. 59.7%) were higher than that of boys. The proportion of the younger group who had an increase in the frequency of meal times (18.2 vs. 16.7%) and who brush their teeth more than twice a day (64.2 vs. 60.2%) was higher than that of the older group.

Tables 5, 6 show parental attitudes toward oral healthcare during and after the epidemic situation. **Table 5** shows a comparison of parental concern on oral health and access to oral treatment during the epidemic with that after the epidemic. A significant difference in the level of concern existed in different periods (P-value of McNemar's test < 0.001). The levels of both concern on oral health and access to treatment after the epidemic were higher than those during the epidemic. **Table 6** shows the relationship of worry on being infected in the process of oral treatment and the attitudes toward dental attendance after the epidemic. The overwhelming majority (93.8%) of the parents worried on being infected in the process of oral treatment after the epidemic, and half of the parents (53.4%) still avoided the dental attendance after the epidemic (no treatment for 9.8%, deal with it by oneself and avoid going to hospital for 13.4%, and avoid dental practice except for emergency cases for 30.2%).

DISCUSSION

This study based on a large sample size with unequal gender distribution, which was resulted from the snowball sampling techniques and consisted with sex ratio imbalance in Wuhan (11).

The results of this study show that some changes happened on children's oral health status, oral healthcare behaviors, and parental attitudes toward oral healthcare in Wuhan during the COVID-19 outbreak. Besides, significant differences were found in oral healthcare between different age groups. What is more, while there was an increasing necessity and concern of oral healthcare because of the epidemic, the outbreak of the epidemic

TABLE 4 | Chi-square test for relationship of gender/age and oral healthcare behaviors during the epidemic.

	Gender					Age					Total	
	Male		Female		*P*-value	6–9 years		10–13 years		*P*-value		
	N	%	*N*	%		*N*	%	*N*	%		*N*	%
Meal times					<0.001					<0.001		
Increase	1,832	18.9%	1,360	15.9%		1,779	18.2%	1,413	16.7%		3,192	17.5%
No change	7,598	78.4%	6,975	81.3%		7,788	79.6%	6,785	80.0%		14,573	79.8%
Decrease	262	2.7%	242	2.8%		222	2.3%	282	3.3%		504	2.8%
Frequency increase of having desserts												
Confectionery	1,736	17.9%	1,635	19.0%	0.053	2,007	20.5%	1,364	16.1%	<0.001	3,371	18.4%
Sweet drinks	1,055	10.9%	824	9.6%	0.004	1,062	10.8%	817	9.6%	0.007	1,879	10.3%
Sugared drinks like milk, yogurts, milk powders, tea, soybean milk, and coffees	2,289	23.6%	1,896	22.1%	0.014	2,355	24.0%	1,830	21.6%	<0.001	4,185	22.9%
Frequency of toothbrushing					<0.001					<0.001		
Twice a day or more	5,822	59.7%	5,635	65.3%		6,318	64.2%	5,139	60.2%		11,457	62.3%
Once a day	3,524	36.1%	2,759	32.0%		3,190	32.4%	3,093	36.2%		6,283	34.2%
Less often than daily	394	4.0%	223	2.6%		325	3.3%	292	3.4%		617	3.4%
Seldom or never	13	0.1%	13	0.2%		13	0.1%	13	0.2%		26	0.1%
Frequency of toothbrushing					<0.001					<0.001		
Increase	707	7.3%	650	7.5%		602	6.1%	755	8.9%		1,357	7.4%
No change	8,447	86.8%	7,591	88.1%		8,688	88.3%	7,350	86.3%		16,038	87.4%
Decrease	578	5.9%	377	4.4%		546	5.6%	409	4.8%		955	5.2%

TABLE 5 | Parental attitudes toward the oral health care compared with that before the epidemic.

	During the epidemic		After the epidemic		*P*-value
	N	%	*N*	%	**(McNemar's test)**
The level of concern on oral health					<0.001
Increase	5,484	30.1%	6,340	35.0%	
No change	12,161	66.7%	11,475	63.4%	
Decrease	589	3.2%	293	1.6%	
The level of concern on access to treatment					<0.001
Extreme	1,783	9.8%	21,66	12.1%	
Severe	2,340	12.9%	2,705	15.1%	
Moderate	1,546	8.5%	1,816	10.1%	
Mild	4,086	22.5%	3,547	19.8%	
Minimal	4,716	26.0%	4,263	23.7%	
Not at all	3,672	20.2%	3,455	19.2%	

brought lots of difficulties for people to have a dental visit even when the epidemic was controlled.

Oral Health Status

On the whole, the school-age children in Wuhan had a poor oral health and dental caries was the most common dental disease among this group. According to some recent reports on dental health among school-age children in China, the prevalence of dental caries was 46.88% for boys and 49.63% for girls among the children aged 6–12 years in Chengdu (12). In Shenzhen, the prevalence of dental caries was 55.7% for 6–9-year-old children and 31.9% for 10–13-year-old children (13). The prevalence of self-reported caries in this survey was 41.1% for children aged 6–9 years and 30.4% for children aged 10–13 years. It is relatively low compared with that in the previous study. A main explanation for this is that it is a result acquired in a self-reported way and it is difficult for people to distinguish whether it was caries or not.

Considering that studies on self-reported oral health and its correlation with clinical evaluation among school-age children were scarce, information about changes on self-reported oral health status during the epidemic was collected to identify what effect the epidemic had on oral health status.

Among the children who suffered pain/discomfort related to teeth and gums during the epidemic, the younger group had

TABLE 6 | Chi-square test for relationship of the level of worry on being infected in the process of oral treatment and the attitudes toward dental attendance after the epidemic.

	The attitudes toward dental attendance after the epidemic																
	No treatment		**Deal with it by oneself and avoid going to hospital**		**Avoid dental practice except for emergency cases**		**Some of dental practice can be performed under adequate protection measures**		**Going to hospital for dental treatment after testing for COVID-9**		**All dental practice can be performed under adequate protection measures**		**All dental practice can be performed without adequate protection measures**		**Total**		***P*-value**
	N	**%**	***N***	**%**	***N***	**%**	***N***	**%**	***N***	**%**	***N***	**%**	***N***	**%**	***N***	**%**	
The level of worry on being infected in the process of oral therapy after the epidemic																	<0.001
Extreme	843	16.3%	873	16.9%	1,534	29.7%	1,162	22.5%	476	9.2%	258	5.0%	11	0.2%	5,157	30.4%	
Severe	404	9.4%	625	14.6%	1,482	34.5%	1,281	29.8%	283	6.6%	209	4.9%	10	0.2%	4,294	25.3%	
Moderate	139	6.6%	254	12.0%	726	34.4%	720	34.1%	149	7.1%	115	5.4%	9	0.4%	2,112	12.5%	
Mild	157	5.0%	313	10.0%	923	29.5%	1,277	40.9%	264	8.5%	179	5.7%	11	0.4%	3,124	18.4%	
Minimal	48	4.0%	92	7.6%	247	20.5%	518	43.0%	128	10.6%	164	13.6%	9	0.7%	1,206	7.1%	
Not at all	72	6.9%	116	11.1%	202	19.3%	353	33.7%	130	12.4%	165	15.7%	10	1.0%	1,048	6.2%	
Total	1,663	9.8%	2,273	13.4%	5,114	30.2%	5,311	31.3%	1,430	8.4%	1,090	6.4%	60	0.4%	16,941	100.0%	

a higher proportion of subjects who had an increased severity than the older group. It indicated that the dental health status of the younger group was more susceptible to the epidemic than the older group. It could be partly explained by the fact that the younger group had a higher proportion of subjects who had a negative change on their diets during the epidemic than the older group.

What interested us is that a significant difference existed in the percentage of subjects who suffered discomfort related to teeth between different groups when the group was divided by age but not gender, while it was quite the opposite in the percentage of subjects who suffered discomfort related to gums. The former result that the younger group had a lower proportion of subjects who suffered discomfort related to teeth than the older group can be explained by the specific timing of tooth replacement (14). The latter result showing that the boys had a lower percentage of subjects who suffered discomfort related to gums than the girls was consistent with some of the previous studies (15), but it was difficult to explain combining the oral healthcare behaviors shown in this study. In this study, girls were more interested in adhering to the oral hygiene behaviors and their parents paid more attention to their children than the boys, which were reflected in the higher prevalence of routine check-up, recommended frequency of toothbrushing, and stable meal times. All of these results indicated that the girls might have a better oral hygiene level than boys. This difference in behaviors was consistent with previous studies. Furthermore, in most of such studies, boys had a worse gum health status (16–19). The result in this study was probably caused by physiological character difference in gender, such as the specific timing of teeth replacement and the fluctuation of hormone levels with stress events (20). Further researches are needed on it.

Oral Healthcare Behaviors

The willingness to use oral healthcare products for the home and oral health services toward prevention had an increase when the epidemic was controlled. Generally, the younger group had a higher proportion of using recommended oral healthcare products and oral health services than the older group during and after the epidemic. It might be because parents tend to put more concern on the younger children.

Parental Attitudes Toward Oral Healthcare

The changes on oral health status and oral healthcare behaviors indicated that there is an increase in the demand for oral healthcare after the epidemic. Besides, a large proportion of parents had an increased level of concern on oral health during and after the epidemic according to the results from parental attitudes toward oral healthcare.

However, 53.4% of them still have a tendency to avoid going to the hospital and the proportion of people who had concern on access to treatment after the epidemic was 80.8%. It can be partly explained by the positive correlation between the level of worry on being infected in the process of oral treatment and the attitudes toward dental attendance considering the large proportion of people who had worry on being infected in the process of oral treatment after the epidemic (93.8%).

Taking all these factors into account, more attention should be paid to spread information about the measures that have been taken to reduce the risk of cross-infection during the treatment.

Strengths and Limitations

This study has both strengths and limitations. A major strength of the current study is that it is the first study to report the oral healthcare of school-age children in Wuhan during the COVID-19 outbreak. Wuhan has its specificity for it was the most serious district in China and has been under the strictest management for the longest time. Besides, it has a large sample size and the data was obtained before the epidemic passed.

There are also some limitations. Firstly, selection bias exists because of the snowballing sampling strategy and the use of an online survey. Secondly, recall bias exists as the oral health condition was reported by the parents. Thirdly, to attract more subjects to fill the questionnaire, the number of the questions was limited. As a result, many items were not able to have a further discussion.

CONCLUSIONS

In conclusion, children's oral health status was affected by the epidemic, especially 6–9-year-old children. More attention should be paid on the eating habits of children aged 6–9 and toothbrushing habits of boys. Parents in Wuhan had more concerns on oral healthcare during and after the epidemic than before the epidemic state. Besides, the findings from this study show a high amount of dental treatment needed among school-age children in Wuhan after the epidemic. However, the worry on being infected in the process of oral treatment after the epidemic might be a major factor which would stop people from dental attendance. Effective measures should be taken to meet people's demands of oral healthcare. What is more, age-specific strategies in prevention are necessary for school-age children.

AUTHOR CONTRIBUTIONS

All authors listed have made a substantial, direct and intellectual contribution to the work, and approved it for publication.

REFERENCES

1. World Health Organization. *Statement on the second meeting of the International Health Regulations 2005 Emergency Committee regarding the outbreak of novel coronavirus (2019-nCoV).* (2020). Available online at: https://www.who.int/news-room/detail/30-01-2020-statement-on-the-second-meeting-of-the-international-health-regulations-2005-emergency-committee-regarding-the-outbreak-of-novel-coronavirus-(2019-ncov) (accessed June 10, 2020).
2. World Health Organization. *Coronavirus Disease 2019. (COVID-19) Situation Report-140.* (2020). Available online at: https://www.who.int/emergencies/diseases/novel-coronavirus-2019/situation-reports (accessed June 10, 2020).
3. Petersen PE. The World Oral Health Report 2003: continuous improvement of oral health in the 21st century–the approach of the WHO Global Oral Health Programme. *Community Dent Oral Epidemiol.* (2003) 31(Suppl. 1):3–23. doi: 10.1046/j.2003.com122.x
4. Hescot P. The new definition of oral health and relationship between oral health and quality of life. *Chin J Dent Res.* (2017) 20:189–92. doi: 10.3290/j.cjdr.a39217
5. Jin LJ, Lamster IB, Greenspan JS, Pitts NB, Scully C, Warnakulasuriya S. Global burden of oral diseases: emerging concepts, management and interplay with systemic health. *Oral Dis.* (2016) 22:609–19. doi: 10.1111/odi.12428
6. General Office of National Health Commission of People's Republic of China, Office of National Administration of Traditional Chinese Medicine. Diagnosis and treatment of corona virus disease-19(7th trial edition). *China Med.* (2020) 15:801–5. doi: 10.3760/j.issn.1673-4777.2020.06.001
7. Yang ZZ. Nosocomial infection risk through aerosol of corona virus disease-19 and preventive measure. *China Med.* (2020) 15:812–5. doi: 10.3760/j.issn.1673-4777.2020.06.003
8. Yang Y, Zhou Y, Liu X, Tan J. Health services provision of 48 public tertiary dental hospitals during the COVID-19 epidemic in China. *Clin Oral Investig.* (2020) 24:1861–4. doi: 10.1007/s00784-020-03267-8
9. Wang C, Pan R, Wan X, Tan Y, Xu L, Ho CS, et al. Immediate psychological responses and associated factors during the initial stage of the 2019. Coronavirus Disease (COVID-19) epidemic among the general population in China. *Int J Environ Res Public Health.* (2020) 17:1729. doi: 10.3390/ijerph17051729
10. National Health Commission of the People's Republic of China. *Distribution of the COVID-19 Outbreak.* (2020). Available online at: http://2019ncov.chinacdc.cn/2019-nCoV/ (accessed June 10, 2020).
11. National Bureau of Statistics of China. *Tabulation on the 2010 Population Census of the Prople's Republic of China.* (2012). Available online at: http://www.stats.gov.cn/tjsj/pcsj/rkpc/6rp/indexch.htm (accessed June 10, 2020).
12. Peng R, Li S, Zhang H, Zeng H, Jiang B, Liu Y, et al. Weight status is associated with blood pressure, vital capacity, dental decay, and visual acuity among school-age children in Chengdu, China. *Ann Nutr Metab.* (2016) 69:237–45. doi: 10.1159/000454888
13. Cheng YH, Liao Y, Chen DY, Wang Y, Wu Y. Prevalence of dental caries and its association with body mass index among school-age children in Shenzhen, China. *BMC Oral Health.* (2019) 19:270. doi: 10.1186/s12903-019-0950-y
14. Nelson SJ, Ash MM. *Wheeler's Dental Anatomy, Physiology, and Occulsion.* 9th ed. Philadelphia: W.B. Saunders Co (2010). p. 36.
15. Gopinath VK, Rahman B, Awad MA. Assessment of gingival health among school children in Sharjah, United Arab Emirates. *Eur J Dent.* (2015) 9:36–40. doi: 10.4103/1305-7456.149636
16. Bashirian S, Seyedzadeh-Sabounchi S, Shirahmadi S, Soltanian AR, Karimi-Shahanjarini A, Vahdatinia F. Socio-demographic determinants as predictors of oral hygiene status and gingivitis in schoolchildren aged 7-12 years old: a cross-sectional study. *PLoS ONE.* (2018) 13:e0208886. doi: 10.1371/journal.pone.0208886
17. Tomazoni F, Vettore MV, Zanatta FB, Tuchtenhagen S, Moreira CH, Ardenghi TM. The associations of socioeconomic status and social capital with gingival bleeding among schoolchildren. *J Public Health Dent.* (2017) 77:21–9. doi: 10.1111/jphd.12166
18. Shiau HJ, Reynolds MA. Sex differences in destructive periodontal disease: a systematic review. *J Periodontol.* (2010) 81:1379–89. doi: 10.1902/jop.2010.100044
19. Natto ZS, Abu Ahmad RH, Alsharif LT, Alrowithi HF, Alsini DA, Salih HA, et al. Chronic periodontitis case definitions and confounders in periodontal research: a systematic assessment. *Biomed Res Int.* (2018) 2018:4578782. doi: 10.1155/2018/4578782
20. Shiau HJ, Reynolds MA. Sex differences in destructive periodontal disease: exploring the biologic basis. *J Periodontol.* (2010) 81:1505–17. doi: 10.1902/jop.2010.100045

6

Public Oral Health Care During COVID-19: Time for Reflection and Action

*Shenuka Singh**

Discipline of Dentistry, School of Health Sciences, University of KwaZulu-Natal (UKZN), Durban, South Africa

Keywords: public sector, oral health promotion, COVID-19, planning, integrated health

Correspondence:
Shenuka Singh
singhshen@ukzn.ac.za

INTRODUCTION

About 2.3 billion people (mainly from upper and lower middle income countries) suffer from untreated dental caries (affecting permanent teeth) while 530 million children have caries involving primary teeth, according to the Global Burden of Disease 2017. This makes dental caries one of the most common global public health concerns (1, 2). Data from the Global Burden of Disease 2017 further suggest a skewed distribution of reported oral diseases across the global platform. Countries with better economic development have a higher burden of tooth loss yet lower rates of untreated caries and severe periodontitis (3). Changes in dietary intake, increased sugar consumption, and limited access to health care could further be attributed to the reported rates of diabetes, obesity, and dental caries (3). Similarly, increasing rates in periodontal disease, oral cancers, oral manifestations of HIV, and oro-dental trauma demand a more committed public health response (1). Oral diseases are considered a major burden on scarce resources, especially from a public health perspective, due to their impact on pain, discomfort, and compromised quality of life (4, 5). Treatment for oral conditions are generally unaffordable and universal health coverage remains a challenge in most parts of the world. Even in high income countries, oral health related care amounts to almost 5% of the total health expenditure and 20% out-of-pocket health expenditure (1).

The COVID-19 pandemic has sharply brought into focus the need to re-examine oral health systems given that virtually every aspect of healthcare delivery has been impacted by the outbreak including oral health care delivery. It can be argued that COVID-19 has completely altered the care landscape with not only new challenges and threats, but also new opportunities. Likewise dentistry and oral care delivery should not be left behind as the entire health delivery systems morphs and evolves along with the times. This paper advocates a review of public oral health systems (both in developed and developing countries) with a renewed focus on improving oral health related outcomes, as a response to the COVID-19 pandemic. A SWOT analysis framework is used to examine strengths, weaknesses, opportunities, and threats related to the current delivery of oral health services. The strengths and weaknesses of oral health systems will first be examined, followed by opportunities to improve oral health care delivery. Possible threats to achieving improved service delivery will also be explored. This analysis is intended to create greater awareness among oral health and health practitioners, oral health planners, policy makers, health decision-makers, researchers, and academics on the value of oral health within general health care. Additionally, this analysis could be used to guide oral health related "decision-making as it is crucial during the current pandemic to work on weaknesses, avoid threats, and utilize all future opportunities" [(6), p.1343].

STRENGTHS AND WEAKNESSES OF ORAL HEALTH SYSTEMS

Oral health systems (both public and private) have been in existence but the challenges of delivering effective oral health care remains a challenge in many parts of the world (4), especially in underserved populations. Given the dependency on the public oral health system, especially in economically challenged countries and in under-served populations (7), it is imperative that the health system is able to respond adequately to unmet oral health needs. While the link between oral health and general health has been widely documented, the challenges of implementing an integrated response to health care also continue to persist in several health settings (8). One of the main shortcomings of oral health care is that it is generally assessed independently of general health outcomes while measures of overall health status tend to exclude oral health determinants (9). Another shortcoming would be a dependency on the formal health system to deliver optimal oral health care, without taking into account other key platforms such as community or facility-based care. This divide between oral health and general health continues to permeate through health policy planning and implementation.

Other weaknesses of the health system became more apparent during COVID-19. The pre-COVID inequities in access to optimal health care have been exacerbated during the pandemic where underserved populations and uninsured as those in the US, have been disproportionately affected by the disease (10). Similarly in Africa and other in developing countries, the rhetoric between saving lives and livelihoods becomes more pronounced as people struggle between disease prevention and earning an income (11). Concurrently, oral health systems appeared to use a "knee jerk" approach in dealing with the pandemic. While oral health authorities in some countries called for a suspension of clinical service delivery while others promoted a more cautious approach with emphasis on increased infection control (12). This sadly suggests that current country specific policies and guidelines on oral health care have failed to plan adequately for a public health emergency.

THE NEED FOR COMMITTED FOCUS ON ORAL HEALTH CARE

A review and re-organization of oral health systems is thus overdue. There is need to ensure equitable and improved access to oral health care with a focus on improving population health outcomes (13). There is need for increased policy discussions on oral health care, research and innovation, monitoring, and surveillance. The primary health care model could provide a viable vehicle (8) to facilitate political commitment from planning to implementation through local legislative efforts.

While there is currently no natural immunity against SARS-CoV-2 infection, studies show that people more at risk of developing COVID-19 related complications include those with diabetes and obesity (14, 15). While vaccines are now available, vaccine nationalism and allegations of stockpiling among high income countries have fuelled global discussions on addressing COVID-19 challenges and low income countries are largely left with little bargaining power (16). The emergence of new variants in COVID-19 has made the disease far more transmissible, thereby placing a greater strain on the health system (17). At the same time, diet and obesity are linked to acquisitions of unhealthy lifestyle practices that are deeply rooted in social and economic circumstances (18–20), that could limit the selection of healthier choices. These determinants could thus impact on oral health status as well (21). Concurrently, access to oral care for people afflicted with COVID-19 disease could be compromised due to ongoing restrictions in social movement during state imposed lockdowns.

Hence a more committed focus is needed on prevention of commonly occurring oral diseases and the promotion of healthier behavioral practices. Isolated individual interventions directed toward modifying specific oral health-related behaviors have not been successful in achieving long-term changes in behavioral practices (5). A population based strategy could include a multi-disciplinary approach for the reduction of risk factors associated with tobacco and alcohol use, healthier dietary intake, and exposure to additional topical fluoride within wider integrated health action. The availability and cost of healthier foods as well as providing information on food labels could influence food choices (22).

OPPORTUNITIES FOR IMPROVED ORAL HEALTH CARE DELIVER

Despite the highlighted challenges, several opportunities exist to optimize a more seamless delivery of oral health services, as outlined below:

Oral Health Promotion

Promotion of oral health care should not be the responsibility of just the health system. From an organizational perspective this requires a shift from health practitioner focus to oral health promotion within a social setting (21, 23). It is known that oral health self-care emanates from the primary socialization period, that is, children engage in activities such general hygiene and taking care of one's oral cavity starts through influences within the family and social setting (22). Oral health self-care can be reinforced at multiple settings such as crèches, schools, workplaces, etc. Oral health action could include efforts to modify oral health behaviors through oral health education, dietary counseling, individual skills development (such as proper toothbrushing and flossing) and access to additional fluoride uptake. In addition, awareness programmes to control risks to oral health such as nutrition intake, tobacco cessation, reduction in alcohol consumption, and avoidance of dental trauma should be considered. Other initiatives could include access to clean water and a safe and supportive environment to develop personal skills for positive oral health outcomes (4, 5, 8, 21, 22). These activities should be integrated into COVID-19 public health measures such as regular handwashing, social distancing, and wearing of face masks. Policy development at the facility or health promotion setting level could assist in ensuing commitments in implementing these initiatives. Oral health promotion delivery needs to occur at multiple levels such as macro level (policy development and agenda setting), meso level (community-based approach), and micro level (interpersonal and intrapersonal). A macro level engagement could also include mass media communications and foster political support for creating supportive environments to address unhealthy behavioral practices (21). Mass media provides opportunities to advocate for integrated health and social messages during COVID-19 that include elements of oral health care (24). However, caution should also be applied to prevent spread of fake news and health-related mis-information (25).

Further investments in oral health could include engagement with technologies to improve the digital interface in health communication (26). Modalities such as tele-dentistry could support the delivery of oral health services, specifically when physical contact or travel to the local clinic is difficult. Tele-dentistry also has potential to link service providers across geographical spaces and ensure continuity in the delivery of expertise in oral health care (26–28). Health or oral health care workers could use these technologies to facilitate support and engagement with service providers in care homes, correctional service facilities and other such settings where public access during COVID-19 is limited. This could ensure that integrated oral health messages and support can still reach these very vulnerable populations. Similarly, remote engagement provides another viable platform for the dissemination of preventive messages. Mobile devices such as smartphones create a personalized platform for the delivery of oral health messages. Although issues such as internet connectivity and availability of data bundles remain a challenge in resource-constrained settings, it is nevertheless valuable to invest in such technologies.

Likewise, stronger collaboration is required between the health system and community based settings for the safe delivery of oral health promotion services (29). These settings provide further opportunities for integrated oral health messages and policy planning (30) such as good oral health habits, positive oral health behaviors, and developing personal oral health skills. Oral health care should be embraced by all stakeholders involved in care provision, and not just the health or oral health worker. Partnerships in health care could also be developed with the private sector and all other stakeholders in community development (29, 30). Thus, the prevention of disease and promotion of healthier lifestyles are integrated into overall community and social development.

Oral health interventions directed at the intrapersonal and interpersonal level should focus on unhealthy behavioral practices such as diet, smoking and alcohol consumption. Smoking has been shown to be linked to a number of health complications such as diminished lung capacity, cardiac complications, and periodontal disease (31). Further complications can linked with COVID-19 (32) given that this a respiratory related disease. Integrated oral health messages could thus be directly beneficial at an individual level. Public health emergency strategies such as isolation and quarantine during COVID-19 places additional strain on the individual's ability to cope with the pandemic (33). Strategies could be developed at the micro-level to help individuals cope with COVID-19, and make healthier behavioral choices. Oral health care workers have a role to play in early recognition of signs of depression in patients and to make the necessary referrals for appropriate care.

Studies have shown that early clinical signs of COVID-19 include a loss of taste and smell (34, 35). COVID-19 provides unique opportunities for oral health care workers to engage in screening services. Thus, oral health workers could play key roles in screening (36) and identifying asymptomatic clients or those presenting with early symptoms; and conduct saliva testing for COVID-19 (37). Oral health care workers could provide integrated health messages such as handwashing, cough etiquette, proper wearing of facial masks/coverings, and oral health related care. Other activities could include infection prevention education and training, reinforcing health and safety measures in client/patient contact, risk management, and program evaluation (12).

Threats

Despite these opportunities some of the possible threats to implementing these strategies could include lack of practitioner skills. There is thus a need for continuing professional and skills development for the oral health care worker as well as a review of undergraduate dental curricula so that appropriate training can provided to better equip the individual practitioner.

Although the notion of integrated oral health care through a multi-disciplinary team approach has been touted as a key strategy to broaden the delivery of oral health promotion services (38), this seemingly uncomplicated patient/client centered initiative continues to face challenges in many parts of the world, as indicated earlier (39, 40). The question begs: why is this so? Perhaps we as dental public health practitioners, academics, health planners, and researchers need to reflect further. Has there been widespread stakeholder engagement to ensure buy-in for these innovative approaches in oral health service delivery? To successfully influence the processes of oral health promotion requires more than simple, document-based policy reforms that are strong on rhetoric, and good ideas, but have not achieved the widespread stakeholder support necessary to carry them through to funding and implementation [(41), p.23]. Simultaneously, we as oral health care workers need to re-examine our roles within a multi-disciplinary team. How can we make more meaningful contribution to overall health outcomes during COVID-19 (42)?

This highlights the need for greater dialogue both within and outside of the health system to explore ways of integrating oral health messages and care within a broader scope of overall community health. This should be supported by ongoing opportunities for health workers to develop skills in oral health promotion activities through training programmes. Further research is required to unpack the barriers and delays in integrated health action.

CONCLUSION

The COVID-19 pandemic has provided opportunities for renewed interest in the oral health agenda. A re-organization of oral health systems with a focus on social orientation of oral health self-care, could see improved oral health gains in the long term. Concurrently, the role of oral health care workers and their preparedness for a public health emergency should be reviewed and addressed through appropriate training platforms.

AUTHOR CONTRIBUTIONS

The author confirms being the sole contributor of this work and has approved it for publication.

REFERENCES

1. World Health Organization 2020. *Oral Health*. (2020). Available online at: https://www.who.int/news-room/fact-sheets/detail/oral-health (accessed August 21, 2020).
2. GBD 2017. Disease and Injury Incidence and Prevalence Collaborators, 2018. Global, regional, national incidence. prevalence, and years lived with disability for 354 diseases and injuries for 195 countries and territories, 1990-2017: a systematic analysis for the Global Burden of Disease Study 2017. *Lancet*. (2018) 392:1789–858. doi: 10.1016/S0140-6736(18)32279-7
3. GBD 2017. Oral Disorders Collaborators, (2020). Global, regional, and national levels and trends in burden of oral conditions from 1990 to 2017: a systematic analysis for the global burden of disease 2017 study. *J Dental Res*. (2020) 99:362–73. doi: 10.1177/0022034520908533
4. Petersen PE. Challenges to improvement of oral health in the 21th century – the approach of the WHO Global Oral Health Programme. *Int Dent J*. (2004) 54:329–43. doi: 10.1111/j.1875-595X.2004.tb00009.x
5. Sheiham A, Watt R. Oral health promotion policy. In: Murray JJ, Nunn JH, Steele JG, editors. *Prevention of Oral Disease*. 4th edn. New York: Oxford University Press (2003). p. 243–56.
6. Gaffar B, Alhumaid J, Alhareky M, Alonaizan F, Almas K. Dental facilities during the new corona outbreak: a SWOT analysis. *Risk Manag Healthc Policy*. (2020) 25:13:1343–52. doi: 10.2147/RMHP.S265998
7. Northridge ME, Kumar A, Kaur R. Disparities in access to oral health care. *Annu Rev Public Health*. (2020) 41:513–35. doi: 10.1146/annurev-publhealth-040119-094318
8. Prasad M, Manjunath C, Murthy AK, Sampath A, Jaiswal S, Mohapatra A. Integration of oral health into primary health care: a systematic review. *J Family Med Prim Care*. (2019) 8:1838–45. doi: 10.4103/jfmpc.jfmpc_286_19
9. Manski RJ, Hoffmann D, Rowthorn V. Increasing access to dental medical care by allowing greater flexibility in scope of practice. *Am J Public Health*. (2015) 105:1755–62. doi: 10.2105/AJPH.2015.302654
10. Clark E, Fredricks K, Woc-Colburn L, Bottazzi ME, Weatherhead J. Disproportionate impact of the COVID-19 pandemic on immigrant communities in the United States. *PLoS Negl Trop Dis*. (2020) 14:e0008484. doi: 10.1371/journal.pntd.0008484
11. United Nations. *Impact of COVID-19 in Africa*. (2020). Available online at: https://unsdg.un.org/sites/default/files/2020-05/Policy-brief-Impact-of-COVID-19-in-Africa.pdf (accessed August 21, 2020).
12. Mallineni SK, Innes NP, Raggio DP, Araujo MP, Robertson MD, Jayaraman J. Coronavirus disease (COVID-19): characteristics in children and considerations for dentists providing their care. *Int J Paediatr Dent*. (2020) 30:245–50. doi: 10.1111/ipd.12653
13. Kassebaum NJ, Smith AGC, Bernabé E, Fleming TD, Reynolds AE, Vos T, et al. Global, regional, national prevalence. incidence, and disability-adjusted life years for oral conditions for 195 countries, 1990-2015: a systematic analysis for the global burden of diseases, injuries, risk factors. *J Dent Res*. (2017) 96:380–7. doi: 10.1177/0022034517693566
14. Petrakis D, Margină D, Tsarouhas K, Tekos F, Stan M, Nikitovic D., et al. Obesity - a risk factor for increased COVID-19 prevalence, severity and lethality (Review). *Mol Med Rep*. (2020) 22:9–19. doi: 10.3892/mmr.2020.11127
15. Muniyappa R, Gubbi S. COVID-19 pandemic, coronaviruses, diabetes mellitus. *Am J Physiol Endocrinol Metab*. (2020) 318:E736–E41. doi: 10.1152/ajpendo.00124.2020
16. Weintraub R, Bitton A, Rosenberg ML. *The Danger of Vaccine Nationalism. Economics & Society May 22*. (2020). Available online at: https://hbr.org/2020/05/the-danger-of-vaccine-nationalism (accessed September 09, 2020).
17. Makoni M. South Africa responds to new SARS-CoV-2 variant. *Lancet*. (2021) 397:267. doi: 10.1016/S0140-6736(21)00144-6
18. Tee JYH, Gan WY, Tan KA, Chin YS. Obesity and unhealthy lifestyle associated with poor executive function among Malaysian adolescents. *PLoS ONE*. (2018)13:e0195934. doi: 10.1371/journal.pone.0195934
19. Jürgensen N, Petersen PE. Oral health and the impact of socio-behavioural factors in a cross sectional survey of 12-year old school children in Laos. *BMC Oral Health*. (2009) 9:29. doi: 10.1186/1472-6831-9-29
20. Lusk JL. Consumer beliefs about healthy foods and diets. *PLoS ONE*. (2019)14:e0223098. doi: 10.1371/journal.pone.0223098
21. Singh. S. Evidence in oral health promotion—implications for oral health planning. *Am J Public Health*. (2012) 102:e15–8. doi: 10.2105/AJPH.2012.300893
22. Locker D, Jokovic A, Stephens M, Kenny D, Tompson B, Guyatt G. Family impact of child oral and oro-facial conditions. *Commun Dent Oral Epidemiol*. (2002) 30:438–48. doi: 10.1034/j.1600-0528.2002.00015.x
23. Bavel JJV, Baicker K, Boggio PS, Capraro V, Cichocka A, Cikara M, et al. Using social and behavioural science to support COVID-19 pandemic response. *Nat Hum Behav*. (2020) 4:460–71. doi: 10.1038/s41562-020-0884-z
24. Sahni H, Sharma H. Role of social media during the COVID-19 pandemic: beneficial, destructive, or reconstructive? *Int J Acad Med*. (2020) 6:70–5. doi: 10.4103/IJAM.IJAM_50_20
25. Budd J, Miller BS, Manning EM, Lampos V, Zhuang M, Edelstein M., et al. Digital technologies in the public-health response to COVID-19. *Nat Med*. (2020) 26:1183–92. doi: 10.1038/s41591-020-1011-4
26. Mascitti M, Campisi G. Dental public health landscape: challenges, technological innovation and opportunities in the 21st century and COVID-19 pandemic. *Int J Environ Res Public Health*. (2020) 17:3636. doi: 10.3390/ijerph17103636
27. Neville P, van der Zande MM. Dentistry, e-health and digitalisation: a critical narrative review of the dental literature on digital technologies with insights from health and technology studies. *Commun Dent Health*. (2020) 37:51–8. doi: 10.1922/CDH_4664Neville08
28. Gray DJ, Kurscheid J, Mationg ML, Williams GM, Gordon C, Kelly M, et al. Health-education to prevent COVID-19 in schoolchildren: a call to action. *Infect Dis Poverty*. (2020) 9:81. doi: 10.1186/s40249-020-00695-2
29. Van den Broucke S. Why health promotion matters to the COVID-19 pandemic, vice versa. *Health Promot Int*. (2020) 35:181–6. doi: 10.1093/heapro/daaa042
30. Bailey W. Public-private partnership: complementary efforts to improve oral health. *J Calif Dent Assoc*. (2014) 42:249–52.
31. Ghanem E, Hage R. Behavior of lung health parameters among smokers and secondhand smokers. *J Environ Public Health*. (2018) 2018:5217675. doi: 10.1155/2018/5217675
32. van Zyl-Smit RN, Richards G, Leone FT. Tobacco smoking and COVID-19 infection. *Lancet Respir Med*. (2020) 8:664–5. doi: 10.1016/S2213-2600(20)30239-3
33. Guan Y, Deng H, Zhou X. Understanding the impact of the COVID-19 pandemic on career development: insights from cultural psychology. *J Vocat Behav*. (2020) 119:103438. doi: 10.1016/j.jvb.2020.103438
34. Klopfenstein T, Zahra H, Kadiane-Oussou NJ, Lepiller Q, Royer P, Toko L, et al. New loss of smell and taste: uncommon symptoms in COVID-19 patients on Nord Franche-Comte cluster, France. *Int J Infect Dis*. (2020) 100:117–22. doi: 10.1016/j.ijid.2020.08.012
35. Samaranayake L, Sadir Fakhruddin K, Panduwawala C. Loss of taste and smell. *Br Dent J*. (2020) 228:813. doi: 10.1038/s41415-020-1732-2

36. Zalewska A, Waszkiewicz N, Lopez-Pintor RM. The use of saliva in the diagnosis of oral and systemic diseases. *Dis Markers.* (2019) 2019:9149503. doi: 10.1155/2019/9149503
37. Azzi, L, Carcano G, Gianfagna F, Grossi P, Gasperina DD, Rossi, A, et al. Saliva is a reliable tool to detect SARS-CoV-2. *J Infect.* (2020) 81:e45–50. doi: 10.1016/j.jinf.2020.04.005
38. Kaufman LB, Henshaw MM, Brown BP, Calabrese JM. Oral health and interprofessional collaborative practice: examples of the team approach to geriatric care. *Dent Clin North Am.* (2016) 60:879–90. doi: 10.1016/j.cden.2016.05.007
39. Harnagea H, Couturier Y, Shrivastava R, Girard F, Lamothe L, Bedos CP, et al. Barriers and facilitators in the integration of oral health into primary care: a scoping review. *BMJ Open.* (2017) 7:e016078. doi: 10.1136/bmjopen-2017-016078
40. Suresh KS, Kumar P, Javanaiah N, Shantappa S, Srivastava P. Primary oral health care in India: vision or dream? *Int J Clin Pediatr Dent.* (2016) 9:228–32. doi: 10.5005/jp-journals-10005-1369
41. Singh S, Myburgh NG, Lalloo R. Policy analysis of oral health promotion in South Africa. *Global Health Promot.* (2010) 17:16–24. doi: 10.1177/1757975909356631
42. Watt RG. COVID-19 is an opportunity for reform in dentistry. *Lancet.* (2020) 396:462. doi: 10.1016/S0140-6736(20)31529-4

7

COVID-19 Related Experience, Knowledge, Attitude and Behaviors Among 2,669 Orthodontists, Orthodontic Residents and Nurses in China

Fang Hua[1,2,3†]*, Danchen Qin*[1†]*, Jiarong Yan*[1]*, Tingting Zhao*[1] *and Hong He*[1*]

[1] Department of Orthodontics, Hubei-MOST KLOS & KLOBM, School & Hospital of Stomatology, Wuhan University, Wuhan, China, [2] Center for Evidence-Based Stomatology, Hubei-MOST KLOS & KLOBM, School & Hospital of Stomatology, Wuhan University, Wuhan, China, [3] Division of Dentistry, Faculty of Biology, Medicine and Health, Manchester Academic Health Science Centre, School of Medical Sciences, University of Manchester, Manchester, United Kingdom

***Correspondence:**
Hong He
drhehong@whu.edu.cn

† These authors have contributed equally to this work

Objectives: To assess the current COVID-19 related experiences, knowledge, attitudes, and behaviors among orthodontists, orthodontic residents, and orthodontic nurses in China, and to identify factors associated with their self-perceived and actual level of knowledge, as well as their willingness to treat/care for COVID-19 patients.

Materials and Methods: A cross-sectional online survey was conducted in China using a 37-item questionnaire developed based on previous research. A professional online survey tool (www.wjx.cn) and a social media platform (WeChat) were used to display and distribute the questionnaire. Data were collected during April 11 to 13, 2020, when most regions of China had resumed dental practice except for high-risk regions such as Wuhan. Then the data were analyzed with multivariable generalized estimating equations.

Results: A total of 2,669 valid questionnaires were collected. Orthodontic services were suspended for nearly all respondents (97.8%) during the epidemic, and 68.0% had resumed work by the time they completed the questionnaire. The majority of respondents (80.2%) were confident that they understood COVID-19 related knowledge, but most of them only correctly answered less than half of the questions testing their actual level of knowledge. About two-thirds (64.1%) were willing to treat/care for patients with confirmed or suspected COVID-19. The completion of relevant training programs was significantly associated with more confidence in knowledge mastery ($P < 0.001$) and a higher actual level of knowledge ($P < 0.001$), but did not increase their willingness to treat/care for patients with COVID-19 ($P = 0.235$).

Conclusions: Before work resumption, COVID-19-related training programs are essential for the improvement of knowledge, confidence, and preparedness of orthodontic professionals. Sufficient and proper protection should also be provided to ensure safety and reduce the psychological burden on them.

Clinical Relevance: The findings can provide evidence for policy-making related to the resumption of elective dental services.

Keywords: COVID-19, coronavirus, infection control, orthodontics, questionnaire

INTRODUCTION

After being discovered in Wuhan, China, last December, the coronavirus disease 2019 (COVID-19), caused by severe acute respiratory syndrome coronavirus 2 (SARS-CoV-2), has spread quickly to most parts of the world (1). The World Health Organization (WHO) officially declared the COVID-19 outbreak a public health emergency of international concern on January 30, 2020 (2), and then a global pandemic on March 11, 2020 (3). As of May 29, 2020, there have been a total of 5,701,337 laboratory-confirmed COVID-19 cases and 357,688 deaths in 217 countries, territories, or areas (4).

Current observations have suggested that people of all ages are generally susceptible to COVID-19. However, those who are in close contact with confirmed cases or asymptomatic carriers, including health care workers (HCWs) and other patients within hospitals and/or clinics, are at higher risk of infection (5). As of February 24, 2020, a total of 3,387 HCWs from 476 medical institutions across China were reported to be infected with SARS-CoV-2 (including 2,055 confirmed cases, 1,070 clinically diagnosed cases, and 157 suspected cases), among whom over 90% were from Hubei province and over 20 had died (6, 7). More recently, the WHO announced that there had been at least 22,073 COVID-19 cases among HCWs from 52 countries by April 8, 2020 (8). However, currently there are no data available for cross-transmission in dental settings or cases reported among dental HCWs (9, 10).

As many dental procedures can generate a large number of droplets and aerosols, standard protective measures used in daily practice are not enough to prevent cross-infection among dental practitioners and dental patients (11). In light of this, most provinces and cities in China released regulations in late January, which explicitly restricted dental services to emergency care only, and suspended all elective treatments until further notice (11). As a result of these regulations, as well as public health interventions such as traffic suspension and home quarantine (12), many dental professionals stayed at home during the epidemic, communicating with existing and potential new patients via smartphones and online consultation platforms (13, 14).

Combined, the above-mentioned changes in work and life due to COVID-19 can have a huge impact on HCWs, including non-frontline workers. Findings of a recent study have suggested that the level of psychological stress among non-frontline nurses could be significantly higher than frontline nurses (15). In addition, as China moves from the 2-month containment phase to the mitigation stage (16), the preparedness of non-frontline HCWs to resume work is of great importance. Two recent studies have investigated the knowledge and attitudes regarding COVID-19 among Chinese HCWs in psychiatric hospitals (17) and Jordanian dentists (18), respectively. However, to our knowledge, similar research has not been carried out among HCWs in the field of orthodontics.

Therefore, the objectives of this study were: (1) to assess the current COVID-19-related experiences, knowledge, attitudes, and behaviors among orthodontists, orthodontic residents, and orthodontic nurses in China; (2) to identify factors associated with the self-perceived and actual level of knowledge; and (3) to explore the association between willingness to treat/care for patients with confirmed or suspected COVID-19 and potentially related factors.

MATERIALS AND METHODS

Ethical Approval

This study was a convenience-sample open online survey, written in accordance with the CHEcklist for Reporting Results of Internet E-Surveys (CHERRIES) guidelines (19). The study protocol was approved by the Ethics Committee of School & Hospital of Stomatology, Wuhan University (No. 2020-B25). Informed consent was obtained from all respondents. A brief introduction to the study was provided in the first part of the questionnaire, including the target population, study objectives, the time needed to complete the questionnaire, as well as the names and contact information of the investigators. Participation in the survey was voluntary, with neither reward nor penalty. All respondents were informed that they were free to continue or quit at any time, and the submission of the questionnaire would be regarded as consent to participate. To protect respondents' privacy, the survey was anonymous, and all the raw data were stored in one author's computer and kept confidential.

Survey Design

A 37-item questionnaire (**Supplementary Material 1**) was developed according to previous research on knowledge, attitudes, and behaviors of HCWs (17, 20). We added several questions for background information of the participants, and rephrased questions to make them relevant to orthodontics; the construction of the measured concepts and scoring methods remained the same. The survey consisted of four aspects: background information, knowledge, attitudes, and behaviors. The first 16 questions were regarding the background characteristics, including seven for demographics, five for workplace information, and four for COVID-related personal experience. Ten questions were in the knowledge section, including three Likert-scale items (#17, #19, and #20) for the self-perceived level of knowledge, one semi-open question (#18) for their source of knowledge, and six (3 single-choice and 3 multiple-choice, #21 to #26) questions for the assessment of actual knowledge level. Among five questions in the attitude section, three were Likert-scale (#27 to #29) to evaluate the attitudes toward personal protective equipment (PPE) in the context of COVID-19. In addition, respondents were asked a yes-no question (#30) about their willingness to treat/care for orthodontic patients with confirmed or suspected COVID-19, and if "no" was selected, they should explain the reasons for this choice (a semi-open question, #31). The behavior section contained six questions. Respondents were required to rate their actual or expected behaviors after the resumption of orthodontic services for five Likert-scale questions (#32, #33, and #35 to #37), and their compliance to PPE on a percentage scale (#34). For all Likert-scale questions, a five-point Likert scale was used ranging from 1 (completely disagree) to 5 (completely agree). In addition, each aspect contained several Likert-scale items to ensure reliability and validity.

Participant Recruitment

Eligible participants were orthodontists, orthodontic residents, orthodontic nurses, and general dental practitioners and nurses offering orthodontic care. The sample size was calculated using an online calculator (www.raosoft.com/samplesize.html). With a 5% margin of error and a 95% confidence level, the required sample size was 377.

Prior to its official release, the questionnaire was sent to a small group of around 20 orthodontic professionals to record the time needed to complete it and check if the questions were clear and unambiguous. After this pilot survey, the questionnaire was distributed and publicized to orthodontic professionals nationwide.

We used purposive and snowball sampling routes to recruit participants. The survey was distributed from April 11 to 13, 2020, when most regions of China had resumed dental practice, except for high-risk regions such as Wuhan. We first disseminated the questionnaire link through orthodontics-related blogs on WeChat (Tencent, Shenzhen, China), which has been the most widely used social media platform in China (21). Then we sent messages to chat groups of orthodontic practitioners and asked them to invite their friends, engaging orthodontics to participate. Also, professor H.H invited her professional network personally.

The questionnaire was collected using a professional online survey platform (www.wjx.cn). Since respondents could submit their answers only when all the questions are finished, this platform guaranteed the completeness of the collected questionnaires. To prevent multiple answers from the same individual, the questionnaire could only be accessed through WeChat, and each WeChat account could only answer once. The respondents could not change their answers once submitted. All valid responses were included, and the expected valid response rate was 90% after excluding invalid answers. As planned *a priori*, questionnaires with incomplete responses, apparent errors, and atypical timestamps (<2 min or more than 30 min) (22) were considered invalid and excluded.

Statistical Analysis

The original data were downloaded from the online survey platform. For the semi-open question, reasons for their unwillingness to treat/care for COVID-19 patients (#31), themes were manually extracted and coded by three authors (F.H., D.Q., and T.Z.), independently and in duplicate, with all discrepancies resolved by discussion. Each response could be coded into multiple themes if containing miscellaneous information, and then the count for each theme were calculated. The self-perceived level of knowledge about COVID-19 was evaluated by averaging the scores of three Likert-scale items (#17, #19, and #20). Regarding the actual level of knowledge, we gave 1 point for each question of #21 to #26 answered correctly, and no point for any item incorrectly answered. Then a total knowledge score (score range: 0 to 6) for each respondent was calculated by totaling the scores of all these six items.

Descriptive statistics were performed to summarize the characteristics and the answers of each question. Categorical data were presented as counts and percentages. Continuous data were expressed as means ± standard deviations (SDs) and range, and skewed data and Likert-scale responses were presented as medians and interquartile ranges. Chi-square tests and Fisher's exact tests were used to analyze categorical data, with pairwise comparisons adjusted by Bonferroni correction. Likert-scale questions were analyzed with Kruskal-Wallis tests, followed by Dunn's tests for *post-hoc* pairwise comparisons. The self-perceived level of knowledge and the total knowledge score were compared using one-way analysis of variance (ANOVA) with Tukey adjustment.

Generalized estimating equations (GEE) regression analyses were performed to explore factors associated with the self-perceived level of knowledge, total knowledge score, and the willingness to treat/care for COVID-19 patients (#30). Robust estimate of covariance and the independent correlation matrix were adopted. For continuous outcomes (the self-perceived level of knowledge and the total knowledge score), we used a GEE with a normal distribution for the response variables and identity link; for the binary outcome (the willingness to treat/care for COVID-19 patients), we used a GEE with a binomial distribution and logit link. As determined *a priori*, all the characteristics in the first part of the questionnaire (#1 to #16) were served as independent variables, namely age, gender, profession, years of practice, academic degree, marital status, cohabitants, location of workplace, settings, provision of online orthodontic consultation, current status of orthodontic services at the workplace, participation in anti-epidemic activities, current status of personal orthodontic practice, completion of any COVID-19-related training program, and experience of treating/caring for COVID-19 patients. In addition, self-perceived level of knowledge and total knowledge score also served as the predictors of the willingness to treat/care for COVID-19 patients. In these analyses, we carried out univariable analyses first, and then entered all significant factors into multivariable analyses. Tolerance and variance inflation factor (VIF) were used to detect multicollinearity, and predictors with tolerance < 0.1 or VIF > 10 were excluded from the final model. Two-sided $P < 0.05$ was considered statistically significant.

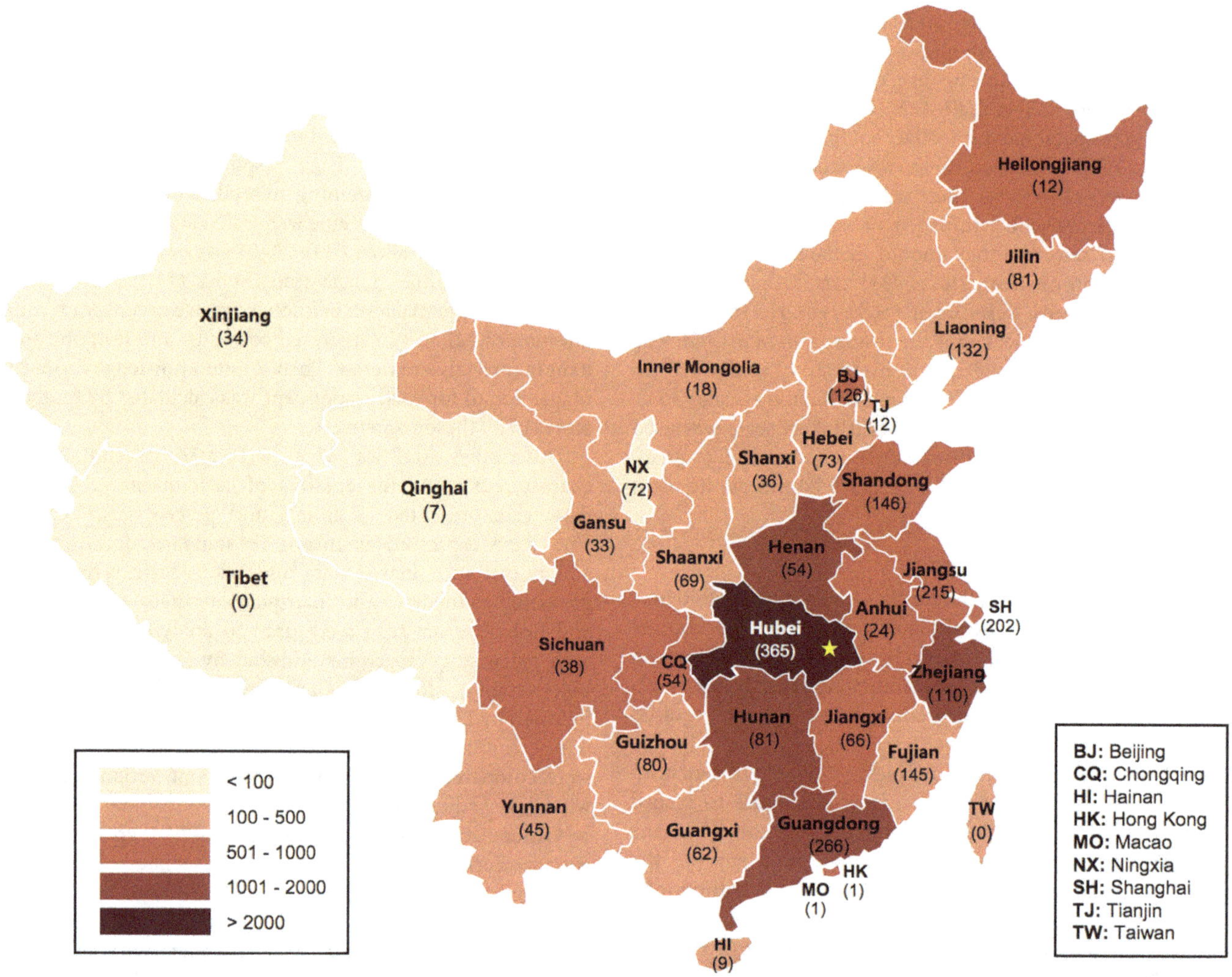

FIGURE 1 | The geographical distribution of respondents to this survey ($n = 2{,}669$). Gradient of colors represents the cumulative number of confirmed COVID-19 cases in each provincial-level administrative region (as of April 10, 2020). Numbers in parentheses indicate the number of respondents from each region. The star marks the location of Wuhan.

RESULTS

Due to the character of our recruitment methods, it was impossible to estimate the total number of orthodontic practitioners who had received our survey invitation. Among the 2,890 questionnaires collected, 221 responses were invalid according to the predetermined eligibility criteria: four failed to complete the survey before the deadline, 15 submitted with an unusual completion time, and 202 questionnaires had obvious mistakes such as abnormal age and contradictory answers to similar questions. After removing these invalid responses, 2,669 questionnaires from 2,669 respondents were included in analyses, resulting in a valid response rate of 92.4%.

General Information

The respondents came from 32 of the 34 provincial-level administrative regions of China. **Figure 1** illustrates the geographical distribution of respondents together with the cumulative number of confirmed COVID-19 cases in each region as of April 10. There were 739 (27.7%) males and 1,930 (72.3%) females between 19 and 62, with an average age of 34.3 (SD, 8.5). The majority of the respondents were orthodontists (64.8%), followed by orthodontic residents/postgraduate students (20.5%) and orthodontic nurses (14.6%). Nearly half (47.7%) of them had a relatively short working experience in orthodontics (≤5 years). The majority (91.0%) lived with other people, and nearly three-fifths (58.2%) lived with their parents and/or children.

As shown in **Table 1**, almost all respondents (97.8%) stated that the dental hospitals or clinics in which they worked had full (49.2%) or partial (48.6%) suspension of orthodontic treatment during the epidemic. Also, a majority of them (87.4%) stated that their workplaces provided online orthodontic consultation to either existing orthodontic patients only (30.9%), or both

TABLE 1 | Demographic and workplace information of the respondents to this survey.

Characteristics	*N*	%
Demographics		
Age§	34.3 ± 8.5	19–62
Gender		
Female	1,930	72.3
Male	739	27.7
Profession		
Orthodontist	1,731	64.8
Orthodontic resident/postgraduate student	547	20.5
Orthodontic nurse	391	14.6
Years of orthodontic practice		
≤5 years	1,274	47.7
5–10 years	620	23.2
10–20 years	516	19.3
>20 years	259	9.7
Highest degree		
PhD	211	7.9
Master	778	29.1
Bachelor	1,371	51.4
Junior college	297	11.1
Technical secondary school	12	0.4
Marital status		
Single	944	35.4
Married, without children	240	9.0
Married, with children	1,465	54.9
Others	20	0.7
Cohabitants		
Live alone	241	9.0
Parents and/or children	1,553	58.2
Others	875	32.8
Workplace information		
Location		
Wuhan	267	10.0
Hubei province (excluding Wuhan)	98	3.7
Others	2,304	86.3
Setting		
Public	1,980	74.2
Private	689	25.8
Orthodontic services during epidemic		
Complete suspension	1,313	49.2
Partial suspension	1,297	48.6
No suspension	59	2.2
Online consultation		
No	337	12.6
Provided, only to existing orthodontic patients	824	30.9
Provided, to both existing and potential new orthodontic patients	1,508	56.5
Current status of orthodontic services		
Not resumed yet	338	12.7
Partially resumed	1,176	44.1
Completely resumed	1147	43.0
No suspension	8	0.3
Total	2,669	100.0

§*Displayed as mean ± SD, and range.*

existing and potential new orthodontic patients (56.5%). In addition, 87.1% of the respondents reported that their workplaces had recently resumed orthodontic services in full (43.0%) or in part (44.1%).

Personal Experience

Table 2 shows the respondents' COVID-19-related personal experience during the epidemic. Although 28.6% of them had participated in anti-epidemic activities, including supporting fever clinics or designated COVID-19 hospitals, and acting as community volunteers, only 3.9% had the experience of treating or caring for patients with confirmed COVID-19. Approximately 80% of the orthodontists and nurses had resumed their orthodontic practice, whereas only one-fifth (19.4%) of the orthodontic residents had returned to work. Additionally, the majority of orthodontists (84.4%) and nurses (90.3%) had finished COVID-19-related training programs, while only 55.2% of orthodontic residents received relevant training.

As listed in **Supplementary Table 1**, the proportion of respondents that had not resumed orthodontic work was significantly different among location groups ($P < 0.001$). The highest proportion occurred in Wuhan (93.3%), followed by other parts of Hubei province (52.0%) and regions outside Hubei (23.8%). Accordingly, the proportion of respondents who had not completed COVID-19-related training programs was significantly higher in Wuhan (29.2%) than places outside Hubei (19.8%). In addition, the experience of treating or caring for COVID-19 patients was more common among respondents from Wuhan (9.0%) and other parts of Hubei (9.2%) than those from areas outside Hubei province (3.1%).

Knowledge

As described in **Supplementary Table 2**, the mean self-perceived level of knowledge of COVID-19 was 4.03 (SD 0.65), which means the respondents agreed that they were confident in their knowledge. Most respondents (80.2%) expressed agreement or complete agreement that they understood COVID-19-related knowledge. In addition, most were confident that they understood the risk of COVID-19 to patients and HCWs (84.1%), as well as how to protect themselves and patients during the epidemic (76.1%). As shown in **Figure 2**, the Internet (92.8%) was the respondents' primary source of knowledge, followed by training programs (74.6%), television (70.5%), medical journals (31.3%), and newspapers (26.0%). However, the mean total knowledge score was 2.74 (SD, 0.85), which suggests the respondents only correctly answered less than half of the six questions testing their actual level of knowledge on average.

Table 3 shows the results of GEE regression analyses for the self-perceived level of knowledge about COVID-19. According to multivariable analysis, respondents who had finished COVID-19-related training programs had significantly more confidence in knowledge mastery than those who had not ($B = 0.406$, 95% CI: 0.341 to 0.471, $P < 0.001$). In addition, a significantly higher self-perceived level of knowledge was also found in orthodontic nurses ($P < 0.001$), older people ($P = 0.008$), male individuals ($P < 0.001$), those who were living with parents and/or children (P

TABLE 2 | Respondents' personal experience during the COVID-19 epidemic by profession.

Personal experience[§]	Total (n = 2,669)	Orthodontists (n = 1,731)	Orthodontic residents (n = 547)	Orthodontic nurses (n = 391)	P-value[†]
Participation in anti-epidemic activities[¶]					**<0.001**
No	1,907 (71.4)	1,150 (66.4)[a]	490 (89.6)[b]	267 (68.3)[a]	
Yes	762 (28.6)	581 (33.6)[a]	57 (10.4)[b]	124 (31.7)[a]	
Current status of orthodontic practice					**<0.001[‡]**
Not resumed yet	849 (31.8)	326 (18.8)[a]	441 (80.6)[b]	82 (21.0)[a]	
Resumed, less than 2 weeks	478 (17.9)	379 (21.9)[a]	46 (8.4)[b]	53 (13.6)[c]	
Resumed, 2 to 4 weeks	725 (27.2)	586 (33.9)[a]	38 (6.9)[b]	101 (25.8)[c]	
Resumed, more than 4 weeks	611 (22.9)	436 (25.2)[a]	22 (4.0)[b]	153 (39.1)[c]	
No suspension	6 (0.2)	4 (0.2)[a]	0 (0.0)[a]	2 (0.5)[a]	
Completion of COVID-19 related training program					**<0.001**
No	553 (20.7)	270 (15.6)[a]	245 (44.8)[b]	38 (9.7)[c]	
Yes	2,116 (79.3)	1,461 (84.4)[a]	302 (55.2)[b]	353 (90.3)[c]	
Experience of treating or caring for COVID-19 patients					**<0.001[‡]**
No	2,564 (96.1)	1,652 (95.4)[a]	543 (99.3)[b]	369 (94.4)[a]	
Yes	105 (3.9)	79 (4.6)[a]	4 (0.7)[b]	22 (5.6)[a]	

[§]Displayed as N (%).
[¶]Including activities in fever clinics or designated hospitals for COVID-19 patients, as community volunteers, and other COVID-19-related works.
[†]P-values in bold are statistically significant (<0.05).
[‡]Fisher' exact test.
[a,b,c]Groups with the same letters in the same row are not statistically different (P > 0.05) according to post hoc tests.

= 0.024), those who suspended their orthodontic practice during the epidemic ($P = 0.029$), and those who had the experience of treating or caring for COVID-19 patients ($P = 0.040$).

However, in terms of the actual level of knowledge, a higher total knowledge score was significantly associated with the completion of COVID-19-related training programs ($B = 0.181$, 95% CI: 0.099 to 0.264, $P < 0.001$), working in a public hospital or clinic ($P < 0.001$), 5 to 10 years of working experience in orthodontics ($P = 0.006$), and having a master's degree ($P = 0.018$). In contrast, male individuals ($P < 0.001$), those who had the experience of treating or caring for COVID-19 patients ($P < 0.001$), as well as those working outside Hubei province ($P = 0.007$) had a significantly lower total knowledge score (**Table 4**). In addition, the current status of personal orthodontic practice was on the borderline statistical significance, and those who had resumed their work <2 weeks before had a significantly higher knowledge score ($P = 0.031$).

Attitude

In general, most respondents agreed about the effectiveness of PPE. They also admitted that it would be somewhat inconvenient to use PPE while treating patients. **Supplementary Table 3** shows the differences in attitude among profession groups. Orthodontic nurses expressed significantly more agreement that PPE could protect orthodontic staff ($P = 0.010$) and orthodontic patients ($P = 0.001$) from COVID-19, and felt less inconvenient to use PPE when treating/caring for patients ($P < 0.001$).

About two-thirds of the participants (64.1%) stated that they were willing to treat or care for patients with confirmed or suspected COVID-19. According to multivariable GEE analysis, the odds of being willing to treat/care for COVID-19 patients were significantly higher among orthodontic nurses ($P < 0.001$), those with a higher self-perceived level of knowledge ($P < 0.001$), those who worked at a public hospital or clinic ($P < 0.001$) that provided online consultation to both existing and potential new orthodontic patients ($P = 0.001$), those with a junior college ($P = 0.011$) or bachelor's degree ($P = 0.019$), and those who had an experience of anti-epidemic activities ($P = 0.022$) (**Table 5**).

As depicted in **Figure 3**, among respondents who were unwilling to treat/care for COVID-19 patients, the most common reasons were concern about the possible infection of their family members (80.2%) and possible infection of themselves (72.0%). Except for the above two choices we provided in this semi-open question, respondents also gave other reasons including concern about possible nosocomial infection (8.8%), the non-emergent nature of orthodontic treatment (6.6%), a lack of COVID-19-related knowledge and experience (5.7%), concern about the possible spread of infection (3.1%), and inadequate protective measures and equipment (2.9%).

Behaviors

In the final part of the questionnaire, respondents were asked about their behaviors after the resumption of orthodontic services (**Supplementary Table 4**). Most respondents (72.3%) agreed that their hospitals/clinics had adequate PPE for them to use, and 61.7% reported that they were 100% sure that after work resumption, they would use the recommended PPE during treatment. In addition, orthodontic nurses reported better compliance with PPE ($P = 0.001$) and were less likely to forget to change PPE between patients ($P < 0.001$).

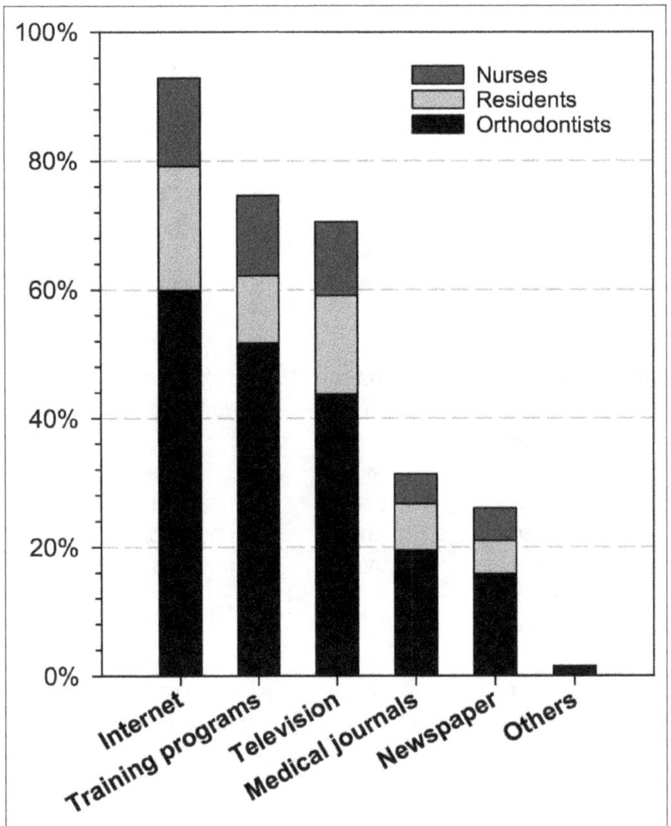

FIGURE 2 | The sources of COVID-19-related knowledge among respondents (semi-open question, #18) (n = 2,669).

DISCUSSION

After the announcement of human-to-human transmission and infections among HCWs on January 20, 2020, China imposed more rigorous public health interventions (e.g., compulsory wearing of face masks in public places, intensive intercity and intracity traffic restriction, social distancing, home isolation, and centralized quarantine) to control the spread of SARS-CoV-2 (12). Since around January 27, 2020, relevant government agencies of most provinces and cities in China began to release their regulations on dental practices during the epidemic, which explicitly suspended all elective dental services, including orthodontic treatment (13, 14). About 1 month later, as the number of daily new cases had decreased substantially in China, provinces and cities began to loosen public health interventions and gradually resume non-emergency dental services, according to their own situation. For instance, as the hardest-hit city in China, Wuhan officially lifted its lockdown on April 8, 2020, and its largest dental care provider—Hospital of Stomatology, Wuhan University, started to provide elective treatments on April 20, 2020. Therefore, with 2,669 responses collected from across China during April 11–13, the present study provides valuable insights into the COVID-19-related experiences, knowledge, attitudes, and behaviors of orthodontic professionals during such a period of transition.

The COVID-19 epidemic had a huge impact on orthodontic practice. In this study, a majority of the respondents stated that, during the epidemic, their workplaces had suspended orthodontic treatment (97.8%) and provided online orthodontic consultation to patients (87.4%). These figures are generally in line with those of a previous study conducted during February 17–23, which found that all of the surveyed 48 public tertiary dental hospitals in China had suspended non-emergent dental services, and 33 of them (68.8%) had been offering online dental consultations during suspension (14). Similarly, some other countries implemented mandatory suspension of dental non-emergencies, including orthodontic treatment to fight against the COVID-19 pandemic and ensure the safety of patients and medical staff (23–25).

With the gradual recovery of normal dental services in China, most of the respondents (87.1%) reported that their workplaces had resumed orthodontic services completely or partially. Compared to orthodontists and nurses, significantly fewer orthodontic residents/postgraduate students had resumed orthodontic work, completed any COVID-19-related training programs, or had experience in anti-epidemic activities or treatment for COVID-19 patients, This could be explained by the fact that they are considered students in China, and had been required by the Ministry of Education to remain at home and not to return to their dental schools until further notice (13). In addition, Wuhan and other parts of Hubei had a significantly lower proportion of people who had resumed work. These results are in accordance with the severe situation in Wuhan and other parts of Hubei during the COVID-19 epidemic, as well as the fact that they were the latest in China to loosen public health interventions.

As part of the preparation before work resumption, nearly 80% of the respondents had finished training; three-quarters reported that the training was their primary source of COVID-19-related information. In addition, most respondents also acquired information from the Internet and television during home quarantine. However, only one-third stated that they obtained the relevant knowledge from medical journals. As COVID-19 was an up-to-date topic and most related articles were published in English, language could be a potential barrier to the knowledge acquisition from medical journals for Chinese practitioners. They could turn to other resources, such as authority websites and official notification, for relevant information.

Responses to our questions regarding knowledge have shown a discrepancy between the self-perceived and actual level of knowledge. Although the majority of respondents stated that they understood COVID-19-related knowledge, risks, and protective measures very well, their total knowledge score was generally suboptimal. According to multivariable analyses, after the adjustment of potential confounding variables, the completion of relevant training programs was significantly associated with both more confidence in knowledge mastery and a higher total knowledge score. This is consistent with previous studies, which suggested additional training and education

TABLE 3 | Results of univariable and multivariable generalized estimating equations (GEE) regression analyses for self-perceived level of knowledge.

Variable	Univariable analysis			Multivariable analysis		
	B	95% CI	*P*-value¶	*B*	95% CI	*P*-value¶
Demographics						
Age	0.012	(0.009, 0.015)	**<0.001**	0.008	(0.002, 0.014)	**0.008**
Gender						
Female	Reference			Reference		
Male	0.112	(0.058, 0.166)	**<0.001**	0.107	(0.054, 0.160)	**<0.001**
Profession			**<0.001**			**<0.001**
Orthodontist	Reference			Reference		
Orthodontic resident/postgraduate student	−0.264	(−0.325, −0.203)	**<0.001**	−0.012	(−0.100, 0.077)	0.797
Orthodontic nurse	0.094	(0.023, 0.164)	**0.009**	0.148	(0.070, 0.225)	**<0.001**
Years of orthodontic practice			**<0.001**			0.370
≤5 years	Reference			Reference		
5–10 years	0.095	(0.033, 0.158)	**0.003**	−0.059	(−0.128, 0.011)	0.099
10–20 years	0.184	(0.119, 0.249)	**<0.001**	−0.051	(−0.137, 0.035)	0.246
>20 years	0.259	(0.178, 0.339)	**<0.001**	−0.030	(−0.162, 0.102)	0.656
Academic degree			0.430			
Marital status			**<0.001**			0.090
Single	Reference			Reference		
Married, without children	0.170	(0.085, 0.255)	**<0.001**	0.078	(−0.011, 0.167)	0.088
Married, with children	0.191	(0.138, 0.245)	**<0.001**	−0.046	(−0.133, 0.042)	0.308
Others	0.095	(−0.247, 0.437)	0.586	0.005	(−0.344, 0.355)	0.976
Cohabitants			**<0.001**			**0.030**
Live alone	Reference			Reference		
Parents and/or children	0.141	(0.045, 0.234)	**0.004**	0.113	(0.015, 0.212)	**0.024**
Others	0.007	(−0.092, 0.106)	0.895	0.048	(−0.047, 0.144)	0.323
Workplace information						
Location			**0.020**			0.191
Wuhan	Reference			Reference		
Hubei province (excluding Wuhan)	0.198	(0.059, 0.338)	**0.005**	0.121	(−0.010, 0.252)	0.069
Others	0.078	(−0.008, 0.164)	0.075	0.056	(−0.052, 0.165)	0.309
Setting			0.612			
Orthodontic services during epidemic			**0.003**			0.130
Complete suspension	Reference			Reference		
Partial suspension	−0.040	(−0.090, 0.010)	0.313	−0.040	(−0.089, 0.010)	0.116
No suspension	0.225	(0.063, 0.387)	**0.032**	0.084	(−0.089, 0.257)	0.342
Online consultation			0.158			
Current status of orthodontic services			**<0.001**			**<0.001**
Not resumed yet	Reference			Reference		
Partially resumed	−0.018	(−0.098, 0.062)	0.658	−0.073	(−0.182, 0.037)	0.193
Completely resumed	0.081	(0.001, 0.161)	**0.047**	−0.045	(−0.163, 0.073)	0.452
No suspension	0.711	(0.388, 1.034)	**<0.001**	0.672	(0.463, 0.881)	**<0.001**
Personal experience						
Participation in anti-epidemic activities						
No	Reference			Reference		
Yes	0.160	(0.107, 0.213)	**<0.001**	−0.073	(−0.182, 0.037)	0.193
Current status of orthodontic practice			**<0.001**			**0.048**
Not resumed yet	Reference			Reference		
Resumed, less than 2 weeks	0.167	(0.096, 0.238)	**<0.001**	0.054	(−0.036, 0.145)	0.241
Resumed, 2 to 4 weeks	0.206	(0.143, 0.270)	**<0.001**	0.056	(−0.033, 0.145)	0.217

(Continued)

TABLE 3 | Continued

Variable	Univariable analysis			Multivariable analysis		
	B	95% CI	*P*-value¶	*B*	95% CI	*P*-value¶
Resumed, more than 4 weeks	0.241	(0.173, 0.309)	**<0.001**	0.073	(−0.024, 0.169)	0.140
No suspension	0.728	(0.335, 1.120)	**<0.001**	−0.402	(−0.762, −0.042)	**0.029**
Completion of COVID-19 related training program						
No	Reference			Reference		
Yes	0.478	(0.417, 0.539)	**<0.001**	0.406	(0.341, 0.471)	**<0.001**
Experience of treating or caring for COVID-19 patients						
No	Reference			Reference		
Yes	0.277	(0.154, 0.399)	**<0.001**	0.137	(0.006, 0.268)	**0.040**

¶*P-values in bold are statistically significant (<0.05).*

improved dental practitioners' knowledge of infection control (26, 27). This finding highlights the importance for dental hospitals, clinics, and relevant professional societies to organize adequate training activities for HCWs before the resumption of dental services. We also found that the time of work resumption was a borderline predictor of the actual level of knowledge; those who had just resumed work performed better. Although COVID-19-related training was required before work resumption in China, orthodontic professionals may forget relevant knowledge as time elapsed. This possibly suggests that regular training is essential to enhance their knowledge mastery. In addition, although respondents with the experience of treating/caring for COVID-19 patients had higher self-perceived knowledge, they performed significantly poorer in the questions that tested their actual knowledge. The possible reason may be that during the epidemic, the highest level of protection was taken in the treatment. However, in this transition period of work resumption, the focus of dental practice shifted from emergencies to routine procedures, and particular caution and different precautions should be taken.

With regard to the respondents' attitude, 64.1% of them were willing to treat/care for patients with confirmed or suspected COVID-19. Eighty percent of those who were reluctant expressed their concern over possible infection of their family members. Researchers found that fear of transmitting the virus to family and coworkers was the top concern of dentists and frontline HCWs (28). Previous studies have shown that knowledge and education could positively affect dentists' attitudes toward the treatment of patients with highly infectious diseases (27, 29). In the present study, however, both the actual knowledge level and the completion of relevant training programs did not increase respondents' willingness to treat COVID-19 patients. Due to the sudden outbreak and quick spread of COVID-19, as well as there being no vaccine or approved treatment, the fear of the unknown and uncertainty about the disease was the main obstacle to the treatment of COVID-19 patients (30). Home quarantine is crucial to the diffusion of coronavirus, but added difficulties to dental treatment and triggered excessive anxiety (31). We also found that respondents from public dental institutions with online consultation were more willing to treat COVID-19 patients. This is probably because these institutions have adequate prevention measures and sufficient medical sources to protect their staff, while the shortage of PPE is strongly associated with the stress and anxiety of HCWs (32).

In the present study, although many respondents had a suboptimal total knowledge score, most of them believed that they could improve their adherence to PPE. A previous study indicated that dental practitioners were generally ill-prepared for COVID-19, as they did not routinely wear recommended respirators during treatment (33). The use of PPE is crucial for protection, and practitioners need to understand which level of protective measures should be used (34). Hand hygiene is also considered a critical measure for infection control, with poor adherence believed to be a major contributor to disease transmission (35). Researchers found that the implementation of recommended infection control measures varied among dentists, and those who were aware of the importance of infection control had better compliance with guidelines (26). This suggests that the use of effective strategies and different modes of training is necessary to enhance dental professionals' awareness of infection control. It has been recommended that the use of a checklist in handy places for repeatable procedures improves the compliance with infection control precautions, including what PPE should be used in certain circumstances, the correct donning and doffing procedures of PPE, and the recommended hand hygiene measures (36).

A questionnaire-based survey is a useful tool to efficiently acquire information regarding opinions and experiences covering wide demographics of participants (37). In the present study, we obtained a sufficiently large sample for data analysis; however, careful interpretation of the results is required. First, this was an online survey and many participants were recruited via one professor's network, which was a potential source of bias. Second, some categories of the respondents' characteristics had a very small sample size, which caused the imprecision of the results and compromised representativeness of certain populations. In addition, a more thorough investigation

TABLE 4 | Results of univariable and multivariable generalized estimating equations (GEE) regression analyses for total knowledge score.

Variable	Univariable analysis			Multivariable analysis		
	B	95% CI	*P*-value¶	*B*	95% CI	*P*-value¶
Demographics						
Age			0.977			
Gender						
Female	Reference			Reference		
Male	−0.171	(−0.244, −0.097)	**<0.001**	−0.151	(−0.226, −0.077)	**<0.001**
Profession			0.887			
Years of orthodontic practice			**0.007**			**0.031**
≤5 years	Reference			Reference		
5–10 years	0.146	(0.062, 0.230)	**0.001**	0.124	(0.035, 0.212)	**0.006**
10–20 years	0.063	(−0.022, 0.147)	0.146	0.054	(−0.038, 0.146)	0.247
>20 years	0.013	(−0.096, 0.122)	0.809	−0.012	(−0.131, 0.107)	0.844
Academic degree			**<0.001**			**0.001**
PhD	Reference			Reference		
Master	0.137	(0.010, 0.265)	**0.035**	0.156	(0.027, 0.284)	**0.018**
Bachelor	−0.028	(−0.148, 0.092)	0.645	0.039	(−0.086, 0.164)	0.539
Junior college	−0.207	(−0.368, −0.067)	**0.005**	−0.081	(−0.242, 0.079)	0.321
Technical secondary school	−0.073	(−0.509, 0.364)	0.744	0.156	(−0.362, 0.523)	0.721
Marital status			0.439			
Cohabitants			0.418			
Workplace information						
Location			**0.016**			**0.002**
Wuhan	Reference			Reference		
Hubei province (excluding Wuhan)	0.044	(−0.169, 0.257)	0.685	0.065	(−0.140, 0.270)	0.535
Others	−0.133	(−0.249, −0.018)	**0.023**	−0.175	(−0.302, −0.048)	**0.007**
Setting						
Public	Reference			Reference		
Private	−0.231	(−0.303, −0.160)	**<0.001**	−0.174	(−0.253, −0.096)	**<0.001**
Orthodontic services during epidemic			0.199			
Online consultation			0.675			
Current status of orthodontic services			0.417			
Personal experience						
Participation in anti-epidemic activities			0.439			
Current status of orthodontic practice			**0.003**			0.050
Not resumed yet	Reference			Reference		
resumed, less than 2 weeks	−0.159	(−0.253, −0.064)	**0.001**	−0.113	(−0.216, −0.010)	**0.031**
resumed, 2 to 4 weeks	0.020	(−0.064, 0.105)	0.640	0.025	(0.124, 0.246)	0.620
resumed, more than 4 weeks	−0.001	(−0.090, 0.089)	0.990	−0.024	(0.081, 0.200)	0.655
No suspension	0.070	(−0.483, 0.623)	0.804	0.109	(0.668, 0.147)	0.701
Completion of COVID−19 related training program						
No	Reference			Reference		
Yes	0.204	(0.125, 0.283)	**<0.001**	0.181	(0.099, 0.264)	**<0.001**
Experience of treating or caring for COVID-19 patients						
No	Reference			Reference		
Yes	−0.265	(−0.429, −0.101)	**0.002**	−0.324	(−0.483, −0.165)	**<0.001**

¶P-values in bold are statistically significant (<0.05).

into the impact of COVID-19 on orthodontists' provision of healthcare services was out of the scope of this study and therefore not included. This could be explored in future research.

CONCLUSIONS

Results of the present study suggest that, during the mitigation stage of the COVID-19 epidemic when orthodontic services

TABLE 5 | Results of univariable and multivariable generalized estimating equations (GEE) regression analyses for willingness to treat/care for patients with COVID-19.

Variable	Univariable analysis			Multivariable analysis		
	OR	95% CI	*P*-value¶	OR	95% CI	*P*-value¶
Demographics						
Age	0.982	(0.973, 0.992)	**<0.001**	1.007	(0.985, 1.030)	0.538
Gender			0.091			
Profession			**<0.001**			**<0.001**
Orthodontist	Reference			Reference		
Orthodontic resident/postgraduate student	1.249	(1.023, 1.526)	**0.029**	1.006	(0.746, 1.357)	0.968
Orthodontic nurse	3.210	(2.429, 4.241)	**<0.001**	1.920	(1.377, 2.678)	**<0.001**
Years of orthodontic practice			**0.001**			0.175
≤5 years	Reference			Reference		
5–10 years	0.836	(0.684, 1.023)	0.082	0.931	(0.725, 1.197)	0.578
10–20 years	0.705	(0.570, 0.870)	**0.001**	0.713	(0.514, 0.989)	**0.043**
>20 years	0.650	(0.495, 0.854)	**0.002**	0.619	(0.372, 1.029)	0.064
Academic degree			**<0.001**			**<0.001**
PhD	Reference			Reference		
Master	0.992	(0.730, 1.349)	0.961	0.967	(0.701, 1.333)	0.837
Bachelor	1.615	(1.203, 2.170)	**0.001**	1.485	(1.069, 2.065)	**0.019**
Junior college	1.801	(1.245, 2.605)	**0.002**	1.781	(1.142, 2.776)	**0.011**
Technical secondary school	1.517	(0.443, 5.193)	0.507	1.952	(0.588, 6.481)	0.274
Marital status			**0.007**			0.273
Single	Reference			Reference		
Married, without children	0.890	(0.660, 1.200)	0.444	0.916	(0.654, 1.283)	0.610
Married, with children	0.754	(0.634, 0.896)	**0.001**	0.824	(0.618, 1.098)	0.186
Others	0.470	(0.194, 1.142)	0.096	0.447	(0.175, 1.141)	0.092
Cohabitants			0.078			
Workplace information						
Location			0.623			
Setting						
Public	Reference			Reference		
Private	0.645	(0.541, 0.771)	**<0.001**	0.643	(0.517, 0.799)	**<0.001**
Orthodontic services during epidemic			0.052			
Online consultation			**<0.001**			**<0.001**
No	Reference			Reference		
Provided, only to existing orthodontic patients	1.031	(0.798, 1.332)	0.817	1.091	(0.827, 1.438)	0.538
Provided, to both existing and potential new orthodontic patients	1.658	(1.302, 2.112)	**<0.001**	1.586	(1.219, 2.063)	**0.001**
Current status of orthodontic services			0.847			
Personal experience						
Participation in anti-epidemic activities						
No	Reference			Reference		
Yes	1.428	(1.193, 1.710)	**<0.001**	1.270	(1.035, 1.559)	**0.022**
Current status of orthodontic practice			0.929			
Completion of COVID-19 related training program						
No	Reference			Reference		
Yes	1.479	(1.222, 1.790)	**<0.001**	1.176	(0.941, 1.470)	0.153
Experience of treating or caring for COVID-19 patients						
No	Reference			Reference		
Yes	2.046	(1.280, 3.272)	**0.003**	1.348	(0.823, 2.208)	0.235
Knowledge						
Self-perceived level of knowledge	1.724	(1.518, 1.957)	**<0.001**	1.705	(1.482, 1.962)	**<0.001**
Total knowledge score	1.026	(0.934, 1.126)	0.595			

¶*P-values in bold are statistically significant (<0.05).*

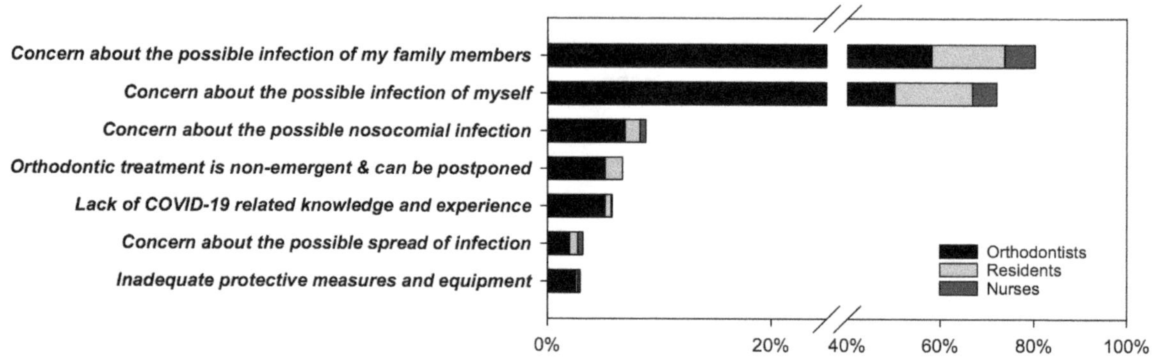

FIGURE 3 | The reasons for being unwilling to treat or care for patients confirmed or suspected with COVID-19 (semi-open question, #31) ($n = 958$).

are gradually resuming, orthodontic professionals in China are generally confident that they understand COVID-19-related risks and knowledge, and about two-thirds of them are willing to treat or care for COVID-19 patients. In addition, COVID-19-related training programs are essential for the improvement of knowledge, confidence, and preparedness of orthodontic professionals before work resumption. Sufficient and proper protection should also be provided to ensure safety and reduce the psychological burden on them.

AUTHOR CONTRIBUTIONS

FH: study conception. FH, DQ, and HH: study design. FH, DQ, JY, TZ, and HH: data collection. FH and DQ: data analysis and manuscript drafting. HH: data interpretation. JY, TZ, and HH: critical revision of the manuscript. All authors: approval of the final version.

ACKNOWLEDGMENTS

The authors would like to thank all the orthodontists, residents, and nurses who responded to this survey.

REFERENCES

1. Wu JT, Leung K, Leung GM. Nowcasting and forecasting the potential domestic and international spread of the 2019-nCoV outbreak originating in Wuhan, China: a modelling study. *Lancet.* (2020) 395:689–97. doi: 10.1016/S0140-6736(20)30260-9
2. Eurosurveillance Editorial Team. Note from the editors: World Health Organization declares novel coronavirus (2019-nCoV) sixth public health emergency of international concern. *Euro Surveill.* (2020) 25:200131e. doi: 10.2807/1560-7917.ES.2020.25.5.200131e
3. Mahase E. COVID-19: WHO declares pandemic because of "alarming levels" of spread, severity, and inaction. *BMJ.* (2020) 368:m1036. doi: 10.1136/bmj.m1036
4. World Health Organization. *Coronavirus Disease 2019 (COVID-19): Situation Report-130.* (2020). Available online at: https://www.who.int/docs/default-source/coronaviruse/situation-reports/20200529-covid-19-sitrep-130.pdf?sfvrsn=bf7e7f0c_4 (accessed May 29, 2020).
5. Wang D, Hu B, Hu C, Zhu F, Liu X, Zhang J, et al. Clinical characteristics of 138 hospitalized patients with 2019 novel coronavirus-infected pneumonia in Wuhan, China. *JAMA.* (2020) 323:1061–9. doi: 10.1001/jama.2020.1585
6. CCTV news. *China-WHO Joint Expert Team: 3387 Health Care Workers Infected With COVID-19, over 90% From Hubei.* (2020). Available online at: https://china.huanqiu.com/article/9CaKrnKpzdJ (accessed April 14, 2020).
7. CGTN. *Colleagues, Family of Deceased Medics in Wuhan Mourn Loss.* (2020). Available online at: https://news.cgtn.com/news/2020-02-25/Colleagues-family-of-deceased-medics-in-Wuhan-mourn-loss-On9XSFmFWM/index.html (accessed April 14, 2020).
8. World Health Organization. *Coronavirus Disease 2019 (COVID-19): Situation Report-82.* (2020). Available online at: https://www.who.int/docs/default-source/coronaviruse/situation-reports/20200411-sitrep-82-covid-19.pdf?sfvrsn$=$74a5d15_2 (accessed April 14, 2020).
9. Carter A. Can orthodontic care be safely delivered during the COVID-19 pandemic? Recommendations from a literature review. *Evid Based Dent.* (2020) 21:66–7. doi: 10.1038/s41432-020-0103-9
10. Centers for Disease Control and Prevention. *Guidance for Dental Settings: Interim Infection Prevention and Control Guidance for Dental Settings During the COVID-19 Response.* (2020). Available online at: https://www.cdc.gov/coronavirus/2019-ncov/hcp/dental-settings.html (accessed July 2, 2020).
11. Meng L, Hua F, Bian Z. Coronavirus disease 2019 (COVID-19): emerging and future challenges for dental and oral medicine. *J Dent Res.* (2020) 99:481–7. doi: 10.1177/0022034520914246
12. Pan A, Liu L, Wang C, Guo H, Hao X, Wang Q, et al. Association of public health interventions with the epidemiology of the COVID-19 outbreak in Wuhan, China. *JAMA.* (2020) 323:1–9. doi: 10.1001/jama.2020.6130
13. Meng L, Hua F, Bian Z. Response to the letter to the editor: how to deal with suspended oral treatment during the COVID-19 epidemic. *J Dent Res.* (2020) 99:988. doi: 10.1177/0022034520920166
14. Yang Y, Zhou Y, Liu X, Tan J. Health services provision of 48 public tertiary dental hospitals during the COVID-19 epidemic in China. *Clin Oral Investig.* (2020) 24:1861–4. doi: 10.1007/s00784-020-03267-8
15. Li Z, Ge J, Yang M, Feng J, Qiao M, Jiang R, et al. Vicarious traumatization in the general public, members, and non-members of medical teams aiding in COVID-19 control. *Brain Behav Immunity.* (2020). doi: 10.1016/j.bbi.2020.03.007. [Epub ahead of print].
16. World Health Organization. *Coronavirus Disease 2019 (COVID-19): Situation Report-76.* (2020). Available online at: https://www.who.int/docs/default-source/coronaviruse/situation-reports/20200405-sitrep-76-covid-19.pdf?sfvrsn$=$6ecf0977_4 (accessed April 14, 2020).
17. Shi Y, Wang J, Yang Y, Wang Z, Wang G, Hashimoto K, et al. Knowledge and attitudes of medical staff in Chinese psychiatric

hospitals regarding COVID-19. *Brain Behav Immun Health.* (2020) 4:100064. doi: 10.1016/j.bbih.2020.100064

18. Khader Y, Al Nsour M, Al-Batayneh OB, Saadeh R, Bashier H, Alfaqih M, et al. Dentists' awareness, perception, and attitude regarding COVID-19 and infection control: cross-sectional study among Jordanian dentists. *JMIR Public Health Surveill.* (2020) 6:e18798. doi: 10.2196/18798
19. Eysenbach G. Improving the quality of web surveys: the Checklist for Reporting Results of Internet E-Surveys (CHERRIES). *J Med Internet Res.* (2004) 6:e34. doi: 10.2196/jmir.6.3.e34
20. Daugherty EL, Perl TM, Rubinson L, Bilderback A, Rand CS. Survey study of the knowledge, attitudes, and expected behaviors of critical care clinicians regarding an influenza pandemic. *Infect Control Hosp Epidemiol.* (2009) 30:1143–9. doi: 10.1086/648085
21. Jao N. *WeChat Now Has Over 1 Billion Active Monthly Users Worldwide.* (2018). Available online at: https://technode.com/2018/03/05/wechat-1-billion-users/ (accessed April 14, 2020).
22. Liu N, Zhang F, Wei C, Jia Y, Shang Z, Sun L, et al. Prevalence and predictors of PTSS during COVID-19 outbreak in China hardest-hit areas: gender differences matter. *Psychiatry Res.* (2020) 287:112921. doi: 10.1016/j.psychres.2020.112921
23. Cotrin P, Peloso RM, Oliveira RC, de Oliveira RCG, Pini NIP, Valarelli FP, et al. Impact of coronavirus pandemic in appointments and anxiety/concerns of patients regarding orthodontic treatment. *Orthod Craniofac Res.* (2020). doi: 10.1111/ocr.12395. [Epub ahead of print].
24. Martina S, Amato A, Rongo R, Caggiano M, Amato M. The perception of COVID-19 among Italian dentists: an orthodontic point of view. *Int J Environ Res Public Health.* (2020) 17:4384. doi: 10.3390/ijerph17124384
25. Saltaji H, Sharaf KA. COVID-19 and orthodontics—a call for action. *Am J Orthodont Dentofacial Orthoped.* (2020) 158:12–13. doi: 10.1016/j.ajodo.2020.04.006
26. Cleveland JL, Foster M, Barker L, Brown GG, Lenfestey N, Lux L, et al. Advancing infection control in dental care settings: factors associated with dentists' implementation of guidelines from the Centers for Disease Control and Prevention. *J Am Dent Assoc.* (2012) 143:1127–38. doi: 10.14219/jada.archive.2012.0044
27. Kumar S, Tadakamadla J, Areeshi A, Tobaigy H. Knowledge and attitudes towards HIV/AIDS among dental students of Jazan University, Kingdom Saudi Arabia. *Saudi Dent J.* (2018) 30:47–52. doi: 10.1016/j.sdentj.2017.10.003
28. Ahmed MA, Jouhar R, Ahmed N, Adnan S, Aftab M, Zafar MS, et al. Fear and practice modifications among dentists to combat novel Coronavirus Disease (COVID-19) outbreak. *Int J Environ Res Public Health.* (2020) 17:2821. doi: 10.3390/ijerph17082821
29. Crossley ML. An investigation of dentists' knowledge, attitudes and practices towards HIV+ and patients with other blood-borne viruses in South Cheshire, UK. *Br Dent J.* (2004) 196:749–54. doi: 10.1038/sj.bdj.4811382
30. Sun N, Shi S, Jiao D, Song R, Ma L, Wang H, et al. A qualitative study on the psychological experience of caregivers of COVID-19 patients. *Am J Infect Control.* (2020) 48:592–8. doi: 10.1016/j.ajic.2020.03.018
31. Bansal P, Bingemann TA, Greenhawt M, Mosnaim G, Nanda A, Oppenheimer J, et al. Clinician wellness during the COVID-19 pandemic: extraordinary times and unusual challenges for the allergist/immunologist. *J Allergy Clin Immunol Pract.* (2020) 8:1781–90.e3. doi: 10.1016/j.jaip.2020.04.001
32. Ehrlich H, McKenney M, Elkbuli A. Protecting our healthcare workers during the COVID-19 pandemic. *Am J Emerg Med.* (2020) 38:1527–8. doi: 10.1016/j.ajem.2020.04.024
33. Ren YF, Rasubala L, Malmstrom H, Eliav E. Dental care and oral health under the clouds of COVID-19. *JDR Clin Transl Res.* (2020) 5:202–10. doi: 10.1177/2380084420924385
34. Peng X, Xu X, Li Y, Cheng L, Zhou X, Ren B. Transmission routes of 2019-nCoV and controls in dental practice. *Int J Oral Sci.* (2020) 12:9. doi: 10.1038/s41368-020-0075-9
35. Boyce JM, Pittet D. Guideline for Hand Hygiene in Health-Care Settings. Recommendations of the Healthcare Infection Control Practices Advisory Committee and the HICPAC/SHEA/APIC/IDSA Hand Hygiene Task Force. Society for Healthcare Epidemiology of America/Association for Professionals in Infection Control/Infectious Diseases Society of America. *Infect Control Hosp Epidemiol.* (2002) 23:S3–40. doi: 10.1086/503164
36. Kohn WG, Collins AS, Cleveland JL, Harte JA, Eklund KJ, Malvitz DM. Guidelines for infection control in dental health-care settings—2003. *MMWR Recomm Rep.* (2003) 52:1–61. doi: 10.14219/jada.archive.2004.0019
37. Kelley K, Clark B, Brown V, Sitzia J. Good practice in the conduct and reporting of survey research. *Int J Qual Health Care.* (2003) 15:261–6. doi: 10.1093/intqhc/mzg031

8

ACE2 and Furin Expressions in Oral Epithelial Cells Possibly Facilitate COVID-19 Infection via Respiratory and Fecal–Oral Routes

Mei Zhong[1†], Bingpeng Lin[1†], Janak L. Pathak[1,2†], Hongbin Gao[3], Andrew J. Young[4], Xinhong Wang[1], Chang Liu[5], Kaibin Wu[1], Mingxiao Liu[1], Jian-ming Chen[1], Jiangyong Huang[1], Learn-Han Lee[6], Cui-ling Qi[7], Linhu Ge[1,2] and Lijing Wang[1,7*]*

[1] Guangzhou Key Laboratory of Basic and Applied Research of Oral Regenerative Medicine, Affiliated Stomatology Hospital of Guangzhou Medical University, Guangzhou, China, [2] Institute of Oral Disease, Guangzhou Medical University, Guangzhou, China, [3] Key Laboratory of Guangdong Laboratory Animals, Guangdong Laboratory Animals Monitoring Institute, Guangzhou, China, [4] Columbus Inpatient Care, Grove City, OH, United States, [5] Stomatology School of Ji'nan University, Guangzhou, China, [6] Novel Bacteria and Drug Discovery Research Group (NBDD), Microbiome and Bioresource Research Strength (MBRS), Jeffrey Cheah School of Medicine and Health Sciences, Monash University Malaysia, Bandar Sunway, Malaysia, [7] School of Life Science and Biopharmaceutics, Vascular Biology Research Institute, Guangdong Pharmaceutical University, Guangzhou, China

***Correspondence:**
Lijing Wang
2018991265@gzhmu.edu.cn
Linhu Ge
gelinhu@yeah.net

†These authors have contributed equally to this work and share first authorship

Background: Coronavirus disease 2019 (COVID-19) is caused by severe acute respiratory syndrome coronavirus 2 (SARS-CoV-2) that mainly transfers from human to human via respiratory and gastrointestinal routes. The S-glycoprotein in the virus is the key factor for the entry of SARS-CoV-2 into the cell, which contains two functional domains: S1 is an angiotensin-converting enzyme 2 (ACE2) receptor binding domain, and S2 is necessary for fusion of the coronavirus and cell membranes. Moreover, it has been reported that ACE2 is likely to be the receptor for SARS-CoV-2. In addition, mRNA level expression of Furin enzyme and ACE2 receptor had been reported in airway epithelia, cardiac tissue, and enteric canals. However, the expression patterns of ACE2 and Furin in different cell types of oral tissues are still unclear.

Methods: In order to investigate the potential infective channel of the new coronavirus via the oropharyngeal cavity, we analyze the expression of ACE2 and Furin in human oral mucosa using the public single-cell sequence datasets. Furthermore, immunohistochemistry was performed in mucosal tissue from different oral anatomical sites to confirm the expression of ACE2 and Furin at the protein level.

Results: The bioinformatics results indicated the differential expression of ACE2 and Furin on epithelial cells from different oral anatomical sites. Immunohistochemistry results revealed that both the ACE2-positive and Furin-positive cells in the target tissues were mainly positioned in the epithelial layers, partly expressed in fibroblasts, further confirming the bioinformatics results.

Conclusions: Based on these findings, we speculated that SARS-CoV-2 could invade oral mucosal cells through two possible routes: binding to the ACE2 receptor and fusion with cell membrane activated by Furin protease. Our results indicated that oral mucosa tissues are susceptible to SARS-CoV-2 that could facilitate COVID-19 infection via respiratory and fecal–oral routes.

Keywords: COVID-19, SARS-CoV-2, ACE2 (angiotensin converting enzyme-2), Furin, oral mucosa, single cell RNA seq

INTRODUCTION

Severe acute respiratory syndrome coronavirus 2 (SARS-CoV-2) causes coronavirus disease 2019 (COVID-19) pandemic and mainly triggers acute respiratory distress syndrome (ARDS) and viral sepsis that bring challenges to the patient's treatment (1, 2). The pandemic infection of COVID-19 confirmed nearly 40,000,000 human cases, including >1,100,000 deaths, and the infection rate is continuously increasing worldwide. The present outbreak of COVID-19 has been labeled as a global pandemic by WHO and has posed critical challenges for public health, research, and medical communities (3). Airborne transmission has been recently reported as a dominant route for COVID-19 infection (4). Similarly, many research groups had reported gastrointestinal manifestation of COVID-19 purposing the fecal–oral route as an alternative route of SARS-CoV-2 transmission (5–8). These findings suggest that the epithelial cells of the oropharyngeal cavity provide the binding site to enter and propagate the SARS-CoV-2. However, the expression of possible receptors of the SARS-CoV-2 in different cell types of the oral cavity has not been investigated yet.

Like patients with SARS and Middle East respiratory syndrome (MERS), the clinical manifestations of COVID-19 at illness onset are fever, dry cough, and myalgia. The patients suffer from dyspnea, shortness of breath, respiratory failure, and even death in later stages (2, 9, 10). Besides, COVID-19 patients show oral manifestations, including oral pain, gingivitis, and ulcers, especially for severe cases (11). Dry mouth and amblygeustia are experienced by a relatively high proportion of COVID-19 patients (12). Also, viral enanthema in the oral mucosa is considered as a possible diagnostic challenge in the COVID-19 pandemic (13). As the oropharyngeal cavity is a route of COVID-19 transmission, it might have adverse impacts on patients' oral health. Since COVID-19 seems to stay longer in our society, the insights in the relationship between oral health and COVID-19 could provide crucial information for decision-making in managing this notorious infectious disease.

SARS-CoV-2 entry into the cell is induced by the binding of viral spike protein to host cellular angiotensin-converting enzyme 2 (ACE2) receptors (14, 15). Previous findings indicated that ACE2 plays an essential role in SARS-CoV-2 entry in the host cells. Thus, ACE2-expressing cells may act as target cells and are susceptible to COVID-19 infection (2, 14–18). Hamming et al. (19) had reported the ACE2 receptor expression in various human tissues, including epithelium of the lung and small intestines. As a co-expressed membrane endopeptidase of the ACE2 receptor, Furin has the potential to cleave the viral envelop glycoprotein, thereby enhancing the viral fusion with host cell membranes (20). Genomic characterization of SARS-CoV-2 has revealed that the Furin enzyme could activate the specific site of its spike protein (21). Meanwhile, Li et al. (22) showed that a putative Furin cleavage site in the spike protein of SARS-CoV-2 facilitates the virus–cell fusion. The Furin cleavage site is absent in SARS-CoV. The presence of the Furin cleavage site in SARS-CoV-2 showed distinct clinical symptoms (23, 24). Furthermore, online single-cell sequence datasets analysis unveiled that Furin was expressed in coronavirus's potential target organs, such as lung, heart, nose, rectum, colon, intestine, and ileum (22). Hence, the expression and distribution of ACE2 and Furin in the epithelium of the oral cavity could be critical for the coronavirus invasion to the host cells. However, information on the expression and distribution of ACE2 and Furin in the human oral cavity is limited.

Single-cell RNA sequencing (scRNA-Seq) technique provides an avenue to understand gene regulation networks and the complexity of cell-to-cell heterogeneity at the single-cell level. scRNA-Seq has diverse applications on bioinformatics, stem cell differentiation, organ development, whole-tissue subtyping, and tumor biology (25–27). scRNA-Seq captures cellular differences underlying tumor biology at a higher resolution than regular bulk RNA-Seq and has revolutionized studies of cancer mechanisms and personalized medicine (28). For a better understanding of the potential COVID-19 infection risk in the oral cavity, we explored whether ACE2 and Furin are expressed and the composition and proportion of their expressing cell in different oral tissues based on the public scRNA-seq profiles from Gene Expression Omnibus (GEO) public databases. Furthermore, we performed immunohistochemistry analysis for ACE2 and Furin in human oral epithelium tissue sections. Oral epithelium showed the expression of ACE2 and Furin in both mRNA and protein levels, indicating the oral cavity as a platform for COVID-19 invasion via the respiratory route and possibly fecal–oral route.

MATERIALS AND METHODS

Public Single-Cell RNA Sequencing Dataset Acquisition

scRNA-Seq datasets (GSE103322), including the gene expression and cell type annotation from human oral squamous cell carcinoma (OSCC) tissue, were downloaded from the GEO database (https://www.ncbi.nlm.nih.gov/geo/). Patient characteristics and demographics for the dataset used are listed in **Supplementary Table 1**.

Single-Cell Sequencing Analysis

scRNA-Seq datasets (GSE103322) were downloaded from the GEO database. Datasets of five patients, which have the closest histological features with normal tissue, were selected for further analysis. The scRNA-Seq datasets of GSE103322_HN_UMI_table.txt were used to subsequently analyze based on R package Seurat (Version 3.6.2). For quality control, we removed cells with <50 genes, as well as the cells with mitochondrial content higher than 5%. Besides, the genes detected in <3 cells were filtered out in the function Create Seurat Object. Subsequently, the data were log-normalized using the function Normalize Data with the default parameters. The Find Variable Genes function was used to determine the highly expressed variable genes, followed by principal component analysis (PCA) dimensionality reduction by RunPCA function. PCA components, which $P < 0.05$, were selected to analyze further using two-dimensional t-distributed stochastic neighbor embedding (tSNE). The setting of k.param was 20 in the function Find Neighbors, and the setting of the resolution was 0.5 in the function Find Clusters. Finally, the cell types were assigned based on their canonical markers. The functions of DotPlot and VlnPlot displayed the gene expression of different cell types. The significant level was set as 0.05.

Human Oral Tissue Specimens

Twelve normal tissues of the oral mucosa (three buccal and gingival tissues, two lip, tongue, and palatal tissues, respectively) were taken from 12 different patients with clinically diagnosed fibrous epithelial polyp or benign tumor (19, 29), whose average age was 53 years. The healthy oral mucosa tissue was collected from a 2-cm distance of the tumor edge. Patient exclusion criteria of this study were patients with a history of smoking, periodontitis, uncompensated diabetes mellitus, immunocompromised status, under radiotherapy and/or chemotherapy, and systemic diseases. Vulnerable populations such as pregnant women, minors (i.e., under 18 years old), and seniors (i.e., over 60 years old) were also excluded. Written informed consent was obtained for each participant, and the study was in accordance with the Declaration of Helsinki and the guidelines and approved by the Clinical Ethics Committee of Affiliated Stomatology Hospital of Guangzhou Medical University (Approval no. KY2020002). Tissue morphology was evaluated in hematoxylin and eosin-stained sections by a qualified pathologist.

Immunohistochemical Staining

The selected tissues were fixed in 10% neutral formalin solution and embedded in paraffin. The paraffin sections (4 μm in thickness) were deparaffinized in xylene, rehydrated in a graded series of alcohol. Human lung bronchi tissue sections were used as positive control of ACE2 and Furin expression. The tissue sections were then incubated in citrate buffer (pH 6.0) for 5 min at 120°C, and the endogenous peroxidase was blocked by 0.3% H_2O_2 for 10 min. Subsequently, the tissue sections were dried and incubated with Rabbit Anti-ACE2 antibody (cat. no. ab15348, Abcam, Cambridge, CB, UK) antibody, Anti-Furin antibody (cat. no. bs-13228R) overnight at 4°C. The negative control sections were incubated with 1% rabbit serum containing phosphate buffered saline (PBS) instead of the primary antibody. The next day, the tissue sections were incubated with the horseradish peroxidase (HRP) (Goat Anti-Rabbit IgG H&L)-conjugated secondary antibody for 1 h at room temperature. Peroxidase activity was developed by using 3,3′-diaminobenzidine (DAB) for 8 min and counterstained with hematoxylin. A qualified pathologist analyzed the staining. The ACE2 and Furin staining intensities were semiquantitatively graded according to the previously described method (30).

RESULTS

Identification of Cell Types in the Oral Mucosal Tissues

We detected the ACE2-expressing cell types in oral tissue by analyzing the scRNA-Seq data. A total of 1,843 individual cells from the oral mucosa of five patients were analyzed. Using the unsupervised graph-based clustering, we found that at least 13 distinct cell clusters existed in the oral tissues (**Figure 1A**), including epithelial cells (clusters 1, 4, 5), fibroblasts (clusters 0, 2, 7), T-cells (clusters 8, 9), and B cells (cluster 12). The heatmap of the main corresponding cell marker gene expression profiles across the cell types can be found in **Figure 1B**. The marker gene of epithelial cells included KRT6B, GJB2, SFN, and KRT14; fibroblasts included THY1, COL1A1, DCN, and ACTA2; B cells included SLAMF7, CD19, CD20, and CD79A; T cells included CD2, CD3, and CD45.

Identification of Angiotensin-Converting Enzyme 2-Expressing Cells in the Oral Mucosa

We explored the online datasets to find out the expression level of ACE2 in the oral mucosa. A single-cell atlas from analysis of scRNA-Seq data of the human oral mucosa identified 13 cell subclusters in the oral mucosal cells, including epithelial cells, fibroblasts, T cells, and B cells (**Figure 1**). The clusters 1, 4, 5, and 6 are epithelial cell clusters. The red dots in the scatter plot (**Figures 2C,D**) showed the expression profiles of ACE2 and Furin in the 13 distinct cell clusters identified from **Figure 1A**. As expected, data from GEO indicated that ACE2 receptor expression level was relatively higher in epithelial cells (clusters 1, 4, 5) (**Figures 2A,C**), while very little cellular expression of ACE2 was found in fibroblasts (cluster 2). Then, we calculated the percentage of ACE2-expressing cells in the dataset (**Figure 2E**). We find that, in oral tissue, the percentage of ACE2-positive cells was 2.2%. Among them, 92% were epithelial cells. The negative control of oral tissue immunohistochemistry (IHC) is listed is **Supplementary Figure 1**.

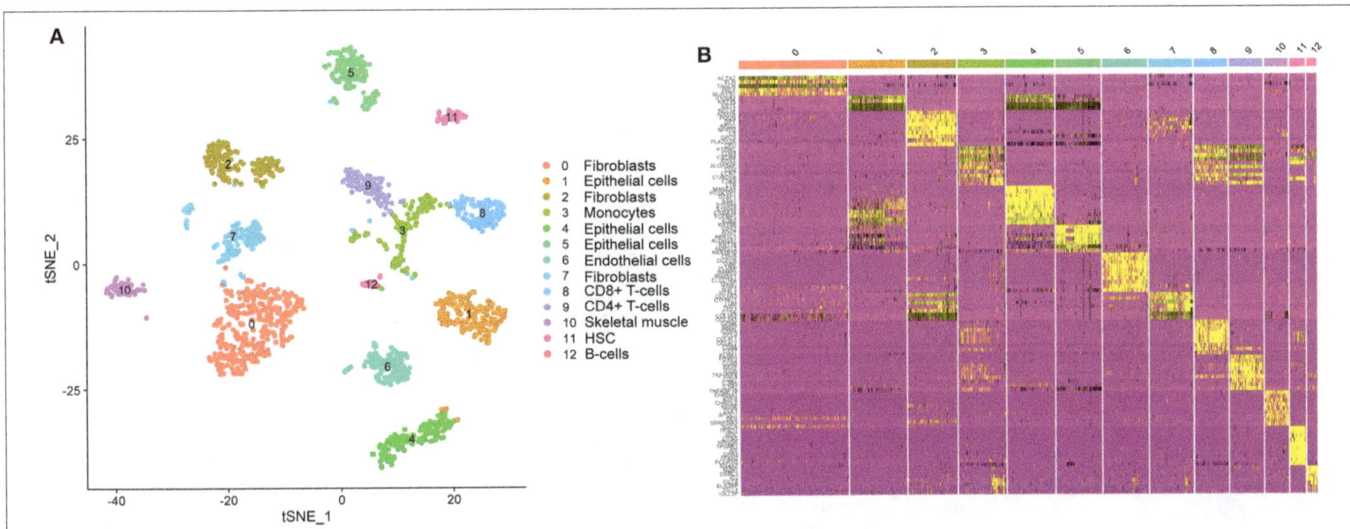

FIGURE 1 | Single-cell atlas of the human oral mucosa. **(A,B)** Analysis of single-cell sequencing data identified 13 cell subclusters in the oral mucosal cells. Thirteen distinct cell clusters existed in the oral tissues **(A)**, including epithelial cells, fibroblasts, T cells, and B cells. The heatmap of the main corresponding cell marker gene expression profiles across the cell types is plotted in **(B)**. The marker gene of epithelial cells included KRT6B, GJB2, SFN, and KRT14.

Identification of Furin-Expressing Cells in the Oral Mucosa

To determine the cell types of expressing Furin, we analyzed the Furin mRNA expression using tSNE method. Violin and scatter plot showed that Furin was highly expressed in epithelial cells, followed by fibroblasts, T cells, and endothelial cells of the oral mucosal tissues, but hardly expressed in B cells (**Figures 2B,D**). Meanwhile, the proportion of Furin expressing cells was ~10%. Among them, epithelial cells make up more than 55% (**Figure 2F**).

Angiotensin-Converting Enzyme 2 Protein Is Highly Expressed in the Epithelial Layer of the Buccal Mucosa, Lip, Palate, Tongue, and Gingiva

IHC analysis further determined the protein level expression of ACE2 in the oral mucosa. ACE2 and Furin were highly expressed in human lung bronchi tissue sections, indicating the specificity of the primary antibodies used in this study. The first remarkable finding was that ACE2 was expressed in epithelial cells in all the tissues studied (**Figure 3**). Results indicated that the expression level of ACE2 protein was significantly higher in the lip, tongue, and buccal mucosa, especially the epithelial cells in the basal layer, although the mRNA expression level is not as high (**Figure 2**). The ACE2-positive cells in the gingival and palatal tissues were limited. The corresponding gingiva and palate epithelial cells showed weak positive ACE2 staining. Systematic ACE2 expression levels in different oral sites are shown in **Figure 5**. Also, we found that ACE2 was expressed in fibroblasts and endothelial cells. These results indicate oral epithelial cells as the potential targets of SARS-CoV-2.

Furin Protein Was Highly Expressed in the Normal Oral Mucosa

Furin mRNA expression has been described mainly in oral epithelial cells through scRNA-Seq technique. To determine whether this differential expression of Furin was maintained at the protein level, oral tissues from different sites were screened. As shown in **Figure 4**, moderate to mild immunostaining in the cytoplasm of epithelial cells was observed in five normal oral tissues. Surprisingly, except for the positive cells in the basal layer of the oral epithelium, the spinous layer in all examined tissues also turned out with large numbers of Furin-positive cells. In addition, the percentage of Furin-positive cells in the lip, tongue, and gingiva was higher than that of buccal and palatal mucosa. Systematic Furin expression levels in different oral sites are shown in **Figure 5**.

DISCUSSION

Highly infectious nature and pandemic spreading of COVID-19 overwhelmed the public health services in the world and have become a global public health problem (31). Studies had reported both the respiratory and gastrointestinal tract manifestations of COVID-19 (4, 32). As mentioned before, the ACE2 receptor in the host cell membrane and Furin cleavage site of SARS-CoV-2 are the key factors that allowed the virus to invade the host cells (22, 23). In this study, we found the expression of ACE2 and Furin in oral epithelial cells in both mRNA and protein levels. Since the oral cavity is connected to both the respiratory and gastrointestinal tract, the ACE2 and Furin in oral mucosal cells could be the possible facilitators of COVID-19 infection *via* respiratory and fecal–oral routes.

Many studies have shown that the ACE2 receptor was highly expressed in respiratory epithelium, kidney, testis, digestive

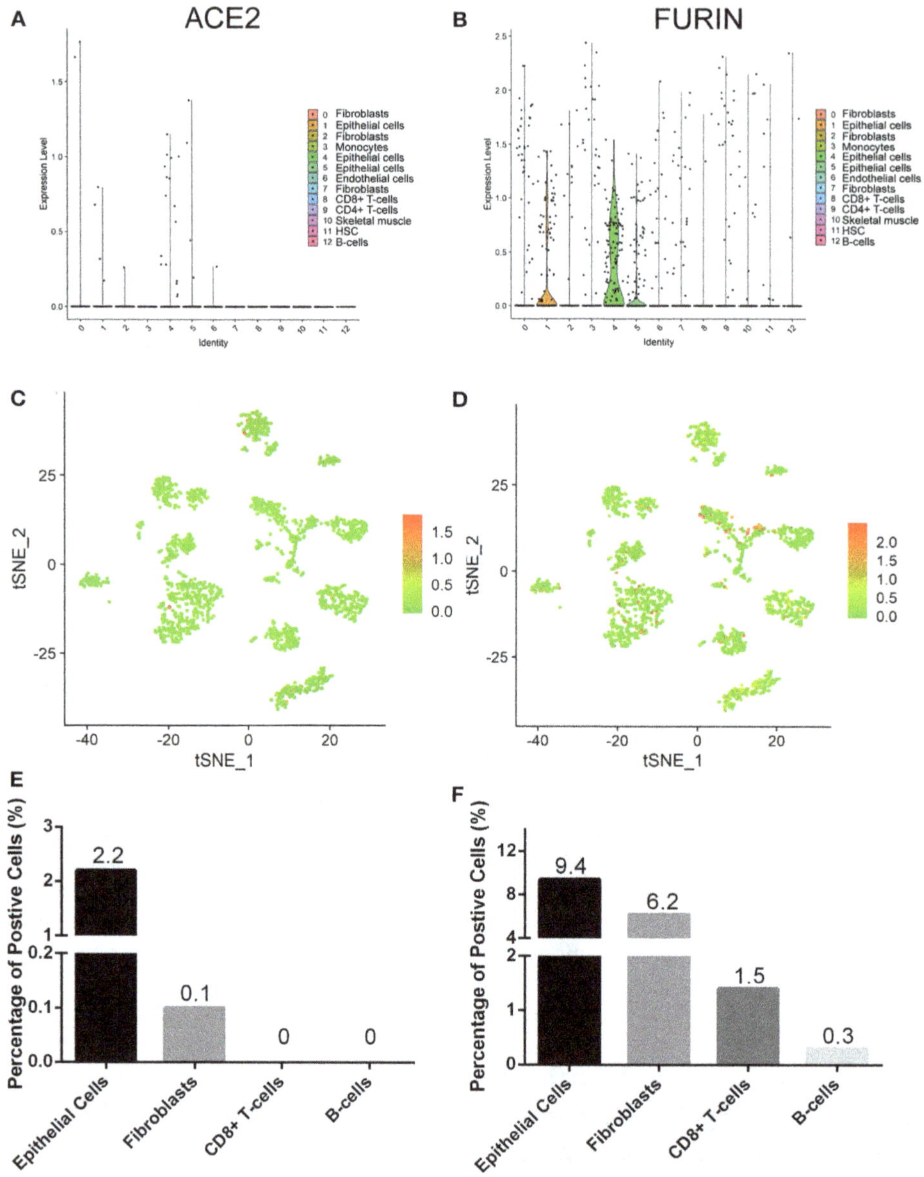

FIGURE 2 | The expression profiles of angiotensin-converting enzyme 2 (ACE2) **(A,C,E)** and Furin **(B,D,F)** in the oral mucosal cells. Violin and scatter plot showed the expression profile of the ACE2 receptor **(A,C)** and Furin **(B,D)** in oral mucosal cells. ACE2 and Furin were mainly expressed in epithelial cells. **(E,F)** The percentage of ACE2- and Furin-positive cells in the oral mucosa.

system, and cardiovascular system (6, 18, 33). Pieces of literature using bulk RNA sequencing data found that ACE2 is expressed in oral tissues, which could not accurately reflect the expression of ACE2 in the single-cell level (29, 34). Chen et al. benefited from the single-cell sequencing data to further prove the expression of ACE2 receptor in the tongue, buccal mucosa, and gingiva (14, 19, 34). However, these studies were based on public databases and did not further analyze the protein level expression. In the current study, we firstly analyzed the ACE2 expression in different cell types present in various oral anatomical sites using the scRNA-Seq public data from five human subjects. We further confirmed the protein level expression of ACE2 in histological tissue sections from different anatomical sites of 12 human subjects by IHC. Results indicated that ACE2 is mainly expressed in epithelial cells in all included oral tissues, especially in the buccal mucosa, lip, and tongue. Our results demonstrated that compared with other oral anatomical sites, buccal mucosa, lip, and tongue showed a higher expression of ACE2, suggesting that these sites are more susceptible to SARS-CoV-2-invasion.

Team of virologists from Cornell University reported another structural analysis of the coronavirus S protein, suggesting that the Furin cutting site allows the SARS-CoV-2 virus to enter cells in a very different way than SARS, and this may regulate the virus stability and infection (35). Other

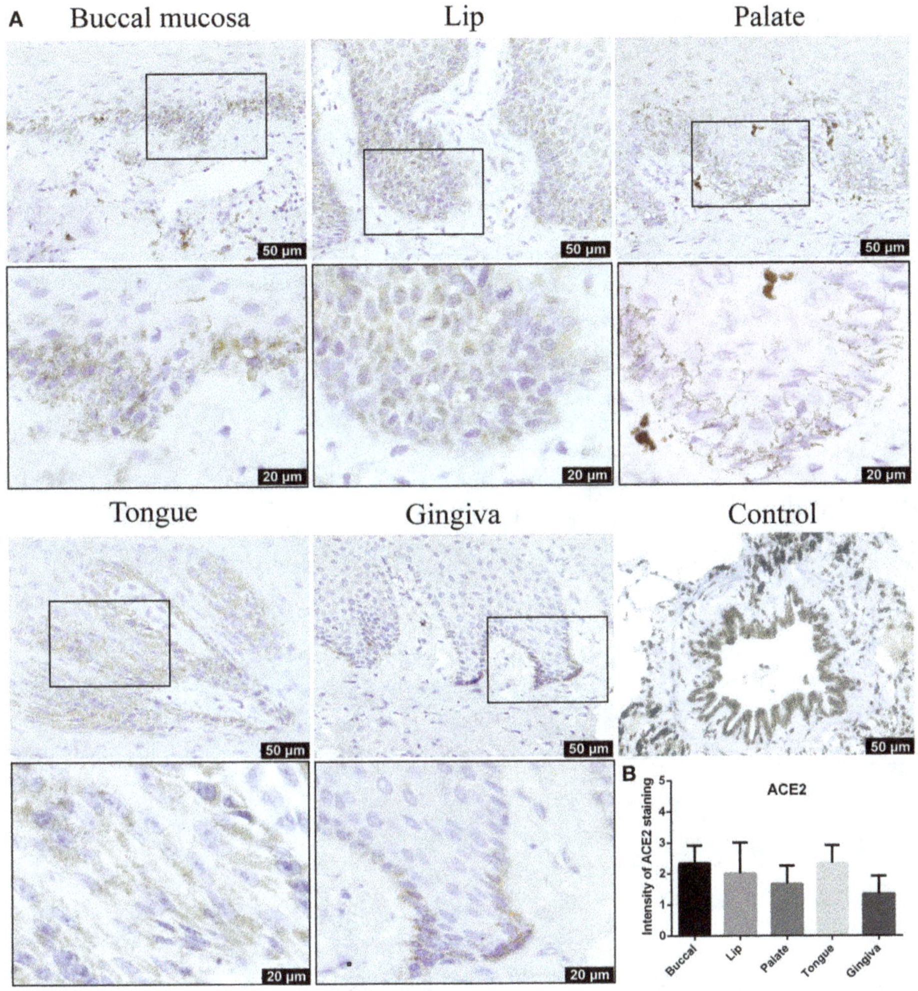

FIGURE 3 | (A) Representative immunohistochemistry (IHC) images of oral tissue showing the expression of angiotensin-converting enzyme 2 (ACE2) protein in buccal, lip, palate, tongue, and gingival mucosa and lung bronchi (positive control). **(B)** Semiquantitative analysis of IHC intensity of ACE2 staining for various oral tissues. Data are presented as mean ± standard deviation (SD).

research teams have also identified this activation site, suggesting that it may enable the virus to spread effectively between humans (21). It has been demonstrated that SARS-CoV-2 could fuse with the cell membrane and then gain entry into the target cells (36, 37). Researchers have found Furin proteases in many tissues, including the lungs, liver, and small intestine (23). However, limited reports were seen regarding the expression of Furin in the oral cavity, and whether the novel coronavirus could spread by the oral cavity is not fully understood. Thus, we reported both gene and protein level expression patterns of Furin enzyme in epithelial cells of five different oral anatomical sites. As expected, Furin was found abundantly enriched in oral mucosa cells, particularly in epithelial cells, and the proportion of Furin-positive cells was higher than that of ACE2-positive cells. Our results would be valuable for the prevention and management of the COVID-19.

Previous reports had demonstrated that Furin protein was expressed in metastasizing OSCCs (38). Besides, Furin was expressed in normal epithelium and upregulated in SCCs from three different organs (30). But the reports of Furin protein expression in the healthy oral cavity are limited. For further validating the results in the gene level, Furin IHC was therefore performed on conventional sections for the first time to assess its expression in oral mucosa obtained from five different sites. It is noteworthy that moderate positive expression of Furin protein was observed in tongue, gingiva, and lip, while weakly positive in the buccal and palatal tissues. Shreds of data from the literature indicate that SARS-CoV-2 enters host cells by binding to ACE2, and the viral S protein is cleaved by transmembrane protease serine 2 (TMPRSS2) (39). Furin cleaves S1/S2 site during the process of S protein transport and virus assembly (40). As a result, we speculated that SARS-CoV-2 could attach to the cell membrane of the oral mucosal cells, then enter into the host

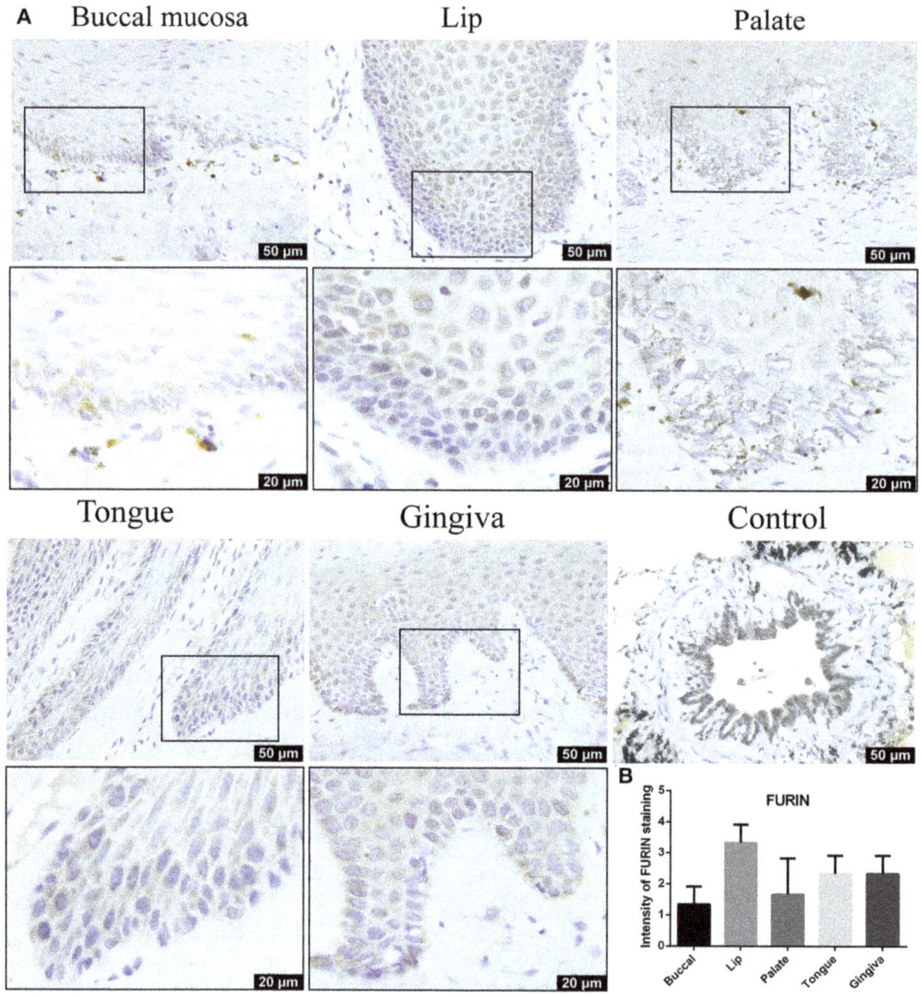

FIGURE 4 | (A) Representative immunohistochemistry (IHC) images of oral tissue showing the expression of Furin protein in buccal, lip, palate, tongue, and gingival mucosa and lung bronchi (positive control). **(B)** Semiquantitative analysis of IHC intensity of Furin staining for various oral tissues. Data are presented as mean ± SD.

cells via the ACE2 and Furin activity. Therefore, Furin could be a possible target to reduce COVID-19 infection.

For entry of SARS-CoV-2 to host cell, viral surface glycoprotein spike (S) must be cleaved at two different sites (S1/S2 and S2) by host cell proteases (41). The S can be cleaved by the Furin at the S1/S2 site and TMPRSS2 at the S2′ site (42). The spread of SARS-CoV-2 also depends on TMPRSS2 activity (43). The Furin-mediated precleavage at the S1/S2 site in infected cells might promote subsequent TMPRSS2-dependent entry into target cells. TMPRSS2 is essential for SARS-CoV-2 activation and multiplication in airway epithelial cells. A combination of TMPRSS2 inhibitor and Furin inhibitor more potently inhibits SARS-CoV-2 replication in human airway epithelial cells compared to any single inhibitor (42). This indicates the important role of Furin and TMPRSS2 proteases in facilitating the entry of SARS-CoV-2 in host cells. The expression of TMPRSS2 in oral tissues should be further investigated.

Strikingly, the scRNA-Seq data analysis and IHC results indicated that ACE2 and Furin were both abundantly expressed in oral mucosa, especially on oral epithelial cells. In other words, two key proteins of SARS-CoV-2 entering the target cell in different routes are both present in oral mucosa, which implied the potential attack and spread of SARS-CoV-2 in the oral tissues. Moreover, the live SARS-CoV-2 was consistently detected in the self-collected saliva of 91.7% (11/12) COVID-19 patients (44). It could be transmitted via saliva, directly or indirectly, even among asymptomatic infected patients. The existence of SARS-CoV-2 in nasal and throats swab samples suggests the strong spreadability of COVID-19 via the oral cavity (45). Thus, it is suggested that all healthcare workers should focus on taking effective measures to prevent the virus from spreading via the oral cavity, and potential impairment of oral tissues should be evaluated after infection with SARS-CoV-2, giving more evidence to the prevention and treatment of COVID-19. Strict precautions

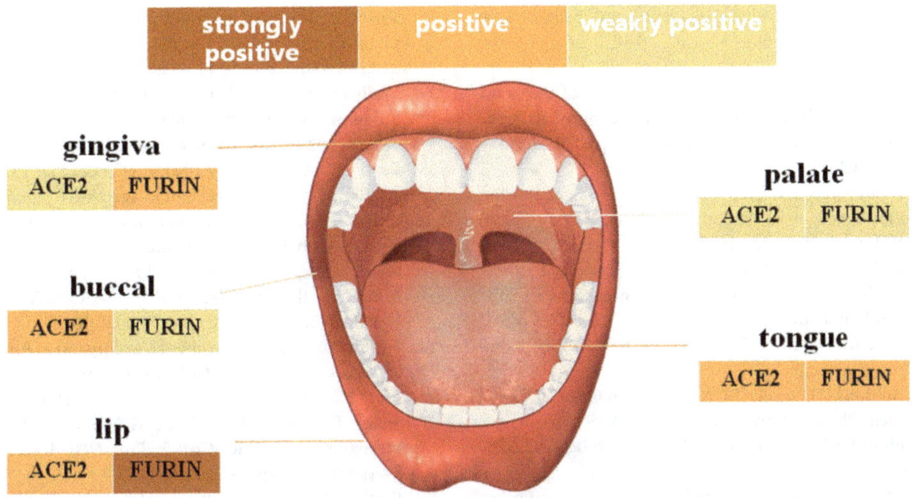

FIGURE 5 | The schematic diagram of angiotensin-converting enzyme 2 (ACE2) and Furin protein expression in different oral anatomical sites.

should be taken to protect from direct exposure of oral tissues to SARS-CoV-2 contamination.

CONCLUSIONS

Our results systematically investigated the expression profiles of Furin enzyme and ACE2 receptor in the oral cavity at the gene and protein levels for the first time. Furthermore, significant expression of Furin and ACE2 was discovered in oral epithelial cells, implying the possibility of COVID-19 transmission through the oral mucosa, which provides new insight into the future prevention strategy and clinical care. More evidence is still needed to reinforce the current findings.

AUTHOR CONTRIBUTIONS

BL, MZ, JP, HG, LW, and LG contributed to the study design. BL, MZ, and HG contributed to the sample collection. XW, CL, KW, and ML contributed to the IHC and analysis. L-HL, C-lQ, JH, and J-mC contributed to the data collection, analysis, and interpretation. MZ, L-HL, and JP contributed to the manuscript preparation. All authors approved the final version of the manuscript.

REFERENCES

1. Huang C, Wang Y, Li X, Ren L, Zhao J, Hu Y, et al. Clinical features of patients infected with 2019 novel coronavirus in Wuhan, China. *Lancet.* (2020) 395:497–506. doi: 10.1016/S0140-6736(20)30183-5
2. Zhou P, Yang XL, Wang XG, Hu B, Zhang L, Zhang W, et al. A pneumonia outbreak associated with a new coronavirus of probable bat origin. *Nature.* (2020) 579:270–3. doi: 10.1038/s41586-020-2012-7
3. Sohrabi C, Alsafi Z, O'Neill N, Khan M, Kerwan A, Al-Jabir A, et al. World Health Organization declares global emergency: a review of the 2019 novel coronavirus (COVID-19). *Int J Surg.* (2020) 76:71–6. doi: 10.1016/j.ijsu.2020.02.034
4. Zhang R, Li Y, Zhang AL, Wang Y, Molina MJ. Identifying airborne transmission as the dominant route for the spread of COVID-19. *Proc Natl Acad Sci USA.* (2020) 117:14857–63. doi: 10.1073/pnas.2009637117
5. Hindson J. COVID-19: faecal-oral transmission? *Nat Rev Gastroenterol Hepatol.* (2020) 17:259. doi: 10.1038/s41575-020-0295-7
6. Zhang H, Kang Z, Gong H, Xu D, Wang J, Li Z, et al. The digestive system is a potential route of 2019-nCov infection: a bioinformatics analysis based on single-cell transcriptomes. *bioRxiv.* (2020) 2020.01.30.927806. doi: 10.1101/2020.01.30.927806
7. Lamers MM, Beumer J, van der Vaart J, Knoops K, Puschhof J, Breugem TI, et al. SARS-CoV-2 productively infects human gut enterocytes. *Science.* (2020) 369:50–4. doi: 10.1126/science.abc1669
8. Zang R, Gomez Castro MF, McCune BT, Zeng Q, Rothlauf PW, Sonnek NM, et al. TMPRSS2 and TMPRSS4 promote SARS-CoV-2 infection of human small intestinal enterocytes. *Sci Immunol.* (2020) 5:eabc3582. doi: 10.1126/sciimmunol.abc3582
9. Wang D, Hu B, Hu C, Zhu F, Liu X, Zhang J, et al. Clinical characteristics of 138 hospitalized patients with 2019 novel coronavirus–infected pneumonia in Wuhan, China. *JAMA.* (2020) 323:1061–9. doi: 10.1001/jama.2020.1585
10. Yang Y, Lu Q, Liu M, Wang Y, Zhang A, Jalali N, et al. Epidemiological and clinical features of the 2019 novel coronavirus outbreak in China. *medRxiv.* (2020) 2020.02.10.20021675. doi: 10.1101/2020.02.10.20021675
11. Vieira AR. Oral manifestations in coronavirus disease 2019 (COVID-19). *Oral Dis.* (2020) 10.1111/odi.13463. doi: 10.1111/odi.13463
12. Ren YF, Rasubala L, Malmstrom H, Eliav E. Dental care and oral health under the clouds of COVID-19. *JDR Clin Transl Res.* (2020) 5:202–10. doi: 10.1177/2380084420924385
13. Rocha BA, Souto GR, Grossmann SMC, de Aguiar MCF, de Andrade BAB, Romanach MJ, et al. Viral enanthema in oral mucosa: a possible diagnostic challenge in the COVID-19 pandemic. *Oral Dis.* (2020) 10.1111/odi.13473. doi: 10.1111/odi.13473
14. Zhang HB, Penninger JM, Li YM, Zhong NS, Slutsky AS. Angiotensin-converting enzyme 2 (ACE2) as a SARS-CoV-2 receptor: molecular mechanisms and potential therapeutic target. *Intens Care Med.* (2020) 46:586–90. doi: 10.1007/s00134-020-05985-9

15. Kai H, Kai M. Interactions of coronaviruses with ACE2, angiotensin II, and RAS inhibitors-lessons from available evidence and insights into COVID-19. *Hypertens Res.* (2020) 43:648–54. doi: 10.1038/s41440-020-0455-8
16. Xu X, Chen P, Wang J, Feng J, Zhou H, Li X, et al. Evolution of the novel coronavirus from the ongoing Wuhan outbreak and modeling of its spike protein for risk of human transmission. *Sci China Life Sci.* (2020) 63:457–60. doi: 10.1007/s11427-020-1637-5
17. Zhao Y, Zhao Z, Wang Y, Zhou Y, Ma Y, Zuo W. Single-cell RNA expression profiling of ACE2, the putative receptor of Wuhan 2019-nCov. *bioRxiv.* (2020) 2020.01.26.919985. doi: 10.1101/2020.01.26.919985
18. Zou X, Chen K, Zou J, Han P, Hao J, Han Z. Single-cell RNA-seq data analysis on the receptor ACE2 expression reveals the potential risk of different human organs vulnerable to 2019-nCoV infection. *Front Med.* (2020) 14:185–92. doi: 10.1007/s11684-020-0754-0
19. Hamming I, Timens W, Bulthuis MLC, Lely AT, Navis GJ, van Goor H. Tissue distribution of ACE2 protein, the functional receptor for SARS coronavirus. a first step in understanding SARS pathogenesis. *J Pathol.* (2004) 203:631–7. doi: 10.1002/path.1570
20. Izaguirre G. The proteolytic regulation of virus cell entry by furin and other proprotein convertases. *Viruses.* (2019) 11:837. doi: 10.3390/v11090837
21. Mallapaty S. Why does the coronavirus spread so easily between people? *Nature.* (2020) 579:183. doi: 10.1038/d41586-020-00660-x
22. Li H, Wu C, Yang Y, Liu Y, Zhang P, Wang Y, et al. Furin, a potential therapeutic target for COVID-19. *ChinaXiv.* (2020) 23:101642. doi: 10.1016/j.isci.2020.101642
23. Ma Y, Hung Y, Wang T, Xiang AP, Huang W. ACE2 shedding and furin abundance in target organs may influence the efficiency of SARS-CoV-2 entry. *ChinaXiv.* (2020) 202002.00082. doi: 10.12074/202002.00082
24. Xin L, GuangYou D, Wei Z, Jinsong S, JiaYuan C, Gao S, et al. A furin cleavage site was discovered in the S protein of the 2019 novel coronavirus. *Chin J Bioinformatics.* (2020) 18:103–08. doi: 10.12113/202002001
25. Navin NE. The first five years of single-cell cancer genomics and beyond. *Genome Res.* (2015) 25:1499–507. doi: 10.1101/gr.191098.115
26. Tanay A, Regev A. Scaling single-cell genomics from phenomenology to mechanism. *Nature.* (2017) 541:331–8. doi: 10.1038/nature21350
27. Zhu S, Qing T, Zheng Y, Jin L, Shi L. Advances in single-cell RNA sequencing and its applications in cancer research. *Oncotarget.* (2017) 8:53763–79. doi: 10.18632/oncotarget.17893
28. Qi Z, Barrett T, Parikh AS, Tirosh I, Puram SV. Single-cell sequencing and its applications in head and neck cancer. *Oral Oncol.* (2019) 99:104441. doi: 10.1016/j.oraloncology.2019.104441
29. Xu H, Zhong L, Deng J, Peng J, Dan H, Zeng X, et al. High expression of ACE2 receptor of 2019-nCoV on the epithelial cells of oral mucosa. *Int J Oral Sci.* (2020) 12:8. doi: 10.1038/s41368-020-0074-x
30. López de Cicco R, Bassi DE, Page R, Klein-Szanto AJ. Furin expression in squamous cell carcinomas of the oral cavity and other sites evaluated by tissue microarray technology. *Acta Odontol Latinoamericana.* (2002) 15: 29–37.
31. Wu Z, McGoogan JM. Characteristics of and important lessons from the coronavirus disease 2019 (COVID-19) outbreak in China: summary of a report of 72 314 cases from the Chinese center for disease control and prevention. *JAMA.* (2020) 323:1239–42. doi: 10.1001/jama.2020.2648
32. Zhou J, Li C, Liu X, Chiu MC, Zhao X, Wang D, et al. Infection of bat and human intestinal organoids by SARS-CoV-2. *Nat Med.* (2020) 26:1077–83. doi: 10.1038/s41591-020-0912-6
33. Fan C, Li K, Ding Y, Lu WL, Wang J. ACE2 expression in kidney and testis may cause kidney and testis damage after 2019-nCoV infection. *medRxiv.* (2020) 2020.02.12.20022418. doi: 10.1101/2020.02.12.20022418
34. Chen L, Zhao J, Peng J, Li X, Deng X, Geng Z, et al. Detection of SARS-CoV-2 in saliva and characterization of oral symptoms in COVID-19 patients. *Cell Prolif.* (2020) e12923. doi: 10.1111/cpr.12923
35. Jaimes JA, Andre NM, Millet JK, Whittaker GR. Structural modeling of 2019-novel coronavirus (nCoV) spike protein reveals a proteolytically-sensitive activation loop as a distinguishing feature compared to SARS-CoV and related SARS-like coronaviruses. *ArXiv.* (2020) 14:arXiv:2002.06196v1. doi: 10.1101/2020.02.10.942185
36. Abassi ZA, Skorecki K, Heyman SN, Kinaneh S, Armaly Z. Covid-19 infection and mortality: a physiologist's perspective enlightening clinical features and plausible interventional strategies. *Am J Physiol-Lung Cell Mol Physiol.* (2020) 318:L1020–L2. doi: 10.1152/ajplung.00097.2020
37. Walls AC, Park Y-J, Tortorici MA, Wall A, McGuire AT, Veesler D. Structure, function, and antigenicity of the SARS-CoV-2 spike glycoprotein. *Cell.* (2020) 181:281–92.e6. doi: 10.1016/j.cell.2020.02.058
38. Bassi DE, Mahloogi H, Al-Saleem L, Lopez De Cicco R, Ridge JA, Klein-Szanto AJ. Elevated furin expression in aggressive human head and neck tumors and tumor cell lines. *Mol Carcinogenesis.* (2001) 31:224–32. doi: 10.1002/mc.1057
39. Drak Alsibai K. Expression of angiotensin-converting enzyme 2 and proteases in COVID-19 patients: a potential role of cellular Furin in the pathogenesis of SARS-CoV-2. *Med Hypotheses.* (2020) 143:109893. doi: 10.1016/j.mehy.2020.109893
40. Hoffmann M, Kleine-Weber H, Pohlmann S. A multibasic cleavage site in the spike protein of SARS-CoV-2 is essential for infection of human lung cells. *Mol Cell.* (2020) 78:779–84.e5. doi: 10.1016/j.molcel.2020.04.022
41. Shang J, Wan Y, Luo C, Ye G, Geng Q, Auerbach A, et al. Cell entry mechanisms of SARS-CoV-2. *Proc Natl Acad Sci USA.* (2020) 117:11727–34. doi: 10.1073/pnas.2003138117
42. Bestle D, Heindl MR, Limburg H, Van Lam van T, Pilgram O, Moulton H, et al. TMPRSS2 and furin are both essential for proteolytic activation of SARS-CoV-2 in human airway cells. *Life Sci Alliance.* (2020) 3:e202000786. doi: 10.26508/lsa.202000786
43. Hoffmann M, Kleine-Weber H, Schroeder S, Kruger N, Herrler T, Erichsen S, et al. SARS-CoV-2 cell entry depends on ACE2 and TMPRSS2 and is blocked by a clinically proven protease inhibitor. *Cell.* (2020) 181:271–80.e8. doi: 10.1016/j.cell.2020.02.052
44. To KK, Tsang OT, Yip CC, Chan KH, Wu TC, Chan JM, et al. Consistent Detection of 2019 Novel Coronavirus in Saliva. *Clin Infect Dis.* (2020) 71:841–3. doi: 10.1093/cid/ciaa149
45. Zou L, Ruan F, Huang M, Liang L, Huang H, Hong Z, et al. SARS-CoV-2 Viral Load in Upper Respiratory Specimens of Infected Patients. *N Engl J Med.* (2020) 382:1177–9. doi: 10.1056/NEJMc2001737
46. Zhong M, Lin BP, Gao HB, Young AJ, Wang XH, Liu C, et al. Significant expression of Furin and ACE2 on oral epithelial cells may facilitate the efficiency of SARS-CoV-2 entry. *BioRxiv.* (2020) doi: 10.1101/2020.04.18.047951

9

Oral Mucosa, Saliva and COVID-19 Infection in Oral Health Care

Devi Sewvandini Atukorallaya and Ravindra K. Ratnayake*

Department of Oral Biology, Dr. Gerald Niznick College of Dentistry, Rady Faculty of Health Sciences, University of Manitoba, Winnipeg, MB, Canada

***Correspondence:**
Devi Sewvandini Atukorallaya
devi.atukorallaya@umanitoba.ca

The SARS-CoV-2 virus has shaken the globe with an ongoing pandemic of COVID-19 and has set challenges to every corner of the modern health care setting. The oral mucosa and saliva are high risk sites for higher viral loads and dental health care professionals are considered a high risk group. COVID-19-induced oral lesions and loss of taste and smell are common clinical complaints in the dental health care setting. The SARS-CoV-2 virus has been found to cause a wide range of non-specific oral mucosal lesions, but the specific diagnosis of these mucocutaneous lesions as COVID-19 lesions will facilitate the prevention of SARS-CoV-2 in dental health care settings and aid in proper patient management. The reported loss of taste and smell needs further investigation at the receptor level as it will give new insights into SARS-CoV-2 pathogenicity. The high yield of virus in the salivary secretion is a common finding in this infection and ongoing research is focusing on developing saliva as a rapid diagnostic fluid in COVID-19. In this review, we discuss the significance of oral mucosa, saliva and the relevance of the COVID-19 pandemic in dentistry.

Keywords: oral epithelial cells, saliva, taste, SARS-CoV-2, ACE2 receptor, COVID-19

INTRODUCTION

Coronavirus disease 2019 (COVID-19) is an infectious disease that was first detected in large numbers in Wuhan, China; it is caused by a newly discovered coronavirus identified as severe acute respiratory syndrome coronavirus 2 (SARS-CoV-2) (1). Coronaviruses are large RNA viruses with beta coronaviruses, including SARS-CoV and SARS-CoV-2, having been shown to be the deadliest viruses, causing respiratory distress syndrome (2, 3). Since 1960, six coronaviruses have been found to cause diseases in humans. In 2002, SARS-CoV caused a major outbreak known as severe acute respiratory syndrome (SARS), which caused about 10,000 fatalities worldwide (4). Only a decade later, another pathogenic coronavirus, known as the Middle East respiratory syndrome coronavirus (MERS-CoV), caused an endemic in Middle Eastern countries (4, 5). SARS-CoV-2 is the seventh member of the coronavirus family to affect humans (4). Interestingly, the genome of SARS-CoV-2 aligned with the genomes of viruses from bats (Bat-CoV and Bat-CoV RaTG13) in *Rhinolophus affinis* species of the Yunnan province with 96% similarity; structural analysis revealed a mutation in the envelope protein (Spike protein) and nucleocapsid protein (6). The coronavirus has a simple structure with few proteins (7). There are 4 major structural proteins: the envelope protein (E), spike protein (S), transmembrane protein (M), and nucleoprotein (N). The E, S, and M proteins facilitate virus entry into the host cells, virion assembly, and viral pathogenesis. The viral genome, is in close association with N protein and also aid the E protein in virion assembly (7).

At present, two modes of transmission for SARS-CoV-2 have been identified: direct and indirect transmission. Direct transmission includes contact with the infected individual's body fluids, respiratory or salivary droplets and, other body fluids such as feces, urine, semen, and tears (8). The signs and symptoms of COVID-19 can be divided into respiratory and extra-respiratory manifestations. The most common reported respiratory signs are cough, fever, and dyspnoea (9–11). There is a wide range of extra-respiratory signs and symptoms, including oral mucosal lesions and neurological dysfunctions, such as loss of smell, loss of taste, headache, and associated myofascial pain; these are now included in the diagnostic criteria of this disease (**Table 1**) (10, 19).

The nasal cavity, nasopharynx, oropharynx and oral cavity are identified as potential replication sites for the SARS-CoV-2 virus (20, 21). The oral cavity, which is rich in saliva and the oral microbiome, is a well-known site harboring various types of respiratory viruses (22, 23). The oral saliva has been found to contain a high yield of viruses, suggesting salivary glands as active proliferating sites for this virus (20, 24). Moreover, xerostomia and loss of taste can be associated with the salivary gland dysfunction associated with COVID-19 (23, 25). However, these signs are often masked by the more life threatening respiratory signs and symptoms, which need emergency medical attention most of the time. This review aimed to provide histological specifications of the oral mucosa and its functional significance in SARS-CoV-2 infection, highlighting the orofacial manifestations and its impacts on the dental health profession.

TABLE 1 | Orofacial manifestations of COVID-19.

Clinical features	References
Headache	(12–15)
Myofacial pain	(13–15)
Oral ulcerations	(14–16)
Burning sensation of the oral mucosa	(14, 16)
Oral vesicle formation	(16, 17)
Loss of taste	(14–16, 18)
Loss of smell	(14–16, 18)
Dry mouth	(14, 15)
Skin discomfort	(16)

ORAL MUCOSA

The oral mucosa is the specialized mucous outer covering layer of the oral cavity which consists of the stratified squamous epithelium and the underlying connective tissue (lamina propria) (**Figure 1**) (26). Apart from the common epithelial functions, such as protection and lining, oral mucosa is regionally specialized to form special functions like taste perception, sensory perception, mastication, and secretion (26). The oral epithelial cells have numerous structural and functional specifications to withstand physical and chemical attacks. Squamous epithelia possess structural properties like stratification and cornification of the keratinocytes and specific cell-to-cell interactions to maintain their barrier functions (26). The epithelial cells are metabolically active and are capable of reacting to external stimuli by synthesizing a number of cytokines, adhesion molecules, growth factors, and chemokines (27). The oral cavity is a dynamic ecosystem that varies over time in ways that influence spatial patterns of microbial community assembly (28). Among

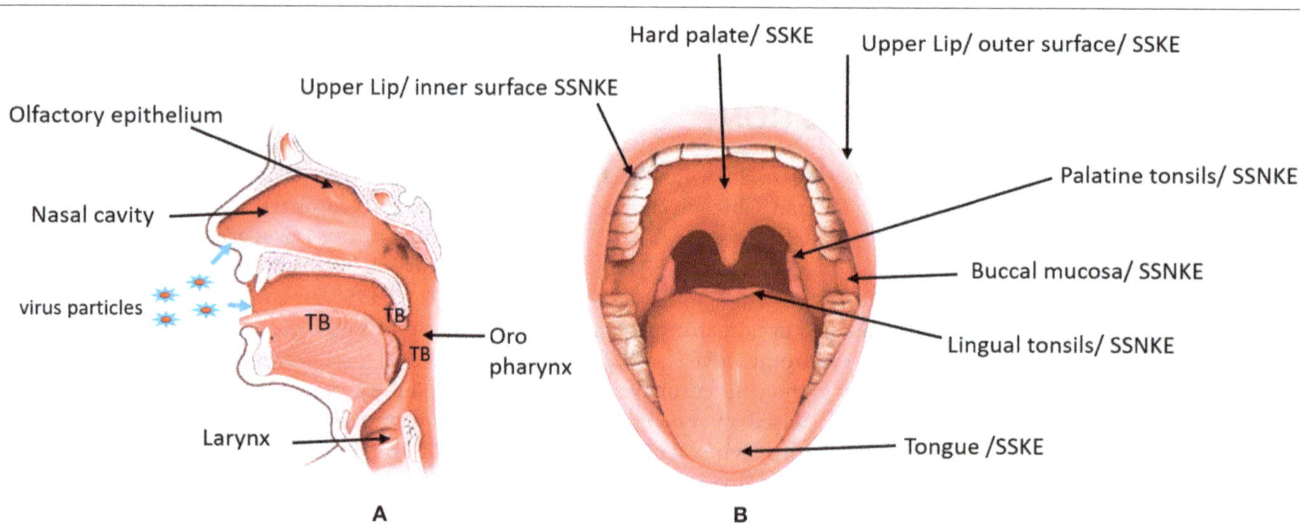

FIGURE 1 | Modified image indicating the location of the entry points of SARS-CoV-2 and the anterior view of the oral cavity labeling different areas of the oral mucosa. **(A)** Blue arrows indicate the nasal and oral entrance of the virus. The location of the olfactory epithelium and taste buds (TB). Olfactory epithelium is located on the roof of the nasal cavity. Taste buds can be found in the tongue, tonsils and oropharynx. **(B)** The specific location of the Stratified squamous keratinized epithelium (SSKE) and Stratified squamous non keratinized epithelium (SSNKE) in the oral cavity. https://www.informedhealth.org/how-do-the-tonsils-work.html, *"How do the tonsils work?"* Institute for Quality and Efficiency in Health Care (IQWiG, Germany), 17 Jan 2019.

the oral microbial community are common commensals that can be opportunistic pathogens when the host immunity is compromised. There are many species of bacteria, fungi and viruses which are either pathogenic or opportunistic, causing common oral diseases such as caries and periodontitis, oral candidiasis and viral mucosal infections (29, 30).

PATHOGENESIS OF SARS-CoV-2 IN ORAL MUCOSA

Oral viral infections are a common clinical complaint in dentistry, which is often associated with oral mucosal lesions. The herpes virus group (herpes simplex 1–8), human immune deficiency virus (HIV) and Zika virus are capable of infecting and replicating in the oral mucosa, leading to painful oral ulcers (22, 27). Viruses like paramyxovirus, HIV, cytomegalovirus and Epstein-Barr virus (EBV) have been found to replicate in salivary glands and negatively affect the normal functioning of the salivary glands (22). Several recent reports have described the oral manifestations of SARS-CoV-2 infection such as vesicular bullous lesions and ulceration (24, 25, 31).

The single cell RNA-seq (scRNA-Seq) studies of ACE2 expression have detected high levels of expression in keratinized epithelial cell surfaces of the oral cavity, such as the dorsum of the tongue and hard palate, rather than buccal or gingival tissues (32). In the human body, the ACE2 receptor is known to be important in regulating blood pressure homeostasis by regulating the renin–angiotensin–aldosterone system (RAAS), where it converts angiotensin I to angiotensin II; this cascades body functions to maintain blood pressure and sodium water retention (33). SARS-CoV-2 enters a host's body and invades host cells via the ACE2 membrane receptor; this binding leads to conformational changes and cleavage of the S protein from the virion, and releases the nucleocapsid into the cytoplasm (7, 34). The S protein is proteolytically cleaved by cellular cathepsin L and the transmembrane protease serine 2 (TMPRSS2) (33). Haga et al. found that SARS-CoV viruses can induce tissue necrosis factor (TNF)-α-converting enzyme (TACE)-dependent shedding of the ectodomain of ACE2, and that process was coupled with TNF-α production (35, 36). TNF-α is an inflammatory cytokine produced by macrophages/monocytes during acute inflammation and is responsible for a diverse range of signaling events within cells, leading to cell necrosis or apoptosis (37). These data suggest that cellular signals triggered by the interaction of SARS-CoV with ACE2 are positively involved in viral entry but lead to tissue damage. The presence of high ACE2 expression in the alveolar tissues, oropharyngeal mucosal cells, gastrointestinal tract, kidneys and endothelial cells, including oral tissues, indicated that those organs with high ACE2-expressing cells should be considered to be potential high risk sites for SARS-CoV-2 (21, 32).

ORAL MANIFESTATION OF COVID-19

The pathology of viral infections is often associated with either cellular destruction due to viral invasion or the consequence of host immune reaction to the viral antigen (23). In the oral mucosa, viral infections disrupt epithelial cells and trigger local inflammatory reactions which typically present with abrupt onset and the association of solitary or multiple blisters or ulcerations (23). Oral vesicles, blisters, macular popular rashes and ulcerations are the common clinical features of viral infections (23). In SARS-CoV-2, epithelial injury causes similar pathogenic features in the oral tissues, such as ulcers, erosions, bullae, vesicles, pustules, fissured or depapillated tongue, macule, papule, plaque, pigmentation, halitosis, whitish areas, haemorrhagic crust, necrosis, petechiae, swelling, erythema, Kawasaki-like angular cheilitis, atypical Sweet syndrome, and Melkerson-Rosenthal syndrome (19, 25, 38). The most common sites of involvement are the tongue (38%), labial mucosa (26%), and palate (22%) (19, 39). Oral lesions were almost equal in both genders (49% female and 51% male). Patients with an older age and higher severity of COVID-19 disease had more widespread and severe oral lesions (25).

The histological analysis of oral SARS-CoV-2 lesions is associated with defects in the vascular arrangement of the oral mucosa (40). Pathogenesis of oral mucosal lesion of COVID-19 are associated with the accumulation of lymphocytes and Langerhans cells in the vasculature of the subcutaneous junctions and virus induce keratinocyte destruction by the cytotoxic lymphocytes (41). Histological examination of biopsies of COVID-19 patients who also had skin manifestations confirmed the vascular ectasia with dilated capillaries, large blood filled spaces and perivascular lymphocytic infiltrate with eosinophilia (40).

A lack of oral hygiene, opportunistic infections, stress, immunosuppression, vasculitis, and hyper-inflammatory response secondary to COVID-19 were found to be the predisposing factors for the onset of oral lesions in COVID-19 patients (19, 39). Stress-induced oral ulceration can be increased among patients due to the unknown fear of the pandemic. It has been already reported that this pandemic has severely affected the mental health of the global community (42). Patients have reported changes in sensation in the tongue, plaque-like changes in the tongue and swelling in the palate, tongue and gums (25). Tongue lesions may be associated with the increasing activity of viral events on the epithelial mucosa of the tongue (39). On the other hand, immune suppression can lead to the harboring of opportunistic pathogens like *Candida albicans,* which can lead to the above observed tongue lesions (19). SARS- CoV-2 oral lesions healed between 3 and 28 days after they appeared. COVID-19-induced oro-mucosal lesions can be treated with mouthwashes, topical or systemic corticosteroids, systemic antibiotics and antivirals (39, 40). Increasing evidences are suggested that the antiseptic mouthwashes such as chlorhexidine, sodium hypochlorite and povidone-iodine found to be effective in reducing the SARS-CoV-2 viral load in the oral cavity and can be prescribed to patients with mucosal lesions as first line of therapy (43, 44). The topical or systemic corticosteroids, systemic antibacterial and antiviral needs to be prescribed according to the individual patient needs. Multidisciplinary team approach is important when prescribing or continuing systemic corticosteroids, antibiotics or antivirals to COVID-19-induced oro-mucosal lesions (39).

COVID-19 INDUCED TASTE AND SMELL LOSS

Taste is a special sensation of the human oral mucosa which plays a vital role in the identification of nutrients and regulation of food intake. Humans are capable of detecting five basic tastes: sweet, sour, salt, bitter and umami. Tastes stimulate specialized cells known as taste receptor cells (TRCs), which contain taste signal transduction proteins. Sour and salty tastes modulate the function of TRCs by the direct activation of specialized membrane channels (45, 46). In contrast, sweet, bitter and umami taste transduction is mediated through the G protein-coupled receptor (GPCR) signaling pathway (47). TRCs are locally organized as taste buds (TBs) which are located in the dorsum of the tongue and extra oral taste buds can be found in the tonsils and oropharynx (**Figure 1A**). TBs are made of receptor cells, support cells and are innervated by branches of the VII (facial), IX (glossopharyngeal), and X (vagal) cranial nerves. Taste information is relayed to the brain and its recognition elicits behavioral responses to the food (48, 49). True loss of taste is extremely rare, and it is usually preceded by the inability to perceive the odor of food due to olfactory dysfunction or the deficiency of saliva to dissolve food molecules to get into the taste receptors (25, 50).

Smells or odorants reach the olfactory epithelium, which covers the cribiform plate and the upper part of the nasal septum and the middle/upper turbinates and dissolve in the mucus layer, binding/activating olfactory receptors (**Figure 1A**). Up to 30 million receptor neurons, which express up to 350 different olfactory receptors, can be found in the olfactory epithelium. A complex combinatorial coding, by which each odorant ligand may be recognized by an olfactory receptor combination, enables humans to detect billions of different odors. Olfactory information, which is processed and integrated in the olfactory bulb, is then projected onto the primary olfactory centers such as the limbic system (emotions) and the hypothalamus (memory), and is finally projected to the olfactory cortex, where humans acquire the consciousness of smelling (50, 51). Smell loss in respiratory infections are multifactorial and are caused by a combination of the mechanical obstruction of odorant transmission in the olfactory cleft due to mucosal type 2 inflammation (oedema or nasal polyps), leading to shedding, and/or degeneration of the olfactory epithelium and the reduction or loss of the sense of smell (51).

The SARS- CoV-2 infection associated sudden loss of taste and smell was reported in several countries in early March, with the rapid increase in COVID-19 patient numbers. Interestingly, a series of sporadic cases, predominantly in health care workers, reporting a sudden, severe, and sometimes isolated loss of smell and/or taste was reported in different countries (50, 52). Nasal congestion was found to be the driving factor for the loss of smell. It is possible that damage to the olfactory neuroepithelium can cause defects in smell detection. Loss of smell is common among females and loss of smell is associated with a loss of taste most of the time (51, 53).

Still, there are a lack of data on a specific loss of different tastants (flavors) (54). In a web-based questionnaire study (n = 128), 67 patients (52%) reported changes in taste sensation. Fifty-two patients reported a change in their spicy taste perception, 54 in salty taste, 53 in sour taste, and 61 in sweet taste. In a comparison between men and women, COVID-19 induce taste changes and changes in taste subgroups were found to be common among women, but this needs further investigations (55, 56). A possible reason for the loss of taste in COVID-19 might be due to the increasing number of ACE-2 receptors on the tongue keratinocytes and the keratinocyte cell death and slough production can block taste buds which can adversely affect taste perception (53, 57). However, the presence of ACE-2 receptor activity on taste receptor cells is unknown at present, hence the specific role of SARS-CoV-2 on specific taste bud cells (receptor cells and supportive cells) needs to be further investigated (57). It has been shown that GPCR can be found in a diverse range of body tissues, not only in the oral cavity but in the lung epithelial cells, blood brain barrier and blood vessels (58). It will be interesting to see the specific role of SARS-CoV-2 and GPCR interactions in terms of COVID-19 pathogenesis. On the other hand, COVID-19 induces salivary gland dysfunction, which leads to dry mouth, and can result in the malfunctioning of taste perception (59). Treatment with artificial saliva can improve the xerostomia-induced taste loss (60). Quantitative smell testing demonstrates that decreased smell function is a major marker of SARS-CoV-2 infection, and suggests the possibility that smell testing may help, in some cases, to identify COVID-19 patients in need of early treatment or quarantine (61). Song et al. found that a loss of taste was more frequent (21%) than a loss of smell (11%) in hospitalized patients, with the loss of taste but not smell being associated with severe COVID-19 (62). Most patients recovered their smell and taste dysfunctions within 2 weeks (50, 62).

Overall, there is no real evidence for any specific pharmacological option for the post-viral loss of smell including COVID-19. Some studies report an improvement in olfactory function following topical or systemic corticosteroid therapy (50, 63). Olfactory training is the only current evidence-based therapeutic option for post-viral olfactory loss, with COVID-19 positive patients reporting an improvement in smell (45.6%) and taste (46.1%) at the time of the survey; in 90.6%, this was within 2 weeks of infection (64). Over 90% of COVID-19 patients with a loss of smell may recover that sense within the first month, and olfactory training is strongly recommended if smell has not recovered after that period of time, but can be started earlier (65).

ROLE OF SALIVA IN COVID-19 PATHOGENICITY AND DISEASE DIAGNOSIS

Human saliva is a unique body fluid of the oral cavity. It is a hypotonic solution of salivary acini, gingival crevicular fluid and oral mucosal exudates (66). Approximately 90% of saliva is secreted from the salivary glands; the major glands include

TABLE 2 | Articles related to COVID-19 and dentistry.

Country	Study overview	Article type	References
Italy	Prevention of spread of SARS-CO-V-2	Review	(72)
Italy	Symptoms/signs, protective measures, awareness, and perception levels regarding COVID-19 among dentists in Lombardy, Italy	Questionnaire survey	(73)
China	COVID-19 and management protocols for dental practitioners and students	Review	(74)
Italy	Prevention of COVID-19 in Pediatric dentistry	Review	(75)
Brazil	Oral Manifestations in Patients with COVID-19	A living systematic review	(76)
Italy	Infection control in Dentistry	Review	(77)
Italy	Oral manifestations of COVID-19	A narrative review	(78)
Spain	Oral lesions of COVID-19	Cross sectional study	(79)
Multicenter study	Endodontic emergency management by endodontists and general dental practitioners in COVID-19 times	Online survey using questionnaire	(80)
USA	Epidemiology, symptoms, and routes of transmission of COVID-19	Review	(81)
India	Safety operative protocols	Commentary	(82)
France	Salivary and Nasal Detection of the SARS-CoV-2 Virus After Antiviral Mouth rinses	Randomized control trial	(83)
Brazil	Mouth wash reducing viral load of COVID-19	Systematic review	(84)
Nigeria	Impact on orthodontic patients	Online questionnaire cross-sectional descriptive study	(85)
India	Appropriate orthodontic appliances during the COVID-19 pandemic	Scoping review	(86)

the parotid glands, submandibular glands and sublingual glands (66). The salivary glands are highly vascular structures, where there is a constant exchange of substances. A normal person produces 600 mL of saliva per day. It is mainly composed of water (94–99%), with organic molecules accounting for ~0.5% and inorganic molecules for 0.2% (66). It has the functions of lubricating the oral mucosa, digesting food, and cleaning and protecting the oral cavity, and is one of the most important factors affecting homeostasis of the oral cavity.

Viral infections are often associated with the infection induced inflammation of the salivary gland (22). Saliva based biomarkers are useful in diagnosis of several viral infections such as hepatitis A virus, hepatitis B virus, hepatitis C virus, HIV-1, measles virus, rubella virus, and mumps virus (66). Several routes of SARS-CoV-2 viral entry into the saliva have being suggested. There is direct entry to the oral cavity from upper and lower respiratory tract secretions, while circulatory viruses in the blood enter the gingival crevicular fluid. Studies reported a high yield of virus particles in the gingival sulcus and crevicular fluid and are suspected to provide favorable conditions for virus replication and maintenance (32). Moreover, SARS-CoV-2 salivary gland infections can produce large amounts of viruses in the salivary gland tissues and release them into the secretions (67). Studies performed on rhesus macaques found that there is a rapid infection in the salivary gland epithelial cells by SARS-CoV, suggesting salivary glands as very early proliferating sites for coronaviruses (68). Hence, increased ACE-2 expression in minor salivary glands compared to the lungs suggestive of salivary glands as an early target organ and saliva can be a vital source in the early diagnosis of disease before the respiratory symptoms appear (20, 31, 68).

In COVID-19, the impaired salivary gland secretions are often associated with xerostomia and taste loss (69). Xerostomia is the subjective complaint of oral dryness, while salivary gland hypofunction is an objective matter characterized by reduced salivary flow (70, 71). In SARS-CoV infections, xerostomia could be aggravated by impaired nasal breathing due to nasal congestion and rhinorrhea, where the oral breathing increase and it can impaired salivary gland function and xerostomia is secondary (25). Similar to COVID-19-induced oral mucosal lesions, pandemic-induced psychosocial factors have a greater impact on normal salivary gland function and quantitative secretions (25, 59).

The saliva-based COVID-19 diagnosis is getting increased attention for several important reasons. First, saliva specimens can be easily obtained, by asking patents to spit into a container, which is not an invasive procedure and minimizes the chance of exposing health care workers to the highly infectious SARS-CoV-2 virus; it is also ideal for testing the elderly vulnerable population, pediatric patients and community settings, where large sample collection is needed (**Table 2**) (87). There is a 92% positive rate of SARS-CoV-2 in saliva compared to nasopharyngeal aspirate and live virus can be successfully cultivated through saliva samples, highlighting the value of saliva in the diagnosis of COVID-19 (88). As discussed previously, the early detection of SARS-CoV-2 in the saliva can be vital in diagnosing COVID-19 patients before respiratory symptoms appear, which greatly aids in controlling public health measures such as the quarantine process (20, 88, 89).

FUTURE PERSPECTIVES WITH REGARD TO THE ORAL HEALTH PROFESSION

On March 11th 2020, the World Health Organization (WHO) declared COVID-19 to be a global pandemic. As of the 20th

January 2021, 96,866,468 cases had been reported globally, with 20,72,466 deaths. The first cases of COVID-19 were seen in Canada on February 10th 2020, and there have since been 723,908 cases and 18,421 deaths (90). The current public health regulations to prevent the spread of this virus have been based on the modes of transmission. Following the strict global (WHO) and Canadian public health guidelines was found to be effective in preventing the spread of COVID-19 (91, 92). Several excellent research and review articles have already been published on the impact of COVID-19 on clinical dentistry and the relevance of the oral cavity in SARS-CoV-2 infection (**Table 2**) (24, 72, 93). The dental regulatory authorities quickly adapted new rules and regulations with regard to patient care and prevention of the spread of SARS-CoV-2 (72, 93). Among the health care professions, dental professionals have a high risk of making contact with diseased individuals and spreading the disease in nosocomial settings.

The American Dental Association has developed guidelines to the patient care during COVID-19 pandemic (94). The dental treatments are divided into the urgent/emergency care and routine/elective procedures. The dental emergencies which needs immediate medical attention includes life threatening conditions uncontrolled bleeding, swelling and fractures which compromise patient's airway. Urgent dental care should focus on minimizing pain, reduce or control infection, and reduce the burden on emergency departments (94). Other than that suture removal, denture adjustment, replacing fillings to alleviate pain and snipping or adjusting orthodontic appliances to prevent trauma also considered as urgent dental care. The non-urgent routine procedures include initial dental visits, routine dental cleaning and preventive therapies, aesthetic dental procedures, and extraction of asymptomatic teeth and orthodontic procedures (94). The ultimate goal is to avoid unnecessary contacts and minimize the contact to prevent the further spread of the virus in the dental care settings. The COVID-19 pandemic opens up a variety of innovative technologies for meetings such as teleconferencing, video calls, and patient photographs. Brian & Weintraub discuss use of communication media such as Teledentistry to educate and consult patients during the pandemic period, where it would greatly facilitate the prevention of unnecessary dental visits for conditions which can be temporarily alleviated at home or postponed for a later date (93). The patients with underlying health conditions such as diabetes, cancer, cardiovascular diseases (CVD) and hypertension are more susceptible to developing COVID-19 thus needs special attention. For instance, diabetes is a metabolic disorder which adversely affect the periodontal health. The periodontal disease (PD) is a chronic inflammatory disease which induce increased cytokine production and the disease severity found to be increased with COVID-19 infection (95). It is important to identify patients with underlying comorbidities and advise them on maintaining good oral hygiene to prevent the further progression of existing PD (**Table 2**).

Dental health care personals should be trained to be familiar with COVID-19 related signs and symptoms. The triage screening is a successful method to identify and separate out patients into three categories: (1) Triage negative (asymptomatic and negative in screening questionnaire and no fever) (2) Triage positive (positive screening questionnaire and /or fever) (3) confirmed COVID-19 cases. However, it is extremely important to take all the necessary precautions when treating the first category (82). The ability to undertake robust patient screening would facilitate the avoidance of COVID-19 transmission in dental clinics. A non-invasive rapid screening test would be of great help to identify positive cases that warrant immediate quarantine or transfer to special clinic for further treatment (88, 93). Current research are focusing on developing biomarkers for early detection, treatment and prevention of COVID-19. In the oral health care settings saliva and mucosal epithelial cells are good candidates to develop the biomarkers to identify the asymptomatic carriers (**Table 2**).

Given the higher viral loads in the oral cavity, it is essential to use personal protective equipment (PPE). Protective goggles or face shields, masks, gloves, and caps should be regularly worn, discarded or properly disinfected between each patient. Salivary aerosols and blood need to be protected against to reduce the risk of infection with COVID-19 (96). The use of rubber dams can significantly minimize the production of saliva-contaminated splatters, droplets and aerosols, particularly when high-speed dental hand pieces and ultrasonic devices are used. The application of a rubber dam can significantly reduce airborne particles in an ~3 foot diameter of the operational field by 70% (97). High-speed dental hand pieces without anti-retraction valves may aspirate and expel debris and fluids during dental procedures; also, the hand instruments used during general dental procedures produce a significant amount of aerosol spread (72). Good ventilation, regular and thorough surface disinfection before and after procedures with alcohol or chlorine and the proper handling of saliva-containing waste are critical in preventing the spread of COVID-19 (96). Recent studies shows that mouth rinses can reduce the SARS-CoV-2 virus load (98). Marui et al. showed that pre-procedural mouth rinses can significantly reduce microbial load in dental aerosols (99). Also, the use of pre-procedural mouth rinses before dental treatment can be advantageous during the pandemic (100).

We are too early to predict the post-pandemic effects of COVID-19. However, COVID-19 has a wide range of impacts on mental health, which can have a negative effect on the oral health of any given community; in particular, a greater impact can be seen in vulnerable populations such as people with low socioeconomic status who lack access to proper health care. On the other hand, this is a challenging time for dental health professionals and it could affect their psychological status, which can adversely affect their overall productivity. For instance, adopting new techniques to minimize the spread of disease, and reduced wages as this is associated with a decline in per capita dental visits (93). The timely vaccination of health care professionals and the vulnerable population is now a strategic priority for the prevention of COVID-19 in many countries. Dai and Gao in their progressive article discussed about the different vaccine candidates against SARS-CoV-2 (i.e., Inactivated virus vaccines, virus like particle or nanoparticle viruses, protein subunit vaccines, virus-vectored vaccines, DNA and mRNA vaccines and live attenuated vaccines) and compare their effectiveness against COVID-19 (101). The world largest vaccination campaign begins with the BioNTech/Pfizer, and Moderna/NIAID vaccines and Oxford-AstraZenca's is now authorized and added to this mass prevention battle against COVID-19. However, the immunization programs needs further investigations for their effectiveness against the novel variants of SARS-CoV-2 (101, 102). Further studies need to be performed to identify the pathogenicity of SARS-CoV-2 on specific epithelial organs of the oral cavity and its effect on oral health. Salivary research can be directed toward designing rapid identification test kits as a chair-side test prior to any dental procedures in order to diagnose SARS-CoV-2 carriers. The use of corticosteroids, antivirals and antibiotics to treat the oral mucosal lesions of COVID-19 needs to be studied further using large samples in different demographic settings. The ongoing COVID-19 pandemic is an eye-opener to all of mankind to be vigilant and prepared to fight future pandemics. Specifically, scientific knowledge gained from this pandemic can be useful in designing public healthcare protocols to prevent future pandemics and vaccines, and therapeutic treatment research will be invaluable in patient management in any virulent coronavirus infections.

AUTHOR CONTRIBUTIONS

DSA and RKR contributed to the conception and critically revised the manuscript. Both authors contributed to the article and approved the submitted version.

ACKNOWLEDGMENTS

We would like to acknowledge University of Manitoba for supporting the research in the Atukorale laboratory.

REFERENCES

1. Bchetnia M, Girard C, Duchaine C, Laprise C. The outbreak of the novel severe acute respiratory syndrome coronavirus 2 (SARS-CoV-2): a review of the current global status. *J Infect Public Health.* (2020) 13:1601–10. doi: 10.1016/j.jiph.2020.07.011
2. Krishnamoorthy S, Swain B, Verma RS, Gunthe SS. SARS-CoV, MERS-CoV, and 2019-nCoV viruses: an overview of origin, evolution, genetic variations. *Virusdisease.* (2020) 31:1–13. doi: 10.1007/s13337-020-00632-9
3. Desforges M, Le Coupanec A, Stodola JK, Meessen-Pinard M, Talbot PJ. Human coronaviruses: viral and cellular factors involved in neuroinvasiveness and neuropathogenesis. *Virus Res.* (2014) 194:145–58. doi: 10.1016/j.virusres.2014.09.011
4. Shereen MA, Khan S, Kazmi A, Bashir N, Siddique R. COVID-19 infection: Origin, transmission, and characteristics of human coronaviruses. *J Adv Res.* (2020) 24:91–8. doi: 10.1016/j.jare.2020.03.005
5. Hasöksüz M, Kiliç S, Saraç F. Coronaviruses and SARS-COV-2. *Turk J Med Sci.* (2020) 50:549–56. doi: 10.3906/sag-2004-127
6. Zhou H, Chen X, Hu T, Li J, Song H, Liu Y, et al. A novel bat coronavirus closely related to SARS-CoV-2 contains natural insertions at the S1/S2 cleavage site of the spike protein. *Current biology : CB.* (2020) 30:2196–2203.e3. doi: 10.1016/j.cub.2020.05.023
7. Neuman BW, Buchmeier MJ. Supramolecular architecture of the coronavirus particle. *Adv Virus Res.* (2016) 96:1–27. doi: 10.1016/bs.aivir.2016.08.005
8. Karia R, Gupta I, Khandait H, Yadav A, Yadav A. COVID-19 and its modes of Transmission. *SN Compr Clin Med.* (2020) 1–4. doi: 10.1007/s42399-020-00498-4. [Epub ahead of print].
9. Richardson S, Hirsch JS, Narasimhan M, Crawford JM, McGinn T, Davidson KW, et al. Presenting characteristics, comorbidities, and outcomes among 5700 patients hospitalized with COVID-19 in the New York City Area. *JAMA.* (2020) 323:2052–9. doi: 10.1001/jama.2020.6775
10. Arentz M, Yim E, Klaff L, Lokhandwala S, Riedo FX, Chong M, et al. Characteristics and outcomes of 21 critically Ill patients with COVID-19 in Washington State. *Jama.* (2020) 323:1612–4. doi: 10.1001/jama.2020.4326
11. Garg S, Kim L, Whitaker M, O'Halloran A, Cummings C, Holstein R, et al. Hospitalization rates and characteristics of patients hospitalized with laboratory-confirmed coronavirus disease 2019 - COVID-NET, 14 States, March 1-30, 2020. *MMWR Morb Mortal Wkly Rep.* (2020) 69:458–64. doi: 10.15585/mmwr.mm6915e3
12. Shi H, Han X, Jiang N, Cao Y, Alwalid O, Gu J, et al. Radiological findings from 81 patients with COVID-19 pneumonia in Wuhan, China: a descriptive study. *Lancet Infect Dis.* (2020) 20:425–34. doi: 10.1016/S1473-3099(20)30086-4
13. Xu XW, Wu XX, Jiang XG, Xu KJ, Ying LJ, Ma CL, et al. Clinical findings in a group of patients infected with the 2019 novel coronavirus (SARS-Cov-2) outside of Wuhan, China: retrospective case series. *BMJ.* (2020) 368:m606. doi: 10.1136/bmj.m606
14. Freni F, Meduri A, Gazia F, Nicastro V, Galletti C, Aragona P, et al. Symptomatology in head and neck district in coronavirus disease (COVID-19): a possible neuroinvasive action of SARS-CoV-2. *Am J Otolaryngol.* (2020) 41:102612. doi: 10.1016/j.amjoto.2020.102612
15. Lechien JR, Chiesa-Estomba CM, De Siati DR, Horoi M, Le Bon SD, Rodriguez A, et al. Olfactory and gustatory dysfunctions as a clinical presentation of mild-to-moderate forms of the coronavirus disease (COVID-19): a multicenter European study. *Eur Arch Otorhinolaryngol.* (2020) 277:2251–61. doi: 10.1007/s00405-020-06024-5
16. Lai C-C, Ko W-C, Lee P-I, Jean S-S, Hsueh P-R. Extra-respiratory manifestations of COVID-19. *Int J Antimicrob Agents.* (2020) 56:106024. doi: 10.1016/j.ijantimicag.2020.106024
17. Guo Y, Yuan C, Wei C. Emergency measures for acute oral mucosa diseases during the outbreak of COVID-19. *Oral Dis.* (2020) 2020:13350. doi: 10.1111/odi.13350
18. Meng X, Deng Y, Dai Z, Meng Z. COVID-19 and anosmia: a review based on up-to-date knowledge. *Am J Otolaryngol.* (2020) 41:102581. doi: 10.1016/j.amjoto.2020.102581
19. Iranmanesh B, Khalili M, Amiri R, Zartab H, Aflatoonian M. Oral manifestations of COVID-19 disease: a review article. *Dermatol Ther.* (2020) 34:e14578. doi: 10.1111/dth.14578. [Epub ahead of print].
20. Wang WK, Chen SY, Liu IJ, Chen YC, Chen HL, Yang CF, et al. Detection of SARS-associated coronavirus in throat wash and saliva in early diagnosis. *Emerg Infect Dis.* (2004) 10:1213–9. doi: 10.3201/eid1007.031113
21. Herrera D, Serrano J, Roldán S, Sanz M. Is the oral cavity relevant in SARS-CoV-2 pandemic?. *Clin Oral Invest.* (2020) 24:2925–30. doi: 10.1007/s00784-020-03413-2
22. Jeffers L, Webster-Cyriaque JY. Viruses and salivary gland disease (SGD): lessons from HIV SGD. *Adv Dent Res.* (2011) 23:79–83. doi: 10.1177/0022034510396882
23. Santosh ABR, Muddana K. Viral infections of oral cavity. *J Family Med Prim Care.* (2020) 9:36–42. doi: 10.4103/jfmpc.jfmpc_807_19
24. Troeltzsch M, Berndt R, Troeltzsch M. Is the oral cavity a reservoir for prolonged SARS-CoV-2 shedding?. *Med Hypoth.* (2020) 146:110419. doi: 10.1016/j.mehy.2020.110419
25. Brandão TB, Gueiros LA, Melo TS, Prado-Ribeiro AC, A.Nesrallah CFA, Prado GVB, et al. Oral lesions in patients with SARS-CoV-2 infection: could the oral cavity be a target organ? *Oral Surg Oral Med Oral Pathol Oral Radiol.* (2020) 131:e45–51. doi: 10.1016/j.oooo.2020.07.014
26. Groeger S, Meyle J. Oral mucosal epithelial cells. *Front Immunol.* (2019) 10:208. doi: 10.3389/fimmu.2019.00208

27. Groeger SE, Meyle J. Epithelial barrier and oral bacterial infection. *Periodontol.* (2015) 69:46–67. doi: 10.1111/prd.12094
28. Proctor DM, Relman DA. The landscape ecology and microbiota of the human nose, mouth, and throat. *Cell Host Microbe.* (2017) 21:421–32. doi: 10.1016/j.chom.2017.03.011
29. Seneviratne CJ, Jin L, Samaranayake LP. Biofilm lifestyle of Candida: a mini review. *Oral Dis.* (2008) 14:582–90. doi: 10.1111/j.1601-0825.2007.01424.x
30. Aas JA, Paster BJ, Stokes LN, Olsen I, Dewhirst FE. Defining the normal bacterial flora of the oral cavity. *J Clin Microbiol.* (2005) 43:5721–32. doi: 10.1128/JCM.43.11.5721-5732.2005
31. Xu J, Li Y, Gan F, Du Y, Yao Y. Salivary glands: potential reservoirs for COVID-19 asymptomatic infection. *J. Dental Res.* (2020) 99:989. doi: 10.1177/0022034520918518
32. Xu H, Zhong L, Deng J, Peng J, Dan H, Zeng X, et al. High expression of ACE2 receptor of 2019-nCoV on the epithelial cells of oral mucosa. *Int J Oral Sci.* (2020) 12:8. doi: 10.1038/s41368-020-0074-x
33. Datta PK, Liu F, Fischer T, Rappaport J, Qin X. SARS-CoV-2 pandemic and research gaps: understanding SARS-CoV-2 interaction with the ACE2 receptor and implications for therapy. *Theranostics.* (2020) 10:7448–64. doi: 10.7150/thno.48076
34. Jin Y, Yang H, Ji W, Wu W, Chen S, Zhang W, et al. Virology, epidemiology, pathogenesis, and control of COVID-19. *Viruses.* (2020) 12:372. doi: 10.3390/v12040372
35. Haga S, Yamamoto N, Nakai-Murakami C, Osawa Y, Tokunaga K, Sata T, et al. Modulation of TNF-alpha-converting enzyme by the spike protein of SARS-CoV and ACE2 induces TNF-alpha production and facilitates viral entry. *Proc Natl Acad Sci USA.* (2008) 105:7809–14. doi: 10.1073/pnas.0711241105
36. Barlow LA. Progress and renewal in gustation: new insights into taste bud development. *Development.* (2015) 142:3620–9. doi: 10.1242/dev.120394
37. Idriss HT, Naismith JH. TNF alpha and the TNF receptor superfamily: structure-function relationship(s). *Microsc Res Tech.* (2000) 50:184–95. doi: 10.1002/1097-0029(20000801)50:3<184::AID-JEMT2>3.0.CO;2-H
38. Carreras-Presas CM, Sanchez JA, Lopez-Sanchez AF, Jane-Salas E, Perez MLS. Oral vesiculobullous lesions associated with SARS-CoV-2 infection. *Oral Dis.* (2020) 3:13382. doi: 10.1111/odi.13382
39. Amorim Dos Santos J, Normando AGC, Carvalho da Silva RL, De Paula RM, Cembranel AC, Santos-Silva AR, et al. Oral mucosal lesions in a COVID-19 patient: new signs or secondary manifestations? *Int J Infect Dis.* (2020) 97:326–8. doi: 10.1016/j.ijid.2020.06.012
40. R.O. Cruz Tapia, Peraza Labrador AJ, Guimaraes DM, Matos Valdez LH. Oral mucosal lesions in patients with SARS-CoV-2 infection. Report of four cases. Are they a true sign of COVID-19 disease? *Spec Care Dentistry.* (2020) 40:555–60. doi: 10.1111/scd.12520
41. Gianotti R, Zerbi P, Dodiuk-Gad RP. Clinical and histopathological study of skin dermatoses in patients affected by COVID-19 infection in the Northern part of Italy. *J Dermatol Sci.* (2020) 98:141–3. doi: 10.1016/j.jdermsci.2020.04.007
42. Heitzman J. Impact of COVID-19 pandemic on mental health. *Psychiatr Pol.* (2020) 54:187–98. doi: 10.12740/PP/120373
43. Carrouel F, Gonçalves LS, Conte MP, Campus G, Fisher J, Fraticelli L, et al. Antiviral activity of reagents in mouth rinses against SARS-CoV-2. *J Dental Res.* (2021) 100:124–32. doi: 10.1177/0022034520967933
44. Yoon JG, Yoon J, Song JY, Yoon SY, Lim CS, Seong H, et al. Clinical Significance of a High SARS-CoV-2 Viral Load in the Saliva. *Journal of Korean medical science.* (2020) 35:e195. doi: 10.3346/jkms.2020.35.e195
45. Horio N, Yoshida R, Yasumatsu K, Yanagawa Y, Ishimaru Y, Matsunami H, et al. Sour taste responses in mice lacking PKD channels. *PLoS ONE.* (2011) 6:e20007. doi: 10.1371/journal.pone.0020007
46. Zhang Y, Hoon MA, Chandrashekar J, Mueller KL, Cook B, Wu D, et al. Coding of sweet, bitter, and umami tastes: different receptor cells sharing similar signaling pathways. *Cell.* (2003) 112:293–301. doi: 10.1016/S0092-8674(03)00071-0
47. Perez CA, Huang L, Rong M, Kozak JA, Preuss AK, Zhang H, et al. A transient receptor potential channel expressed in taste receptor cells. *Nat Neurosci.* (2002) 5:1169–76. doi: 10.1038/nn952
48. Okada S. The taste system of small fish species. *Biosci Biotechnol Biochem.* (2015) 79:1039–43. doi: 10.1080/09168451.2015.1023251
49. de Araujo ie, Simon SA. The gustatory cortex and multisensory integration. *Int J Obes (Lond).* (2009) 33 (Suppl 2):S34–43. doi: 10.1038/ijo.2009.70
50. Mullol J, Alobid I, Mariño-Sánchez F, Izquierdo-Domínguez A, Marin C, Klimek L, et al. The loss of smell and taste in the COVID-19 outbreak: a tale of many countries. *Curr Allergy Asthma Rep.* (2020) 20:61. doi: 10.1007/s11882-020-00961-1
51. Mullol J, Mariño-Sánchez F, Valls M, Alobid I, Marin C. The sense of smell in chronic rhinosinusitis. *J Allergy Clin Immunol.* (2020) 145:773–776. doi: 10.1016/j.jaci.2020.01.024
52. Lechner M, Chandrasekharan D, Jumani K, Liu J, Gane S, Lund VJ, et al. Anosmia as a presenting symptom of SARS-CoV-2 infection in healthcare workers - A systematic review of the literature, case series, and recommendations for clinical assessment and management. *Rhinology.* (2020) 58:394–9. doi: 10.4193/Rhin20.189
53. Glezer I, Bruni-Cardoso A, Schechtman D, Malnic B. Viral infection and smell loss: the case of COVID-19. *J Neurochem.* (2020). doi: 10.1111/jnc.15197. [Epub ahead of print].
54. Risso D, Drayna D, Morini G. Alteration, reduction and taste loss: main causes and potential implications on dietary habits. *Nutrients.* (2020) 12:3284. doi: 10.3390/nu12113284
55. Biadsee A, Biadsee A, Kassem F, Dagan O, Masarwa S, Ormianer Z. Olfactory and oral manifestations of COVID-19: sex-related symptoms-a potential pathway to early diagnosis. *Otolaryngol Head Neck Surg.* (2020) 163:722–8. doi: 10.1177/0194599820934380
56. Elkholi SMA, Abdelwahab MK, Abdelhafeez M. Impact of the smell loss on the quality of life and adopted coping strategies in COVID-19 patients. *Europ Arch Oto-Rhino-Laryngol.* (2021). doi: 10.1007/s00405-020-06575-7. [Epub ahead of print].
57. Cooper KW, Brann DH, Farruggia MC, Bhutani S, Pellegrino R, Tsukahara T, et al. COVID-19 and the chemical senses: supporting players take center stage. *Neuron.* (2020) 107:219–33. doi: 10.1016/j.neuron.2020.06.032
58. Jaggupilli A, Singh N, Upadhyaya J, Sikarwar AS, Arakawa M, Dakshinamurti S, et al. Analysis of the expression of human bitter taste receptors in extraoral tissues. *Mol Cell Biochem.* (2017) 426:137–47. doi: 10.1007/s11010-016-2902-z
59. da Silva Pedrosa M, Sipert CR, Nogueira FN. Altered taste in patients with COVID-19: the potential role of salivary glands. *Oral Dis.* (2020). doi: 10.1111/odi.13496. [Epub ahead of print].
60. Baghizadeh Fini M. Oral saliva and COVID-19. *Oral Oncol.* (2020) 108:104821. doi: 10.1016/j.oraloncology.2020.104821
61. Moein ST, Hashemian SM, Mansourafshar B, Khorram-Tousi A, Tabarsi P, Doty RL. Smell dysfunction: a biomarker for COVID-19. *Int Forum Allergy Rhinol.* (2020) 10:944–50. doi: 10.1002/alr.22587
62. Song J, Deng Y-K, Wang H, Wang Z-C, Liao B, Ma J, et al. Self-reported taste and smell disorders in patients with COVID-19:distinct features in China. *medRxiv [Preprint].* (2020). doi: 10.1101/2020.06.12.20128298
63. Abdelalim AA, Mohamady AA, Elsayed RA, Elawady MA, Ghallab AF. Corticosteroid nasal spray for recovery of smell sensation in COVID-19 patients: a randomized controlled trial. *Am J Otolaryngol.* (2021) 42:102884. doi: 10.1016/j.amjoto.2020.102884
64. Izquierdo-Domínguez A, Rojas-Lechuga MJ, Chiesa-Estomba C, Calvo-Henríquez C, Ninchritz-Becerra E, Soriano-Reixach M, et al. Smell and taste dysfunction in COVID-19 is associated with younger age in ambulatory settings: a multicenter cross-sectional study. *J Investig Allergol Clin Immunol.* (2020) 30:346–57. doi: 10.18176/jiaci.0595
65. Bousquet J, Akdis C, Jutel M, Bachert C, Klimek L, Agache I, et al. Intranasal corticosteroids in allergic rhinitis in COVID-19 infected patients: an ARIA-EAACI statement. *Allergy.* (2020) 75:2440–4. doi: 10.1111/all14302
66. Zhang CZ, Cheng XQ, Li JY, Zhang P, Yi P, Xu X, et al. Saliva in the diagnosis of diseases. *Int J Oral Sci.* (2016) 8:133–7. doi: 10.1038/ijos.2016.38
67. Sabino-Silva R, Jardim ACG, Siqueira WL. Coronavirus COVID-19 impacts to dentistry and potential salivary diagnosis. *Clin Oral Invest.* (2020) 24:1619–21. doi: 10.1007/s00784-020-03248-x
68. Liu L, Wei Q, Alvarez X, Wang H, Du Y, Zhu H, et al. Epithelial cells lining salivary gland ducts are early target cells of severe acute respiratory syndrome

coronavirus infection in the upper respiratory tracts of rhesus macaques. *J Virol.* (2011) 85:4025–30. doi: 10.1128/JVI.02292-10
69. Sinjari B, D'Ardes D, Santilli M, Rexhepi I, D'Addazio G, Di Carlo P, et al. SARS-CoV-2 and oral manifestation: an observational, human study. *J Clin Med.* (2020) 9:3218. doi: 10.3390/jcm9103218
70. Thomson WM, Chalmers JM, Spencer AJ, Williams SM. The Xerostomia Inventory: a multi-item approach to measuring dry mouth. *Community Dent Health.* (1999) 16:12–7.
71. Mortazavi H, Baharvand M, Movahhedian A, Mohammadi M, Khodadoustan A. Xerostomia due to systemic disease: a review of 20 conditions and mechanisms. *Ann Med Health Sci Res.* (2014) 4:503–10. doi: 10.4103/2141-9248.139284
72. Spagnuolo G, De Vito D, Rengo S, Tatullo M. COVID-19 outbreak: an overview on dentistry. *Int J Environ Res Public Health.* (2020) 17:2794. doi: 10.3390/ijerph17062094
73. Cagetti MG, Cairoli JL, Senna A, Campus G. COVID-19 outbreak in North Italy: an overview on dentistry. A questionnaire survey. *Int J Environ Res Public Health.* (2020) 17:3835. doi: 10.3390/ijerph17113835
74. Meng L, Hua F, Bian Z. Coronavirus Disease 2019 (COVID-19): emerging and future challenges for dental and oral medicine. *J Dent Res.* (2020) 99:481–7. doi: 10.1177/0022034520914246
75. Ferrazzano GF, Ingenito A, Cantile T. COVID-19 disease in children: what dentists should know and do to prevent viral spread. The Italian point of view. *Int J Environ Res Public Health.* (2020) 17:3642. doi: 10.3390/ijerph17103642
76. Amorim Dos Santos J, Normando AGC, Carvalho da Silva RL, Acevedo AC, De Luca Canto G, Sugaya N, et al. Oral manifestations in patients with COVID-19: a living systematic review. *J Dent Res.* (2021) 100:141–54. doi: 10.1177/0022034520957289
77. Amato A, Caggiano M, Amato M, Moccia G, Capunzo M, De Caro F. Infection control in dental practice during the COVID-19 pandemic. *Int J Environ Res Public Health.* (2020) 17:4769. doi: 10.3390/ijerph17134769
78. Capocasale G, Nocini R, Faccioni P, Donadello D, Bertossi D, Albanese M, et al. How to deal with coronavirus disease 2019: a comprehensive narrative review about oral involvement of the disease. *Clin Exp Dent Res.* (2021) 7:101–8. doi: 10.1002/cre2.332
79. Nuno-Gonzalez A, Martin-Carrillo P, Magaletsky K, Martin Rios MD, Herranz Mañas C, Artigas Almazan J, et al. Prevalence of mucocutaneous manifestations in 666 patients with COVID-19 in a field hospital in Spain: oral and palmoplantar findings. *Br J Dermatol.* (2021) 184:184–5. doi: 10.1111/bjd.19564
80. Ates AA, Alomari T, Bhardwaj A, Tabnjh A, Gambarini G. Differences in endodontic emergency management by endodontists and general dental practitioners in COVID-19 times. *Braz Oral Res.* (2020) 34:e122. doi: 10.1590/1807-3107bor-2020.vol34.0122
81. Ather A, Patel B, Ruparel NB, Diogenes A, Hargreaves KM. Coronavirus Disease 19 (COVID-19): implications for clinical dental care. *J Endod.* (2020) 46:584–95. doi: 10.1016/j.joen.2020.03.008
82. Gugnani N, Gugnani S. Safety protocols for dental practices in the COVID-19 era. *Evid Dent.* (2020) 21:56–57. doi: 10.1038/s41432-020-0094-6
83. Carrouel F, Viennot S, Valette M, Cohen JM, Dussart C, Bourgeois D. Salivary and nasal detection of the SARS-CoV-2 virus after antiviral mouthrinses (BBCovid): a structured summary of a study protocol for a randomised controlled trial. *Trials.* (2020) 21:906. doi: 10.1186/s13063-020-04846-6
84. Cavalcante-Leão BL, de Araujo CM, Basso IB, Schroder AG, Guariza-Filho O, Ravazzi GC, et al. Is there scientific evidence of the mouthwashes effectiveness in reducing viral load in Covid-19? A systematic review. *J Clin Exp Dent.* (2021) 13:e179–89. doi: 10.4317/jced.57406
85. Umeh OD, Utomi IL, Isiekwe IG, Aladenika ET. Impact of the coronavirus disease 2019 pandemic on orthodontic patients and their attitude to orthodontic treatment. *Am J Orthod Dentofacial Orthop.* (2021). doi: 10.1016/j.ajodo.2020.11.030
86. Kaur H, Kochhar AS, Gupta H, Singh G, Kubavat A. Appropriate orthodontic appliances during the COVID-19 pandemic: a scoping review. *J Oral Biol Craniofac Res.* (2020) 10:782–7. doi: 10.1016/j.jobcr.2020.10.014
87. To KK, Tsang OT, Yip CC, Chan KH, Wu TC, Chan JM, et al. Consistent detection of 2019 novel coronavirus in Saliva. *Clin Infect Dis.* (2020) 71:841–3. doi: 10.1093/cid/ciaa149
88. Michailidou E, Poulopoulos A, Tzimagiorgis G. Salivary diagnostics of the novel coronavirus SARS-CoV-2 (COVID-19). *Oral Dis.* (2020). doi: 10.1111/odi.13729. [Epub ahead of print].
89. To KKW, Chan KH, Ho J, Pang PKP, Ho DTY, Chang ACH, et al. Respiratory virus infection among hospitalized adult patients with or without clinically apparent respiratory infection: a prospective cohort study. *Clin Microbiol Infect.* (2019) 25:1539–45. doi: 10.1016/j.cmi.2019.04.012
90. European Centre for Disease Prevention and Control, A.a.o.t.E.U. *COVID-19 Situation Update.* Solna (2020).
91. Organization WH. *Coronavirus Disease (COVID-19) Advice for the Public.* Geneva (2020).
92. Canada Go. *Coronavirus Disease (COVID-19): Measures to Reduce COVID-19 in Your Community.* Ottawa, ON (2020).
93. Brian Z, Weintraub JA. Oral Health and COVID-19: increasing the need for prevention and access. *Prev Chronic Dis.* (2020) 17:E82. doi: 10.5888/pcd17.200266
94. Association AD. COVID19 Dental Emergency (2020).
95. Pitones-Rubio V, Chávez-Cortez EG, Hurtado-Camarena A, González-Rascón A, Serafín-Higuera N. Is periodontal disease a risk factor for severe COVID-19 illness? *Med Hypoth.* (2020) 144:109969. doi: 10.1016/j.mehy.2020.109969
96. Li Y, Ren B, Peng X, Hu T, Li J, Gong T, et al. Saliva is a non-negligible factor in the spread of COVID-19. *Mol Oral Microb.* (2020) 35:141–5. doi: 10.1111/omi.12289
97. Samaranayake LP, Reid J, Evans D. The efficacy of rubber dam isolation in reducing atmospheric bacterial contamination. *ASDC J Dent Child.* (1989) 56:442–4.
98. Seneviratne CJ, Balan P, Ko KKK, Udawatte NS, Lai D, Ng DHL, et al. Efficacy of commercial mouth-rinses on SARS-CoV-2 viral load in saliva: randomized control trial in Singapore. *Infection.* (2020). doi: 10.1007/s15010-020-01563-9. [Epub ahead of print].
99. Marui VC, Souto MLS, Rovai ES, Romito GA, Chambrone L, Pannuti CM. Efficacy of preprocedural mouthrinses in the reduction of microorganisms in aerosol: a systematic review. *J Am Dental Assoc.* (2019) 150:1015–1026.e1. doi: 10.1016/j.adaj.2019.06.024
100. Vergara-Buenaventura A, Castro-Ruiz C. Use of mouthwashes against COVID-19 in dentistry. *Br J Oral Maxillofac Surg.* (2020) 58:924–7. doi: 10.1016/j.bjoms.2020.08.016
101. Dai L, Gao GF. Viral targets for vaccines against COVID-19, Nature reviews. *Immunology.* (2021) 21:73–82. doi: 10.1038/s41577-020-00480-0
102. Abdel-Moneim AS, Abdelwhab EM, Memish ZA. Insights into SARS-CoV-2 evolution, potential antivirals, and vaccines. *Virology.* (2021) 558:1–12. doi: 10.1016/j.virol.2021.02.007

10

Remote Management of Prosthodontic Emergencies in the Geriatric Population During the Pandemic Outbreak of COVID-19

Sami Aldhuwayhi [1†], *Saquib Ahmed Shaikh* [1†], *Amar Ashok Thakare* [1†], *Mohammed Ziauddeen Mustafa* [1†] and *Sreekanth Kumar Mallineni* [2,3*†]

[1] Department of Prosthodontics, College of Dentistry, Majmaah University, Al-Majmaah, Saudi Arabia, [2] Department of Preventive Dental Science, College of Dentistry, Majmaah University, Al-Majmaah, Saudi Arabia, [3] Department of Pediatric and Preventive Dentistry, Saveetha Dental College and Hospital, Saveetha Institute of Medical and Technical Science, Saveetha University, Chennai, India

***Correspondence:**
Sreekanth Kumar Mallineni
s.mallineni@mu.edu.sa;
drmallineni@gmail.com

†ORCID:
Sami Aldhuwayhi
orcid.org/0000-0002-0695-0889
Saquib Ahmed Shaikh
orcid.org/0000-0003-0794-8104
Amar Ashok Thakare
orcid.org/0000-0001-7225-100X
Mohammed Ziauddeen Mustafa
orcid.org/0000-0003-1090-1200
Sreekanth Kumar Mallineni
orcid.org/0000-0002-9432-2590

The global pandemic outbreak of coronavirus disease 2019 (COVID-19) has put the world in a panic situation. It has been evident that the geriatric population is more susceptible to acquire this infection. Thus, due to this ongoing crisis, geriatric individuals cannot visit a dental operatory, and there is the possibility of their dental needs and emergencies to remain unattended. Partial or complete edentulism is very prevalent among the geriatric population, and prosthodontic management of these patients is essential for their well-being. However, the prosthesis can lead to various emergencies of the oral and its supporting structures. There are currently no available recommendations to address these prosthodontic emergencies in geriatric individuals during this pandemic period. Hence, the aims of this minireview were to discuss the common prosthodontic emergencies in the geriatric population and provide recommendations to manage these issues during the COVID-19 pandemic outbreak.

Keywords: COVID-19, geriatric dentistry, prosthodontics, portable equipment, teledentistry

INTRODUCTION

The public health crisis has evolved rapidly with the outbreak of novel coronavirus disease 2019 (COVID-19) in Wuhan, China (1), and exponentially, it has spread to all parts of the world. Healthcare providers are at a higher risk of transmission susceptibility of COVID-19 (2, 3); among them, oral healthcare professionals are at the front line. Oral health problems are more likely to be seen in the geriatric age groups than in the other age groups (4, 5). The geriatric population is prone to increased risk from COVID-19 because of psychological and pathological changes, decreased immune function, and existing comorbidity making them more susceptible to COVID-19 (6, 7). The geriatric population and people with severe underlying medical conditions such as diabetes and cardiac or respiratory diseases are at higher risk of developing symptoms of COVID-19 (1, 6). A Chinese study reported that a case fatality was more in older adults of 50 years of age or above (8). Similarly, an Italian study (9) reported that case fatality was more in geriatric patients (36%) compared with younger patients (15%). On the other hand, Ningthoujam and Khomdram (10) postulated that people with chronic health conditions are at the highest risk from COVID-19 and stated that immunity is the key to defense against COVID-19. According to the Malaysian national oral health survey of adults, it has been reported that 50.8% of the elderly aged 60 years and older geriatric patients had some form of oral prosthesis (11). The majority of prosthodontic procedures require direct contact with the patients and indirect contact with dental technicians and dental laboratories for the procedures which include dental casts, dental impressions, fabrication of removable prosthesis, and mock trials (4, 5). The provision of prosthodontic care in geriatric patients could be urgent and/or emergency, depending on the procedure. Some of the emergencies in prosthodontics include provisional restoration debonding, denture adjustments or repairs, prosthetic fractures, and screw loosening in implant prostheses (12–14). There is an impending need to formulate specific guidelines/protocols for managing the geriatric population in the backdrop of COVID-19, considering the physiological, psychological, and treatment needs of geriatric patients, which are unique (4, 5). Nonetheless, the aims of this minireview were to gain an overview of prosthodontic emergencies in the geriatric population and provide recommendations for their management during this pandemic outbreak of COVID-19.

PATIENTS' CLINICAL HANDLING PROTOCOLS

The emergency dental intervention for a COVID-19 suspected patient, when warranted, is that the clinical setup should have negative pressure treatment rooms. The prosthodontist should be aware of the American Dental Association (ADA) recommendations (15). It is mandatory to follow standard airborne and contact protocol by appropriate use of personal protective equipment (PPE) and hand hygiene practices[1]. Prior to the beginning of prosthodontic treatments, 0.23% of povidone-iodine solution mouth rinse for at least 15 s is recommended, and this will help in the reduction of viral load in the patient's saliva (16). The use of single-use and/or disposable instruments and devices is recommended to minimize the cross-contamination of COVID-19 in the dental operatory. The use of a rubberdam will significantly reduce the spread of microbes. Radiographs are generally avoided, and if mandated, the sensor should be double covered to prevent cross-contamination (17). The emphasis on minimally invasive and non-aerosol generating procedures is recommended wherever possible in the dental operatory. The commonly seen prosthodontic emergencies in the geriatric population areas are represented in **Table 1**.

EMERGENCIES RELATED TO PROSTHESIS

Removable Partial Prosthesis

The partial prosthesis can either be made of acrylic resin, cobalt chrome, or a combination. Dentures can fracture in various ways, including the acrylic part, metal substructure, and/or clasps. The patient might present with emergencies when the broken prosthesis causes noticeable discomfort and impingement to the underlying tissues upon wearing. Prosthodontists are recommended to repair the fracture components by laboratory technicians (previous dental master casts if available or with the help of digital impressions); otherwise, the use of prosthesis is suspended if extensive work is required during this pandemic outbreak of COVID-19 to avoid any further emergency (**Table 1**).

Complete Denture Prosthesis

Complete dentures are the most common prosthesis offered to edentulous geriatric patients worldwide (18). Acrylic resin (polymethylmethacrylate) is the material of choice used to manufacture complete dentures, and fracture of the denture is the most common complication associated with it (19). Fracture complete partial dentures may occur due to various reasons such as ill-fit, poor fabrication and design, accidental dropping, parafunction leading to unfavorable stresses, and lack of balanced occlusion (20). Depending on how and where the denture has fractured, the emergency can be managed in various ways. The use of a prosthesis that can cause complications might be avoided till the end of the pandemic period. The virulent effect on acrylic components of the prosthesis is not clearly understood; however, it is better to avoid collecting the prosthesis from the affected geriatric people, and dentists are recommended to send it directly to the dental laboratory for repair. If the denture has a clean break with proper fit and fracture segments are well-located, a laboratory-based repair can be undertaken, provided that the denture is thoroughly disinfected. Sodium hypochlorite exhibited to be the most superior to all the other denture cleansers, and it was suggested that the soaking period is not more than 10 min (21). The dental laboratory technicians should strictly follow the laboratory biosafety protocols (18, 21) and guidelines related to biosafety in surgical pathology (22) while receiving the prosthesis.

Fixed Partial Denture

Cantilever bridges and resin-bonded fixed partial denture (FPD) that are loosened or dislodged can be managed after the pandemic period if the patient is asymptomatic. The hypersensitivity of exposed abutment tooth can be governed by the self-application of silver diamine fluoride (SDF) or casein phosphopeptide amorphous calcium phosphate (CPP-ACP) to the exposed vital abutment tooth (23). Conventional fixed bridge designs that have dislodged on one abutment or one retainer are challenging to diagnose. The patient is aware of the prosthesis movement, but clinically, it is not easy to diagnose for that reason for dislodgement can be parafunction, poor retention form, resistance form and framework design, and incorrect cementation procedure. If one abutment gets dislodged, it can be assessed by informing the patient and caretaker through video communication to gently tie floss underneath the bridge and pull the prosthesis away from the individual abutment teeth. If the patient is asymptomatic, removing the prosthesis can be made after the pandemic period. If the patient is symptomatic, this condition needs to be attended to, and the patient may consult the dentist either by going to his dental practice or *via* portable dentistry where the dentist can offer his services at the patient's residence. The fractured fixed partial prosthesis can cause emergency conditions if the geriatric patient presents with underlying tissue impingement and pain (24). It leads to disturbance in sleep, anxiety and

[1]https://www.cdc.gov/coronavirus/2019-ncov/hcp/infection-control-recommendations.html.

TABLE 1 | Prosthodontic emergency scenarios in the geriatric population and recommendations.

Type of prosthesis	Prosthodontic emergencies	Recommendation
Removable partial denture	If broken or does not fit	• Triaging and teledentistry and suspend the use of the prosthesis to avoid future emergencies
Complete denture	A clean break with reasonably fitting fracture segment	• Triaging and teledentistry and laboratory-based repair by strictly following laboratory biosafety guidelines related to COVID-19
Cantilever bridges resin-bonded fixed partial denture	• Dislodged prostheses usually come out in the hand of a patient • Patient symptomatic with hypersensitivity	• Teledentistry and management after the pandemic period • Application of silver diamine fluoride (SDF) to the exposed vital abutment tooth using the applicator tip
Conventional fixed prosthesis	• Fractured and asymptomatic • Fractured and impinging underlying tissue	• Teledentistry and if asymptomatic the situation can be managed after a pandemic period • Adhering to the American Dental Association, interim guidance for managing emergency dental care and careful removal of the bridge with crown remover
Single or multiple implants supported fixed prosthesis	**Biological emergencies** • Acute peri-implantitis • Asymptomatic failed implants • Symptomatic failed implant	• Pus drainage and debridement under local anesthesia • Managed therapeutically by the AAA protocol (advice, antibiotic, and analgesic) • If symptoms remain, use a local anesthetic to prevent any infection and further bone loss
	Mechanical emergencies Screw loosening and screw fracture	• Retightened with the corresponding screwdriver to the correct torque and retrieving the fractured screw portion is laborious and if possible should be postponed till the deferment period
Implant-supported removable prosthesis	**Biological emergencies** Gingival hyperplasia beneath a bar	• Triaging and teledentistry • Temporarily topical astringents in combination with anesthetic can be used for local application and discontinuation of denture until definitive treatment is done
	Mechanical emergencies • Loosening of attachments • Fracture of acrylic denture	• Can be retightened with specific screwdrivers at the appropriate torque • A fractured acrylic denture is temporarily repaired with repair resins until a new prosthesis can be fabricated later on

depression, a decrease in socialization, cognitive dysfunction, multimedications, malnutrition, and increased healthcare costs that affect the quality of life. If the decision to remove the fracture prosthesis is made, the patient should be informed of the findings and discussed options. An appropriate plan should be put in place to ensure the replacement of the fractured prosthesis with temporization. The dental setup should strictly adhere to the ADA interim guidance to manage emergency dental care (24). The precautionary measures that can be taken when dealing with a prosthodontic emergency are as follows:

- Use of anti-retraction functional dental handpiece, four-handed dentistry with high vacuum saliva ejectors.
- Cleaning of handpieces after each patient to remove debris followed by autoclave.
- Prior to treatment, mouth rinse with 0.2% povidone-iodine or 1.5% hydrogen peroxide.
- Frequently clean and disinfect the reception areas, including waiting rooms, door handles, chairs, and washrooms.
- Accompanying persons of the patient should be made to wait outside the reception area or in the car parking.
- Clinic staff should maintain a list of patients who are suspected of COVID-19 infection.
- The following techniques can be used for removing fracture FPD or partially dislodged bridges causing tissue impingement:
- Gentle tapping of the fractured prosthesis using crown removers and avoid using ultrasonic scalers or WAM key to loosen the cement as it generates aerosol.
- Partially dislodged resin-bonded FPD can be removed by placing the sharp chisel's tip.
- The prosthesis should be secured with dental floss held outside the dental assistant's mouth to reduce the risk of inhalation or swallowing the prosthesis.
- FPD can be sectioned with an anti-retraction functional dental handpiece using special diamond cutting burs and removed.

Before planning for removing the fractured prosthesis, the putty index is made to facilitate the fabrication of temporization. Once the dislodged prosthesis is removed, the underlying abutment tooth and tissue are assessed to ensure they are sound and suitable for temporization.

Single or Multiple Implant-Supported Fixed Prostheses

The often occurring biological emergency after prosthesis fabrication includes peri-implantitis and mobile implant fixtures. Acute peri-implantitis usually presents as painful and fluctuant swelling in the dental implant region, which is an emergency and often is managed by careful debridement under local anesthesia and antibiotic coverage (25, 26). Asymptomatic failed implants can be managed primarily by the AAA protocol (advice, antibiotic, and analgesic) until a substantial diagnosis, and treatment planning should be formulated in the clinical setup after the pandemic period (27, 28). Symptomatic failed implants are recommended to be removed under local anesthesia to prevent further infection and bone loss (29). The common mechanical emergencies include suprastructure prosthesis components such as fixed restorations including lost access cavity restoration and loose implant-supported crown/bridge. In lost access cavity restoration, the patient complains of food entrapment, halitosis, and unesthetic appearance of the prosthesis. Although this situation does not warrant an immediate dental clinic visit, especially during a pandemic outbreak, it can lead to much discomfort to the patient. The patient can procure a temporary restoration on an e-commerce platform such as Amazon, which still allows fast shipment or can be supplied by the dentist. Utilizing teledentistry, the patients' accompanying person can be guided by the dentist. Loose implant-supported crown/bridge mainly happens most commonly because of screw loosening and screw fracture (30). It is classified under emergencies as the patient experiences functional impairment and pain due to the impingement of underlying tissues. Screw loosening can be retightened with the corresponding screwdriver. Worn-out screws are a frequent problem with a screw-retained prosthesis; hence, it is advisable to use a new screw to reduce further fracture risk. The process of retrieving the fractured screw portion is laborious (29) and, if possible, should be postponed. In the event of failure of a luting agent, the previous cement from the crown and abutment can be removed, and the abutment' screw hole can be protected with polytetrafluoroethylene (PTFE) tape or cotton wool, followed by recementation of the crown (30).

Removable Implant-Supported Prosthesis

Prosthodontic complications commonly occur with a removable implant-supported prosthesis, ranging from loss of retention of attachment systems to loosening of screws (31). Biological emergencies usually include gingival hyperplasia beneath a bar, which can lead to failure of the denture to the seat. It often requires a comprehensive clinical and radiographical examination followed by removal of excessive soft tissue surgically. However, for a temporary measure, topical astringents combined with anesthetic can be used for local application and discontinuation of denture until definitive treatment is done. Mechanical emergencies prevent a patient from using their prosthesis due to loss of retention of the attachment system (25) caused by problems with the components in the denture and fracture of the acrylic denture base. Loose attachments present with significant discomfort for the patients due to the attachment system's mobile male counterpart. It can be simply managed by retightening with specific screwdrivers at appropriate torque. Loss of retention due to worn-out female counterparts of the attachment system usually requires replacing the female component. The replacement procedure is not an emergency and can be postponed until normalcy returns in dental practice. A fractured acrylic denture is another complication that commonly occurs and can be temporarily repaired with repair resins until a new prosthesis can be fabricated later.

Maxillofacial Prosthesis

Geriatric patients using maxillofacial prosthesis are relatively less compared with other age groups (32). However, the maxillofacial prosthesis significantly impacts the quality of life in the geriatric population (33). The common complications with such prosthesis are loss of retention and prosthesis ill-fit due to surgical site remodeling. Patients who have recently undergone maxillofacial surgery usually have a prefabricated obturator or get a temporary obturator immediately after the surgery in the hospital setup. Such patients can be advised to continue using the same until the pandemic ends (34). A recently inserted definitive obturator may cause discomfort; in such cases, a telephone consultation can help. If the problem persists, it is advised limiting the use of prostheses only while eating. In severe discomfort, it is advised to discontinue the use. Maxillofacial prosthesis requires adhesives for retention, and it can be purchased online. Any other issue related to wear and tear of the prosthesis can be addressed after the pandemic.

Role of Teledentistry for the Management of Dental Problems in Geriatric Patients

It is essential to use a teledentistry model prior to planning an appointment with geriatric patients. A choice can be made to postpone the routine prosthodontic appointment, but the patient needs to be assured and followed up for experiencing discomfort or problems related to their prosthesis. The first step of managing prosthodontic problems encountered in geriatric emergencies during these COVID-19 situations should always be virtual assistance by "WhatsApp" or "Messenger" or "Instagram" or "Skype." A message with photographs, a video recording, or a video call could be the best option for an initial evaluation in the present COVID-19 pandemic situation (**Figure 1**). This model was adopted and developed base don using a model proposed recently by Nuvvula and Mallineni (35). The healthcare provider should be trained to use modern web-based communication with patients' assessment using a teledentistry model to avoid potential transmission of COVID-19 (15). After the geriatric patients' virtual screening, it is planned to divide the patients into five groups based on COVID-19 and five groups based on treatment needs. Based on signs and symptoms, patients are divided into five groups (See Footnote 1) [(i) asymptomatic/unsuspected/unconfirmed COVID-19 cases, (ii) symptomatic and suspected/unconfirmed COVID-19 cases, (iii) stable confirmed COVID-19 cases, (iv) unstable confirmed COVID-19 cases, and (v) recovered confirmed COVID-19 cases].

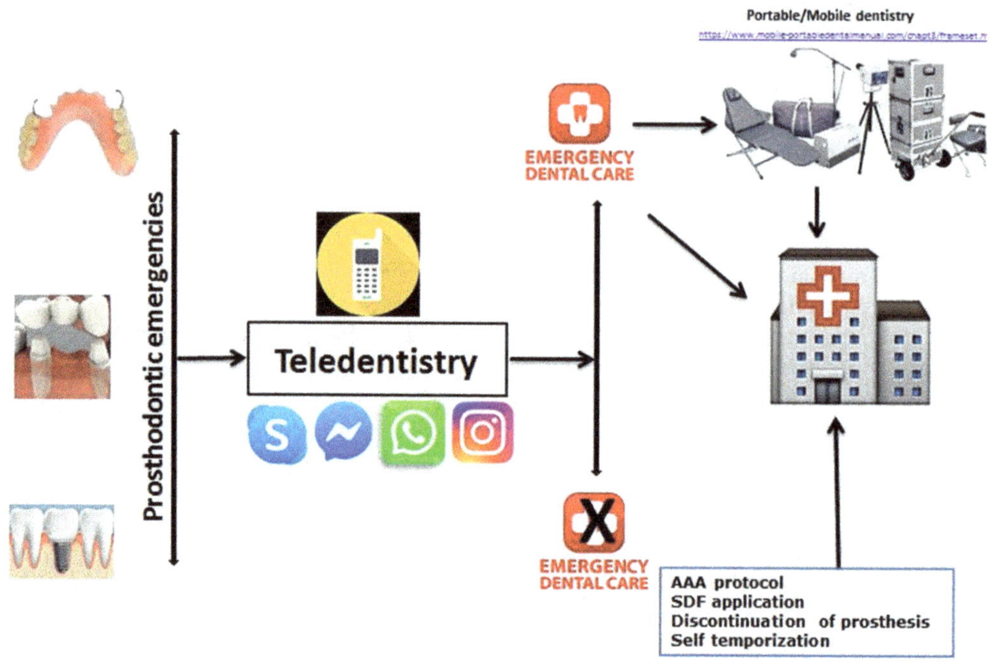

FIGURE 1 | Proposed model for the management of prosthodontic problems in geriatric patients.

DISCUSSION

The global pandemic outbreak of COVID-19 has increased the likelihood that the dental care professional should also take precautionary measures to minimize the spread. These measures include careful prescreening of the patient in a confirmed COVID-19 patient is highly obligatory. The common complications are discomfort due to faulty or fractured prosthesis in geriatric patients. On appointments, there may be a higher chance that clinicians might encounter asymptomatic/symptomatic patients. To assess and manage such patients, it might be possible to use a teledentistry model with the suggested questions as described in this short communication. Advancement in technology and social media has made communication easy, and it can be used as an appropriate tool in such pandemic outbreak situations to manage geriatric patients. Furthermore, the use of the recommended questionnaire *via* the teledentistry model has a vital role in approaching geriatric patients (**Figure 1**). The incubation period of COVID-19 ranges from 2 to 24 days, and most of the patients develop only mild symptoms (15). Consequently, all patients visiting for the management of such emergencies are potential carriers, and the clinicians are advised to follow standard infection control protocols. Radiographs are essential aids in diagnosing dental problems along with clinical examination (36). Radiography should be kept very simple to diminish patient-to-staff contact while providing diagnostic quality radiographs[2] Intraoral radiographs could be avoided to prevent potential aerosol exposure, and extraoral bitewings were suggested to be appropriate substitutes to the sectional panoramic radiographs as they offer quality images with low radiation (36). However, the authors opine that radiographs are based on essential, but the majority of the emergencies in prosthodontics other than the emergencies related to implants could be solved with recommendations discussed in this minireview. The teledentistry approach plays an essential role in the management of prosthodontic emergencies.

Geriatric patients staying in nursing homes, private homes, or institutions have practical difficulties in reaching the dental office. Henceforth, domiciliary dental care services like mobile dentistry could be used for treating such patients (37–39) by following PPE guidelines (2, 7). In mobile dentistry, the instruments, materials, and equipment can be transferred from the dental office to the patients' location to offer timely care (38). This approach, coupled with meticulous attention to instrument disinfection and application of barrier protection, can be considered a viable treatment option for handling dental emergencies in the geriatric population. Care can be limited to the basic requirements to ensuring that the patient should be pain- and infection-free, which includes treating the emergency, affecting their quality of life (40, 41). Management of biological emergencies, as discussed, can be managed with the help of this portable dentistry approach. Similarly, denture repairs, adding teeth to existing complete or partial dentures, and relining of dentures do not require extensive equipment and can be performed at the patient's residence (40, 41). In this work, the guidelines put forward are general, prosthodontic recommendations, and

[2]https://www.fgdp.org.uk/implications-covid-19-safe-management-general-dental-practice-practical-guide.

the final decision will always be the critical insight into the practitioner's judgment to manage geriatric patients during this pandemic outbreak. On the other hand, treatment can be postponed, and pharmacologic management (AAA protocol) for the pain (27, 28) and infection can always be considered (42). The practitioner should always consider the case and treatment categorization based on the recommendations that were suggested. The prosthodontic emergencies in the geriatric population cause an additional burden to those who are already suffering from one or other comorbidities. It is always advisable for the prosthodontist to evaluate these emergencies case by case and use the clinical acumen to aid in decision-making. Therefore, these recommendations help oral healthcare providers treat prosthodontic emergencies in geriatric patients during this pandemic period. Negative ion generators and high-efficiency particulate air (HEPA) filters have also shown a potential reduction of viral load in the dental operatory. The use of these two aids in dental practice may not reduce 100% of the risk of COVID-19 disease transmission in the dental operatory. However, it can assuredly minimize the chance of aerosols generated by dental procedures. In comparison with other dental clinical specialties, very nominal emergency situations occur in the prosthodontics department, and specific treatment could be delayed and does not necessarily need hurried attention. Therefore, the recommendations that are provided in this paper could serve as a guide for older adults with prosthodontic problems and also for general dental practitioners that practice prosthodontics. Consequently, the prosthodontist must visualize the clinic's protective needs as a general dentist and not just as a specialist. This present review gives awareness to the dentists to provide recommendations to prepare them with PPE and the provision of essential emergency treatments to geriatric populations with prosthesis issues.

CONCLUSIONS

The prudent method to manage prosthodontic emergencies in geriatric individuals during a pandemic is to reassure, comfort, motivate, and follow the patient remotely while they are in their home through web-based communications.

Teledentistry and/or mobile dentistry could be considered in the remote management of all prosthodontic non-emergency and emergencies. In emergency cases, teledentistry, along with portable or mobile dentistry, can be recommended with PPE managing geriatric individuals during this pandemic to avoid potential transmission of COVID-19.

AUTHOR CONTRIBUTIONS

SA and SS developed the concept. MM, AT, and SM wrote the first draft. SM designed the figure. All authors were involved in reviewing and editing the manuscript.

ACKNOWLEDGMENTS

The authors would like to thank the Deanship of Scientific Research at Majmaah University for supporting this work under Project Number No. R-2021-147.

REFERENCES

1. Dong E, Du H, Gardner L. An interactive web-based dashboard to track COVID-19 in real time. *Lancet Infect Dis.* (2020) 20:533–4. doi: 10.1016/S1473-3099(20)30120-1
2. Peng X, Xu X, Li Y, Cheng L, Zhou X, Ren B. Transmission routes of 2019-nCoV and controls in dental practice. *Int J Oral Sci.* (2020) 12:9. doi: 10.1038/s41368-020-0075-9
3. Bhumireddy J, Mallineni SK, Nuvvula S. Challenges and possible solutions in dental practice during and post COVID-19. *Environ Sci Pollut Res Int.* (2020) 28:1275–7. doi: 10.1007/s11356-020-10983-x
4. Sa Y, Lin WS, Morton D, Huang C. Coronavirus disease 2019 (COVID-19): experiences and protocols from the Department of Prosthodontics at the Wuhan University. *J Prosthet Dent.* (2020) S0022-3913(20)30374-7. doi: 10.1016/j.prosdent.2020.06.004. [Epub ahead of print].
5. Sivaraman K, Chopra A, Narayana A, Radhakrishnan RA. A five-step risk management process for geriatric dental practice during SARS-CoV-2 pandemic. *Gerodontology.* (2020) 38:17–26. doi: 10.1111/ger.12499
6. Gill TM, Allore HG, Holford TR, Guo Z. Hospitalization, restricted activity, and the development of disability among older persons. *J Am Geriatr Soc.* (2004) 292:2115–24. doi: 10.1001/jama.292.17.2115
7. Mallineni SK, Innes NP, Raggio DP, Araujo MP, Robertson MD, Jayaraman J. Coronavirus disease (COVID-19): characteristics in children and considerations for dentists providing their care. *Int J Paediatr Dent.* (2020) 30:245–50. doi: 10.1111/ipd.12653
8. Porcheddu R, Serra C, Kelvin D, Kelvin N, Rubino S. Similarity in case fatality rates (CFR) of COVID-19/SARS-COV-2 in Italy and China. *J Infect Dev Ctries.* (2020) 14:125–8. doi: 10.3855/jidc.12600
9. Grasselli G, Zangrillo A, Zanella A, Antonelli M, Cabrini L, Castelli A, et al. COVID-19 Lombardy ICU Network. Baseline characteristics and outcomes of 1591 patients infected with SARS-CoV-2 admitted to ICUs of the Lombardy region, Italy. *JAMA.* (2020) 323:1574–81. doi: 10.1001/jama.2020.5394
10. Ningthoujam R, Khomdram D. WHO statement - "Older people are at highest risk from COVID-19": should the hypothesis be corroborated or rejected? *Med Hypotheses.* (2020) 144:109896. doi: 10.1016/j.mehy.2020.109896
11. Oral Health Division and Oral Healthcare in Malaysia. Ministry of Health Malaysia. (2005). Available online at: https://www.mah.se/upload/FAKULTETER/OD/Avdelningar/who/WPRO/Malaysia/data/oral_healthcare_in_malaysia_05.pdf (accessed September 7, 2020).
12. Issrani R, Ammanagi R, Keluskar V. Geriatric dentistry – meet the need. *Gerodontology.* (2012) 29:e1–5. doi: 10.1111/j.1741-2358.2010.00423.x
13. Barenghi L, Barenghi A, Cadeo C, Di Blasio A. Innovation by computer-aided design/computer-aided manufacturing technology: a look at infection prevention in dental settings. *BioMed Res Int.* (2019) 2019:6092018. doi: 10.1155/2019/6092018
14. Batista AUD, Silva PLPD, Melo LA, Carreiro ADFP. Prosthodontic practice during the COVID-19 pandemic: prevention and implications. *Braz Oral Res.* (2021) 35:e049. doi: 10.1590/1807-3107bor-2021.vol35.0049
15. *ADA Recommending Dentists Postpone Elective Procedures* (2021). Available online at: https://www.ada.org/en/publications/ada-news/2020-archive/march/adarecommending-entists-postpone-elective-procedures (accessed April 20, 2021).
16. Eggers M, Koburger-Janssen T, Eickmann M, Zorn J. *In vitro* bactericidal and virucidal efficacy of povidone-iodine gargle/mouthwash against respiratory and oral tract pathogens. *Infect Dis Ther.* (2018) 7:249–59. doi: 10.1007/s40121-018-0200-7
17. *Disinfectants for Coronavirus (COVID-19)* (2020). Available online at: https://www.epa.gov/pesticide-registration/list-n-disinfectants-coronavirus-covid-19 (accessed November 24, 2020).

18. Roessler DM. Complete denture success for patients and dentists. *Int Dent J.* (2003) 53:340–5. doi: 10.1111/j.1875-595X.2003.tb00908.x
19. Huggett R, Harrison A, Darbar UR. Denture fracture–a survey. *Br Dent J.* (1994) 176:342–5. doi: 10.1038/sj.bdj.4808449
20. Vallittu PK. An overview of development and status of fiber-reinforced composites as dental and medical biomaterials. *Acta Biomater Odontol Scand.* (2018) 4:44–55. doi: 10.1080/23337931.2018.1457445
21. Felton D, Cooper L, Duqum I, Minsley G, Guckes A, Haug S, et al. Evidence based guidelines for the care and maintenance of complete dentures: a publication of the American College of Prosthodontists. *J Prosthodont.* (2011) 20:S1–12. doi: 10.1111/j.1532-849X.2010.00683.x
22. Barbareschi M, Ascoli V, Bonoldi E, Cavazza A, Colombari R, Cozzi I, et al. Biosafety in surgical pathology in the era of SARS-Cov2 pandemia. A statement of the Italian Society of Surgical Pathology and Cytology. *Pathologica.* (2020) 112:59–63. doi: 10.32074/1591-951X-14-20
23. Nuvvula S, Mallineni SK. Silver diamine fluoride in pediatric dentistry. *J South Asian Assoc Pediatr Dent.* (2019) 2:73–80. doi: 10.5005/jp-journals-10077-3024
24. Kaye AD, Baluch A, Scott JT. Pain management in the elderly population: a review. *Ochsner J.* (2010) 10:179–87.
25. Zitzmann NU, Berglundh T. Definition and prevalence of peri-implant diseases. *J Clin Periodontol.* (2008) 35:286–91. doi: 10.1111/j.1600-051X.2008.01274.x
26. Kalsi H, Rodriguez JM, Darbar U, Bavisha K. The emergency dental appointment: restorative emergencies Part 2 - dental implant related problems. *Prim Dent J.* (2017) 6:62–70. doi: 10.1308/205016817821281792
27. *British Endodontic Society Information and Advice on Triage and Management for Primary Dental Care and Other Healthcare Providers During the COVID-19 Pandemic.* Available online at: https://www.nhsggc.org.uk/media/259571/bes-aaa-document-final-document-29-march-2020.pdf (accessed on 15th April, 2021)
28. Modgill O, Patel G, Akintola D, Obisesan O, Tagar H. AAA: a rock and a hard place. *Br Dent J.* (2021) 21:1–5. doi: 10.1038/s41415-020-2594-3
29. Goodacre CJ, Bernal G, Rungcharassaeng K, Kan JY. Clinical complications with implants and implant prostheses. *J Prosthet Dent.* (2003) 90:121–32. doi: 10.1016/S0022-3913(03)00212-9
30. Guzaitis KL, Knoernschild KL, Viana MA. Effect of repeated screw joint closing and opening cycles on implant prosthetic screw reverse torque and implant and screw thread morphology. *J Prosthet Dent.* (2011) 106:159–69. doi: 10.1016/S0022-3913(11)60115-7
31. Ülkü SZ, Acun Kaya F, Uysal E, Gulsun B. Clinical evaluation of complications in implant-supported dentures: a 4-year retrospective study. *Med Sci Monit.* (2017) 23:6137–43. doi: 10.12659/MSM.907840
32. Mozafari PM, Amirchaghmaghi M, Moeintaghavi A, Khajedaluee M, Dorri M, Koohestanian N, et al. Oral health related quality of life in a group of geriatrics. *J Clin Diagn Res.* (2015) 9:ZC52–5. doi: 10.7860/JCDR/2015/14345.6816
33. Nemli SK, Aydin C, Yilmaz H, Bal BT, Arici YK. Quality of life of patients with implant-retained maxillofacial prostheses: a prospective and retrospective study. *J Prosthet Dent.* (2013) 109:44–52. doi: 10.1016/S0022-3913(13)60010-4
34. Pruthi G, Parkash H, Bharathi PV, Jain R, Gupta A, Rai S. Comprehensive review of guidelines to practice prosthodontic and implant procedures during COVID-19 pandemic. *J Oral Biol Craniofac Res.* (2020) 10:768–75. doi: 10.1016/j.jobcr.2020.10.010
35. Nuvvula S, Mallineni SK. Remote management of dental problems in children during and post the COVID-19 pandemic outbreak: a teledentistry approach. *Dent Med Probl.* (2021). doi: 10.17219/dmp/133182
36. Little R, Howell J, Nixon P. COVID-19 and beyond: implications for dental radiography. *Br Dent J.* (2020) 229:105–9. doi: 10.1038/s41415-020-1842-x
37. Henry RG, Ceridan B. Delivering dental care to nursing home and homebound patients. *Dent Clin North Am.* (1994) 38:537–51.
38. Bee JF. Portable dentistry: a part of general dentistry's service mix. *Gen Dent.* (2004) 52:520–6.
39. Mallineni SK, Bhumireddy JC, Nuvvula S. Dentistry for children during and post COVID-19 pandemic outbreak. *Child Youth Serv Rev.* (2021) 120:105734. doi: 10.1016/j.childyouth.2020.105734
40. Lee EE, Thomas CA. Mobile and portable dentistry: alternative treatment services for the elderly. *Spec Care Dentist.* (2001) 21:153–5. doi: 10.1111/j.1754-4505.2001.tb00245.x
41. Nazliel HE, Hersek N, Ozbek M, Karaagaoglu E. Oral health status in a group of the elderly population residing at home. *Gerodontology.* (2012) 29:e761–7. doi: 10.1111/j.1741-2358.2011.00556.x
42. Papi P, Di Murro B, Penna D, Pompa G. Digital prosthetic workflow during COVID-19 pandemic to limit infection risk in dental practice. *Oral Dis Suppl.* (2021) 3:723–6. doi: 10.1111/odi.13442

11

The Role of Dentists in COVID-19 is Beyond Dentistry: Voluntary Medical Engagements and Future Preparedness

Chaminda Jayampath Seneviratne [1,2], Matthew Wen Jian Lau [1] and Bee Tin Goh [1,2]*

[1] National Dental Research Institute Singapore, National Dental Centre Singapore, Singapore, Singapore, [2] Duke-NUS Graduate Medical School, Singapore, Singapore

***Correspondence:**
Chaminda Jayampath Seneviratne
jaya.seneviratne@ndcs.com.sg

The emergence of the highly infectious novel coronavirus SARS-CoV-2 has led to a global COVID-19 pandemic. Since the outbreak of COVID-19, worldwide healthcare systems have been severely challenged. The rapid and explosive surge of positive cases has significantly increased the demand for medical care. Herein we provide a perspective on the role dentists can play in voluntary medical assistance and future preparedness for a similar pandemic. Though dentists and physicians have different scopes of practice, their trainings share many similarities. Hence, dental professionals, with their knowledge of basic human science and sterile surgical techniques, are an invaluable resource in the COVID-19 pandemic response. Overall, it is commendable that many dentists have risen to the challenge in the fight against COVID-19. For example, in Singapore, National Dental Centre Singapore (NDCS) deployed dental clinicians as well as volunteers from research laboratories to screen for suspected cases, provide consultations as well as conduct swabbing operations. Dental practice will be considerably changed in the post-COVID-19 era. There is a greater need to have refresher courses for practicing dentists on new infection control strategies. Moreover, the curriculum in dental schools should be expanded to include competencies in pandemic and disaster relief. In addition, voluntary medical work should be made a part of the community dentistry curriculum. This volunteerism will leave a positive impact on developing the careers of young dentists. Hence, the contribution of dentists beyond dental practice in this pandemic situation will be appreciated by future generations.

Keywords: COVID-19, dentistry, voluntary work, preparedness, infection control

BACKGROUND

The emergence of the highly infectious novel coronavirus has led to a global pandemic in a span of just 3 months. It was only on 31 December 2019 that first reports of pneumonia of an unknown cause detected in Wuhan, China, began to surface to the World Health Organization (WHO). Provisionally named as 2019 novel coronavirus (2019-nCoV), there was evidence of exponential human-to-human transmission in the early outbreak stage (1–3). Consequently, on 30 January 2020, the WHO declared the outbreak a Public Health Emergency of International Concern (PHEIC). Subsequently, assessment by the Coronavirus Study Group (CSG) of the International

Committee on Taxonomy of Viruses found that SARS-CoV-2 clusters phytogenetically with the species *Severe acute respiratory syndrome-related coronavirus* (SARS-CoVs) and genus *Betacoronavirus*, and formally designated it as *Severe acute respiratory syndrome coronavirus 2* (SARS-CoV-2) (4). CSG also emphasized that the name SARS-CoV-2 has no relationship to the name of the SARS disease caused by SARS CoV-1. In fact, the SARS CoV-2 genome shares only 79.6% similarity to that of SARS-CoV-1 (5). The initial sequencing of the new coronavirus revealed that it is closely related to betacoronaviruses of bat origin i.e., bat-SL-CoVZC45 (87.99% similarity) and bat-SL-CoVZXC21 (87.23% similarity) (5). More recent genome sequencing showed that a bat coronavirus BatCoV RaTG13 originally found in the bat *Rhinolophus affinis* from Yunnan Province, China has 96.2% genome similarly to that of SARS CoV-2 (6). These foregoing studies indicate that the bats are the likely zoonotic reservoir host for SARS CoV-2. Although bats may be the original source of the new coronavirus, it is assumed to be transmitted to humans via an intermediate host, possibly pangolins or wild animals currently yet unknown (7). On 11 February 2020, the WHO announced coronavirus disease 2019 (COVID-19) to be the disease caused by SARS-CoV-2. Subsequently, many countries continued to experience clusters of cases and community transmissions. This led the WHO to declare the COVID-19 outbreak a pandemic on 12 March 2020.

GLOBAL HAVOC CAUSED BY COVID-19

As of 26 July 2020, more than 15.78 million confirmed cases of COVID-19 and 640,016 associated deaths have been reported worldwide (8). With the number of infected cases surging each day, researchers are racing to understand what makes it spread so easily. From the evidence so far, the transmission of SARS-CoV-2 can occur via respiratory droplets, contact and aerosols (9). A major factor facilitating the transmission of COVID-19 is the high level of SARS-CoV-2 shedding in the upper respiratory tract, even among pre-symptomatic patients (10). It has been reported that pharyngeal virus shedding of SARS-CoV-2 reaches its peak on day 4 of symptoms onset, and it can be over 1,000 times higher than SARS-CoV-1 (11). Numerous cases have been reported wherein patients who had positive test results were asymptomatic at testing (12). Moreover, the asymptomatic incubation period for infected individuals could be ~1–14 days in general, although longer incubation periods as long as 24 days have been reported. Thus, symptom-based screening alone may have failed to detect a high number of COVID-19 positive cases and most likely contributed to the rampant transmission.

IMPACT OF COVID-19 ON HEALTHCARE PROVIDERS

Since the outbreak of COVID-19, worldwide healthcare systems have been severely challenged. The rapid and explosive surge of positive cases have led to a significant increase in the demand for medical care. On the infrastructure front, hospitals have actively scaled up their capacity of basic and critical care beds. However, global medical manpower resources are finite. Consequently, many hospital-based healthcare workers have had to work overhours and take on extra shifts. Such stressors have been associated with reduced job performance and fatigue-related errors which could harm patients (13). In responding to this crisis with a multi-sectorial, equitable and human-rights focused approach, the United Nations entities have called for voluntary support from professionals with medical backgrounds for various job capacities to manage the pandemic (14).

ARE DENTISTS EQUIPPED TO SUPPORT WORKFORCE WORKING AGAINST COVID-19?

Though dentists and physicians have different scopes of practice, their trainings share many similarities. The dental student, like his medical counterpart, has to attain proficiency in his understanding of the basic sciences such as anatomy, physiology, pharmacology, and microbiology. This is essential given that dentists are expected to competently manage dental issues of medically compromised patients. Moreover, dentists must be able to expeditiously and effectively manage medical emergencies that may arise in routine dental practice. To this end, many dental practitioners would have undergone basic cardiac life support training. Thus, the robust training of clinical medicine in dentistry strengthens the candidature of dentists to volunteer services for COVID-19 control and spread.

The outbreak of COVID-19 has significantly affected the practice of dentistry. Dental treatment can generate large amounts of aerosols and droplets mixed with the patient's saliva or blood (15). This poses a risk to dental professionals as SARS-CoV-2 has been detected in saliva of infected individuals (16). Many dentists have therefore discontinued the provision of elective dental treatment, in accordance with guidelines released by national-level government healthcare authorities such as the Centers for Disease Control and Prevention (CDC) in the US and National Health Service (NHS) in the UK. Only limited cases that require urgent or emergency dental care continue to be seen. The significantly reduced workload during this time, coupled with robust training in a medical setting, makes the dentist a prime candidate to volunteer in the fight against COVID-19.

HOW CAN THE DENTAL FRATERNITY PLAY THEIR PART IN THE CURRENT CRISIS?

Dental professionals, with their knowledge of basic human science and sterile surgical techniques, are an invaluable resource in the COVID-19 pandemic response. Licensed dentists are eligible to administer COVID-19 diagnostic tests such as nasopharyngeal and oropharyngeal swabs. With their detailed understanding of head and neck anatomy, dentists are well placed to perform such procedures accurately and atraumatically. This is imperative as irritation to the oral or nasal mucosa while swabbing risks the patient sneezing or coughing, potentially releasing contaminated droplets and aerosols to the environment.

TABLE 1 | Key considerations and recommendations on how dental fraternity can play their part in the current crisis and recommendations for dental implementation in post-COVID-19 era.

Key considerations	Recommendations
How dental fraternity can play their part in the current crisis	Administer COVID-19 diagnostic tests • Nasopharyngeal swabs • Oropharyngeal swabs • Salivary sampling
	Volunteer appropriately equipped dental clinics as screening facility • Negative pressure rooms • High-volume excavators
	Assist medical counterparts in the inpatient setting
	Develop online platforms to promote oral hygiene and oral health maintenance
Recommendations for dental implementation in post-COVID-19 era	Revise and strengthen education on infection control measures in dental practice
	Dental education should include competencies in pandemic and disaster relief • Training to administer COVID-19 diagnostic tests • Training to be part of an effective surveillance network
	Include voluntary medical work in the community dentistry curriculum
	Organize refresher courses for practicing dentists on infection control and best practices

Unlike negative-pressure rooms, many makeshift medical screening facilities are unable to limit the aerosol spread of SARS-CoV-2. This may lead to contamination of open-air healthcare facilities. In this context, dental clinics that are well equipped with facilities to control aerosol spread of infections, such as negative pressure rooms and high-volume excavators, can offer help to augment the capacity for COVID-19 screening. In this regard, global health authorities as well as health ministries from the respective countries have provided clear standard infection control procedures for dentists (17–19).

Dentists can also assist their medical counterparts in the inpatient setting. Such duties include patient triage, monitoring vital signs, administering oxygen and injectables, and writing prescriptions. Should emergency procedures need to be performed, dentists are capable of administering local anesthesia and suturing. In addition, oral surgeons and dentist anesthesiologists are competent in performing intubation, deep sedation and general anesthesia services (20).

The COVID-19 outbreak as well as harsh lock down practices worldwide have created a stressful environment for many people globally. Such stressful situations have been shown to lead to poor oral health (21, 22). Therefore, oral healthcare professionals should consider developing online platforms to provide information on oral hygiene and oral health maintenance. Digitalized healthcare services can be implemented with a qualified team of dentists being available online to provide reliable oral healthcare solutions in an accessible, affordable and appropriate manner and allay patients' dental concerns during the lockdown period. Oral healthcare professionals can also engage in voluntary service for residents in community housing to promote good oral health. The recommendations on how the dental fraternity can play their part in the current crisis are summarized in **Table 1**.

EVIDENCE REPORTS OF VOLUNTEERING ACTS BY DENTISTS ON THE GLOBAL FOREFRONT

In Singapore, while limited community transmission of COVID-19 remains, there has been a rapid surge in the number of infected cased among foreign workers living in dormitories. Such facilities become conducive for rapid spread of SARS-CoV-2 as residents are housed in close proximity and share many common amenities. In a whole-of-government approach to isolate and eradicate the virus, the Singapore government implemented aggressive mass-scale testing for COVID-19 for foreign workers residing in dormitories. This major operation was undertaken by multiple agencies including Singapore Health Services (SingHealth), Singapore Police Force and Singapore Armed Forces. Supporting this move, National Dental Centre Singapore (NDCS) deployed dental clinicians as well as volunteers from research laboratories to the foreign worker dormitories to conduct swab operations. All patients were treated as suspect cases, and all volunteers observed universal precautions and donned appropriate personal protective equipment (PPE). The use of specially manufactured swab booths further minimized the risk of cross-infection between patients and volunteers (**Figure 1**). In this massive operation, NDCS staff worked collaboratively with colleagues across various professional backgrounds including clinicians, nurses, pharmacists, radiographers, and medical social workers (**Figure 2**). Without the cohesive and coordinated effort, it would have been a considerable task to successfully establish and staff the field swab clinics within a short period of time.

In the UK, dentists, dental support teams as well as clinical academics have played a vital role in supporting the NHS (23). For instance, there are news reports that dental staff from Bath Health NHS Trust and QMUL Institute of Dentistry are helping in maternity, critical care, and emergency units. Dental hospitals have undergone reconfiguration to support medical care. In the US, dentist volunteers in states such as Virginia and California have responded to appeals to assist with critical emergency care needs, and have been redeployed to the frontlines. Importantly, states such as California have made changes to their law to allow greater flexibility in scope and licensure in the time of a catastrophic emergency. The law provides immunity from liability for care provided "in good faith" during an emergency for a person who "voluntarily and without compensation or expectations of compensation, and consistent with the dental education and emergency training that he or she has received,

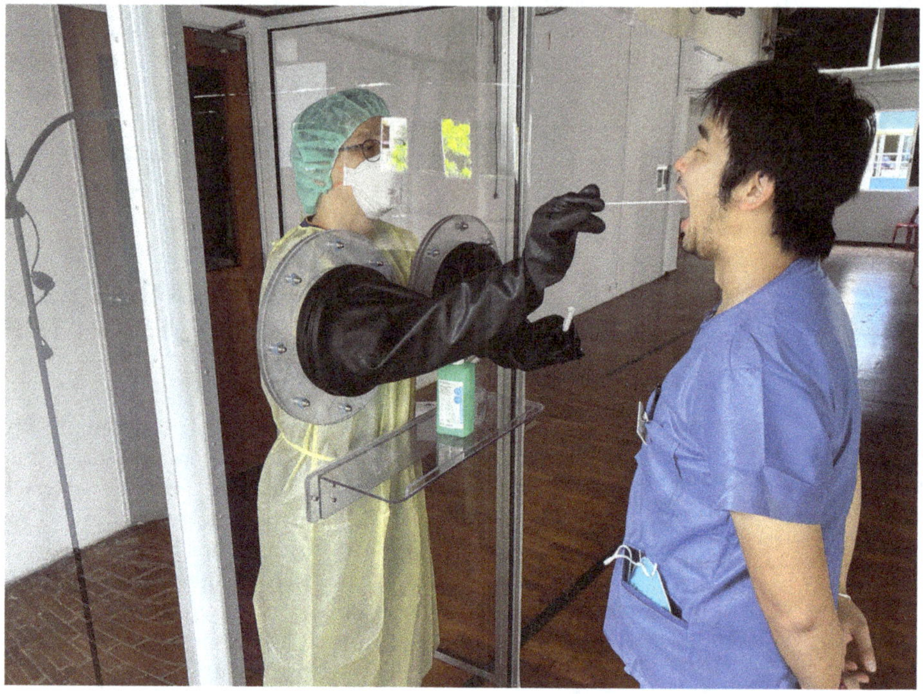

FIGURE 1 | Dental clinicians from National Dental Centre Singapore were trained to conduct swab procedure using swab booths manufactured in Singapore (Photo credit: National Dental Centre Singapore).

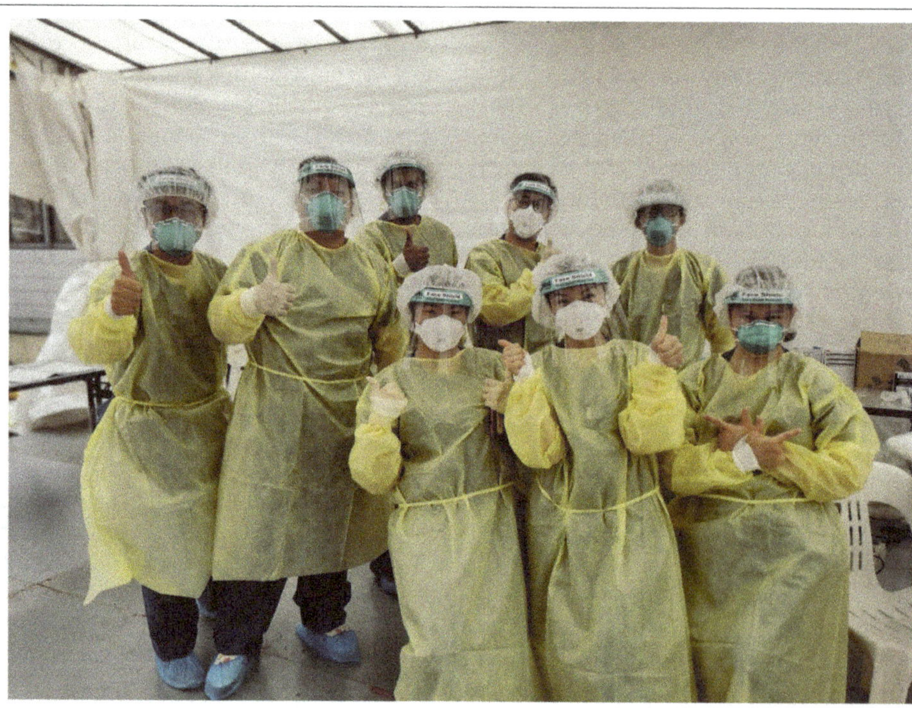

FIGURE 2 | A team of Singapore Health Services (SingHealth) volunteers assigned to manage a medical clinic at a foreign workers' dormitory in Singapore. This team included a neurologist, a dental scientist, a pharmacologist, a cancer patient service associate, a radiographer and nurses (Photo credit: National Dental Centre Singapore).

provides emergency medical care to a person during a state of emergency." This would be an important consideration for other countries to follow.

RECOMMENDATIONS FOR DENTAL IMPLEMENTATION IN POST-COVID-19 ERA

COVID-19 has been an unprecedented experience for mankind. The scale and extent of the pandemic has forced many governments to take drastic and decisive action, resulting in considerable disruption in daily life and damage to global economies. This episode has revealed the need to be better prepared for future pandemics. To this end, educational institutions can take the lead. Dental schools should revise and strengthen education on infection control measures in dental practice. Some areas where universal precaution protocols can be re-evaluated and strengthened include hand hygiene, donning and doffing of PPE, respiratory hygiene/cough etiquette, sterilization of instruments and devices, and disinfection of workplaces. Additionally, with the growing evidence of asymptomatic transmission of COVID-19, infection control practices should be re-examined and improved to prevent cross-infection in a dental setting. Notwithstanding, recent attempts have been made to review the current literature on precautions when providing dental care during the current pandemic, and make recommendations for dental practitioners (24, 25).

The curriculum in dental schools should also be expanded to include competencies in pandemic and disaster relief. Such exposure enable dentists and their dental auxiliaries to augment the existing medical professionals in response to declared medical emergencies. Dentists have already been trained to undertake oral swab procedures and biopsies as part of oral cancer screening. However, in the wake of a pandemic outbreak, dental students should be additionally trained to perform nasopharyngeal and oropharyngeal swabs, as well as saliva sampling procedures. Dentists can also be a part of an effective surveillance network by notifying public health authorities about unusual oral symptoms or clinical presentations detected in questionable frequency in a population. Thus, dentists can facilitate the early detection of a disease outbreak or bioterrorism attack, and prevent mass casualties by prompt interventions.

In addition, voluntary medical work should be made a part of the community dentistry curriculum. In dentistry, clinical outreach programs during undergraduate training are still in their infancy. Such programs should be quickly scaled up. Several studies have reported that overseas voluntary outreach programs are a fulfilling and life-changing experience for dentists (26), and that community-based learning experience brings significant positive outcomes in terms of productivity and higher professional standards of dental students (27). With the expanded level of contact with patients from various strata of society, students will have additional opportunities to see the complexities of social and cultural aspects of their future patients. In addition, students are likely to gain appreciation for alternative career paths in public health as well as volunteer work. These experiences also have a positive impact on their understanding of ethical and social issues related to oral health care (28).

Some dental schools have already included community engagement programs as a part of the dental curriculum. Such engagements instill a sense of voluntarism in the minds of the dental graduates and prepare them to contribute in future disease outbreaks. A study looking at Stony Brook University's humanitarian dental mission to rural Madagascar found that all dental students who participated gained experience and confidence in their clinical ability and increased their speed in performing procedures under demanding conditions (29). Beyond medical training, such programs also nurture team work, communication skills and leadership qualities in young dentists.

Moving forward, it is likely that dental practice will be considerably changed in the post-pandemic era. Therefore, there is a greater need for refresher courses for practicing dentists on infection control in order to adjust with patients' apprehension in the post-COVID-19 world. Dental authorities and dental schools should urgently look into this need and appoint taskforces to develop protocols and appropriate courses for dental practitioners. Concurrently, research on infection control in the dental setting needs to be advanced. In order to formulate best practices, new research should be conducted across all disciplines of dentistry covering all procedures and their respective infection control strategies. The field of public oral health should find new research avenues on community oral health that can provide an insight on the perception and apprehension of patients during hospital visits. Such information would help to revive the financial viability of public hospitals and private clinics. The recommendations for dental implementation in the post-COVID-19 era are summarized in **Table 1**.

OCCUPATIONAL HEALTH AND SAFETY

Volunteers are being selfless in providing services amid crisis. However, it should be borne in mind that similar with medical staff, volunteers are also a vulnerable group. Preparation and medical support for volunteers during their placement is a significant aspect of any overseas voluntary work. Lack of understanding and preparation may expose volunteers to certain diseases during community engagement as well as subject them to psychological problems (30). Hence, it is highly advisable that proper training is provided to the volunteers. Volunteers should be trained on proper donning and doffing of PPE. It is important not just to minimize cross-infection but to keep it to zero. Therefore, strict infection control measures such as correct use of gloves and hand hygiene steps should be practiced. Volunteers working in close contact with COVID-19 positive patients should check for proper fit and size of N95 masks. It is very likely for cross-contamination to occur during public mass-scale swabbing operations. A single breach of the chain of infection control will put the whole team in jeopardy leading to quarantine of its members and closure of the medical facility.

Not all volunteers have the same physical and mental strength and the amount of volunteering work that one can engage must be monitored by group leaders and higher level authority. Frequent breaks in between and off days are necessary, in particular for a longer engagement, to support mental and psychosocial well-being of the volunteers. It is also important to provide an understanding of the precautionary safe-distancing measures to be taken with family during and after engagement in risk activities. It is essential that volunteers are mindful of their own and their family's health while serving others.

CONCLUSION

Overall, it is commendable that many dentists have risen to the challenge in the fight against COVID-19. The role of the dentist in a pandemic can be beyond dentistry. By virtue of their training and practical experience, dentists can provide services in various ways to reduce the strain on the healthcare sector. Volunteerism in such a time also leaves a positive impact on the individual. Pandemics rarely occur, and practical experience gained will be a lifelong lesson for the volunteer. In fact, the fighting spirit of a volunteer working in risky operations instills a high moral esteem and self-confidence. The rejuvenated personality of the volunteer can prove to be valuable in developing his career in future. The selfless voluntary service will be appreciated by the larger community and future generations. Together we will be able to pull through this crisis and emerge stronger than before.

AUTHOR CONTRIBUTIONS

CJS and ML contributed to the conception. CJS, ML, and BTG drafted and critically revised the manuscript. All authors contributed to the article and approved the submitted version.

REFERENCES

1. Huang C, Wang Y, Li X, Ren L, Zhao J, Hu Y, et al. Clinical features of patients infected with 2019 novel coronavirus in Wuhan, China. *Lancet.* (2020) 395:497–506. doi: 10.1016/S0140-6736(20)30183-5
2. Li Q, Guan X, Wu P, Wang X, Zhou L, Tong Y, et al. Early transmission dynamics in wuhan, china, of novel coronavirus-infected pneumonia. *N Engl J Med.* (2020) 382:1199–207. doi: 10.1056/NEJMoa2001316
3. Chen N, Zhou M, Dong X, Qu J, Gong F, Han Y, et al. Epidemiological and clinical characteristics of 99 cases of 2019 novel coronavirus pneumonia in Wuhan, China: a descriptive study. *Lancet.* (2020) 395:507–13. doi: 10.1016/S0140-6736(20)30211-7
4. Gorbalenya AE, Baker SC, Baric RS, de Groot RJ, Drosten C, Gulyaeva AA, et al. Severe acute respiratory syndrome-related coronavirus: the species and its viruses – a statement of the Coronavirus Study Group. *bioRxiv.* (2020). doi: 10.1101/2020.02.07.937862. Available online at: https://digital.csic.es/handle/10261/212994
5. Lu R, Zhao X, Li J, Niu P, Yang B, Wu H, et al. Genomic characterisation and epidemiology of 2019 novel coronavirus: implications for virus origins and receptor binding. *Lancet.* (2020) 395:565–74. doi: 10.1016/S0140-6736(20)30251-8
6. Zhou P, Yang XL, Wang XG, Hu B, Zhang L, Zhang W, et al. A pneumonia outbreak associated with a new coronavirus of probable bat origin. *Nature.* (2020) 579:270–3. doi: 10.1038/s41586-020-2012-7
7. Lam TT, Shum MH, Zhu HC, Tong YG, Ni XB, Liao YS, et al. Identifying SARS-CoV-2 related coronaviruses in Malayan pangolins. *Nature.* (2020) 583:282–5. doi: 10.1038/s41586-020-2169-0
8. World Health Organisation. *Coronavirus disease (COVID-19) Situation Report - 188.* (2020). Available online at: https://www.who.int/docs/default-source/coronaviruse/situation-reports/20200726-covid-19-sitrep-188.pdf?sfvrsn=f177c3fa_2 (accessed July 27, 2020).
9. Peng X, Xu X, Li Y, Cheng L, Zhou X, Ren B. Transmission routes of 2019-nCoV and controls in dental practice. *Int J Oral Sci.* (2020) 12:9 doi: 10.1038/s41368-020-0075-9
10. Gandhi M, Yokoe DS, Havlir DV. Asymptomatic transmission, the achilles' heel of current strategies to control Covid-19. *N Engl J Med.* (2020) 382:2158–60. doi: 10.1056/NEJMe2009758
11. Wolfel R, Corman VM, Guggemos W, Seilmaier M, Zange S, Muller MA, et al. Virological assessment of hospitalized patients with COVID-2019. *Nature.* (2020) 581:465–9. doi: 10.1038/s41586-020-2196-x
12. Arons MM, Hatfield KM, Reddy SC, Kimball A, James A, Jacobs JR, et al. Presymptomatic SARS-CoV-2 infections and transmission in a skilled nursing facility. *N Engl J Med.* (2020) 382:2081–90. doi: 10.1056/NEJMoa2008457
13. Caruso CC. Negative impacts of shiftwork and long work hours. *Rehabil Nurs.* (2014) 39:16–25. doi: 10.1002/rnj.107
14. UN Volunteers. *Volunteers for Novel Coronavirus (COVID-19) Pandemic Response.* (2020). Available online at: http://www.unv.org/Volunteers-for-Novel-Coronavirus-COVID-19-pandemic-response (accessed May 10, 2020).
15. Harrel SK, Molinari J. Aerosols and splatter in dentistry: a brief review of the literature and infection control implications. *J Am Dent Assoc.* (2004) 135:429–37. doi: 10.14219/jada.archive.2004.0207
16. Azzi L, Carcano G, Gianfagna F, Grossi P, Gasperina DD, Genoni A, et al. Saliva is a reliable tool to detect SARS-CoV-2. *J Infect.* (2020) 81:e45–50. doi: 10.1016/j.jinf.2020.04.005
17. Centers for Disease Control and Prevention. *Guidance for Dental Settings.* (2020). Available at: https://www.cdc.gov/coronavirus/2019-ncov/hcp/dental-settings.html (accessed July 27, 2020).
18. National Health Service. *COVID-19 Guidance and Standard Operating Procedure.* (2020). Available online at: https://www.england.nhs.uk/coronavirus/wp-content/uploads/sites/52/2020/06/C0581-covid-19-urgent-dental-care-sop-update-16-june-20-.pdf (accessed July 27, 2020).
19. Ministry of Health Singapore. *Gradual Resumption of Dental Services after COVID-19 Circuit Breaker Period.* (2020). Available online at: https://www.healthprofessionals.gov.sg/docs/librariesprovider11/default-document-library/moh-cir-no-132_2020_21may20_dental-services-after-cb-period67b93be2bc2542d18c675325ab75f730.pdf (accessed July 27, 2020).
20. California Dental Association. *Dentists Can Register to Help With State's COVID-19 Pandemic Response.* (2020). Available online at: http://www.cda.org/Home/News-and-Events/Newsroom/Article-Details/dentists-can-register-to-help-with-states-covid-19-pandemic-response (accessed May 10, 2020).
21. Renzaho AM, de Silva-Sanigorski A. The importance of family functioning, mental health and social and emotional well-being on child oral health. *Child Care Health Dev.* (2014) 40:543–52. doi: 10.1111/cch.12053
22. Vasiliou A, Shankardass K, Nisenbaum R, Quinonez C. Current stress and poor oral health. *BMC Oral Health.* (2016) 16:88 doi: 10.1186/s12903-016-0284-y
23. Coulthard P. Dentistry and coronavirus (COVID-19) - moral decision-making. *Br Dent J.* (2020) 228:503–5. doi: 10.1038/s41415-020-1482-1
24. Ge ZY, Yang LM, Xia JJ, Fu XH, Zhang YZ. Possible aerosol transmission of COVID-19 and special precautions in dentistry. *J Zhejiang Univ Sci B.* (2020) 21:361–8. doi: 10.1631/jzus.B2010010
25. Shi AH, Guo W, Chng CK, Chan BH. Precautions when providing dental care during Coronavirus Disease 2019 (COVID-19) pandemic. *Ann Acad Med Singapore.* (2020) 49:312–9.
26. Perkins N, Jones L. Dental mission for children–Vietnam. *Br Dent J.* (2009) 206:109–11. doi: 10.1038/sj.bdj.2009.50
27. Bean CY, Rowland ML, Soller H, Casamassimo P, Van Sickle R, Levings K, et al. Comparing fourth-year dental student productivity and experiences in a dental school with community-based clinical

education. *J Dent Educ.* (2007) 71:1020–6. doi: 10.1002/j.0022-0337.2007.71.8.tb04368.x

28. Bean CY. Community-based dental education at the Ohio State University: the OHIO Project. *J Dent Educ.* (2011) 75(10 Suppl.):S25–35. doi: 10.1002/j.0022-0337.2011.75.10_suppl.tb05192.x
29. Wynn LA, Krause DW, Kucine A, Trehan P, Goren AD, Colosi DC. Evolution of a humanitarian dental mission to Madagascar from 1999 to 2008. *J Dent Educ.* (2010) 74:289–96. doi: 10.1002/j.0022-0337.2010.74.3.tb04874.x
30. Bhatta P, Simkhada P, van Teijlingen E, Maybin S. A questionnaire study of Voluntary Service Overseas (VSO) volunteers: health risk and problems encountered. *J Travel Med.* (2009) 16:332–7. doi: 10.1111/j.1708-8305.2009.00342.x

12

Association of Viral Infections with Oral Cavity Lesions: Role of SARS-CoV-2 Infection

Giusy Rita Maria La Rosa [1*], *Massimo Libra* [2], *Rocco De Pasquale* [1], *Sebastiano Ferlito* [1] *and Eugenio Pedullà* [1]

[1] *Department of General Surgery and Medical-Surgical Specialties, University of Catania, Catania, Italy,* [2] *Department of Biomedical and Biotechnological Sciences, Oncologic, Clinic and General Pathology Section, University of Catania, Catania, Italy*

Correspondence:
Giusy Rita Maria La Rosa
g_larosa92@live.it

Different viral agents, such as herpesviruses, human papillomavirus, and Coxsackie virus, are responsible for primary oral lesions, while other viruses, such as human immunodeficiency virus, affect the oral cavity due to immune system weakness. Interestingly, it has been reported that coronavirus disease 2019 (COVID-19) patients can show cutaneous manifestations, including the oral cavity. However, the association between oral injuries and severe acute respiratory syndrome coronavirus 2 (SARS-CoV-2) infection is still unclear. This narrative review aimed to summarize the available literature and provide an overview of oral lesions associated with COVID-19. An online literature search was conducted to select relevant studies published up to November 2020. The results of 17 studies showed variability in oral lesions associated with COVID-19, including ulcerations, aphthous-like lesions, and macules. The tongue, lips, and palate were the most frequent anatomical locations. According to current knowledge, the etiopathogenesis of multiple COVID-19-associated lesions seems to be multifactorial. The appearance of such lesions could be related to the direct or indirect action of SARS-CoV-2 over the oral mucosa cells, coinfections, immunity impairment, and adverse drug reactions. Nevertheless, COVID-19-associated oral lesions may be underreported, mainly due to lockdown periods and the lack of mandatory dispositive protection. Consequently, further research is necessary to determine the diagnostic and pathological significance of oral manifestations of COVID-19. All medical doctors, dentists, and dermatologists are encouraged to perform an accurate and thorough oral examination of all suspected and confirmed COVID-19 cases to recognize the disease's possible early manifestations.

Keywords: COVID-19, novel coronavirus, oral health, oral lesions, oral mucosa, SARS-CoV-2, viral infection

INTRODUCTION

The oral cavity is particularly susceptible to viral infections because of its conformation, particularly its soft tissue and salivary glands. Several viruses, including herpes simplex virus (HSV) and human papillomavirus (HPV), are associated with oral disease-causing primary lesions. Furthermore, oral mucosa can be affected by the secondary pathological processes of a bacterial or fungal nature due to viral immunosuppression, such as the human immunodeficiency virus (HIV).

Consequently, the oral cavity could be considered a "biological barometer" of the viral immunosuppression advancement. Moreover, an implication of certain viral agents has been seen in dysplastic and neoplastic transformations of squamous epithelium (i.e., HPV) (1, 2). General and specialist dentists play a crucial role in evaluating, diagnosing, and managing such lesions, particularly considering the impacts of oral diseases on overall health and quality of life.

A new coronavirus, known as severe acute respiratory syndrome coronavirus 2 (SARS-CoV-2), responsible for coronavirus disease 2019 (COVID-19), was identified in Wuhan, Hubei Province, China, at the end of 2019. It then spread worldwide, becoming a global pandemic (3).

The main transmission route is via large respiratory droplets, even though the virus has also been identified in the stool and urine of affected individuals. It presents great variability in the severity of clinical manifestations, such as dry cough, shortness of breath, and fever (4, 5), passing from a mild flu-like illness to severe respiratory syndrome. Mortality rates vary according to region and change as the number of affected individuals is updated (6). Angiotensin-converting enzyme 2 (ACE2) receptor is considered the main functional receptor through which SARS-CoV-2 infects cells. The wide expression of ACE2 receptors in different anatomical sites, including the respiratory and gastrointestinal tracts, could explain the variability of reported clinical manifestations (7).

Interestingly, dermatological manifestations have also been observed in some patients affected by COVID-19. The most common skin lesions in these subjects include erythematous rash, urticaria, and vesicle formation, especially localized on the trunk, which seems to be the anatomic region most involved (5, 8). Oral lesions, such as unspecific ulceration, desquamative gingivitis, petechiae, and coinfections, such as candidiasis (9–13), have also been reported. Moreover, Xu et al. (14) reported a high level of expression of ACE2 receptors in epithelial cells of the oral mucosa, particularly tongue epithelial cells. These results suggest that oral mucosa could be a target of SARS-CoV-2 infection. Nevertheless, it is still unclear whether these manifestations are a specific clinical pattern derived from direct SARS-CoV-2 infection or a consequence of systemic involvement because of the possibility of coinfections, a compromised immune system, and adverse reactions to medical treatment (13, 15, 16). Because the prevalence of clinical oral manifestations is still unknown, the range of COVID-19 manifestations in the oral mucosa is of broad and current interest.

Therefore, after a brief excursus into the main viral agents associated with oral mucosa lesions, this review aims to summarize the updated literature on oral lesions in patients with COVID-19 and emphasize their clinical implications.

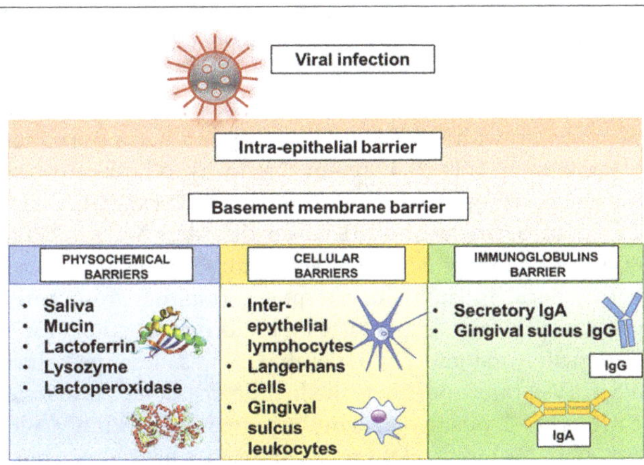

FIGURE 1 | The principal host defense mechanisms in the oral cavity.

The Host Defense of Mouth and Viral Diseases

The oral cavity possesses a series of physicochemical, cellular, and immunoglobulin barriers that prevent the entrance of harmful substances and microorganisms (2) (**Figure 1**). However, physicochemical barriers within the oral mucosa, including saliva and oral epithelium, are not absolute. The saliva secreted by the major and minor salivary glands contains many non-specifically protective agents, such as mucin, lysozyme, lactoperoxidase, and lactoferrin. In particular, lactoferrin, an iron-binding glycoprotein of the transferrin family, can inactivate many deoxyribonucleic acid (DNA) and ribonucleic acid (RNA) viruses, including cytomegalovirus, HSV, and rotavirus (17, 18). Cellular barriers involve the cells of the gingival sulcus, inter-epithelial lymphocytes, and Langerhans cells. In particular, Langerhans cells, which are dendritic inter-epithelial cells and act as mucosa "sentinels," are localized in the mouth inverse to the degree of oral mucosa keratinization and are primarily implicated in immune reactions (2, 19, 20). Despite these defense mechanisms, the oral mucosa is particularly subjected to viral infections (**Figure 2**). A virus is a sub-microscopic entity formed by a protein shell (known as a capsid) surrounding a single nucleic acid, DNA or RNA, only able to replicate in bacterial, animal, and vegetal cells (21). Viral genetic material is distinguishable from human genetic material due to its unique chemical and/or physical features. Also, a lipid envelope derived from the host cell membrane can be identified in some viruses (22, 23). Even though viral infection can involve any human cell, the oral cavity offers an ideal entry into a new host (24). Some of the most well-known viral agents associated with oral lesions are HSVs and HPVs. HSVs contain a double-stranded linear DNA molecule enveloped by an icosahedral capsid and a lipid casing (25). Initially involved in primary infections, they then remain dormant but can later cause secondary or recurrent infections. Eight types of HSV have been identified as human pathogens, and most are responsible for oral diseases (1, 23, 25–35). HPVs are non-enveloped viruses containing double-stranded DNA (36). Over 100 subtypes of HPV have been identified, with at least 13 correlated to an insurgence of oral lesions (37–42). The oral wart is a generic term used to identify all papillary and verrucal proliferations. Squamous papilloma is one of the most represented papillary lesions in the oral cavity (1, 36). Oral lesions can also be secondary due to an immunosuppression state, such as occurs in HIV

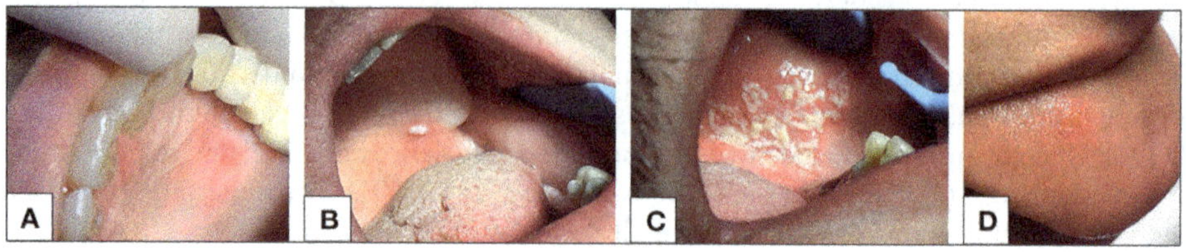

FIGURE 2 | (A) Herpetic-like oral lesion. **(B)** Oral mucosal verruca lesion. **(C)** Opportunistic infection (candidiasis) in patient affected by HIV. **(D)** Unspecific ulcerous lesion in a SARS-CoV-2 infected patient. Image 2D is a case courtesy of Chaux-Bodard et al. (9).

infection (43, 44). HIV is part of the *Lentivirus* genus, part of the *Orthoretroviridae* subfamily of the *Retroviridae* family. Two identical single-stranded RNA molecules form the HIV genome. The most frequent oral manifestations of HIV infection are opportunistic infections, such as candidiasis (45, 46), and malignancies, such as Kaposi's sarcoma (47, 48). The other most important viral agents associated with oral lesions are reported in **Table 1**. The association between oral lesions and SARS-CoV-2 remains controversial.

MATERIALS AND METHODS

An electronic search was conducted in PubMed, Scopus, and Web of Science for literature updated to November 20, 2020. A combination of the following keywords was used: "oral mucosal lesions" OR "oral lesions" AND "COVID-19" OR "SARS-CoV-2" OR "novel coronavirus disease." The full-text articles of all potential studies were evaluated, and the references cited by the relevant studies were manually searched for further studies. Given the lack of available data, all types of studies reporting oral mucosal lesions in patients with laboratory-confirmed COVID-19 were included; only literature reviews were excluded. However, we decided to include only those with laboratory-confirmed COVID-19 when evaluating the reported cases; suspected COVID-19 were excluded. Other exclusion criteria were articles for which the full text was not accessible or not available in English. Duplicate articles were removed, and a first screening was performed by reading only the titles and abstracts of the studies.

RESULTS

From the 86 studies retrieved, only 17 satisfied the inclusion criteria, of which 11 were letters to the editor, 3 were case reports, 2 were case series, and 1 was a short communication. **Table 2** provides a detailed description of the cases included. Given that the studies were published between April and November 2020, the results were listed in the table in alphabetical order of the first author's surname. Excluding the only study in which the gender and age of the participants were not reported (58), 33 cases were female and 24 cases were male. The mean age of reported cases was 42.92 ± 18.05.

The documented manifestations of oral mucosa were quite heterogeneous, varying in the kind of lesion and the location. The most frequent findings were ulcerations (9, 50, 60–62), sometimes associated with necrotic areas (50, 51), aphthous-like lesions (51, 55, 56, 58), and petechiae (51, 52, 54). Maculae (53, 60), blisters (10, 57), lingual papillitis or depapillation (58), and erythema or red plaques (52, 63) were also among the described oral lesions. Besides, a case of dark brown hyperpigmentation was documented by Corchuelo and Ulloa (63).

Tongue (9, 51, 54, 55, 58–62), lips (10, 50, 51, 57, 59, 60, 63) and palate (52, 54, 60) were the most frequently described anatomical locations.

DISCUSSION

An increasing number of atypical clinical presentations have been reported during SARS-CoV-2 infection, including dermatological and oral manifestations (16, 64–67). The pathogenesis of skin damage during COVID-19 is not well known, but some hypotheses have been formulated. For example, the presence of viral particles in cutaneous blood vessels could induce lymphocytic vasculitis through cytokine production, i.e., interleukin-1 (IL-1), interferon gamma (IFN-γ), and tumor necrosis factor alfa (TNF-α) by CD4+ T helper lymphocytes and the migration of eosinophils, CD8+ cytotoxic T cells, B cells, and natural killer (NK) cells (68, 69). Another possible explanation of cutaneous disturbances correlated to SARS-CoV-2 is the formation and accumulation of microthromboses, which could reduce the blood flow to the cutaneous microvasculature (70), and the presence of deoxygenated blood in venous plexi could further contribute to these cutaneous lesions. Moreover, the deposition of complement components C5b-9 and C4d in pauci-inflammatory thrombogenic vasculopathy and their co-localization with COVID-19 spike glycoproteins were shown by Magro et al. (71). It is reasonable to hypothesize that skin involvement is due to a combination of these mechanisms rather than a single one (5). Taste disorders were the most common oral symptom in patients with COVID-19, probably due to a local inflammatory response resulting from rhinitis triggers, which can hamper taste buds' normal function (15, 72). Additionally, oral mucosa involvement was described during SARS-CoV-2 infection. Since the first description of oral lesions in SARS-CoV-2 positive patients, reported by Martín Carreras-Presas et al. (10), several more recent studies have also reported oral mucosa lesions in COVID-19, such as ulcers (50, 60–62),

TABLE 1 | Viruses associated with oral lesions.

Viral family	Virus	Oral disease	Oral lesion
Herpesvirus (HSV)	HSV-1	Primary herpetic gingivostomatitis Herpes labialis (recurrent infection)	Vesicles Erosions Ulcers
	HSV-2	Similar to HSV-1 but rare	
	HSV-3 (Varicella zoster)	Primary infection (rare) Recurrent infection	
	HSV-4 (Epstein Barr)	Mononucleosis Burkitt's lymphoma Nasopharyngeal carcinoma	
	HSV-5 (Citomegalovirus)	Sialadenopathy Aphthae	
	HSV-6	-	
	HSV-7	-	
	HSV-8	Kaposi's sarcoma	
Papillomavirus (HPV)	More than 100 subtypes: HPV-2,−6,−11,−57 HPV-6 and−11	Squamous papillomas Verruca vulgaris Condyloma acuminatum	Exophytic papillary lesions Multiple, pink, soft tissue masses
	HPV-13 and−32	Focal epithelial hyperplasia (Heck's disease)	
	HPV-16 and−18	Dysplastic and neoplastic transformations of squamous epithelium	
Poxvirus	Variola Molluscum contagiosum (MCV)	Smallpox Molluscum contagiosum	Maculopapular lesions Erythematous papules
Picornavirus	Coxsackie virus: A16, A6 A1-A6, A8, A10, A22	Hand, foot, and mouth disease Herpangina	Vesicles Ulcers
Paramyxovirus	Measles virus (MV) Mumps virus	Rubeola Mumps	Small erythematous macules with white necrotic center (Koplik's spots) Ulcers
Retrovirus	Human immunodeficiency virus (HIV)	Opportunistic infections (viral, bacterial, fungal) Malignancies	Not typical lesions but dependent on the secondary lesion

aphthae (51, 55), and maculae (53, 60). The clinical significance of oral mucosa involvement during SARS-CoV-2 infection remains controversial.

As previously reported (14), the high expression of ACE2 on oral epithelial cells, especially on the tongue, suggests that the oral cavity might be an anatomical site particularly susceptible to SARS-CoV-2 infection. Consequently, as suggested by Brandão et al. (51), the interaction between SARS-CoV-2 and ACE2 might disrupt the oral keratinocytes' function, resulting in painful oral ulcers. Furthermore, oral mucosa lesions during COVID-19 could be justified by the variable inflammatory reaction, which can induce vascular inflammation, as observed for cutaneous manifestations (5, 73). The most recent publications on oral mucosa lesions in patients affected by COVID-19 support an association with organic damage and/or complications for thrombocytopenia, anticoagulant therapy, disseminated intravascular coagulation, and systemic inflammation (60, 62, 63). According to Cruz Tapia et al. (54), clinical manifestations and histological findings suggest the possibility that the oral cavity presents the primary or secondary alterations of vascular-hematologic damage associated with COVID-19. Nevertheless, as reported by Martín Carreras-Presas et al. (10) and Hedou et al. (74), ulcers or vesiculobullous lesions can occur as in other viral infections. It is largely documented that high levels of fatigue and stress can increase the risk of the reactivation of HSV (75).

Moreover, oral damage could also be a manifestation of an immunosuppression state and microbiome dysbiosis caused by a viral infection (76). According to Bezerra et al. (50), it is reasonable to think that COVID-19 systemic immune deregulation may cause a more prolonged immune imbalance, which could predispose these late, secondary oral lesions. In addition, as stated by de Sousa et al. (13), most patients developed oral mucosal injury during the hospitalization period, which supports the hypothesis of coinfections, immunity impairment, and adverse reactions to COVID-19 treatment medications.

Interestingly, Martín Carreras-Presas et al. (10) suggested that oral lesions, such as ulcers, could be an inaugural symptom of COVID-19. According to Amorim Dos Santos et al. (15), in mild cases, oral mucosal lesions occurred before or at the same time as the initial respiratory symptoms; however, in those who required medication and hospitalization, the lesions developed approximately 7–24 days after the onset of symptoms. Limited to the cases reported, the time to onset was variable, ranging from 4 to 90 days; however, the time on onset was unavailable in several reported studies, confirming the necessity to verify this data in larger patients' cohorts.

Regarding the age of patients presenting with oral injuries, Brandão et al. (51) reported two distinct oral lesions patterns. One was represented by aphthous-like ulcers in young patients with mild cases of COVID-19, and the other resembled HSV-1 necrotic ulcers in more severe cases of immunosuppressed older patients. Again, the lack of data available from a large sample of participants makes further investigations necessary to support these hypotheses.

Another interesting fact emerging from the reported cases is how online professional consultation using photography (telemedicine) could be a very useful, additional tool to support clinicians in the early diagnosis of oral lesions, especially when direct observation is not possible (57, 63). Indeed, an early clinical diagnosis and the development of sensitive diagnostic tools are essential for a correct management of the disease (77, 78).

There are some limitations to underline in this study. First, almost all the reports were published as letters to the editor, thus imposing editorial limitations that reduce reporting

TABLE 2 | General aspects of the included studies.

Study	Design	Sample (n)	Age and gender	Oral lesion	Localization	Time on onset (days)[a]
Amorim Dos Santos et al. (62)	Case report	1	67 (M)	White plaque; pinpoint yellowish ulcers	Tongue dorsum	24
Ansari et al. (49)	Letter to the Editor	2	75 (M) and 56 (F)	Ulcer	Hard palate and tongue	6 ± 1.41
Bezerra et al. (50)	Letter to the Editor	1	33 (M)	Ulceration; ulcer with necrotic background	Floor of mouth; retromolar region and lip mucosa	70 (first appearance) and 90 (second)
Brandão et al. (51)	Case series	8	53.87 ± 24.86; 5 (M) and 3 (F)	Aphthous-like + necrosis; hemorrhagic ulceration with necrotic areas; aphthous-like; petechia	Upper and lower lip mucosa; anterior dorsal tongue; lateral borders of the tongue; ventral portion of tongue; upper and lower labial mucosa; tonsillar pilar	6 ± 2.56
Carreras-Presas et al. (10)	Short communication	1	65 (F)	Blisters; desquamative gingivitis	Internal lip mucosa	22
Cebeci Kahraman et al. (52)	Letter to the Editor	1	51 (M)	Erythema; petechia; pustular enanthema	Hard palate; soft palate border	10
Chaux-Bodard et al. (9)	Letter to the Editor	1	45 (F)	Erythematous macula evolved into ulcer	Tongue	8 days before the laboratory-confirmed COVID-19
Ciccarese et al. (53)	Letter to the Editor	1	19 (F)	Erosion; ulceration and petechia	Palate and lips	7
Corchuelo and Ulloa (63)	Case report	1	40 (F)	Reddish plaque; dark brown hyperpigmentation	Lower lip; gum	21
Cruz Tapia et al. (54)	Case series	4	47 ± 7.11; 1 (M) and 3 (F)	Bulla; macula; papule-plaque	Hard palate; tongue	N.A.
Díaz Rodríguez et al. (55)	Letter to the Editor	3	58 ± 18.02; 1 (M) and 2 (F)	Aphthous-like; tongue depapillation; fissures; red plate	Dorsum of the tongue; labial commissure; palate	N.A.
Dominguez-Santas et al. (56)	Letter to the Editor	4	33 ± 10.19; 3 (M) and 1 (F)	Minor aphthae	Buccal and labial mucosa; tongue	3 ± 2.16
Kitakawa et al. (57)	Case report	1	20 (F)	Vesicle	Median lower lip semimucosa	7
Nuno-Gonzalez et al. (58)	Research letter	78	N.A.	Lingual papillitis; glossitis; aphthous-like	Tongue; oral mucosa	N.A.
Riad et al. (61)	Letter to the Editor	26	36.81 ± 15.65; 9 (M) and 17 (F)	Ulcer	Tongue	4.12 ± 1.39
Sakaida et al. (59)	Letter to the Editor	1	52 (F)	Erosion	Lips; buccal mucosa	N.A.
Soares et al. (60)	Letter to the Editor	1	42 (M)	Ulceration and reddish macula	Hard palate, tongue and lips	N.A.

n = 17. M, Male; F, Female; N.A., Not available.
[a]The time on onset refers to days passed after the laboratory-confirmed diagnosis of COVID-19.

comprehensibility (12). Moreover, the oral manifestations' real incidence could have been underestimated due to exposure and contamination risk while conducting photographic imaging (15) and the limited data available on oral lesion injuries in asymptomatic patients. Another important aspect to consider is the limited availability of microscopic and histological data of oral mucosa lesions in COVID-19. The only accessible data referred to histological characterizations performed by Soares et al. (60) and Ansari et al. (49), which confirmed the presence of an inflammatory infiltrate, suggesting that the patients' lesions could be associated with COVID-19 disease. It is auspicious that the characterization of the oral lesions of COVID-19 infected patients should include incisional biopsies, followed by direct viral testing for SARS-CoV-2, as suggested by Brandão et al. (51).

Further research is necessary to determine the diagnostic and pathological significance of oral manifestations during COVID-19. Indeed, oral mucosa involvement during viral infection may assume differing clinical significance: it could represent either the first sign of viral disease or coexist as a co-symptom or represent a unique sign of the viral infection (26). In this context, the importance of the clinical oral examination of patients with confirmed or suspicious COVID-19 infection should be emphasized, given the need for support, pain control, and quality of life. In addition, dental operators are potentially exposed to a high degree of contamination with SARS-CoV-2 because of dental procedures that produce aerosols (79, 80). Consequently, an accurate inspection of the oral cavity, always with the mandatory dispositive protection (79), could be crucial in the dental setting to perform a more accurate triage of patients and improve safety operator, avoiding underestimation and misdiagnoses of oral signs and symptoms.

CONCLUSIONS

The new SARS-CoV-2 responsible for the global COVID-19 pandemic has become a sanitary emergency of primary importance. Although the typical symptoms include fever, shortness of breath, and a dry cough, cutaneous manifestations have also been reported, including some oral lesions. An association between oral diseases and SARS-CoV-2 infection is still unclear and currently poorly investigated. The appearance of such lesions could be related to the direct or indirect action of SARS-CoV-2 over the oral mucosa cells, coinfections, immunity impairment, and adverse drug reactions. Nevertheless, oral manifestations of this disease seem to be underreported, especially due to lockdown periods and the lack of mandatory dispositive protection. Consequently, based on these outcomes, we can conclude that (1) further studies are necessary to establish the diagnostic and pathological significance of oral manifestations during COVID-19; (2) the oral examination in patients with COVID-19 should not be unattended but rather promote a specialist multidisciplinary approach, including especially dental practitioners; (3) early recognition of oral lesions associated to COVID-19 could be crucial in the dental setting to perform a more accurate triage of patients and improve operator safety, avoiding underestimation and misdiagnosis of oral manifestations.

AUTHOR CONTRIBUTIONS

GL, ML, and EP contributed to all steps of manuscript preparation. RD and SF participated in editing and critical revision of article. All authors contributed to the article and approved the submitted version.

ACKNOWLEDGMENTS

The authors thank Dr. Chaux-Bodard for authorizing to use the **Figure 2D**.

REFERENCES

1. Lynch DP. Oral manifestations of viral diseases. In: Tyring S, editor. *Mucosal Immunology and Virology*. Cham: Springer (2006). p. 99–156.
2. Dolby AE. The host defence system of the mouth. In: Ivanyi L, editor. *Immunological Aspects of Oral Diseases*. London: MTP Press Limited (1986). p. 1–11.
3. Wu Z, McGoogan JM. Characteristics of and important lessons from the coronavirus disease 2019 (COVID-19) outbreak in China: summary of a report of 72 314 cases from the Chinese Center for Disease Control and Prevention. *JAMA*. (2020) 323:1239–42. doi: 10.1001/jama.2020.2648
4. Huang C, Wang Y, Li X, Ren L, Zhao J, Hu Y, et al. Clinical features of patients infected with 2019 novel coronavirus in wuhan, china. *Lancet*. (2020) 395:497–506. doi: 10.1016/S0140-6736(20)30183-5
5. Sachdeva M, Gianotti R, Shah M, Lucia B, Tosi D, Veraldi S, et al. Cutaneous manifestations of COVID-19: report of three cases and a review of literature. *J Dermatol Sci*. (2020) 98:75–81. doi: 10.1016/j.jdermsci.2020.04.011
6. Gupta R, Ghosh A, Singh AK, Misra A. Clinical considerations for patients with diabetes in times of COVID-19 epidemic. *Diabetes Metab Syndr*. (2020) 14:211–2. doi: 10.1016/j.dsx.2020.03.002
7. Li MY, Li L, Zhang Y, Wang XS. Expression of the SARS-CoV-2 cell receptor gene ACE2 in a wide variety of human tissues. *Infect Dis Poverty*. (2020) 9:45. doi: 10.1186/s40249-020-00662-x
8. Recalcati S. Cutaneous manifestations in COVID-19: a first perspective. *J Eur Acad Dermatol Venereol*. (2020) 34:e212–3. doi: 10.1111/jdv.16387
9. Chaux-Bodard AG, Deneuve S, Desoutter A. Oral manifestation of Covid-19 as an inaugural symptom? *J Oral Med Oral Surg*. (2020) 26:18. doi: 10.1051/mbcb/2020011
10. Martín Carreras-Presas C, Amaro Sánchez J, López-Sánchez AF, Jané-Salas E, Somacarrera Pérez ML. Oral vesiculobullous lesions associated with SARS-CoV-2 infection. *Oral Dis*. (2020). doi: 10.1111/odi.13382. [Epub ahead of print].
11. Capocasale G, Nocini R, Faccioni P, Donadello D, Bertossi D, Albanese M, et al. How to deal with coronavirus disease 2019: a comprehensive narrative review about oral involvement of the disease. *Clin Exp Dent Res*. (2020). doi: 10.1002/cre2.332. [Epub ahead of print].
12. Riad A, Klugar M, Krsek M. COVID-19-related oral manifestations: early disease features? *Oral Dis*. (2020). doi: 10.1111/odi.13516. [Epub ahead of print].
13. de Sousa FACG, Paradella TC. Considerations on oral manifestations of COVID-19. *J Med Virol*. (2020). doi: 10.1002/jmv.26451
14. Xu H, Zhong L, Deng J, Peng J, Dan H, Zeng X, et al. High expression of ACE2 receptor of 2019-nCoV on the epithelial cells of oral mucosa. *Int J Oral Sci*. (2020) 12:8. doi: 10.1038/s41368-020-0074-x
15. Amorim Dos Santos J, Normando AGC, Carvalho da Silva RL, Acevedo AC, De Luca Canto G, Sugaya N, et al. Oral manifestations in patients with COVID-19: a living systematic review. *J Dent Res*. (2020). doi: 10.1177/0022034520957289. [Epub ahead of print].
16. Halboub E, Al-Maweri SA, Alanazi RH, Qaid NM, Abdulrab S. Orofacial manifestations of COVID-19: a brief review of the published literature. *Braz Oral Res*. (2020) 34:e124. doi: 10.1590/1807-3107bor-2020.vol34.0124
17. Ng TB, Cheung RCF, Wong JH, Wang Y, Ip DTM, Wan DCC, et al. Antiviral activities of whey proteins. *Appl Microbiol Biotechnol*. (2015) 17:6997–7008. doi: 10.1007/s00253-015-6818-4
18. Wakabayashi H, Oda H, Yamauchi K, Abe F. Lactoferrin for prevention of common viral infections. *J Infect Chemother*. (2014) 20:666–71. doi: 10.1016/j.jiac.2014.08.003
19. Upadhyay J, Upadhyay RB, Agrawal P, Jaitley S, Shekhar R. Langerhans cells and their role in oral mucosal diseases. *N Am J Med Sci*. (2013) 5:505–14. doi: 10.4103/1947-2714.118923
20. Sistig S, Vucićević-Boras V, Lukac J, Kusić Z. Salivary IgA and IgG subclasses in oral mucosal diseases. *Oral Dis*. (2002) 8:282–6. doi: 10.1034/j.1601-0825.2002.20844.x
21. Kiselev NA, Sherman MB, Tsuprun VL. Negative staining of proteins. *Electron Microsc Rev*. (1990) 3:43–72. doi: 10.1016/0892-0354(90)90013-I
22. Caspar DL, Klug A. Physical principles in the construction of regular viruses. *Cold Spring Harb Symp Quant Biol*. (1962) 27:1–24. doi: 10.1101/SQB.1962.027.001.005
23. Ramesh N, Don KR. Oral manifestations of viral diseases. *Drug Invent Today*. (2019) 12:321–30.
24. Grinde B, Olsen I. The role of viruses in oral disease. *J Oral Microbiol*. (2010) 2:2127. doi: 10.3402/jom.v2i0.2127

25. Pellett PE, Roizman B. The family herpesviridae: a brief introduction. In: Knipe DM, Howley PM, editors. *Fields Virology*. 5th ed. Philadelphia, PA: Lippincott, Williams and Wilkins (2007) p. 2479–99.
26. Santosh A, Muddana K. Viral infections of oral cavity. *J Family Med Prim Care*. (2020) 9:36–42. doi: 10.4103/jfmpc.jfmpc_807_19
27. Scully C. Ulcerative stomatitis, gingivitis, and skin lesions. An unusual case of primary herpes simplex infection. *Oral Surg Oral Med Oral Pathol.* (1985) 59:261–3. doi: 10.1016/0030-4220(85)90163-X
28. Nahmias AJ, Roizman B. Infection with herpes simplex viruses 1 and 2. III. *N Engl J Med.* (1973) 289:781–9. doi: 10.1056/NEJM197310112891505
29. Weller T. Varicella and herpes zoster. *N Engl J Med.* (1983) 309:1362–8. doi: 10.1056/NEJM198312013092205
30. Sampathkumar P, Drage LA, Martin DP. Herpes zoster (shingles) and postherpetic neuralgia. *Mayo Clin Proc.* (2009) 84:274–80. doi: 10.4065/84.3.274
31. Lambore S, McSherry J, Kraus AS. Acute and chronic symptoms of mononucleosis. *J Fam Pract.* (1991) 33:33–7.
32. Mach M, Stamminger T, Jahn G. Human cytomegalovirus: recent aspects from molecular biology. *J Gen Virol.* (1989) 70:3117–46. doi: 10.1099/0022-1317-70-12-3117
33. Bagg J. Human herpesvirus-6: the latest human herpes virus. *J Oral Pathol Med.* (1991) 20:465–8. doi: 10.1111/j.1600-0714.1991.tb00404.x
34. De Araujo T, Berman B, Weinstein A. Human herpesviruses 6 and 7. *Dermatol Clin.* (2002) 20:301–6. doi: 10.1016/S0733-8635(01)00008-0
35. Cannon M, Cesarman E. Kaposi's sarcoma-associated herpes virus and acquired immunodeficiency syndrome-related malignancy. *Semin Oncol.* (2000) 27:409–19.
36. Handisurya A, Schellenbacher C, Kirnbauer R. Diseases caused by human papillomaviruses (HPV). *J Dtsch Dermatol Ges.* (2009) 7:453–66. doi: 10.1111/j.1610-0387.2009.06988.x
37. Garlick JA, Taichman LB. Human papillomavirus infection of the oral mucosa. *Am J Dermatopathol.* (1991) 13:386–95. doi: 10.1097/00000372-199108000-00010
38. Kellokoski J, Syrjanen S, Syrjanen K, Yliskoski M. Oral mucosal changes in women with genital HPV infection. *J Oral Pathol Med.* (1990) 19:142–8. doi: 10.1111/j.1600-0714.1990.tb00813.x
39. Ficarra G, Adler-Storthz K, Galeotti F, Shillitoe E. Focal epithelial hyperplasia (Heck's disease): the first reported case from Italy. *Tumori.* (1991) 77:83–5. doi: 10.1177/030089169107700119
40. Morrow DJ, Sandhu HS, Daley TD. Focal epithelial hyperplasia (Heck's disease) with generalized lesions of the gingiva. A case report. *J Periodontol.* (1993) 64:63–5. doi: 10.1902/jop.1993.64.1.63
41. Miller CS, Johnstone BM. Human papillomavirus as a risk factor for oral squamous cell carcinoma: a meta-analysis, 1982-1997. *Oral Surg Oral Med Oral Pathol Oral Radiol Endod.* (2001) 91:622–35. doi: 10.1067/moe.2001.115392
42. Hennessey PT, Westra WH, Califano JA. Human papillomavirus and head and neck squamous cell carcinoma: recent evidence and clinical implications. *J Dent Res.* (2009) 88:300–6. doi: 10.1177/0022034509333371
43. German Advisory Committee Blood (Arbeitskreis Blut), Subgroup 'Assessment of Pathogens Transmissible by Blood'. Human Immunodeficiency Virus (HIV). *Transfus Med Hemother.* (2016) 43:203–22. doi: 10.1159/000445852
44. Mbopi-Keou FX, Belec L, Teo CG, Scully C, Porter SR. Synergism between HIV and other viruses in the mouth. *Lancet Infect Dis.* (2002) 2:416–24. doi: 10.1016/S1473-3099(02)00317-1
45. Warrier SA, Sathasivasubramanian S. Human immunodeficiency virus induced oral candidiasis. *J Pharm Bioallied Sci.* (2015) 7:S81214. doi: 10.4103/0975-7406.163577
46. Shetti A, Gupta I, Charantimath SM. Oral candidiasis: aiding in the diagnosis of HIV-a case report. *Case Rep Dent.* (2011) 2011:929616. doi: 10.1155/2011/929616
47. Curtiss P, Strazzulla LC, Friedman-Kien AE. An update on Kaposi's Sarcoma: epidemiology, pathogenesis and treatment. *Dermatol Ther.* (2016) 6:465–70. doi: 10.1007/s13555-016-0152-3
48. Cesarman E, Damania B, Krown SE, Martin J, Bower M, Whitby D. Kaposi sarcoma. *Nat Rev Dis Primers.* (2019) 5:9. doi: 10.1038/s41572-019-0060-9
49. Ansari R, Gheitani M, Heidari F, Heidari F. Oral cavity lesions as a manifestation of the novel virus (COVID-19). *Oral Dis.* (2020). doi: 10.1111/odi.13465. [Epub ahead of print].
50. Bezerra TMM, Feitosa SG, Carneiro DTO, Costa FWG, Pires FR, Pereira KMA. Oral lesions in COVID-19 infection: is long term follow-up important in the affected patients? *Oral Dis.* (2020). doi: 10.1111/odi.13705. [Epub ahead of print].
51. Brandão TB, Gueiros LA, Melo TS, Prado-Ribeiro AC, Nesrallah A, Prado G, et al. Oral lesions in patients with SARS-CoV-2 infection: could the oral cavity be a target organ? *Oral Surg Oral Med Oral Pathol Oral Radiol.* (2020). doi: 10.1016/j.oooo.2020.07.014. [Epub ahead of print].
52. Cebeci Kahraman F, Çaşkurlu H. Mucosal involvement in a COVID-19-positive patient: a case report. *Dermatol Ther.* (2020) 33:e13797. doi: 10.1111/dth.13797
53. Ciccarese G, Drago F, Boatti M, Porro A, Muzic SI, Parodi A. Oral erosions and petechiae during SARS-CoV-2 infection. *J Med Virol.* (2020). doi: 10.1002/jmv.26221. [Epub ahead of print].
54. Cruz Tapia RO, Peraza Labrador AJ, Guimaraes DM, Matos Valdez LH. Oral mucosal lesions in patients with SARS-CoV-2 infection. Report of four cases. Are they a true sign of COVID-19 disease? *Spec Care Dentist.* (2020) 40:555–60. doi: 10.1111/scd.12520
55. Díaz Rodríguez M, Jimenez Romera A,Villarroel M. Oral manifestations associated with COVID-19. *Oral Dis.* (2020). doi: 10.1111/odi.13555. [Epub ahead of print].
56. Dominguez-Santas M, Diaz-Guimaraens B, Fernandez-Nieto D, Jimenez-Cauhe J, Ortega-Quijano D, Suarez-Valle A. Minor aphthae associated with SARS-CoV-2 infection. *Int J Dermatol.* (2020). doi: 10.31128/AJGP-COVID-32. [Epub ahead of print].
57. Kitakawa D, Oliveira FE, Neves de Castro P, Carvalho LFCS. Short report - Herpes simplex lesion in the lip semimucosa in a COVID-19 patient. *Eur Rev Med Pharmacol Sci.* (2020) 24:9151–3. doi: 10.26355/eurrev_202009_22863
58. Nuno-Gonzalez A, Martin-Carrillo P, Magaletsky K, Martin Rios MD, Herranz Mañas C, Artigas Almazan J, et al. Prevalence of mucocutaneous manifestations in 666 patients with COVID-19 in a field hospital in Spain: oral and palmoplantar findings. *Br J Dermatol.* (2020). doi: 10.1111/bjd.19564. [Epub ahead of print].
59. Sakaida T, Tanimoto I, Matsubara A, Nakamura M, Morita A. Unique skin manifestations of COVID-19: is drug eruption specific to COVID-19? *J Dermatol Sci.* (2020) 99:62–4. doi: 10.1016/j.jdermsci.2020.05.002
60. Soares CD, Carvalho RA, Carvalho KA, Carvalho MG, Almeida OP. Letter to editor: oral lesions in a patient with Covid-19. *Med Oral Patol Oral Cir Bucal.* (2020) 25:e563–4. doi: 10.4317/medoral.24044
61. Riad A, Kassem I, Hockova B, Badrah M, Klugar M. Tongue ulcers associated with SARS-CoV-2 infection: a case series. *Oral Dis.* (2020). doi: 10.1111/odi.13635. [Epub ahead of print].
62. Amorim Dos Santos J, Normando AGC, Carvalho da Silva RL, De Paula RM, Cembranel AC, Santos-Silva AR, et al. Oral mucosal lesions in a COVID-19 patient: New signs or secondary manifestations? *Int J Infect Dis.* (2020) 97:326–8. doi: 10.1016/j.ijid.2020.06.012
63. Corchuelo J, Ulloa FC. Oral manifestations in a patient with a history of asymptomatic COVID-19: case report. *Int J Infect Dis.* (2020) 100:154–7. doi: 10.1016/j.ijid.2020.08.071
64. Guan WJ, Ni ZY, Hu Y, Liang WH, Ou CQ, He JX, et al. Clinical characteristics of coronavirus disease 2019 in china. *N Engl J Med.* (2020) 382:1708–20. doi: 10.1056/NEJMoa2002032
65. Aziz M, Perisetti A, Lee-Smith WM, Gajendran M, Bansal P, Goyal H. Taste changes (dysgeusia) in Covid-19: a systematic review and metaanalysis. *Gastroenterology.* (2020) 159:1132–3. doi: 10.1053/j.gastro.2020.05.003
66. Gianotti R, Zerbi P, Dodiuk-Gad RP. Clinical and histopathological study of skin dermatoses in patients affected by COVID-19 infection in the Northern part of Italy. *J Dermatol Sci.* (2020) 98:141–3. doi: 10.1016/j.jdermsci.2020.04.007
67. Xue X, Mi Z, Wang Z, Pang Z, Liu H, Zhang F. High expression of ACE2 on the keratinocytes reveals skin as a potential target for SARS-CoV-2. *J Invest Dermatol.* (2020) 141:206–9.e1. doi: 10.1016/j.jid.2020.05.087
68. Lee JS, Kossard S, McGrath MA. Lymphocytic thrombophilic arteritis: a newly described medium-sized vessel arteritis of the skin. *Arch Dermatol.* (2008) 144:1175–82. doi: 10.1001/archderm.144.9.1175

69. Gianotti, R. *COVID 19 and the Skin-Heuristic Review.* Milan: DermoSprint (2020).
70. Manalo IF, Smith MK, Cheeley J, Jacobs R. A dermatologic manifestation of COVID-19: transient livedo reticularis. *J Am Acad Dermatol.* (2020) 83:700. doi: 10.1016/j.jaad.2020.04.018
71. Magro C, Mulvey JJ, Berlin D, Nuovo G, Salvatore S, Harp J, et al. Complement associated microvascular injury and thrombosis in the pathogenesis of severe COVID-19 infection: a report of five cases. *Transl Res.* (2020) 220:1–13. doi: 10.1016/j.trsl.2020.04.007
72. Finsterer J, Stollberger C. Causes of hypogeusia/hyposmia in SARS- CoV2 infected patients. *J Med Virol.* (2020) 92:1793–4. doi: 10.1002/jmv.25903
73. Madjid M, Safavi-Naeini P, Solomon SD, Vardeny O. Potential effects of coronaviruses on the cardiovascular system: a review. *JAMA Cardiol.* (2020) 5:831–40. doi: 10.1001/jamacardio.2020.1286
74. Hedou M, Carsuzaa F, Chary E, Hainaut E, Cazenave-Roblot F, Masson Regnault M. Comment on 'Cutaneous manifestations in COVID-19: a first perspective' by Recalcati S. *J Eur Acad Dermatol Venereol.* (2020) 34:e299–300. doi: 10.1111/jdv.16519
75. Forbes H, Warne B, Doelken L, Brenner N, Waterboe T, Luben R, et al. Risk factors for herpes simplex virus type-1 infection and reactivation: cross-sectional studies among EPIC- Norfolk participants. *PLoS ONE.* (2019) 14:e0215553. doi: 10.1371/journal.pone.0215553
76. Santacroce L, Charitos IA, Ballini A, Inchingolo F, Luperto P, De Nitto E, et al. The human respiratory system and its microbiome at a glimpse. *Biology.* (2020) 9:318. doi: 10.3390/biology9100318
77. Pham VH, Gargiulo Isacco C, Nguyen KCD, Le SH, Tran DK, Nguyen QV, et al. Rapid and sensitive diagnostic procedure for multiple detection of pandemic Coronaviridae family members SARS-CoV-2, SARS-CoV, MERS-CoV and HCoV: a translational research and cooperation between the Phan Chau Trinh University in Vietnam and University of Bari "Aldo Moro" in Italy. *Eur Rev Med Pharmacol Sci.* (2020) 24:7173–91. doi: 10.26355/eurrev_202006_21713
78. Charitos IA, Ballini A, Bottalico L, Cantore S, Passarelli PC, Inchingolo F, et al. Special features of SARS-CoV-2 in daily practice. *World J Clin Cases.* (2020) 8:3920–33. doi: 10.12998/wjcc.v8.i18.3920
79. Bordea IR, Xhajanka E, Candrea S, Bran S, Oni?or F, Inchingolo AD, et al. Coronavirus (SARS-CoV-2) pandemic: future challenges for dental practitioners. *Microorganisms.* (2020) 8:1704. doi: 10.3390/microorganisms8111704
80. Cantore S, Ballini A. Coronavirus disease 2019 (COVID-19) pandemic burst and its relevant consequences in dental practice. *Open Dent J.* (2020) 1:111–2. doi: 10.2174/18742106020140111

13

Effectiveness of Pre-Procedural Mouth Rinses in Reducing Aerosol Contamination During Periodontal Prophylaxis

*Shahida Mohd-Said[1], Tuti Ningseh Mohd-Dom[1], Nawal Suhaimi[1], Haslina Rani[1] and Colman McGrath[1,2]**

[1] *Faculty of Dentistry, Universiti Kebangsaan Malaysia (The National University of Malaysia), Kuala Lumpur, Malaysia,* [2] *Faculty of Dentistry, The University of Hong Kong, Sai Ying Pun, Hong Kong*

Correspondence:
Colman McGrath
mcgrathc@hku.hk

Background: Aerosol-producing dental procedures are of concern in the spread of infections, especially during the COVID-19 pandemic. Periodontal prophylaxis is the most common aerosol-producing procedure conducted in dental practice globally. During COVID-19, many national and international organizations advocated the use of pre-procedural mouth rinsing to prevent the spread of infections from aerosol-generating procedures in the dental setting; however, many questioned the scientific basis for such recommendations.

Objective: This systematic review aimed to evaluate the effectiveness of pre-procedural rinsing when preforming periodontal prophylaxis in reducing aerosol contamination in the dental setting.

Methods: A comprehensive standardized search strategy was employed, informed by a defined PICO question across four electronic databases. The review of the literature was conducted using the PRISMA framework. Agreement between assessors was determined throughout. Synthesis of study characteristics and key outcomes were conducted. Cochrane's risk-of-bias tool for randomized trials (RoB 2) was employed to assess the quality/bias among studies.

Results: The initial search yielded 731 citations across the four databases; 95 potentially effective studies were identified, with 56 effective studies found. Thirty randomized control trial studies were identified, 21 with a focus on effectiveness of pre-procedural mouth rinsing, involving 984 participants (aged 18–70). Agreement between assessors was high (Kappa >0.80). Various pre-procedural mouth rinses were tested, most frequently chlorhexidine (CHX) in 18 studies. The concentrations, volume, and prescribed duration of rinsing varied among studies, hampering meta-analyses. Nonetheless, all studies identified significant reductions in bacterial contamination, as measured by colony forming units (cfu). The effectiveness of CHX over other agents was evident with more than half of the studies (7/15) reporting over a 70% reduction in bacterial contamination (cfu). There were concerns over the risk of bias in most studies (76.2%); 19.0% had a high risk of bias and 4.8% were of low risk of bias.

Conclusion: There is substantial evidence to support pre-procedural mouth rinsing, such as with chlorohexidine, to effectively reduce aerosol contamination when performing periodontal prophylaxis compared to mouth rinsing with water or not rinsing.

Keywords: COVID-19, periodontics, splatter, bioaerosol, air polishing, debridement, periodontal scaling

INTRODUCTION

The cornerstone for maintaining periodontal health is effective dental plaque control. This may be achieved through a combination of diligent home care practices and compliance to scheduled dental visits, whereby the dentist or hygienist undertakes the necessary scaling, polishing, and root debridement using ultrasonic scalers and air polishers. For individuals who have been affected with periodontitis, it is particularly crucial that they comply with scheduled dental visits regardless if they are in the active or maintenance phase of periodontal therapy.

Interruptions to regular dental services have been unexpectedly imposed due to the COVID-19 pandemic as part of the collective efforts to reduce the risk of transmission within dental clinics. Around the globe, the dental fraternity resolved that only urgent and emergency dental care should be permitted during the pandemic. Amidst dynamic health and community-related updates of the pandemic, the dental profession developed various guidelines to assist dentists to make appropriate clinical decisions in the management of their patients (1–3). These guidelines were necessary, although in some instances the available evidence to support them was questioned.

For patients with periodontal concerns, this disruption to scheduled periodontal therapy may not cause immediate pain or discomfort. Nonetheless, postponement of regular care can aggravate or be detrimental to their oral health status, may increase their risk of non-communicable diseases, or worsen their health status, particularly those with underlying systemic conditions (4). Non-surgical periodontal therapy like scaling, polishing, and root debridement are aerosol-generating procedures (AGP) and carry a high risk for aerosol contamination (5, 6). This causes concern for increased risk of infectious disease transmission during these procedures during the COVID-19 pandemic. There is an urgent need to reduce or eliminate the risk of aerosol contamination from AGPs given the necessity to carry out treatment to avoid periodontal disease progression (7).

One of the most widely advocated methods to reduce the level of contamination in the aerosol during dental procedures is pre-procedural mouth rinsing (8). The aim of our review was to investigate the effect of mouth rinsing before periodontal prophylaxis (pre-procedural mouth rinsing) on aerosol contamination in dental clinics. The findings from this review have implications in providing evidence to support or refute current guidelines for pre-procedural mouth rinsing.

METHODOLOGY

Search Strategy

The PICO strategy (9) was employed in focusing the review questions: What is the effectiveness of pre-procedural rinsing in periodontal prophylaxis in reducing aerosol contamination and what are the factors attributing to its effectiveness? The study population (**P**) was periodontitis patients receiving interventions (**I**) for reducing aerosol contaminations during non-surgical prophylaxis including dental scaling and tooth polishing, root planning or debridement, and air polishing using powered instruments with/without use of adjunctive antimicrobials. Findings from the relevant studies were to be compared (**C**) to the subjects or patients that did not receive similar interventions, with the primary outcomes (**O**) of interventions being reduced aerosol contamination.

Selection Criteria

Electronic database searches were conducted on Scopus, MEDLINE via PubMed, Cochrane Library, and Web of Science up to 8th April 2020 using the predefined keywords "aerosol" and "dental prophylaxis" (Appendix 1 in **Supplementary Material**). Selection of key words and terms for search strategy were informed by Medical Subject Headings (MeSH) and previous related reviews (8, 10–19). No time limit was set in this search. Our initial search did not find any references for viral contamination in aerosol; hence the review is limited to bacterial contamination only.

Data Selection and Extraction

The reviewers in this study were consulting specialists in Periodontology (S.M-S.) and Dental Public Health (T.N.M., H.R., and C.M.), and a dental graduate (N.S.). Initially, titles and abstracts were independently screened by two reviewers (S.M-S. and N.S.) to identify potential effective studies. Then, full-text articles were retrieved for the secondary screening by two additional reviewers (T.N.M., H.R., C.M.) for consensus on the eligibility. Disagreement between reviewers were resolved with the supervising author (C.M.) and Kappa statistics was used to assess the agreement between assessors throughout.

In synthesis of evidence from 'effective' studies, details included authors, article publication year, design of study, sampling size and allocation of test and control groups, details of intervention, type and description of periodontal prophylaxis procedures, and primary outcomes in terms of statistically significant findings and reduction of aerosol contamination between groups measured by colony forming units (cfu) using means and percentages. If permissible, mean cfu reduction % was

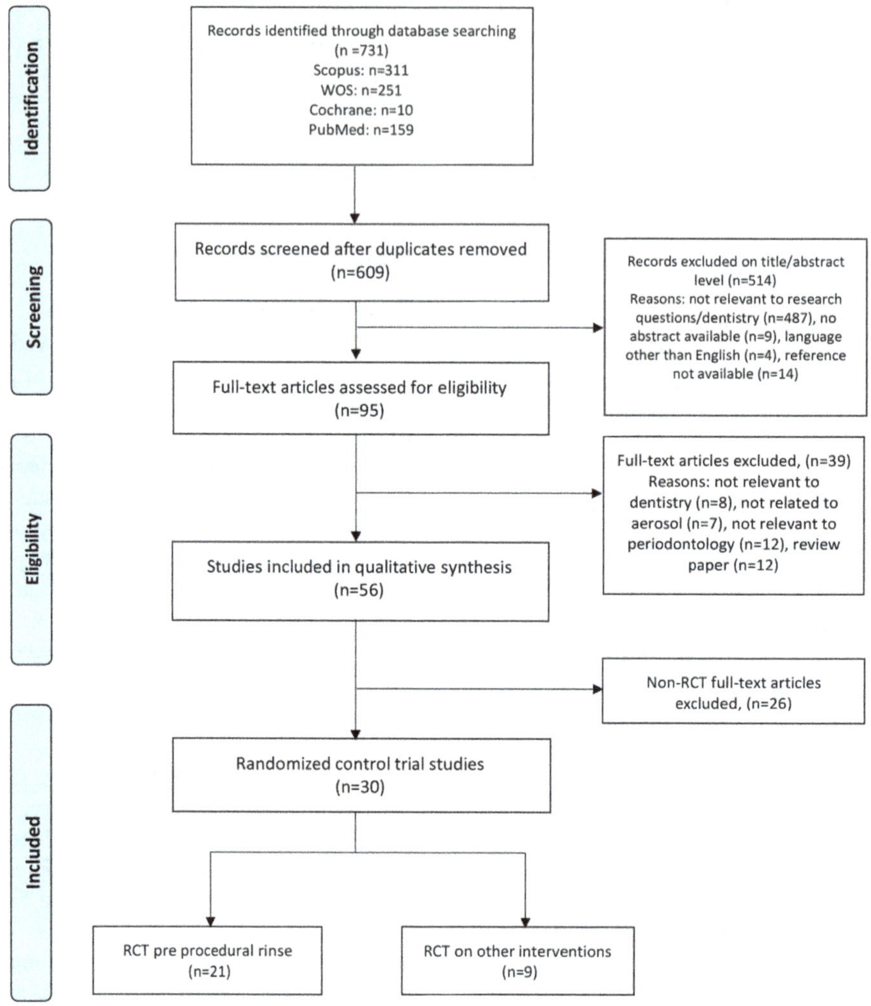

From: Moher D, Liberati A, Tetzlaff J, Altman DG, The PRISMA Group (2009). *P*referred *R*eporting *I*tems for *S*ystematic Reviews and *M*eta-*A*nalyses: The PRISMA Statement. PLoS Med 6(7): e1000097. doi:10.1371/journal.pmed1000097

For more information, visit www.prisma-statement.org.

FIGURE 1 | Summary of the selection process for systematic review.

calculated by Mean cfu reduction (%) = [(total amount of mean cfu at baseline—total amount of mean cfu after prophylaxis)/total amount of mean cfu at baseline] x 100%. When baseline data were not provided in the articles, mean reduction percentage was calculated as Mean cfu reduction (%) = (total amount of mean cfu for control group—total amount of mean cfu for test group)/total amount of mean cfu for control group] x 100%.

Quality and Risk of Bias Assessment

An assessment of quality and risk of bias assessment was conducted on effective studies that informed the review employing the revised Cochrane risk-of-bias tool for randomized trials (RoB 2) (20). Domains evaluated were: Domain 1—risk of bias arising from the randomization process, Domain 2—risk of bias due to deviation from the intended interventions, Domain 3—risk of bias due to missing outcome data, Domain 4—risk of bias in measurement of outcomes, and Domain 5—risk of bias in the selection of the reposted results. Using specific signaling questions for each domain, response options including **Yes** (Y), **Probably yes** (PY), **Probably no** (PN), **No** (N), and **No information** (NI) available were made. Finally, the overall risk-of-bias judgement was made for each article based on the criteria for **Low Risk**, judged to raise **Some Concerns**, or **High Risk** of bias. Agreement between evaluators for this section (S.M-S., T.N.M., and H.R.) were discussed with the supervising author (C.M.) and the inter-evaluator reliability was calculated using Kappa statistics.

RESULTS

Identification and Screening

The initial search yielded 731 articles across four databases. After removal of duplicates, the "title and abstract" of 609 articles were assessed, identifying 95 "potentially effective" studies (Agreement between assessors was high, **K** = 0.96). The full texts of potentially effective studies were then assessed, and 56 studies were identified as "effective studies" (Agreement between assessors was high **K** = 0.88). No additional studies were identified through "reference linkage" and among the effective studies 30 randomized control trial (RCT) studies were identified, 21 with a specific focus on pre-procedural rinsing (21–41) (**Figure 1**).

Characteristics of the Studies

The study characteristics and periodontal procedures undertaken to generate aerosol in the studies included in this review are described in **Table 1**. Studies were published between 1992 and 2020. Approximately a quarter (6/21) were split-mouth design RCTs (21–25), 13 were full-mouth design (27–40), and one did not provide details of study design (41). The vast majority were parallel-arm TCTs (19/21) and two were RCTs of cross-over design. Over a third of studies (8/21) were identified as double-blinded interventions, and one claimed to be a single-blind study. The total number of participants among the studies was 984, ranging from 18 to 120 among studies, and of varying ages (18 to 70 years old). Participation was high among studies, except in one study where a subject received/ initiated antibiotics during the course of the study (36).

In eleven studies there were three experimental groups; nine studies had two or four experimental groups. One study had all participants as their own controls (41). Of the 21 RCTs, 18 used chlorhexidine (CHX)-containing mouth rinse as either a test (21, 22, 24, 26, 28–41) or as a positive control group (27). Other agents tested were novel antiseptics (four studies) (22, 23, 25, 36), herbal essential oils, EO (two studies) (28, 37), cetylpyridinium chloride, CPC (three studies) (32, 35, 38), povidone iodine (two studies) (30, 31), chlorine dioxide (one study) (24), aloe vera (one study) (30), and herbal extract (two studies) (34, 40). Controls used were saline, sterile water, distilled water, hydro alcohol, or no rinse at all.

Apart from using pre-rinses, some studies added other interventions to examine the impact on reducing bacterial load, namely the use of high-volume evacuation, HVE (three studies) (21, 22, 26) and irrigation using ozone (one study) (31). The protocol for pre-procedural rinsing varied: participants were instructed to rinse between 30 s and 2 min, the amount of mouth rinse used range between 10–20 ml, and participants waited between 2 and 40 min before they were given periodontal prophylaxis. Most studies (19/21) used ultrasonic scaling as the periodontal prophylaxis procedure, and two studies used polishing devices (29, 37). The duration of the periodontal prophylaxis ranged from 3 to 30 min.

Effectiveness of Pre-procedural Rinse

Among the 21 studies, the majority (95.2%, 20) assessed bacterial contamination for aerosols (**Table 2**). For the most part, the key outcome measured was bacterial count expressed as colony forming units (cfu) on blood agar plates; however, incubation protocol differed among studies. One study assessed bacterial count per ml of blood, from blood drawn from the antecubital fossa (23); another study, in addition to aerosol bacterial contamination, assessed bacterial contamination from salivary samples (40). The sites of data collection differed among studies in terms of number of samples obtained, position, direction, and distance from subjects' mouth. However, there were no notable differences in the reduction of cfu from the aspects of periodontal prophylaxis devices used nor location of aerosol sampling collection from these studies. Approximately half of the studies (52.4%, 11/21) obtained the sample at or near the operator and dental assistant. Mostly, CHX rinse were tested (80.9%, 17/21), with various concentrations and volumes. Among studies comparing CHX with other agents (71.4%, 15/21), the effectiveness of CHX over other agents was evident, with more than half of the studies (7/15) reporting over a 70% reduction in cfu.

Assessment of Bias

Risk of bias varied among studies, **Figure 2**. For the most part (90.5% of studies), there was of unclear risk of bias in terms of the randomization process (domain 1) with 9.5% being of low risk of bias. There was generally a low risk of bias in terms of deviation from the intended interventions (95.2% of studies, domain 2) and the remaining were of questionable risk of bias (4.8%). There was a high risk of bias regarding missing outcome data in approximately 1 in 20 studies (4.8%), although 95.2% of studies in this regard were of low risk of bias (95.2%). For a third of studies (33.3%) there was a low risk of bias regarding the measurement of outcome; approximately half (52.4%) had an unclear risk of bias and 14.3% were of high risk of bias. In terms of selection of reported results, all studies were of low risk of bias.

DISCUSSION

As the number of fatalities and morbidities due to COVID-19 continues to rise it is important to acknowledge that oral health remains an integral element of overall health and well-being (42). Despite the uncertainties associated with the exact characteristics for SARS-Cov-2 transmission in dental settings, the dental team and administration must ensure safety of all personnel and patients, as well as other related parties involved in providing dental care to the public, such as cleaning and services. Reducing contamination of aerosol produced in dental clinics is a simple way to minimize and prevent cross-infections and has been increasingly reviewed during this pandemic (8, 43). The majority of these reviews focus on recommendations for general precautions in dental practice, but do not emphasize the aerosol contamination from periodontal prophylaxis, as one of the most common AGPs in dental clinics.

Our review is limited to aerosol contamination. Although our search was focused on microbial contamination in dental aerosol, there was no literature found on virus, which would provide more insight on possible COVID-19 cross-contamination in dental clinics. A majority of these studies included the use of CHX as

TABLE 1 | Pre-procedural rinse study characteristics (Ctd).

No.	References	Design	Subject size (N)	Pre-rinse intervention groups	Additional intervention group	Control group	Duration of rinse and interval before procedure	Periodontal procedure
1	Devker et al. (21)	Split mouth, parallel	90 patients, 30 per group 18 - 45y/o	0.2% CHX	Scaling with HVE (140mmHg), CHX + scaling with HVE	No CHX pre-rinse/no HVE/no combination	2 min pre-rinse 10 ml *interval:NA*	Piezoelectric ultrasonic, 10 min scaling
2	Sawhney et al. (22)	Split mouth, parallel	60 patients, 20 per group 25–54y/o	0.2% CHX (1:1 in water), antiseptic (*contents: NA*) (1:1 in water)	With / without HVE	Water	2 x 30 sec pre-rinse 15ml CHX / 20ml antiseptic, *interval:NA*	Piezoelectric ultrasonic, *duration: NA*
3	Fine et al. (23)	Split mouth, crossover, double blind	18 patients, 9 per group *age: NA*	Antiseptic mouthwash (*contents and concentration: NA*)		5% hydro alcohol	30 sec pre-rinse 20 ml *interval:NA*	Magnetostrictive (Cavitron) ultrasonic, 5 min scaling
4	Saini (24)	Split mouth, parallel, double blind, placebo controlled	120 patients, 40 per group 18 - 55y/o	Chlorine dioxide, 0.2% CHX		Water	1 min pre-rinse, 10 ml *interval:NA*	Piezoelectric ultrasonic 10 min scaling, power medium 15ml/min flow
5	Fine et al. (25)	Split mouth cross over, double blind, repeated at 1 week after	18 patients, 9 per group >18y/o	Antiseptic mouthwash (*contents and concentration: NA*)		5% hydro alcohol	30 sec pre-rinse, 20 ml, 10 min before scaling	Ultrasonic, 10 min scaling
6	Narayana et al. (26)	Split mouth parallel	45 patients, 15 per group *age: NA*	0.12% CHX	With HVE (30 - 40 psikg/cm2)	No rinse, no HVE	30 sec pre-rinse 10 ml *interval:NA*	Piezoelectric (EMS) ultrasonic, 20 min scaling
7	Rajachandrasekaran et al. (27)	Full mouth, parallel	50 patients, 25 per group 20 - 50y/o	Herbal oral rinse (*contents and concentration: NA*)		0.12% CHX	1 min pre-rinse 15 ml 10 min before scaling	Magnetostrictive (Cavitron Bobcat Pro) ultrasonic, 10 min scaling
8	Shetty et al. (28)	Full mouth, parallel	60 patients, 20 per grp 25 - 45y/o	0.2% CHX, Tea tree oil (*concentration: NA*)		Distilled water	*Duration: NA* 10 ml 2 min before scaling	Ultrasonic 10 min scaling
9	Santos et al. (29)	Full mouth, parallel	23 patients, 23 per group 10-40y/o	0.12% CHX		Distilled water	1 min pre-rinse, 15 ml 10 min before prophylaxis	Jet hand I, sodium bicarbonate, 4 min polishing
10	Paul et al. (30)	Full mouth, parallel	60 patients, 20 per group 18 - 35y/o	0.2% CHX, 1% Povidone iodine, 94.5% aloe vera extract		None	1 min pre-rinse, *volume: NA* 10 min before scaling	Piezoelectric ultrasonic, 20 min scaling

(Continued)

TABLE 1 | Continued

No.	References	Design	Subject size (N)	Pre-rinse intervention groups	Additional intervention group	Control group	Duration of rinse and interval before procedure	Periodontal procedure
11	Kaur et al. (31)	Full mouth, parallel, double blind	60 patients, 20 per group 20 - 50yold	0.2% CHX, 1% Povidone iodine	Irrigation with ozone(0.082mg/h)	None	1 min pre-rinse, *volume: NA interval:NA*	Ultrasonics, 10 min scaling
12	Retamal-Valdes et al. (32)	Full mouth, parallel, single blind	60 patients, 15 per group 18 - 70y/o	0.075% CPC + 0.28% Zn lactate + 0.05% NaF, 0.12% CHX + 10% alcohol		Water, no rinsing	1 min pre-rinse, 20 ml *interval: NA*	Magnetostrictive ultrasonic, 10 min scaling, frequency 25k Hz, power <50%
13	Reddy et al. (33)	Full mouth, parallel	30 patients, 10 per group *age: NA*	Non-tempered CHX 0.2%, tempered CHX 0.2%		Sterile water	1 min pre-rinse, *volume: NA interval:NA*	Ultrasonic scaling *duration: NA*
14	Gupta et al. (34)	Full mouth, parallel, double blind, placebo controlled	24 patients, 8 per group 25 - 55y/o	0.2% CHX, herbal extracts (*contents and concentration: NA*)		Water	1 min pre-rinse, 10 ml, 10min before scaling	Piezoelectric ultrasonic, 30 min scaling
15	Joshi et al. (35)	Full mouth, parallel, double blind	40 patients, 10 per group mean age 32.5	0.05% CPC (47°C), 0.2% CHX (47°C), 0.05% CPC (18°C), 0.2% CHX (18°C)			1 min pre-rinse 10 ml 10 min before scaling	Ultrasonic, 30 min scaling
16	Fine et al. (36)	Full mouth, crossover, double blind	18 patients, (1 initiated antibiotic, data excluded at the end) *per group: NA age:NA*	Antiseptic mouthwash (*contents and concentration: NA*)		5% hydro alcohol	30 s pre-rinse 20 ml 40 min before scaling	Magnetostrictive (Cavitron 3000) ultrasonic, 5 min scaling at each phase
17	Logothetis et al. (37)	Full mouth, parallel	18 patients 6 per group 25–54y/o	0.12% CHX, EO (*contents and concentration: NA*)		Distilled water	2 x 30 s pre-rinse 15 cc each rinse 10 min before air polishing	Polishing device, 3 min polishing
18	Feres et al. (38)	Full mouth, parallel, double blind, placebo controlled	60 patients, 15 per group 30 - 70y/o	0.05% CPC, 0.12% CHX		Water, no rinsing	1 min pre-rinse 15 ml *interval:NA*	Magnetostrictive (Cavitron Select) ultrasonic, 10 min scaling
19	Mohan et al. (39)	Full mouth parallel	20 patients, 10 per group 25 - 40y/o	0.2% CHX		Saline	1 min pre-rinse *volume: NA interval:NA*	Ultrasonic scaling *duration: NA*
20	Swaminathan et al. (40)	Full mouth, parallel	30 patients 10 per group 18–50y/o	0.2% CHX, herbal rinse (*concentration: NA*)		Saline	60 s pre-rinse 15 ml *interval:NA*	Ultrasonic scaling *duration: NA*
21	Serban et al. (41)	*NA*	80 patients, 40 per group 20–65y/o	0.1% CHX		Sterile water	*Duration: NA volume: NA interval:NA*	Ultrasonic scaling *duration: NA*

HVE, high volume evacuator; CHX, chlorhexidine; CPC, cetylpyridinium chloride; PI, povidone iodine, EO, essential oil; NA, information not available inarticles.

TABLE 2 | Pre-procedural rinse study main findings (Ctd).

No.	References	Outcome (unit)	Microbiological evaluation	Site of collection	Significant results (p values)	% of reduction of cfu
1	Devker et al. (21)	Bacterial count (cfu)	Bacterial contamination in aerosol, cultured on blood agar, incubated at 37°C for 24 h,	From patient's mouth: 1. 6in - operator's nose, 2. 6in - assistant's nose, 3. 12in - patient's chest, 4. 36in - patient's right side	Significant cfu count/reduction: - in all groups, in all location (Student's paired t-test, - $p < 0.01$), - in HVE alone was better than CHX alone, - in combine CHX + HVE was better than CHX or HVE alone	Mean cfu reduction between CHX - no CHX, HVE - no HVE, CHX+HVE - scaling only at: - operator's nose: 59.2%, 83.2%, 88.1% - assistant's nose: 60.7%, 81.6%, 87.7% - patient's chest: 55.9%, 83.1%, 87.9% - patient's right side: 48.0%, 65.0%, 79.3%
2	Sawhney et al. (22)	Bacterial count (cfu)	Bacterial contamination in aerosol, cultured on blood agar plates incubated at 37°C for 24 h	1. Patient's chest 2. Dental unit tray, 3. 6in away from patients' mouths	Significant cfu count/reduction: - in all groups (ANOVA, $p < 0.05$) - between CHX-water (Student's t-test, $p = 0.001$) and CHX-Listerine (Student's t-test, $p = 0.025$)	Mean aerobic cfu reduction between CHX, antiseptic and water: - with use of HVE: 95%, 70%, 40% - without use of HVE: 65%, 45%, 20%
3	Fine et al. (23)	Bacterial count per ml blood (cfu/ml)	Blood drawn from antecubital fossa then incubated on agar plates at 37°C for 24 h (aerobically), or 5 days (anaerobically)		Significant cfu count/reduction between antiseptic and control both aerobic and anaerobic colonies ($p = 0.00001$)	Mean cfu reduction between antiseptic-control for: - aerobic: 92.3% - anaerobic: 87.8%
4	Saini (24)	Bacterial count (cfu)	Bacterial contamination in aerosol, cultured on blood agar, incubated at 37°C for 48 h	From patient's mouth: 1. 1 feet - patient's chest 2. 1 feet - operator 3. 1 feet - assistant 4. 2 feet - 12 o'clock 5. 8 feet - 6 o'clock	Significant cfu count/reduction: - in ClO2 and CHX compared to water (ANOVA, $p < 0.001$) in all positions, - highest at patient's front, and almost the same in all other areas (ANOVA, $p < 0.001$)	Mean cfu reduction between water, ClO2, CHX at: - patient's chest: 2.1%, 85.4%, 88.0% - operator position: 2.1%, 85.7%, 87.7% - assistant position: 2.3%, 85.3%, 88.1% - 12 o'clock: 3.8%, 85.7%, 87.6% - 6 o'clock: 3.4%, 89.2%, 92.8%
5	Fine et al. (25)	Bacterial count (cfu)	Bacterial contamination in aerosol, cultured on blood agar, incubated at 37°C for 24–72 h	From patient's mouth: 1. 1 feet - patient's chest 2. 1 feet - operator's chest 3. 1 feet - assistant' chest 4. 2 feet - 12 o'clock 5. 8 feet - 6 o'clock	Significant cfu count/reduction: - in CHX compared to control (Student's t test, $p < 0.001$)	Mean cfu reduction between CHX and control at was 94.1% and 33.9%
6	Narayana et al. (26)	Bacterial count (cfu)	Bacterial contamination in aerosol, cultured on on blood agar incubated at 37°C for 48 h	Left of patient (between patient and assistant)	Significant cfu count/reduction: - in CHX pre-rinse group compared to no rinse (ANOVA, $p < 0.001$) - when HVE was used compared to no HVE (ANOVA, $p < 0.001$) - when both CHX and HVE were used (ANOVA, $p < 0.001$)	Mean cfu reduction between test-control groups for use of: - CHX: 61.4% - HVE: 67.0% - combination of CHX+HVE: 86.0%
7	Rajachandrasekaran et al. (27)	Bacterial count (cfu)	Bacterial contamination in aerosol, cultured on MeReSa with supplements agar plates, incubated at 37°C for 48 h	From patient's mouth: 1. 2 feet - patient's right 2. 2 feet - behind patient 3. 2 feet - patient's left 4. 3 feet - patient's right 5. 3 feet - patient's left 6. 5 feet - patient's right 7. 5 feet - patient's left 8. 9 feet	Significant cfu count/reduction: - in CHX (control) compared to herbal for MRSA (One way ANOVA, $p = 0.0001$) - in herbal group compared to CHX for MRSA colony compared to Actinobacter in all 8 locations (One way ANOVA, $p = 0.0001$)	Mean cfu reduction between herbal - CHX: - for MRSA: 55.6% - for Actinobacter: 17.5%

(Continued)

TABLE 2 | Continued

No.	References	Outcome (unit)	Microbiological evaluation	Site of collection	Significant results (*p* values)	% of reduction of cfu
8	Shetty et al. (28)	Bacterial count (cfu)	Bacterial contamination in aerosol, cultured on Trypticase soy agar plates	1. 6in - operator's nose 2. 6in - dental assistant's nose 3. 12in - patient's chest level	Significant cfu count/reduction: - between CHX-water, CHX-TTO, TTO-water, (Kruskal-Wallis, Mann-Whitney U, p <0.001)	Mean cfu reduction between CHX-water, TTO-water, CHX-TTO at all positions were 20.8%, 6.7%, 27.7%
9	Santos et al. (29)	Bacterial count (cfu)	Bacterial contamination in aerosol, cultured on Brain heart infusion (BHI) agar, incubated at 37°C, 48 h	1. operator's forehead 2. 10cm from operator's mouth (vertical downward) 3. 15cm from patient's mouth - patient's chest	Significant cfu count/reduction: - between interval T1 - T2 for both CHX and water (Wilconxon test comparing within groups; p <0.001) - in al 3 positions (Kruskal-Wallis): i- clinicians forehead: p = 0.0074 ii- clinician's chest: p = 0.0051 iii- patient's chest: p = 0.0035	Mean cfu reduction following CHX rinse at 1month at: - operator's forehead: 36.1% - operator's chest: 35.8% - patient's chest: 40.5%
10	Paul et al. (30)	Bacterial count (cfu)	Bacterial contamination in aerosol, cultured on blood agar, incubated at 37°C for 48 h	From patient's mouth: 1. 12in - patient's chest 2. 12in - operator's chest	Significant cfu count/reduction: - in all groups, in both location (one-way ANOVA, p = 0.001) - highest in CHX, AV then PVO-I (independent *t* test, p = 0.001) - between CXH - PVP-I and PVP-I - AV (ANOVA, *post hoc* comparison, p = 0.001)	Mean cfu reduction between CHX - PVP-I, CHX - AV and PVP-I - AV at: - operator's chest: 69.1%, 9.3%, 66.0% - patient's chest: 60.4%, 8.3%, 56.8%
11	Kaur et al. (31)	Bacterial count (cfu)	Bacterial contamination in aerosol, cultured on blood agar, incubated at 37°C for 48h	1. operator's chest, 2. 9feet behind patient's head	Significant cfu count/reduction: - in all groups, in all locations (paired t test, *post-hoc* Tukey's test) for aerobic (p <0.01) and anaerobic bacteria (*p* <0.001) - for aerobic bacteria at patient's chest between CHX-PI and PI-Ozone (*p* <0.01) - for anaerobic at patient's chest between CHX-Ozone (*p* <0.05)	Aerobic cfu reduction between CHX, PI, Ozone at: - operator's mask: 57%, 54%, 47% - patient's chest: 35%, 37% 29% - behind patient: 36%, 47%, 29% - anaerobic cfu reduction between CHX, PI, ozone at: - patient's chest: 43%, 36%, 35% - behind patient: 44%, 32%, 38%
12	Retamal-Valdes et al. (32)	Bacterial count (cfu)	Bacterial contamination in aerosol, cultured on enriched TSA blood agar, incubated at 37°C for 72 h	1. support board in front of patient 2. operator's forehead 3. patient's chest	Significant cfu count/reduction: - in CPC+Zn+F and CHX compared to water and those who did not rinse (Kruskall-Wallis and Dunn tests, p<0.05) at operator's forehead and patient's chest	Mean cfu reduction between CPC+Zn+F / CHX - no rinsing at: - all areas: 70%, 77% - operator's forehead: 89%, 94% - patient's chest: 55%, 60% - support board: 70%, 81% Mean cfu reduction between CPC+Zn+F / CHX - water at: - all areas: 61%, 70% - operator's forehead: 78%, 87% - patient's chest: 55%, 60% - support board: 59%, 75%
13	Reddy et al. (33)	Bacterial count (cfu)	Bacterial contamination in aerosol, cultured on blood agar, incubated at 37°Cfor 48 h	4 feet from patient's mouth: 1. 3 o'clock 2. 6 o'clock 3. 12 o'clock	Significant cfu count/reduction: - in tempered and non-tempered CHX compared to water (ANOVA, *p* <0.001) - in all positions as a cumulative data	Mean cfu reduction between water, non-tempered, tempered CHX at: 19.3%, 83.2%, 90.0%

(Continued)

TABLE 2 | Continued

No.	References	Outcome (unit)	Microbiological evaluation	Site of collection	Significant results (p values)	% of reduction of cfu
14	Gupta et al. (34)	Bacterial count (cfu)	Bacterial contamination in aerosol, cultured on blood agar, incubated at 37°C for 48 h	1. patient's chest 2. operator's chest 3. assistant's chest	Significant cfu count/reduction: - among all 3 groups (ANOVA, p <0.001) in all 3 locations - CHX significantly reduced cfu compared to herbal mouthwash (independent t test, p <0.001) in all 3 locations	Mean cfu reduction between CHX - water, herbal - water, CHX - herbal at: - patient's chest: 71.3%, 38.4%, 35.2% - operator's chest: 71.6%, 35.0%, 36.6% - assistant's chest: 16.1%, 6.9%, 9.3%
15	Joshi et al. (35)	Bacterial count (cfu)	Bacterial contamination in aerosol, cultured on blood agar plates, *details of incubation: NA*	From patient's mouth: 1. 12in - neck of patient 2. 12in - operator's chest 3. 12in - assistant's chest	Significant cfu count/reduction: - patient's chest had highest contamination ($p = 0.02$) - between cold CPC - cold CHX (unpaired t-tests, $p = 0.0284$) - equally in CPC and CHX (ANCOVA, p <0.001) - greater in warm CPC and CHX (p <0.001)	Mean cfu reduction CPC - CHX at: - all positions: 0.68% - 21.8% (not significant) - patient: warm CPC - cold CPC 26.3%, warm CHX - cold CHX 31.8% - operator: warm CPC - cold CPC 18.2%, warm CHX - cold CHX 31.4% - assistant: warm CPC - cold CPC 13.0%, warm CHX - cold CHX 20.9%
16	Fine et al. (36)	Bacterial count (cfu)	Bacterial contamination in aerosol, cultured on enriched soy agar, incubated at 37°C for 24–72 h	2 in from patient's mouth	Significant cfu reduction between antiseptic and water ($p = 0.0001$)	Mean cfu reduction between test - control was 93.6% and 32.1%
17	Logothetis et al. (37)	Bacterial count (cfu)	Bacterial contamination in aerosol, cultured on blood agar plates incubated at 37°C for 48h	From patient's mouth: 1. operator's mask 2. 2 feet - assistant 3. 3 feet - 12 o'clock 4. 3 feet - 9 o'clock 5. 3 feet - 3 o'clock 6. 5 feet 8in - 4 o'clock 7. 6 feet - 6 o'clock 8. 9 feet - 6 o'clock	Significant cfu reduction: - in all locations by CHX compared to others ($p = 0.001$)	Mean cfu reduction between CHX-water, EO-water and CHX-EO at: - operator's mask: 69%, 1%, 70% - 2 feet - assistant: 60%, 7%, 67% - 3 feet - 12 o'clock: 43%, 8%, 51% - 3 feet - 9 o'clock: 42%, 0%, 42% - 3 feet - 3 o'clock: 42%, 0%, 42% - 5 feet 8in - 4 o'clock: 35%,–5%, 30% - 6 feet - 6 o'clock: 30%,–5%, 25% - 9 feet - 6 o'clock: 25%,–5%, 20%
18	Feres et al. (38)	Bacterial count (cfu)	Bacterial contamination in aerosol, cultured on blood agar incubated with 10% CO_2 at 37°C for 72 h	From patient's mouth: 1. 12in - clinician's forehead 2. 12in - support board 3. 12in - patient's chest	Significant cfu count/reduction: - in CPC and CHX compared to water and no rinsing - equally in CPC and CHX in all locations (Kruskal-Wallis and Mann-Whitney U tests, p <0.05)	Mean cfu reduction between CPC - water / no rinsing and CHX - water / no rinsing at: - all: CPC: 68% / 77%, CHX: 70% / 78% - operator: CPC: 79% / 78%, CHX: 73% / 72% - board: CPC: 79% / 82%, CHX: 76% / 79% patient: CPC: 61% / 65%, CHX: 66% / 78%
19	Mohan et al. (39)	Bacterial count (cfu)	Bacterial contamination in aerosol, cultured on blood agar incubated at 37°C for 24 h	3 feet from patient (6 o'clock)	Significant cfu count/reduction: - within CHX ($p = 0.0049$) - between CHX and saline ($p = 0.0037$)	Mean cfu reduction between CHX - saline was 66.6% and 2.0%

(Continued)

TABLE 2 | Continued

No.	References	Outcome (unit)	Microbiological evaluation	Site of collection	Significant results (*p* values)	% of reduction of cfu
20	Swaminathan et al. (40)	Bacterial count (cfu) in saliva and aerosol	Bacterial contamination in aerosol, cultured on BHI agar incubated anaerobically at 37°C for 24 h	From patient's mouth: 1. 1 feet 2. 2 feet 3. 3 feet	Significant cfu count/reduction in: - aerosol at 3feet and saliva in all locations (Kruskal-Wallis, p <0.001) - between CHX-saline, herbal-saline, CHX-herbal (p <0.001)	Mean cfu reduction between CHX - saline and herbal – saline at: In aerosol: - 1 feet: 56.2%, 24.9% - 2 feet: 50.6%, 17.5% - 3 feet: 62.7%, 37.7% In saliva: - saline / CHX / herbal:–182% / 64.7% / 0.4% - CHX – saline: 103.0%, - herbal – saline: 47.7%
21	Serban et al. (41)	Total number of bacteria (cfu/m3).	Bacterial contamination in aerosol, cultured on blood agar, *details of incubation: NA*	Dentist's mask	Significant cfu count/reduction: - in CHX compared to water for bacteria (p <0.001) and haemolytic bacteria (p <0.001)	Mean cfu reduction between CHX - water for: - bacteria: 83.2% - haemolytic bacteria: 74.8%

HVE, high volume evacuator; CHX, chlorhexidine; CPC, cetylpyridinium chloride; PI, povidone iodine; EO, essential oil; NA, information not available in articles.

the main antiseptic agent to reduce aerosol contamination, as it is a well-established antimicrobial agent used in dentistry. CPC has also been widely tested in anti-plaque and anti-gingivitis studies (44, 45) as well as infection control in the dental clinic for disinfection of hands and surfaces (46, 47). Its potential to reduce microbial load after dental scaling is promising and, in this review, CPC had been included in three of the studies.

The key outcome measure among studies was bacterial contamination, which is predominantly related to associated aerosol contaminations. Given the importance of viruses such as COVID-19, there is a need to investigate the effectiveness of mouth rinses on viral counts. The lack of *in vivo* viricidal studies in part relates to the challenges and associated risk in culturing the virus (17). *In vitro* studies have shown chlorhexidine (0.12%) to be effective against most viruses, in as little as 30 s (48). Difference in effectiveness is thought to be due to physical/chemical structures of viruses' envelopes. In addition, several mouth rinses have been shown to be effective against standard strains of fungi *in vitro* (49). Whilst evidence of aerosol contamination and evidence of growth from such does suggest, at least theoretically, the risk of transmission, evidence from blood, saliva, or other samples can confirm actual transmission and potentially the reduction in risk following use of mouth rinses (50, 51). All studies demonstrated some degree of effectiveness of the mouth rinses, although their effectiveness varied widely. This is in part related to differences in study design (i.e., split mouth vs. subject level randomisation), differences in mouth rinses agent, differences in concentration among the same agent, differences in number and where assessments were conducted (i.e., distance from patient's mouth), and the use of other preventive measures (such as use of high-volume suctions). Such heterogeneity among studies precludes the ability to perform a meta-analysis. Nonetheless, the evidence suggests that mouth rinses are effective in reducing bacterial contamination and there is a need to consider their role in preventing viral infections, such as COVID-19.

A recent publication by Meister et al. (52) reported potential *in vitro* antiviral efficacy of some commercially available oral rinses against strains of SARS-CoV-2 when exposed within 30 s in saliva. Reasonably, strains of the virus reacted differently in many levels of susceptibility depending on the formulation prepared and contents of active ingredients in these rinses. Nevertheless, this finding may mark a turning point in efforts to lower the transmission of viruses, such as COVID-19, through use of oral rinses in the near future. Also noteworthy are the new trials being conducted to study the efficacy of oral mouthwashes on COVID-19 patients (https://clinicaltrials.ucsf.edu/trial/NCT04409873, https://clinicaltrials.gov/ct2/show/NCT04341688) that could help provide safe alternatives to dental practices and healthcare for the public at large.

Continuous periodontal care for periodontitis patients is of the utmost importance and must be done in a timely manner to prevent progression and reinfection of the disease, especially among high-risk individuals (53–56). Progression and reinfection of periodontal pockets does not only have implications for oral health, but also systemic health, given the bidirectional link between periodontal disease and

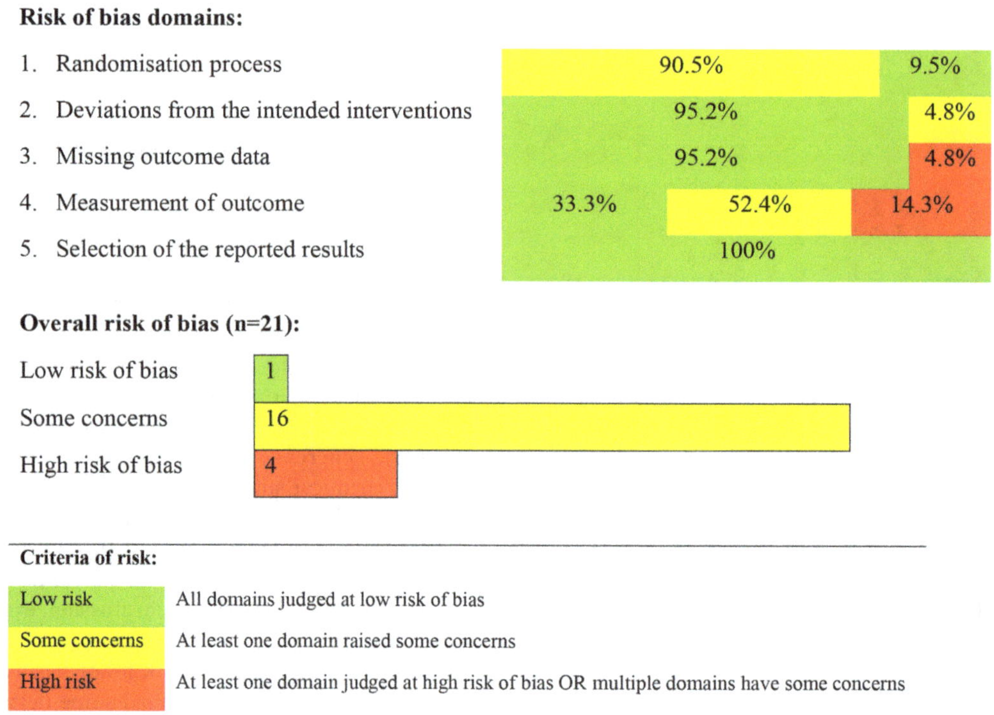

FIGURE 2 | Risk of bias criteria for the literature studied.

common non-communicable diseases such as diabetes mellitus, rheumatoid arthritis, and hypertension, and those who are immune suppressed. The treatment needs of the patients should not be hampered during this pandemic, but instead should be further prioritized, as there are restrictions of movement, limited access to dental care, and fear of cross-infections from dental clinics. Resolving this issue would offer more benefits than containing the progression of periodontal disease in the population, as it would also improve the quality of life of patients (57, 58) with long-term supportive care (55).

Pre-procedural rinsing for clinical dental procedures has long been advocated for and, during the current pandemic, its importance to practice is more relevant than ever. A number of acceptable quality RCTs of pre-procedural mouth rinsing have been conducted. The focus has been on bacterial contamination rather than viral or fungal assay. A range of different pre-procedural mouth rinses have been tested (mostly chlorhexidine), of varying concentrations and amounts, and for dental procedures of different durations and using different techniques with and without additional means. We acknowledge that these systematic review findings do not differ much from the previous reviews, nevertheless it emphasizes on the importance of pre-rinsing particularly in periodontal prophylaxis procedures. This is especially important during the current pandemic where transmission bacterial-borne diseases could well be avoided by reducing the risk on dental personnel as well as the patients. This also supports the need to include the pre-rinsing procedure for dental patients as one of the mandatory SOP in current practice.

CONCLUSION

Our systematic review found no remarkable new evidence on the effectiveness of pre-procedural rinse in periodontal prophylaxis, but it highlights the importance of the procedure to be given a mandatory emphasis in the current pandemic SOP in dental clinics. Pre-procedural rinsing for 30 s to 2 min with selected antimicrobial solutions compared to water or no rinsing were found to effectively reduce aerosol contamination in periodontal prophylaxis on dental patients. There is evidence that chlorhexidine (either 0.12 or 0.2%) is an effective antimicrobial solution for this purpose. The use of HVE during the procedure also helps to reduce the aerosol contamination.

AUTHOR CONTRIBUTIONS

CM, TM-D, and SM-S: conceptualization. CM, TM-D, and SM-S: methodology. SM-S, HR, TM-D, and CM: analysis. SM-S, NS, and TM-D: writing—original draft preparation. SM-S, HR, TM-D, and CM: writing—review and editing. CM: supervision. All authors contributed to the article and approved the submitted version.

ACKNOWLEDGMENTS

The authors wish to thank the Deans of both Universiti Kebangsaan Malaysia and The University of Hong Kong for their support in our collaborative effort in adopting measures to improve dental education and oral health care in teaching institutions during the 2020 COVID-19 pandemic.

REFERENCES

1. Centre for Disease Control. *Interim Infection Prevention and Control Guidance for Dental Settings During the Coronavirus Disease 2019 (COVID-19) Pandemic.* Available online at: https://www.cdc.gov/coronavirus/2019-ncov/hcp/dental-settings.html (accessed April 15, 2020)
2. National Health Service, NHS England & NHS Improvement. *COVID-19 Guidance and Standard Operating Procedure Urgent Dental Care Systems in the Context of Coronavirus.* Delay Phase NHS England. Version 1. 15 April 2020. Available on at: http://www.essexldc.org.uk/C0282-covid-19-urgent-dental-care-sop.pdf (accessed June 16, 2020).
3. World Health Organisation. *Considerations for the Provision of Essential oral Health Services in the context of COVID-19.* Available online at: https://www.who.int/publications/i/item/who-2019-nCoV-oral-health-2020.1 (accessed August 3, 2020).
4. Huang KC, Lai CH, Huang CF, Lu HK. A comprehensive periodontal treatment project: The periodontal status, compliance rates, and risk factors. *J Dent Sci.* (2016) 11:182–8. doi: 10.1016/j.jds.2015.07.006
5. Kumar PS, Subramanian K. Demystifying the mist: Sources of microbial bioload in dental aerosols. *J Periodontol.* (2020) 91:1113–22. doi: 10.1002/JPER.20-0395
6. Chuang CY, Cheng HC, Yang S, Fang W, Hung PC, Chuang SY. Investigation of the spreading characteristics of bacterial aerosol contamination during dental scaling treatment. *J Dent Sci.* (2014) 9:294–6. doi: 10.1016/j.jds.2014.06.002
7. Ge ZY, Yang LM, Xia JJ, Fu XH, Zhang YZ. Possible aerosol transmission of COVID-19 and special precautions in dentistry. *J Zhejiang Univ Sci B.* (2020) 21:361–68. doi: 10.1631/jzus.B2010010
8. Marui VC, Souto ML, Rovai ES, Romito GA, Chambrone L, Pannuti CM. Efficacy of preprocedural mouthrinses in the reduction of microorganisms in aerosol: a systematic review. *J Am Dent Assoc.* (2019) 150:1015–26. doi: 10.1016/j.adaj.2019.06.024
9. Santos CM, Pimenta CA, Nobre MR. The PICO strategy for the research question construction and evidence search. *Rev Latino-Am Enfermagem.* (2007). 15:508–11. doi: 10.1590/S0104-11692007000300023
10. Tran K, Cimon K, Severn M, Pessoa-Silva CL, Conly J. *Aerosol-Generating Procedures and Risk of Transmission of Acute Respiratory Infections: A Systematic Review [Internet].* Ottawa, ON: Canadian Agency for Drugs and Technologies in Health (2011). Available online at: https://www.cadth.ca/media/pdf/M0023__Aerosol_Generating_Procedures_e.pdf
11. Tran K, Cimon K, Severn M, Pessoa-Silva CL, Conly J. Aerosol generating procedures and risk of transmission of acute respiratory infections to healthcare workers: a systematic review. *PLoS ONE.* (2012) 7:e35797. doi: 10.1371/journal.pone.0035797
12. Tran K, Cimon K, Severn M, Pessoa-Silva C, Conly J. Aerosol-generating procedures and risk of transmission of acute respiratory infections: a systematic review. *CADTH Technol Overv.* (2013) 3:e3201.
13. Needleman I, McGrath C, Floyd P, Biddle A. Impact of oral health on the life quality of periodontal patients. *J Clin Periodontol.* (2004) 31:454–7. doi: 10.1111/j.1600-051X.2004.00498.x
14. Smiley CJ, Tracy SL, Abt E, Michalowicz BS, John MT, Gunsolley J, et al. Systematic review and meta-analysis on the nonsurgical treatment of chronic periodontitis by means of scaling and root planing with or without adjuncts. *J Am Dent Assoc.* (2015) 146:508–24. doi: 10.1016/j.adaj.2015.01.028
15. Trombelli L, Franceschetti G, Farina R. Effect of professional mechanical plaque removal performed on a long-term, routine basis in the secondary prevention of periodontitis: a systematic review. *J Clin Periodontol.* (2015) 42:S221–36. doi: 10.1111/jcpe.12339
16. Bühler J, Amato M, Weiger R, Walter C. A systematic review on the patient perception of periodontal treatment using air polishing devices. *Int J Dent Hyg.* (2016) 14:4–14. doi: 10.1111/idh.12119
17. Zemouri C, de Soet H, Crielaard W, Laheij A. A scoping review on bio-aerosols in healthcare and the dental environment. *PLoS ONE.* (2017) 12:e0178007. doi: 10.1371/journal.pone.0178007
18. Robertson S, Douglas P, Jarvis D, Marczylo E. Bioaerosol exposure from composting facilities and health outcomes in workers and in the community: a systematic review update. *Int J Hyg Environ Health.* (2019) 222:364–86. doi: 10.1016/j.ijheh.2019.02.006
19. Zhang J, Liu J, Li J, Chen B, Li H, Yan F. The clinical efficacy of subgingival debridement by ultrasonic instrumentation compared with subgingival air polishing during periodontal maintenance: a systematic review. *J Evid Based Dent Pract.* (2019) 19:101314. doi: 10.1016/j.jebdp.2019.02.001
20. Higgins JP, Thomas J, Chandler J, Cumpston M, Li T, Page MJ, et al. *Cochrane Handbook for Systematic Reviews of Interventions.* Hoboken, NJ: John Wiley & Sons (2019).
21. Devker NR, Mohitey J, Vibhute A, Chouhan VS, Chavan P, Malagi S, et al. A study to evaluate and compare the efficacy of preprocedural mouthrinsing and high volume evacuator attachment alone and in combination in reducing the amount of viable aerosols produced during ultrasonic scaling procedure. *J Contemp Dent Pract.* (2012) 13:681–9. doi: 10.5005/jp-journals-10024-1209
22. Sawhney A, Venugopal S, Babu GR, Garg A, Mathew M, Yadav M, et al. Aerosols how dangerous they are in clinical practice. *J Clin Diagn Res.* (2015) 9:ZC52–7. doi: 10.7860/JCDR/2015/12038.5835
23. Fine DH, Korik I, Furgang D, Myers R, Olshan A, Barnett ML, et al. Assessing pre-procedural subgingival irrigation and rinsing with an antiseptic mouthrinse to reduce bacteremia. *J Am Dent Assoc.* (1996) 127:641–6. doi: 10.14219/jada.archive.1996.0276
24. Saini R. Efficacy of preprocedural mouth rinse containing chlorine dioxide in reduction of viable bacterial count in dental aerosols during ultrasonic scaling: a double-blind, placebo-controlled clinical trial. *Dent Hypotheses.* (2015) 6:65. doi: 10.4103/2155-8213.158479
25. Fine DH, Mendieta C, Barnett ML, Furgang D, Meyers R, Olshan A, et al. Efficacy of preprocedural rinsing with an antiseptic in reducing viable bacteria in dental aerosols. *J Periodontol.* (1992) 63:821–4. doi: 10.1902/jop.1992.63.10.821
26. Narayana TV, Mohanty L, Sreenath G, Vidhyadhari P. Role of preprocedural rinse and high volume evacuator in reducing bacterial contamination in bioaerosols. *J Oral Maxillofac Surg Med Pathol.* (2016) 20:59–65. doi: 10.4103/0973-029X.180931
27. Rajachandrasekaran Y, Valiathan M, Jayaraman BG, Mahalakshmi K, Padmavathy K. An herbal alternative to control nosocomial pathogens in aerosols and splatter during ultrasonic scaling. *Pesqui Bras Odontopediatria e Clin Integr.* (2019) 19:e4807, 1–9. doi: 10.4034/PBOCI.2019.191.106
28. Shetty SK, Sharath K, Shenoy S, Sreekumar C, Shetty RN, Biju T. Compare the efficacy of two commercially available mouthrinses in reducing viable bacterial count in dental aerosol produced during ultrasonic scaling when used as a preprocedural rinse. *J Contemp Dent Pract.* (2013) 14:848–51. doi: 10.5005/jp-journals-10024-1414
29. Santos IR, Moreira AC, Costa MG, Barbosa MD. Effect of 0.12% chlorhexidine in reducing microorganisms found in aerosol used for dental prophylaxis of patients submitted to fixed orthodontic treatment. *Dental Press J Orthod.* (2014) 19:95–101. doi: 10.1590/2176-9451.19.3.095-101.oar
30. Paul B, Baiju RM, Raseena NB, Godfrey PS, Shanimole PI. Effect of aloe vera as a preprocedural rinse in reducing aerosol contamination during ultrasonic scaling. *J Indian Soc Periodontol.* (2020) 24:37. doi: 10.4103/jisp.jisp_188_19
31. Kaur R, Singh I, Vandana KL, Desai R. Effect of chlorhexidine, povidone iodine, and ozone on microorganisms in dental aerosols: Randomized double-blind clinical trial. *Indian J Dent Res.* (2014) 25:160. doi: 10.4103/0970-9290.135910
32. Retamal-Valdes B, Soares GM, Stewart B, Figueiredo LC, Faveri M, Miller S, et al. Effectiveness of a pre-procedural mouthwash in reducing bacteria in dental aerosols: randomized clinical trial. *Braz Oral Res.* (2017) 31:e21. doi: 10.1590/1807-3107bor-2017.vol31.0021
33. Reddy S, Prasad MS, Kaul S, Satish K, Kakarala S, Bhowmik N. Efficacy of 0.2% tempered chlorhexidine as a pre-procedural mouth rinse: a clinical study. *J Indian Soc Periodontol.* (2012) 16:213–17. doi: 10.4103/0972-124X.99264

34. Gupta G, Mitra D, Ashok KP, Gupta A, Soni S, Ahmed S, et al. Efficacy of preprocedural mouth rinsing in reducing aerosol contamination produced by ultrasonic scaler: a pilot study. *J Periodontol.* (2014) 85:562–8. doi: 10.1902/jop.2013.120616
35. Joshi AA, Padhye AM, Gupta HS. Efficacy of two pre-procedural rinses at two different temperatures in reducing aerosol contamination produced during ultrasonic scaling in a dental set-up-A microbiological study. *J Int Acad Periodontol.* (2017) 19:138–44.
36. Fine DH, Yip J, Furgang D, Barnett ML, Olshan AM, Vincent J. Reducing bacteria in dental aerosols: pre procedural use of an antiseptic mouthrinse. *J Am Dent Assoc.* (1993) 124:56–8. doi: 10.14219/jada.archive.1993.0122
37. Logothetis DD, Martinez-Welles JM. Reducing bacterial aerosol contamination with a chlorhexidine gluconate pre-rinse. *J Am Dent Assoc.* (1995) 126:1634–9. doi: 10.14219/jada.archive.1995.0111
38. Feres M, Figueiredo LC, Faveri M, Stewart B, de Vizio W. The effectiveness of a preprocedural mouthrinse containing cetylpyridinium chloride in reducing bacteria in the dental office. *J Am Dent Assoc.* (2010) 141:415–22. doi: 10.14219/jada.archive.2010.0193
39. Mohan M, Jagannathan N. The efficacy of pre-procedural mouth rinse on bacterial count in dental aerosol following oral prophylaxis. *Dent Med Probl.* (2016) 53:78–82. doi: 10.17219/dmp/60694
40. Swaminathan YO, Thomas JT, Muralidharan NP. The efficacy of preprocedural mouth rinse of 0.2% chlorhexidine and commercially available herbal mouth containing salvadora persica in reducing the bacterial load in saliva and aerosol produced during scaling. *Asian J Pharm Clin Res.* (2014) 7:71–4.
41. Serban D, Banu A, Serban C, Tută-Sas I, Vlaicu B. Predictors of quantitative microbiological analysis of spatter and aerosolization during scaling. *Rev Med Chir Soc Med Nat lasi.* (2013) 117:503–8.
42. Herrera D, Serrano J, Roldán S, Sanz M. Is the oral cavity relevant in SARS-CoV-2 pandemic? *Clin Oral Invest.* (2020) 24:2925–30. doi: 10.1007/s00784-020-03413-2
43. Koletsi D, Belibasakis GN, Eliades T. Interventions to reduce aerosolized microbes in dental practice: a systematic review with network meta-analysis of randomized controlled trials. *J Dent Res.* (2020) 99:1228–38. doi: 10.1177/0022034520943574
44. Teng F, He T, Huang S, Bo CP, Li Z, Chang JL, et al. Cetylpyridinium chloride mouth rinses alleviate experimental gingivitis by inhibiting dental plaque maturation. *Int J Oral Sci.* (2016) 8:182–90. doi: 10.1038/ijos.2016.18
45. Haps S, Slot DE, Berchier CE, Van der Weijden GA. The effect of cetylpyridinium chloride-containing mouth rinses as adjuncts to toothbrushing onplaque and parameters of gingival inflammation: a systematic review. *Int J Dent Hyg.* (2008) 6:290–303. doi: 10.1111/j.1601-5037.2008.00344.x
46. Millns B, Martin MV, Field EA. The sensitivity to chlorhexidine and cetyl pyridinium chloride of staphylococci on the hands of dental students and theatre staff exposed to these disinfectants. *J Hosp Infect.* (1994) 26:99–104. doi: 10.1016/0195-6701(94)90051-5
47. Ziskind D, Gleitman J, Rotstein I, Friedman M. Evaluation of cetylpyridinium chloride for infection control in storage solution. *J Oral Rehabil.* (2003) 30:477–81. doi: 10.1046/j.1365-2842.2003.01091.x
48. Baqui AA, Kelley JI, Jabra-Rizk MA, DePaola LG, Falkler WA, Meiller TF. *In vitro* effect of oral antiseptics on human immunodeficiency virus-1 and herpes simplex virus type 1. *J Clin Periodontol.* (2001) 28:610–6. doi: 10.1034/j.1600-051x.2001.028007610.x
49. Moroz J, Kurnatowski P. The *in vitro* activity of selected mouthrinses on standard strains of fungi. *Ann Parasitol.* (2017) 63:331–9. doi: 10.17420/ap6304.120
50. Guo ZD, Wang ZY, Zhang SF, Li X, Li L, Li C, et al. Aerosol and surface distribution of severe acute respiratory syndrome coronavirus 2 in hospital wards, Wuhan, China, 2020. *Emerg Infect Dis.* (2017) 26:1586–91. doi: 10.3201/eid2607.200885
51. Cheng VC, Wong SC, Chan VW, So SY, Chen JH, Yip CC, et al. Air and environmental sampling for SARS-CoV-2 around hospitalized patients with coronavirus disease 2019 (COVID-19). *Infect Control Hosp Epidmiol.* (2020) 41:1258–65. doi: 10.1017/ice.2020.282
52. Meister TL, Brüggemann Y, Todt D, Conzelmann C, Müller JA, Groß R, et al. Virucidal efficacy of different oral rinses against SARS-CoV-2. *J Infect Dis.* (2020) 222:1289–92. doi: 10.1093/infdis/jiaa471
53. Pennington M, Heasman P, Gaunt F, Güntsch A, Ivanovski S, Imazato S, et al. The cost-effectiveness of supportive periodontal care: a global perspective. *J Clin Periodontol.* (2011) 38:553–61. doi: 10.1111/j.1600-051X.2011.01722.x
54. Mohd-Dom TN, Wan-Puteh SE, Muhd-Nur A, Ayob R, Abdul-Manaf MR, Abdul-Muttalib K, et al. Cost-effectiveness of periodontitis management in public sector specialist periodontal clinics: a societal perspective research in Malaysia. *Value Health.* (2014) 3:117–23. doi: 10.1016/j.vhri.2014.04.012
55. Graetz C, Schwalbach M, Seidel M, Geiken A, Schwendicke F. Oral health-related quality of life impacts are low 27 years after periodontal therapy. *J Clin Periodontol.* (2020) 47:952–61. doi: 10.1111/jcpe.13324
56. Sanz M, Herrera D, Kebschull M, Chapple I, Jepsen S, Berglundh T, et al. Treatment of stage I–III periodontitis—The EFP S3 level clinical practice guideline. *J Clin Periodontol.* (2020) 47(Suppl. 22):4–60. doi: 10.1111/jcpe.13290
57. Needleman I, Nibali L, Di Iorio A. Professional mechanical plaque removal for prevention of periodontal diseases in adults–systematic review update. *J Clin Periodontol.* (2015) 42:S12–35. doi: 10.1111/jcpe.12341
58. Ferreira MC, Dias-Pereira AC, Branco-de-Almeida LS, Martins CC, Paiva SM. Impact of periodontal disease on quality of life: a systematic review. *J Periodontal Res.* (2017) 52:651–65. doi: 10.1111/jre.12436

14

Management of the Oral Health of Children During the COVID-19 Pandemic in Poland

Aneta Olszewska [1†], Elzbieta Paszynska [2†], Magdalena Roszak [3] and Agata Czajka-Jakubowska [4]*

[1] Department of Developmental Facial Malformation, Poznan University of Medical Sciences, Poznań, Poland, [2] Department of Integrated Dentistry, Community Dentistry Section, Poznan University of Medical Sciences, Poznań, Poland, [3] Department of Computer Science and Statistics, Poznan University of Medical Sciences, Poznań, Poland, [4] Department of Temporomandibular Joint Disorders, Poznan University of Medical Sciences, Poznań, Poland

***Correspondence:**
Aneta Olszewska
anetaol@ump.edu.pl

† These authors have contributed equally to this work and share first authorship

Managing the oral health of children during the time of a health emergency linked to the current COVID-19 pandemic presents specific problems. A high number of non-specific effective infection control protocols are available in dental settings. It is of fundamental importance to implement specific protocols relating to those clinical situations that normally do not represent an emergency but which now fall into that category. The aim of this study was the comparison of data obtained from the Regional National Health Fund (NFZ) relating to the number and the type of procedures in the oral health management of children aged 0–18 years from the Wielkopolska region, with the months of March and April of 2019 being compared with those of the, respective, pandemic period of 2020. The results showed statistical differences in the number of performed procedures when comparing 2019 and 2020; especially in April (n = 53,077 in 2019 but only n = 2,287 in 2020), when lockdown restrictions reached their highest level and when only 30% of the dental clinics for children were open for patients in the Wielkopolska region of Poland. Regarding surgical cases, there were no differences in percentage frequency between April 2019 and 2020 in terms of extractions. However, an increase was observed in abscess incisions (3.5–17.8%) and surgical dressings (1.5–10.07%). There was a decrease in the total number of performed conservative dentistry procedures in April 2020, but temporary fillings in primary and permanent teeth showed a prominent increase: from 6.4% in 2019 to 19.3% in 2020; and 5.8–11.4%, respectively. Pulp treatment and mucosal lesions therapy fall into the dental emergency category during this COVID-19 pandemic. These cases have shown an increase from 3.2% in 2019 to 12.8% in 2020 for pulp treatment, and from 2.3 to 4.3% for the treatment of oral mucosal lesions. As suspected, after the lockdown was implemented, the number of pediatric dental cases were low. Moreover, the analysis revealed differences in the profile of clinical situations that represented the emergency cases and the pandemic treatment protocols. Future implications suggest that dental prophylactic procedures be included in pandemic protocols with even dental services being limited to a form of urgent treatment. New approaches and treatment models should be implemented in the control of the infectious spread of the disease in the management of the oral health of children in this pandemic period.

Keywords: oral health, children, COVID-19 pandemic, dentistry, protocols

INTRODUCTION

During the new SARS-CoV-2 virus pandemic, countries implemented different measures for the delivery of dental care for adult and pediatric patients (1). Many dental procedures have been associated with the transmission of SARS-Cov-2 via droplets and splatter from blood and saliva through direct and indirect contact. Direct transmission occurs through respiratory droplets by coughing or sneezing, or in the course of dental procedures between the dentist, the assistant, and the patients. The risk of indirect transmission can occur when a patient or the dental team are in contact with surfaces contaminated with the virus (dental chair, spittoons, floor, etc.). Some procedures, such as using a high-speed turbine, ultrasonic scaler and spray gun, produce a large amount of aerosol, which can remain suspended in the air for long periods of time, increasing the risk of transmission (2, 3).

Because children can be asymptomatic or present with non-specific symptoms, it has been recommended that all pediatric patients and their parents/caregivers should be considered as possible carriers of SARS-CoV-2. This potentially puts pediatric dentists at a high risk of infection (4–7). The management of pediatric patients can also be influenced by behavioral problems connected with greater dental anxiety due to the use of personal protective equipment (mask, goggles, face shield) which makes conversation and adaptation to the dental environment very difficult (8).

During the COVID-19 epidemic (March/April 2020), according to the national recommendations for medical specialties, the routine dental treatment for children in Poland was suspended and limited to emergency cases only. It was reported that only 30% of the dental clinics for children were open for patients in the Wielkopolska region of Poland.

Therefore, the objective of this study was to compare a number dental cases performed in both children and adolescents with national insurance before (March and April 2019 y) and during the actual phase of COVID-19 (March and April 2020 y).

MATERIALS AND METHODS

Approval by the Ethics Committee has been revised by the project protocol at the Poznan University of Medical Sciences (9/06/2020). The analysis was based on data from dental offices in Wielkopolska, which have signed a contract for medical services agreed to be performed in dental care in pediatric dentistry. The data collection was obtained from the National Health Fund (NFZ) under its administrative agreement as well as freedom in access to information guaranteed by national law regulations. The patient status was obviously kept anonymous. One of the examiners involved in data extraction holds the function of a qualified consultant in pediatric dentistry (A.O.). A comparison of the dental service from March/April 2019 vs. March/April 2020 was conducted. The above-mentioned period of time was chosen as a blow up of the first SARS-CoV-2 pandemic lockdown in relation to community activities. Dental service procedures for surgery (S) and conservative dentistry (CD) were divided into the following categories: tooth extraction: single-root (category S), tooth extraction: multiple-root (S), surgical dressing (S), abscess incision (S) and temporary filling of secondary teeth (category CD), temporary filling of primary teeth (CD), restoration of primary teeth (CD), restoration of secondary teeth (CD), post-trauma reconstruction of tooth (CD), trepanation (CD), devitalization (CD), and other procedures (CD). It is noteworthy that during the severe phase of the SARS-CoV-2 pandemic, regular prosthodontic, orthodontic, and periodontal procedures were suspended and they were not considered as marginal in the analyzed period of time.

In 2019, 97 dental clinics in Wielkopolska provided dental services for children and adolescents up to the age of 18. In 2020, this number increased to 99 offices that were dedicated to treating children.

The dental offices are required to submit a report each month for counter-work. The work done during the pandemic period did not release these dental offices from the obligation to submit these reports.

Only correctly filled forms of the reports were accepted in the study and these served as a sources of data. In this study, we have not analyzed data according to age, sex, location of dental practice, specialty of dental practitioners, or any level subject to satisfaction with the provided dental services.

According to the information provided by the Central Statistical Office (GUS), the population of children and adolescents (up to 18 years of age) in Wielkopolska in 2019 stood at 744,228.

Statistical Analysis

The data are presented as absolute numbers and/or percentages, as appropriate. The categorical data (2 × 2 or larger contingency tables) were analyzed using the Chi-squared test for independence and/or as the difference between the two proportions. All results were considered significant at $p < 0.05$. All statistical analyses were performed with InStat 3.06 (GraphPad Inc.) and Statistica 13.0 (StatSoft Inc.).

RESULTS

The results showed statistical differences in the number of performed procedures when comparing 2019 and 2020; especially in April ($n = 53,077$ in 2019 but only $n = 2,287$ in 2020), when lockdown restrictions reached their highest level and when only 30% of dental clinics for children were open for patients in the Wielkopolska region of Poland (**Table 1**).

The statistical analysis revealed changes in the profiles of clinical situations that represented emergency cases and pandemic treatment protocols (**Figures 1, 2**).

Regarding the surgical cases, there were no differences in percentage frequency between April 2019 and 2020, in terms of extractions.

No correlation was seen between the month/year and the number of extractions in both single-rooted and multi-rooted teeth, and the distribution of services was similar in all the periods analyzed, namely March 2019, April 2019, March 2020, and April 2020 ($p = 0.9186$), despite the fact that fewer surgical procedures were performed in 2020.

TABLE 1 | The statistical comparison in the number of dental service procedures for surgery and conservative dentistry (primary and secondary dentition) performed in March and April 2019 and 2020 y.

	2019	2019	2020	2020	Differences between months*
	March	**April**	**March**	**April**	**Multiple comparisons (*p*-value)**
Dental surgery procedures	$n = 1,440$	$n = 1,283$	$n = 564$	$n = 112$	
Tooth extraction: single-root	556	487	204	31	April 19 vs. April 20 ($p = 0.031$)
Tooth extraction: multi-root	829	731	326	49	April 19 vs. April 20 ($p = 0.007$) March 20 vs. April 20 ($p = 0.007$)
Surgical dressing	28	19	17	12	April 19 vs. April 20 ($p < 0.001$) March 20 vs. April 20 ($p = 0.001$)
Abscess incision	27	46	17	20	April 19 vs. April 20 ($p < 0.001$) March 19 vs. April 19 ($p = 0.009$) March 20 vs. April 20 ($p < 0.001$)
Conservative dentistry procedures	$n = 8,127$	$n = 7,517$	$n = 3,501$	$n = 352$	**Multiple comparisons (*p*-value)****
Temporary filling of secondary teeth	462	433	199	40	April 19 vs. April 20 ($p < 0.001$) March 20 vs. April 20 ($p < 0.001$)
Temporary filling of primary teeth	525	480	205	68	April 19 vs. April 20 ($p < 0.001$) March 20 vs. April 20 ($p < 0.001$)
Restoration primary teeth	4,074	3,847	1,709	12ggz6	April 19 vs. April 20 ($p < 0.001$) March 20 vs. April 20 ($p < 0.001$)
Restoration of secondary teeth	1,999	1,840	915	50	April 19 vs. April 20 ($p < 0.001$) March 20 vs. April 20 ($p < 0.001$)
Post-trauma reconstruction of tooth	70	62	36	2	ns
Trepanation	265	241	100	45	April 19 vs. April 20 ($p < 0.001$) March 20 vs. April 20 ($p < 0.001$)
Devitalization	236	169	99	15	April 19 vs. April 20 ($p = 0.016$) March 19 vs. April 19 ($p = 0.048$)
Other procedures	496	445	238	6	April 19 vs. April 20 ($p < 0.001$) March 20 vs. April 20 ($p < 0.001$)

*n, number of total procedures; *statistical significance difference using the χ^2-test $p < 0.05$; **statistical significance difference using the χ^2-test except post-trauma reconstruction of toot; non-significance $p > 0.05$ (ns).*

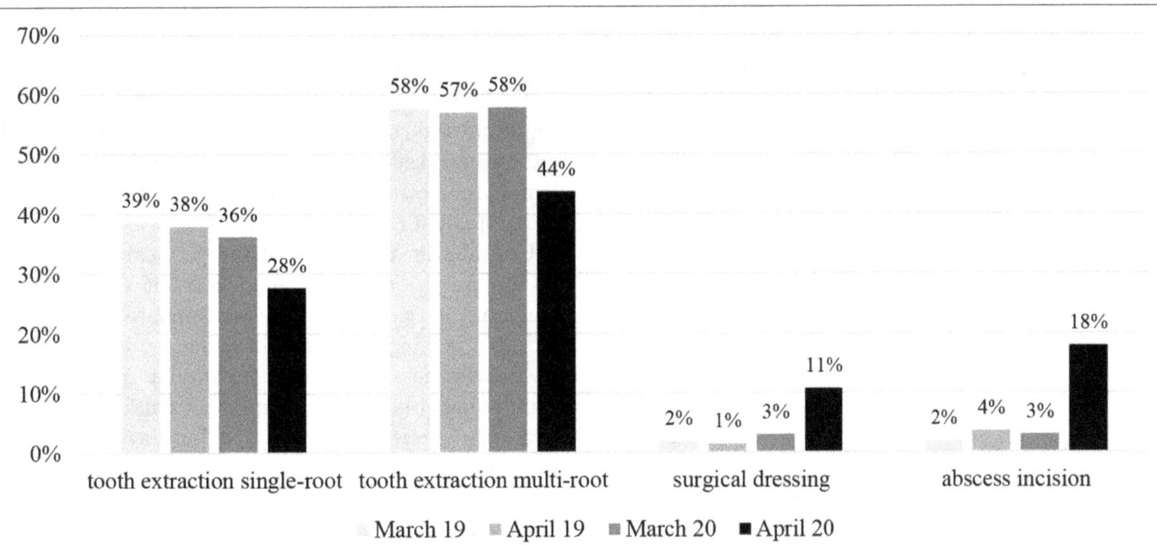

FIGURE 1 | The Statistical comparison showing the percentage of the dental service procedures for surgical procedures (primary and secondary dentition) conducted in March and April 2019 and 2020 y.

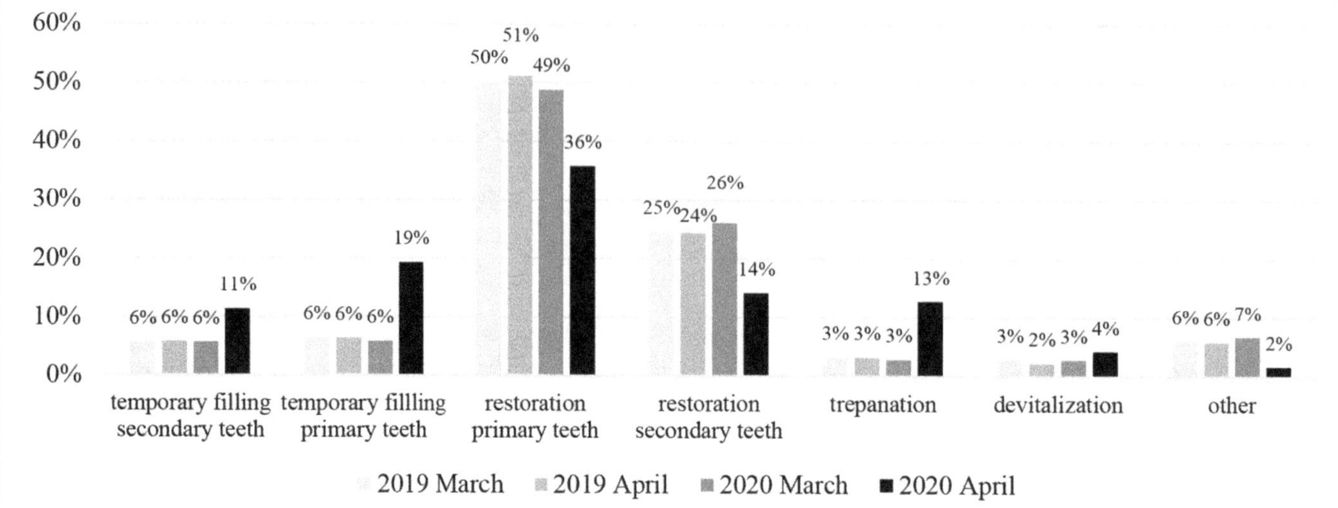

FIGURE 2 | The Statistical comparison showing the percentage of dental service procedures for conservative dentistry (primary and secondary dentition) performed in March and April 2019 and 2020 y.

However, an increase was observed in abscess incisions (3.5–17.8%) and surgical dressings (1.5–10.07%) (**Table 1**, **Figure 1**).

There was a decrease in the total number of performed conservative dentistry procedures in April 2020, but temporary fillings in primary and permanent teeth showed a prominent increase: from 6.4% in 2019 to 19.3% in 2020; and 5.8–11.4%, respectively.

For deciduous and permanent teeth, in March 2019, April 2019, and March 2020, the distribution of the number of therapeutic dressings and fillings was similar and there were no statistical differences. Only April 2020 was different, where the number of fillings decreased in relation to an increased number of dressings ($p < 0.0001$) (**Table 1**).

Taking into consideration the relationship between the time period (month/year) and the performance of the trepanation/devitalization procedures, there was a different distribution of trepanation/devitalization in the month of April 2020 when compared to the other months analyzed ($p < 0.002$): more trepanation was performed in relation to devitalization, with the ratio changing to 75/25% (previously it was 52.9/47.1%; 58.8/41.2%; 50.3/49.7%) (**Figure 2**).

Pulp treatment and mucosal lesions therapy fall into the dental emergency category in this COVID-19 pandemic. These cases showed an increase from 3.2% in 2019 to 12.8% in 2020 for pulp treatment and from 2.3 to 4.3% for the treatment of oral mucosal lesions.

DISCUSSION

As suspected after the lockdown was implemented, the number of pediatric dental cases were low. Moreover, the analysis revealed differences in the profile of clinical situations that represented emergency cases and pandemic treatment protocols.

During the first phase of the COVID-19 pandemic, restricting dental interventions to urgent and emergency cases showed that pediatric dentists have to reassess the benefits of treatment and the risks for the patient associated with potential infection. In this context, good cooperation with the parents/guardians of the child with regard to assessing the health condition and the observed symptoms as well as the measures that can be taken if a visit to the office of the dentist is not essential, as minor issues can be managed at home, makes it possible for pediatric dentists to effectively diagnose and treat patients through the use of "teledentistry."

Based on information from the literature, clinical conditions that are not classified as urgent dental interventions and can be managed by parents/guardians at home include, among others, loss of temporary fillings in deciduous and permanent teeth which is not accompanied by pain; delayed exfoliation of deciduous teeth; and pericoronitis around the erupting permanent molars (2).

The new experience of the COVID-19 pandemic shows how important the roles played by the development of information and communication technology and the ability to remotely solve dental problems that do not require a visit to a dental office are in doctor–patient communication (9).

Considering the effects of the pandemic-related restrictions on the provision of dental services, it seems that when the pandemic is over it will be necessary to adapt to preventive and therapeutic procedures in pediatric dentistry based on the new challenges and greater treatment needs. The effects of abandoning preventive treatment in children is likely to result in a rapid increase in the need for therapeutic intervention, and reinstating regular preventive visits ought to be the first stage in the post-pandemic resumption of operations of pediatric dental offices.

During the SARS-CoV-2 pandemic, the new epidemic situation requires the implementation of special protocols and precautions, in line with the recommendations and the guidelines issued by local and global health authorities.

The safety and health of children is always a priority, especially in the dynamic conditions of the pandemic. The concerns of parents on the potential risks associated with the visit of their child to the office of the dentist can often be the reason for refraining from making an appointment, which in turn may lead to the worsening of the original problem accompanied by complications and severe pain (2).

A child who comes to the dentist with severe pain, especially during the pandemic, is at a high risk of internalizing the unpleasant sensations associated with a dental visit. In the future, this may lead to anxiety that may make it impossible for them to cooperate during dental treatment, requiring sedation via inhalation or general anesthesia.

The role of a pediatric dentist is to educate the parents/guardians of the children about the safety of the procedures performed at the office of the dentist during this particularly difficult pandemic period, while at the same time making them aware of the risks associated with abandoning or delaying dental interventions (10).

It is noteworthy that regular prosthodontic, periodontal, and orthodontic procedures were suspended due to risk of bioaerosol contamination risk at the dental clinics and, hence they were not performed. The reason for this decision lies in significant exposure to infection to pathogens from the mouth and respiratory tract of the patients (11). When working with rotary burs that require water cooling, bioaerosol is formed and the water drops act as carriers of infectious microorganisms. In 2020, the Ministry of Health completed the group of the highest risk factors for infection with biological material by including the Sars-CoV-2 virus transmitted by droplets on the list. The dynamic COVID-19 pandemic forced changes in the organization of work in dental offices based on infection prevention protocols. It is assumed that the longer bioareosol treatment, the higher the risk of COVID-19 infection in the operating areas in dental clinics. Therefore, it is believed that exposure is one of the highest cause of infection among all medical professions. Additionally, if the patient is a child who cries or screams, the risk increases significantly due to the speed of the bioaerosol trajectory. The present COVID-19 time has forced the implementation of safe work procedures with the recommendation to use effective personal protective equipment. For example, use of disposable PPE kits, face shields, masks, caps, protective materials in clothing resistant to fluids, and moisture with hermetic eye protection are recommended for dental personnel.

The recommendations of dental teams with regard to the dental visits of children during the pandemic include the presence of only one parent/caregiver in the office of the dentist; the use of oxidizing rinses (H_2O_2) or chlorhexidine (CHX) before examining the mouth of the child; isolating the treatment area with rubberdam; four-handed work; and the use of high-power suction systems.

The procedure should include all the necessary interventions aimed at relieving the pain of the patient at the given moment, as well as those aimed at preventing the development of other potential ailments; therefore, it is recommended that a dental clearance examination of the mouth of the child should be performed during the same visit (12).

Similar approaches to dental patients may include rinsing with commercial mouthrinses to reduce oral viremia from saliva and oral mucosa. There are several active ingredients of mouthwash that have been tested for their anticovid efficacy. These include chlorhexidine gluconate, cetylpyridine chloride, povidone iodine, hydrogen peroxide, cyclodextrin, and essential oils (13). Other reports confirm the effective protection against the transmission of SARS-CoV-2 due to the content of zinc and stannous fluoride in mouthrinses and toothpastes. In all cases, it is indicated that the exposure to the oral cavity of the patient and the concentration of an active ingredient may have a crucial role in reducing virus transmission (14).

Work safety against the spread of infectious bioaerosols has significantly increased the amount of medical wastes. Currently these materials are not biodegradable, not recyclable, and require radical disposal by complete incineration. This form of waste reduction is not ecological and burdens our environment with harmful gas compounds. Therefore, there is a need to improve protective materials, both for the safety of the natural environment and to provide better protection for medical personnel as well. The search for new solutions will also ensure a sense of security and verify the readiness of stationary dental care. Moreover, it is important for the academic education in all medical professions, which is currently a great challenge (15–19).

To assume, the end of the pandemic will have to mean the beginning of new methods of management in pediatric dentistry. Intelligent technology systems would prefer a remote dentist–patient communication as a standard tool for projecting oral health education in children, especially in the school age. Virtual contact as teleprophylaxis or dental tele-advice will be helpful in strengthening healthy habits and motivating children to follow hygienic and dietary recommendations. As recommended, minimally invasive procedures should be employed, but also strenuous efforts should be made to promote preventive measures.

The pandemic has exacerbated inequalities in health care access. Changing the financing of services for children and adolescents and shifting funds from the model of reimbursement of reconstructive treatments to prophylaxis are currently the expected models in dental care.

CONCLUSIONS

During the first phase of the COVID-19 pandemic, restricting dental interventions to urgent and emergency cases showed that pediatric dentists had to reassess the benefits of treatment and the risks for the patients associated with potential infection.

The analysis revealed changes in the profile of clinical situations that represented emergency cases and pandemic treatment protocols. Future implications suggest that dental prophylactic procedures be included in pandemic protocols with even dental services being limited to a form of urgent treatment.

AUTHOR CONTRIBUTIONS

MR is responsible for statistics analyzes. AC-J for ideas and revisions of the research. All authors contributed to the article and approved the submitted version.

REFERENCES

1. Del Rio C, Malani PN. 2019 novel coronavirus-important information for clinicians. *JAMA*. (2020) 323:1339–40. doi: 10.1001/jama.2020.1490
2. Peng X, Xu X, Li Y, Cheng L, Zhou X, Ren B. Transmission routes of 2019-nCoV and controls in dental practice. *Int J Oral Sci.* (2020) 12:9. doi: 10.1038/s41368-020-0075-9
3. Liu W, Zhang Q, Chen J, Xiang R, Song H, Shu S, et al. Detection of Covid-19 in children in early January 2020 in Wuhan, China. *N Engl J Med.* (2020) 382:1370–1. doi: 10.1056/NEJMc2003717
4. The Chinese Preventive Medicine Association. An update on the epidemiological characteristics of novel coronavirus pneumonia (COVID-19). *Zhonghua Liu Xing Bing Xue Za Zhi.* (2020). 41:139–44. doi: 10.3760/cma.j.issn.0254-6450.2020.02.002
5. Meng L, Hua F, Bian Z. Coronavirus disease 2019. (COVID-19): emerging and future challenges for dental and oral medicine. *J Dent Res.* (2020) 99:481–7. doi: 10.1177/0022034520914246
6. Henry BM, Oliveira MHS. Preliminary epidemiological analysis on children and adolescents with novel coronavirus disease 2019 outside Hubei Province, China: an observational study utilizing crowdsourced data. *medRxiv [Preprint].* (2020) doi: 10.1101/2020.03.01.20029884
7. Liu T, Yuan WJ, Wang XD, Xiao Y, Yu L-Y. [Nursing strategy of oral and maxillofacial trauma emergency during epidemic situation of the novel coronavirus pneumonia]. *China J Oral Maxillofac Surg.* (2020) 18:198–203.
8. Lu X, Zhang L, Du H, Zhang J, Li YY, Qu J, et al. SARS-CoV-2 infection in children. *N Engl J Med.* (2020) 382:1663–5. doi: 10.1056/NEJMc 2005073
9. Sun P, Lu X, Xu C, Sun W, Pan B. Understanding of COVID 19 based on current evidence. *J Med Virol.* (2020) 92:548–51. doi: 10.1002/jmv. 25722
10. Chen J. Pathogenicity and transmissibility of 2019-nCoV—a quick overview and comparison with other emerging viruses. *Microb Infect.* (2020) 22:69–71. doi: 10.1088/1475-7516/2020/01/004
11. Wang C, Horby PW, Hayden FG, Gao GF. A novel coronavirus outbreak of global health concern. *Lancet.* (2020). 395:470–3. doi: 10.1016/S0140-6736(20)30185-9
12. Fox C. Evidence summary: what 'cost of illness' evidence is there about cross-infection related infections in dental practice? *Br Dent J.* (2010) 209:87–8. doi: 10.1038/sj.bdj.2010.651
13. Seneviratne CJ, Balan P, Ko KKK, Udawatte NS, Lai D, Ng DHL, et al. Efficacy of commercial mouth-rinses on SARS-CoV-2 viral load in saliva: randomized control trial in Singapore. *Infection.* (2020) 49:305–11. doi: 10.1101/2020.09.14.20186494
14. Carrouel F, Gonçalves LS, Conte MP, Campus G, Fisher J, Fraticelli L, et al. Antiviral Activity of Reagents in Mouth Rinses against SARS-CoV-2. *J Dent Res.* (2021) 100:124–32. doi: 10.1177/0022034520967933
15. Mizumoto K, Omori R, Nishiura H. Age specificity of cases and attack rate of novel 2 coronavirus disease (COVID-19). *medRxiv [Preprint].* (2020) doi: 10.1101/2020.03.09.20033142
16. Trottini M, Bossù M, Corridore D, et al. Assessing risk factors for dental caries: a statistical modeling approach. *Caries Res.* (2015) 49:226–35. doi: 10.1159/000369831
17. Tang A, Xu W, Shen M, Chen P, Li G, Liu Y, et al. A retrospective study of the clinical characteristics of COVID-19 infection in 26 children. *medRxiv [Preprint].* (2020) doi: 10.1101/2020.03.08.20029710
18. Ji LN, Chao S, Wang YJ, Li XJ, Mu XD, Lin MG, et al. Clinical features of pediatric patients with COVID-19: a report of two family cluster cases. *World J Pediatr.* (2020) 16:267–70. doi: 10.1007/s12519-020-00356-2
19. Hammel J Fischel J. Dental emergencies. *Emerg Med Clin North Am.* (2019) 37:81–93. doi: 10.1016/j.emc.2018.09.008

15

A Risk-Based Approach to the COVID-19 Pandemic: The Experience in National Dental Centre Singapore

John Rong Hao Tay [1], Ethan Ng [1], Marianne Meng Ann Ong [1,2], Chelsia Sim [3], Ken Tan [2] and Chaminda Jayampath Seneviratne [2,4]*

[1] Department of Restorative Dentistry, National Dental Centre Singapore, Singapore, Singapore, [2] Oral Health Academic Clinical Programme, Duke-NUS Medical School, Singapore, Singapore, [3] Department of Oral and Maxillofacial Surgery, National Dental Centre Singapore, Singapore, Singapore, [4] National Dental Centre Singapore, National Dental Research Institute Singapore, Singapore, Singapore

***Correspondence:**
Chaminda Jayampath Seneviratne
jaya.seneviratne@ndcs.com.sg

The emergence of a highly infectious coronavirus strain, severe acute respiratory syndrome coronavirus 2 (SARS-CoV-2), has led to a major global public health emergency. The increasing number of infected cases and fatalities worldwide forced several countries into lockdown in a bid to control virus transmission. The practice of dentistry is considered high-risk due to the generation of aerosols associated with most dental procedures, and healthcare professionals must take appropriate precautions whilst working in this challenging environment. This review aims to provide an overview on transmission routes and shares a risk-based approach to coronavirus disease 2019 (COVID-19) in a specialty tertiary center. Risk assessment and mitigation focussed on staff and patient safety, adopting a wide safety margin, and responding dynamically to the level of risk at the workplace. As the severity of the pandemic depends on many still-unknown factors and shows little sign of abating, the routine practice of dentistry will continue to be disrupted in the near future. We describe a color-coded framework to maximize safety and to minimize disease spread. Areas covered include healthcare team management, personal protective equipment, clinical work, and dental education. Guidelines in each category change with the corresponding severity of the situation, and we believe it will be useful for the safer practice of dentistry in this current climate and can be modified for future similar disease outbreaks.

Keywords: communicable diseases, emerging/epidemiology/therapy/virology, disease outbreaks, dental care/standards, infection control, dental, coronavirus infections/epidemiology/prevention & control/transmission, COVID-19

INTRODUCTION

Coronaviruses are single-stranded RNA viruses with an envelope. They were first identified around 70 years ago, and are capable of causing respiratory, gastrointestinal, and central nervous system diseases in humans and animals (1). The name "corona" implies a crown-like structure with spikes on the surface. These spike proteins are critical for binding of host cells receptors to facilitate entry, they may undergo evolutionary changes over time (2). Notable coronavirus infections in human history include severe acute respiratory syndrome-related coronavirus (SARS-CoV) in 2003 and Middle East Respiratory syndrome-related coronavirus (MERS-CoV) in 2012. SARS-CoV and

MERS-CoV were highly virulent and deadly, causing ~10 and 35% mortality in infected individuals (3, 4).

The first confirmed cluster of patients with pneumonia associated with a novel strain of coronavirus virus emerged in December 2019 (5). Since then, next-generation sequencing of the virus genome has found it to be around 79% similar to SARS-CoV and 50% similar to MERS-CoV, although sufficiently divergent to be considered a novel virus (6). The official name of the disease has been termed "COVID-19," with SARS-CoV-2 announced as the virus causing this disease (7). The announcement of COVID-19 as a pandemic by the World Health Organization (WHO) in March 2020 marked a turning point in the containment of this disease.

COVID-19 IS A GLOBAL AND NATIONAL PUBLIC HEALTH EMERGENCY

COVID-19 was declared to be a public health emergency of international concern on 30 January 2020 (8). On 6 October 2020, WHO reported over 35 million cases globally, with over one million deaths and rising each day (9).

At the time of writing (6 October 2020) Singapore had 57,792 confirmed cases and 27 fatalities. A large majority of the confirmed cases were clinically well and were isolated and cared for at community facilities. There were 153 cases are at community facilities, 42 cases are hospitalized but are medically stable, none of the cases are in critical condition, and 57,597 cases have been discharged after successful recovery (10). A total of 88 healthcare workers and support staff were infected with COVID-19 between January and April 2020, representing 1.7% of total confirmed COVID-19 cases during the same period (11). Most of these infected healthcare workers and support staff were in the public sector (68.2%) or served at the frontlines with frequent patient contact (63.6%) (11). While most of these healthcare workers acquired COVID-19 infection locally, epidemiological links of cross-infection between healthcare workers and COVID-19-positive patients have not been demonstrated (11, 12). Singapore's management of this crisis has been based on a structured nation-wide strategy for global infectious disease outbreaks termed Disease Outbreak Response System Condition (DORSCON). This is a four-tiered color-coded crisis management plan and ranges from green, yellow, orange and red (13). The color code is based on the nature of the disease (severity and degree of spread locally and abroad) and amount of disruption to daily life on a community and individual level. The current status in Singapore since 7 February 2020 has been DORSCON orange. Accordingly, various measures such as daily health checks at workplaces, temperature screening at hospitals, and suspension of inter-school and external activities for schools were put in effect. As part of its early containment strategy, Singapore was already conducting contact tracing for confirmed cases, quarantining close contacts, issuing stay-home notices for citizens recently arriving from China, and issuing travel bans into the country to reduce the risk of imported cases into the community (14). Stay home notices were later broadened to anyone who had traveled outside Singapore, with travel bans imposed for all short-term visitors from any country (15, 16). As the transmission of COVID-19 progressed, anyone coming in from abroad were given stay-home notices or issued with quarantine orders, depending on their exposure to the virus. Others were instructed to take a leave of absence from their employers. If they presented with respiratory symptoms, they were given a mandatory 5 days of medical leave and were not allowed to leave their place of residence.

In March 2020, a suspect case was defined as one who presented with an acute respiratory illness of any degree of severity, who, within the last 14 days before onset of illness had traveled abroad to high-risk areas, or had close contact with a COVID-19-positive patient. Any person with clinical signs and symptoms suggestive of pneumonia or severe respiratory infection with breathlessness was also considered a suspect case. A close contact was defined as anyone who provided care for the COVID-19-positive patient, including a healthcare worker or a family member, or who had other similarly close physical contact; anyone who had stayed (e.g., household members) at the same place with the patient; or anyone who had close (< 2 m) and prolonged contact (30 min or more) with the patient (15). Suspect cases who were medically stable were referred to a medical general practitioner for further evaluation immediately. Suspect cases who required urgent dental treatment such as the need to alleviate oral infection or pain were referred to the national specialty centers for management.

From 7 April to 1 June 2020 Singapore entered a "circuit breaker" period (**Table 1**) due to a surge in locally transmitted

TABLE 1 | Different stages of the national response in Singapore to COVID-19.

Disease Outbreak Response System Condition (DORSCON): a four-tiered color-coded crisis management plan for an infectious disease outbreak and ranges from green, yellow, orange, and red. Singapore has been under DORSCON orange since February 2020 at the time of writing (6 October 2020). At NDCS, all non-essential dental review appointments were rescheduled for at least 4 months at the onset of DORSCON orange. Patients on active therapy had their treatment deferred if they presented with a specific set of respiratory symptoms, contact history, or travel history.

Safe distancing measures: These measures were implemented in March 2020 where seats were to be separated by at least a meter apart in public venues; places where people gathered in close contact for long periods of time such as bars, cinemas, places of worship were closed; and gatherings outside school and work were limited to 10 or fewer people. These measures were adopted at NDCS.

"Circuit breaker" period: A 2-month period (7 April to 1 June 2020) where heightened restrictions to community movement was imposed nationwide to further prevent community spread of SARS-CoV-2. This included the closure of non-essential workplaces and schools. Food establishments were not allowed to offer dine-in options, and all members of the public were to leave their homes only for essential needs. At NDCS, only essential services requiring urgent or emergency care were performed.

Singapore has since transited from the "circuit breaker" period to a **phased staged of reopening**. Phase 1 lasted from 2 June to 19 June 2020. Singapore is currently in Phase 2 as of 6 October 2020. Schools and business have gradually been allowed to re-open, with social gatherings of up to five people allowed. Since Phase 1 till the time of writing, NDCS requires patient appointments to be booked 15 min apart from each other. This has reduced the number of patients seen each day, reducing the potential risk of transmission between patients and staff.

cases, new clusters developing among large groups of people housed together, and to mitigate the risk of widespread community transmission. As a result, heightened measures were implemented to minimize further community spread of the virus. Residents were prohibited from leaving their homes except for essential purposes (17). The wearing of masks was made compulsory outside one's home, and all workplaces were closed except for essential services. Elderly people and those with co-morbidities were advised to stay home as much as possible. Similarly, all elective dental procedures were halted during this period, except for essential services. Essential services were defined as procedures "if not provided or performed, would result in significant or rapid deterioration of the patient's condition, potentially threatening their health and well-being" (18). Hence, only patients requiring urgent/emergency dental care were seen.

The practice of dentistry is considered high-risk due to the close proximity between patients and dental practitioners and the generation of aerosols associated with most dental procedures (19). The potential for unknown interaction with COVID-19 patients due to asymptomatic spread is a concern as well. In this paper we provide an overview on transmission routes of COVID-19 and describe a risk mitigation approach during the period of DORSCON orange at National Dental Centre Singapore (NDCS), a referral tertiary center for patients needing specialist oral healthcare in Singapore. A color-coded framework to maximize safety and minimize disease spread is also described.

TRANSMISSION ROUTES

The transmissibility of COVID-19 remains poorly understood. Droplet transmission from respiratory secretions is the postulated principal mechanism of spread of COVID-19. Coughing consists not only of short-range semiballistic emission, but also consists of a turbulent gas cloud and may travel as far as 7–8 m (20). Droplets may vary in size, with small particles dehydrating and existing as droplet nuclei or aerosolised forms (21). Droplet generation into the surroundings decreases significantly to background levels when a cloth is placed over the mouth during speech (22). Virus particles have been found in air exhaust outlets in a Singapore study, demonstrating airflow displacement of the virus and spread through ventilation systems (23). Airborne transmission was also shown to occur in closed spaces with air re-circulation with no evidence of contact between patients (24, 25). SARS-CoV-2 has been shown to be suspended in the air as aerosols in crowded places and may also be resuspended from medical staff personal protective equipment while they are being removed (26). The virus has also been found to be viable in aerosols for a duration of 3 h (27). The transmission distance of the virus in aerosolised form has been detected up to 4 m from COVID-19-positive patients (28). In addition, the conjunctival mucosa and bronchial epithelium appear to be portals of entry in getting infected with COVID-19 (29). This underscores the need for healthcare workers to be socially responsible and ensure that they remain appropriately masked during work, even with 1–2-m safe distancing advisories. It also implies that many routine procedures performed in dentistry are potentially hazardous due to the aerosol generation from handpieces and ultrasonic scaler tips.

Environmental contact is another possible mode of transmission. Human coronaviruses can survive on inanimate objects and can remain viable for up to 5–9 days at temperatures of 22–25°C and relative humidity of 40–50% (30, 31). Surface type seems to play a role in the viability of the virus. An experimental study using a SARS-CoV-2 strain reported viability on plastic for up to 72 h, for 48 h on stainless steel and up to 8 h on copper (27). Another study showed that the virus could still be detected on glass and banknotes after 4 days, and surgical masks, stainless steel and plastic after 7 days (32). The virus has also been found on the floor, computer mice, trash cans, and doorknobs, emphasizing the need for thorough decontamination of surfaces (28). The persistence on surfaces is particularly worrying because inadvertent self-inoculation may be possible after touching such contaminated surfaces. Some of these studies used samples of the virus that were several orders of magnitude higher than those in droplets in real-life scenarios and it may be argued that the risk of transmission of COVID-19 through surfaces is extremely small (33). However, as environmental transmission remains a theoretical possibility, disinfection of the clinical environment with prescribed workflows and trained dental personnel is prudent in reducing transmission. SARS-CoV-2019 is susceptible to standard disinfectants such as 70% alcohol, 0.5% hydrogen peroxide, 0.1% sodium hypochlorite, 7.5% povidone-iodine, 0.05% chloroxylenol, 0.05% chlorhexidine, and 0.1% benzalkonium chloride (30, 32). Decontamination can also be achieved with a combined detergent/disinfectant solution at a dilution of 1,000 parts per million available chlorine (31).

The last postulated mode of transmission is the fecal-oral route. Digestive symptoms have been found in 50% of patients with COVID-19, they may present before respiratory symptoms (34). Indeed, viable virus has been isolated from stool samples, testing positive although respiratory tract tests were negative (35). Therefore, fecal-oral transmission may occur even after viral clearance from the respiratory tract. SARS-CoV-2 has also shown to be present in toilet bowl samples in another Singapore study, strengthening the hypothesis of possible transmission through fecal matter (36).

It was initially suggested that patients with COVID-19 are not infectious until the onset of symptoms, and that the infectivity depends on the severity of their symptoms and illness (31). However, from an analysis of a group of seven clusters in Singapore it appears that transmission of SARS-CoV-2 can occur even before patients develop symptoms (37). While there are also case reports of asymptomatic transmission where patients remain asymptomatic throughout the course of infection, its exact risk of transmission is unclear, and the prevalence and detection of asymptomatic infection is not well-understood (38–40). Emerging evidence suggests that 20% of subjects that test positive for COVID-19 remain asymptomatic throughout the course of infection, and asymptomatic individuals have a relative risk of 0.35 in transmitting the disease when compared to symptomatic individuals (41). SARS-CoV-2 has an incubation period of up to 14 days, with a median time of 4–5 days before onset of symptoms (42, 43). In another study, 97.5% of persons develop symptoms within 11.5 days (44). The time for recovery after onset of symptoms generally takes 2 weeks for mild cases, and 3–6 weeks for severe cases (8, 45).

HEALTHCARE TEAM MANAGEMENT

In Singapore, public provision of health services (medical and dental) is through three integrated clusters, divided according to geographical location. Each cluster comprises of primary care centers, general hospitals, community hospitals and specialty centers (46). National Dental Centre Singapore (NDCS) is a tertiary dental specialist center in the Singapore Health Services cluster, and is located in the Singapore General Hospital campus, together with four other national specialty centers.

At the beginning of the COVID-19 outbreak, an important consideration was the risk of transmission unknowingly between patients and staff as there were concerns of local clusters of infection, unlinked cases, and the risk of widespread community transmission. Evidence has since shown that asymptomatic individuals that are infected with COVID-19 can have a high viral load similar to symptomatic individuals (47, 48). Both infected individuals who never develop symptoms ("asymptomatic") or infected individuals who later develop symptoms ("pre-symptomatic") have shown to be able to transmit the disease, with a relative risk of 0.35 and 0.63, respectively, in transmitting the disease when compared to symptomatic individuals (41). A staff member getting infected or exposed to the virus could lead to clinic downtime in its provision of core services. Movement of healthcare workers across different healthcare institutions was limited in order to mitigate this. At NDCS, dental operatories are located on the first, second, fourth, fifth and sixth levels of the building (**Figure 1**). The first, fifth, and sixth levels consist of closed operatories or separate rooms, while the second and fourth levels consist of both open and closed operatories. The open operatories have walls between them that are just high enough to screen patients from each other when seated upright. Day ambulatory surgeries are located on the first, third and fourth levels. Since DORSCON orange, dental specialists and general dentists were segregated to work in three independent teams, and each team had access to two levels and a day ambulatory surgery (i.e., the first team worked on first and sixth levels, the second team worked on second and third levels, and the third team worked on fourth, and fifth levels). Each team was self-contained with the complement of clinicians (specialists and general dentists), dental surgery assistants, lab technicians, patient service associate executives and health attendants. Administrative staff were similarly divided into teams during this period. Other mitigation measures included twice daily temperature taking with checks on compliance, and safe distancing of at least 1 m during all meetings and meals. Any staff member with a fever and/or acute respiratory symptoms was not allowed entry into the workplace and was advised to seek medical treatment at the staff clinic immediately. These staff members would be issued stay home notices during their medical leave period. Staff feeling unwell during the course of the day were told to stop work immediately and to seek medical attention.

To support the government's stricter measures for social and physical distancing during the "circuit breaker" period (7 April to 1 June), dental procedures were limited to emergency and urgent dental care services. The three teams in NDCS took turns to be deployed out of the center to support whole-of-government COVID-19 efforts as needed.

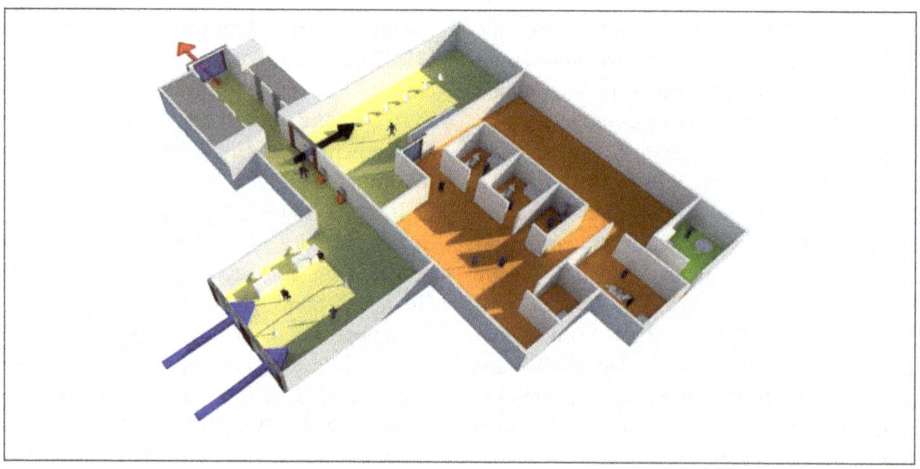

FIGURE 1 | Schematic layout of the first level of National Dental Centre Singapore. Patients and staff enter through two separate centralized entrances (blue arrow on left for patients, blue arrow on right for staff). A thermal scanner is used to screen staff and patients for any signs of fever. Queues are demarcated such that patients stand at least 1 m apart. Patients are screened immediately for travel history, contact history, and for any respiratory symptoms. Known suspect cases requiring urgent or emergency care would be received and isolated at a separate holding area and treated in an isolated dental operatory unit (not shown). Patients head to the Level 1 clinic reception (black arrow) or take the lifts (demarcated gray) to clinics on the other levels. Self-check-in counters outside the clinic minimizes contact between staff and patients. Yellow floor: triage and waiting area. Orange floor: clinical area which include dental operatories (simplified as two units in this schematic), radiographic unit, decontamination room for dental instruments, and day ambulatory surgery. Green floor: pantry area for staff only. All staff and patients in the building exit through a centralized door (red arrow).

TABLE 2 | PPE use in different settings in NDCS.

Setting	Personal Protective Equipment (PPE)
Triage Staff	Surgical mask
Performing or assisting in aerosol-generating procedures	Full PPE: N95 mask, gown, gloves, and eyewear protection Powered air purifying respirators were used by healthcare workers where N95 masks were found to be ineffective during mask fitting
Performing or assisting in non-aerosol-generating procedures	Surgical mask, gown, gloves, and eyewear protection
Non-clinical areas with no direct patient contact (e.g., administrative offices, storerooms, and pantry)	Surgical masks and hand hygiene with alcohol-based hand rub if handling items from a patient environment (e.g., forms and patient files) Employees to put on surgical masks immediately after meals, conversations between staff minimized

PERSONAL PROTECTIVE EQUIPMENT (PPE)

A risk-based approach was adopted for the use of personal protective equipment. This depended on the risk areas in NDCS, the exposure risk, and the type of procedure performed.

At the onset of DORSCON orange, nation-wide guidelines did not advise the use of PPE for non-clinical areas with no patient contact, e.g., administrative offices and storerooms. In clinical areas (i.e., triage, reception, and operatories), the same nation-wide guidelines advised that staff members were to wear a surgical mask, and protective eyewear or a face shield for dental procedures. Treatment of suspect cases referred to national specialty centers required the use of gloves, an N95 mask, gown, and eyewear protection. A wider safety margin was adopted as a further precaution in NDCS, with all aerosol-generating procedures requiring the use of at least an N95 mask and eyewear protection, irrespective of patient status (**Table 2**). N95 masks had to be tested for fit prior to use as improper fits may lead to unintentional exposure of aerosols. Facial hair, in particular, may interfere with the mask seal, and in general, hair must not cross the sealing surface (31). These masks were not to be touched once put on, changed once soiled with blood or any other splash contaminants, and worn only for up to 6 h, which were similar to CDC guidelines (49).

These precautions were similar to other national guidelines regarding the use of PPE. In the United Kingdom, when caring for a patient with a suspected or confirmed case of COVID-19, dental procedures such as high-speed drilling required the use of a filtering face piece (class 3) (FFP3) respirator, a long-sleeved disposable gown, gloves, and disposable eye protection. Close patient contact of within 1 m only or in a cohorted area did not require an FFP3 respirator, but at least a fluid resistant (type IIR) surgical face mask (31). In the United States, the Centres for Disease Control and Protection recommended the use of N95 respirators or respirators that provided a higher level of protection when performing or present during aerosol-generating procedures. Furthermore, if reusable respirators such as powered air purifying respirators (PAPRs) are used, they had to be disinfected prior to reusing them (50). The use of PAPRs may provide more reliable protection, but training in putting them on and removing them without contaminating surfaces is necessary, and whether it is necessary for treating COVID-19-positive patients is unknown (51). However, others have recommended its use for other high-risk procedures such as intubation of patients (52).

Besides donning of appropriate PPE, staff members were also reminded to practice the five moments of hand hygiene, i.e., use an alcohol-based hand rub or wash hands with soap and water, (1) before touching a patient; (2) before engaging in clean/aseptic procedures; (3) after body fluid exposure risk; (4) after touching a patient; (5) after touching patient surroundings (53).

When treating suspect cases, the clinicians and dental assistant would don a full PPE consisting of an N95 mask, gown, gloves, and eyewear protection. Staff would then self-monitor for a period of 14 days for any respiratory symptoms, with twice-daily temperature monitoring. As the risk of transmission was deemed to be low due to the appropriate usage of PPE, the staff was not required to stop work.

However, staff could have unknowingly treated COVID-19-positive patients where they were later found to have the infection. If the staff members had donned appropriate PPE during treatment, the same self-monitoring guidelines were followed. However, if there was close contact without appropriate PPE, the staff would then be placed on quarantine for 14 days. If there was only casual contact (<30 min face-to-face interaction without a high risk procedure *i.e.*, consultation, making impressions, and radiographs) the staff was not required to stop work but monitored by a Ministry of Health Staff for 14 days over the phone.

CLINICAL CARE AND PATIENT MANAGEMENT

At the onset of DORSCON orange in February 2020, in order to review PPE supply and the classification of urgent and essential dental procedures, all aerosol generating procedures were rescheduled for 3 days. A centralized patient triage and temperature screening for staff, visitors and patients was created at the ground floor of NDCS where all patients entered through one entrance before going to the waiting areas at their respective levels (**Figure 1**). Queues were kept fast-moving by ensuring that there were adequate staff to carry out the triage. Visitors were limited to one per patient to reduce overcrowding areas, and essential ones such as the patient's caregiver or a pediatric patient's parents took priority.

In NDCS, a wide safety margin was used in patient management. All non-essential dental review appointments were rescheduled for at least 4 months to reduce clinical workload and risk of disease transmission. Patients on active therapy that presented with any of the following were asked to have their dental procedures deferred for 2 weeks or until recovery of their symptoms if they did not present with a dental emergency: (1) any travel history in the last 14 days; (2) contact history with any known positive cases; (3) respiratory symptoms such as cough and fever. Travel and contact history were confirmed, and patients re-assessed for symptoms by the attending clinician. Suspect cases requiring urgent care were isolated at a designated holding area and managed accordingly by the dentist in an isolation room with appropriate PPE. Patients with pre-existing movement restrictions (stay-home notice, quarantine orders, leave of absence, medical leave) who presented to NDCS but had respiratory symptoms were also referred to the Department of Emergency Medicine at Singapore General Hospital for further assessment. Patients without respiratory symptoms were informed to have their treatment deferred unless they presented with a dental emergency.

On 20 March 2020, Singapore implemented stricter safe distancing measures which included separation of at least a meter between seats at public venues (54). These measures were also similarly employed at NDCS at queues and waiting areas. Patients were also encouraged to use existing self-check-in counters, in order to minimize contact with counter staff. These self-check-in counters were disinfected after every use. Alcohol-based hand rubs and posters that reminded visitors and patients to practice good respiratory and hand hygiene were also placed at these triaging and waiting room areas. This included encouraging frequent hand washing with soap and water or alcohol-based hand rubs, covering one's mouth and nose, keeping a distance of at least 1 m from someone who is coughing, sneezing, or has a fever, and to avoid touching one's eyes, nose and mouth. Precautionary measures were further heightened on 14 April 2020, and anyone leaving their homes were mandated to don a mask (55).

When Singapore entered its "circuit breaker" period, further mitigations were employed. In order to reduce the risk of non-essential commuting by patients and visitors to NDCS, only treatment requiring urgent or emergency care was continued according to specialty-determined guidelines. This included dental clearance for patients referred from other departments in the hospital receiving oncological treatment, general anesthesia, intravenous, or intramuscular antiresorptive medications. Other essential treatment included biopsies for oral pathological cases, treatment for dental trauma, periodontal abscesses, cracked teeth, and irreversible pulpitis. All non-essential cases such as orthodontic therapy, implant therapy, and asymptomatic endodontic lesions and third molars were deferred. A medication delivery system was also set up to minimize patient visits. These were patients who only required a refill of prescription for the management of chronic dental conditions, recurrent oral disorders or orofacial pain. A tele-consultation with the patient was done, and medications would be delivered to patients' homes where necessary. "Last-mile" procedures were also performed to complete ongoing treatment so as to minimize unscheduled returns arising from complications with treatment delay. For cases that required treatment, a high suction evacuator was always used during procedures that were aerosol generating, and a dental assistant was always present to ensure the practice of four-handed dentistry.

New or existing patients who had their treatment canceled or deferred also faced risks in their dental condition and overall prognoses deteriorating, such as malnutrition in frail patients awaiting denture treatment. To mitigate this, clinicians were also informed to scan through their appointment lists to identify patients who required urgent reviews and to prioritize their care concurrent to the gradual easing of restrictions of people movement and reopening of workplaces after the "circuit breaker" period.

It has to be noted that the extended suspension of routine dentistry leaves the risk of an increase in emergency or urgent cases occurring. In events where healthcare supplies (such as PPE) and manpower are strained, decision making in dentistry can be challenging. For example, it has been suggested that extractions of teeth over restorative treatment take priority in cases of acute swelling as a means of early and definitive intervention in order to reduce aerosol generation and for antibiotic stewardship (56).

EDUCATION

Lectures, seminars, and journal clubs usually takes place within the center for dental officers, residents and staff. These are held in seminar rooms or lecture halls. When DORSCON orange started, an online refresher class on infection prevention practices was implemented for all staff. Dental education that involved different team members was conducted through video conferencing. Staff within the same teams could meet but in reduced group sizes with safety distances observed between each other. During the "circuit breaker" period, and with several staff not required to be at work, all meetings were held online.

In Singapore, large classes have been postponed in schools, including universities, due to disease transmission concerns. This has led to teaching interruptions especially for final year students. School closures have coincided with key assessment periods where internal and external assessments have been rescheduled. Medical and dental training has been disrupted in the same regard, with clinical postings for medical students suspended (57). It is crucial that continued education takes place, and amidst a time where many workplaces are closed and social distancing measures are in effect, digitized education or distance learning provides a means to mitigate the loss of learning.

Preparedness has been paramount in containing and mitigating this present pandemic, and this posture should remain so for future disease outbreaks. Singapore had a previous experience with medical and dental school disruptions during the SARS epidemic in 2003. During that period, videotaped vignettes and audiotaped webcasts for medical students were used (58). In what was novel at that time, the first fully online module was also implemented (59). Technological advances have been made since then, and with the past familiarity of the SARS epidemic, and with improved technological infrastructure, it has enabled education to continue as seamlessly as possible within the given limitations of school closures.

DENTAL PRACTICE: QUO VADIS?

There remain challenges to the practice of dentistry during this pandemic. In the absence of pharmaceutical options to treat or prevent COVID-19 cases, the only viable options for the healthcare team at large include thorough contact tracing, postponing non-urgent dental appointments for patients who are suspect cases, reducing the number of patients seen each day, and social distancing.

Implementation of these safety measures in NDCS have largely been adhered to due to strong teamwork and cooperation amongst staff members. However, the protracted nature of the COVID-19 pandemic globally has affected staff morale negatively due to restrictions in social gatherings and the inability to travel abroad to visit family members. Staff fatigue to safety measures are of concern too. Furthermore, some staff members have chosen to remain abroad to be with their families and this poses potential manpower issues in terms of work allocation. Lectures and seminars are still conducted online and its impact on the quality of dental education remains to be seen.

The severity of this pandemic depends on several still-unknown factors such as duration of acquired immunity to the virus, and seasonal variations in transmission. A gradual exit strategy from the "circuit breaker" period with long-term

TABLE 3 | Proposed color-coded framework for dental practice during the COVID-19 pandemic.

Status	Green	Yellow	Orange	Red
Nature of SARS-CoV-2	Virus has mutated into a mild form and/or does not spread easily	Virus spreads easily but: (i) has mutated into a mild form; and/or (ii) is being contained and treated effectively	Virus spreads easily and: (i) infected patients have a high morbidity/mortality rate; and/or (ii) is not being contained or treated effectively	Virus is not being contained with exponential increases of outbreaks in the community, and infected patients have a high morbidity/mortality rate
Healthcare team management	Normal deployment of staff	Normal deployment of staff	Divide staff into teams and segregate to different clinics/levels (if possible) Reduce social contact with other teams with safe distancing observed within the same team	Alternate teams on duty
Personal protective equipment	Surgical masks to be worn in operatories	Surgical masks to be worn at all times in clinical areas (i.e., triage, reception, and operatories)	N95 masks and protective eyewear for aerosol generating procedures (e.g., use of ultrasonic scalers and surgical handpieces) Surgical masks to be worn at all times in clinical areas (i.e., triage, reception, operatories, and pantry except when eating)	N95 masks and protective eyewear for aerosol generating procedures (e.g., use of ultrasonic scalers and surgical handpieces) Surgical masks to be worn at all times in clinical areas (i.e., triage, reception, operatories, and pantry except when eating)
Clinical care and patient management	Normal workload	Normal workload with heightened precautions, i.e., thorough screening at triage, monitoring temperature of patients and staff, maintain good personal hygiene Defer all suspect cases and refer to a medical GP (if medically stable) or hospital via ambulance for further management	Implement centralized patient triage Defer non-emergency cases for patients with a travel history, contact history to a known case, or respiratory symptoms Reduce patient bookings and postpone recalls Isolated holding areas and operatories for suspect cases All suspect cases and high-risk patients requiring urgent/emergency care to be treated at selected tertiary institutions or in-house hospital dental team Defer non-emergency treatment for COVID-19-positive patients	Defer all new/ongoing elective procedures Emergency cases only (e.g., swelling of the face, neck, and mouth; uncontrolled hemorrhage) Treat urgent cases (e.g., abscesses, pericoronitis, and pulpitis) with minimized aerosol generation Defer non-emergency treatment for COVID-19-positive patients Tele-consultation and medication delivery to patients' homes
Education	Normal classroom-/lecture hall-based interactions	Normal classroom-/lecture hall-based interactions	Online conferences/classes and/or classroom-based interactions with reduced group sizes, surgical masks, and social distancing	Online conferences/classes

ASA, American Society of Anesthesiologists physical status classification system; PAPR, powered air-purifying respirator.

safe distancing measures in Singapore has been shown to be effective when compared to an immediate lifting of restrictions using an epidemic simulation model (60). However, reopening the country and its national borders for international travel risks having new community outbreaks of COVID-19. A single episode of a complete lockdown in a state or country to restrict non-essential movement and social interactions that was introduced by many countries may not be sufficient to contain the pandemic, and intermittent lockdowns of varying degrees to limit social interactions may need to continue until 2022 to prevent national critical care capacities from being exceeded, even in high-income countries (61).

With this in mind, **Table 3** outlines a color-coded framework for the practice of dentistry in COVID-19. This framework offers guidelines for each specific color-code and corresponds to different suggested severities of an outbreak. This may be modified further for future similar disease outbreaks.

CONCLUSION

The COVID-19 pandemic is a rapidly evolving situation that is causing great disruption to daily life. Dental practice is no exception and protocols have to be adjusted to continue operation in a way that maximizes safety and reduces disease spread. SARS-CoV-2 can be transmitted through droplets, aerosols, environmental contact and oral-faecally, outlining the importance of upholding hygiene standards and minimizing contact with one another. A risk-based approach to the pandemic that is focussed on staff and patient safety, adopting a wide safety margin, and responding dynamically to the level of risks involved in the workplace is also outlined for areas in healthcare team management, personal protective equipment, clinical work, and dental education. This in turn leads to the safer practice of dentistry in the current climate.

AUTHOR CONTRIBUTIONS

JT and EN contributed to conception, data acquisition and drafted, and critically revised the manuscript. CJS contributed to the conception, drafted and critically revised the manuscript. MO, CS, and KT contributed to the data acquisition and drafted and critically revised the manuscript. All authors gave their final approval and agree to be accountable for all aspects of the work.

ACKNOWLEDGMENTS

The authors would like to thank the NDCS Taskforce, QSM Department, and NDCS Infection Control Committee for providing and updating NDCS' guidelines in response to the COVID-19 pandemic. The authors are also grateful to Michelle Kustamin for designing and illustrating **Figure 1**.

REFERENCES

1. Perlman S, Netland J. Coronaviruses post-SARS: update on replication and pathogenesis. *Nat Rev Microbiol.* (2009) 7:439–50. doi: 10.1038/nrmicro2147
2. Li F. Structure, function, and evolution of coronavirus spike proteins. *Annu Rev Virol.* (2016) 3:237–61. doi: 10.1146/annurev-virology-110615-042301
3. Peiris JS, Guan Y, Yuen KY. Severe acute respiratory syndrome. *Nat Med.* (2004) 10:S88–97. doi: 10.1038/nm1143
4. Arabi YM, Arifi AA, Balkhy HH, Najm H, Aldawood AS, Ghabashi A, et al. Clinical course and outcomes of critically ill patients with Middle East respiratory syndrome coronavirus infection. *Ann Intern Med.* (2014) 160:389–97. doi: 10.7326/M13-2486
5. Chen N, Zhou M, Dong X, Qu J, Gong F, Han Y, et al. Epidemiological and clinical characteristics of 99 cases of 2019 novel coronavirus pneumonia in Wuhan, China: a descriptive study. *Lancet.* (2020) 395:507–13. doi: 10.1016/S0140-6736(20)30211-7
6. Lu R, Zhao X, Li J, Niu P, Yang B, Wu H, et al. Genomic characterisation and epidemiology of 2019 novel coronavirus: implications for virus origins and receptor binding. *Lancet.* (2020) 395:565–74. doi: 10.1016/S0140-6736(20)30251-8
7. World Health Organisation. *Naming the Coronavirus Disease (COVID-19) and the Virus That Causes it.* (2020). Available online at: https://www.who.int/emergencies/diseases/novel-coronavirus-2019/technical-guidance/naming-the-coronavirus-disease-(covid-2019)-and-the-virus-that-causes-it (accessed April 15, 2020).
8. World Health Organisation. *Statement on the Second Meeting of the International Health Regulations (2005) Emergency Committee Regarding the Outbreak of Novel Coronavirus (2019-nCoV).* (2020). Available online at: https://www.who.int/news-room/detail/30-01-2020-statement-on-the-second-meeting-of-the-international-health-regulations-(2005)-emergency-committee-regarding-the-outbreak-of-novel-coronavirus-(2019-ncov) (accessed April 16, 2020).
9. World Health Organisation. *Coronavirus Disease (COVID-19) Situation Reports.* (2020). Available online at: https://www.who.int/emergencies/diseases/novel-coronavirus-2019/situation-reports/ (accessed October 6, 2020).
10. Ministry of Health. *Updates on COVID-19 (Coronavirus Disease 2019) Local Situation.* (2020). Available online at: https://www.moh.gov.sg/covid-19 (accessed October 6, 2020).
11. Wong LY, Tan AL, Leo YS, Lee VJM, Toh M. Healthcare workers in Singapore infected with COVID-19: 23 January-17 April 2020. *Influenza Other Respir Viruses.* (2020). doi: 10.1111/irv.12803
12. Jalelah AB. *66 COVID-19 Cases Among Healthcare Workers and Support Staff: Gan Kim Yong.* Channel News Asia (2020). Available online at: https://www.channelnewsasia.com/news/singapore/66-covid-19-cases-among-healthcare-workers-and-support-staff-gan-12700342 (accessed May 14, 2020).
13. Ministry of Health. *Being Prepared for a Pandemic.* (2019). Available online at: https://www.moh.gov.sg/diseases-updates/being-prepared-for-a-pandemic (accessed April 16, 2020).
14. Ministry of Health. *Extension of Precautionary Measures to Minimise Risk of Community Spread in Singapore.* (2020). Available online at: https://www.moh.gov.sg/news-highlights/details/extension-of-precautionary-measures-to-minimise-risk-of-community-spread-in-singapore (accessed April 26, 2020).
15. Ministry of Health. *Revision of Suspect Case Definition for Coronavirus Disease 2019 (COVID-19).* (2020). Available online at: https://www.ams.edu.sg/view-pdf.aspx?file=media%5C5316_fi_62.pdf&ofile=2.$+$MOH$+$SUSPECT$+$CASE$+$DEFINITION$+$FOR$+$CORONAVIRUS$+$DISEASE$+$54A-2020_1$+$9$+$March.pdf (accessed April 27, 2020).
16. Ministry of Health. *Additional Border Control Measures to Reduce Further Importation of COVID-19 cases: 22nd Mar 2020.* (2020). Available online at: https://www.moh.gov.sg/news-highlights/details/additional-border-control-measures-to-reduce-further-importation-of-covid-19-cases (accessed April 26, 2020).

17. Government of Singapore. *What you can and cannot do during the circuit breaker period.* (2020). Available online at: https://www.gov.sg/article/what-you-can-and-cannot-do-during-the-circuit-breaker-period/ (accessed November 5, 2020).
18. Ministry of Health. *Continuation of Essential Healthcare Services During Period of Heightened Safe Distancing Measures.* (2020). Available online at: https://www.moh.gov.sg/news-highlights/details/continuation-of-essential-healthcare-services-during-period-of-heightened-safe-distancing-measures (accessed April 16, 2020).
19. Harrel SK, Molinari J. Aerosols and splatter in dentistry: a brief review of the literature and infection control implications. *J Am Dent Assoc.* (2004) 135:429–37. doi: 10.14219/jada.archive.2004.0207
20. Bourouiba L. Turbulent gas clouds and respiratory pathogen emissions: potential implications for reducing transmission of COVID-19. *JAMA.* (2020) 323:1837–8. doi: 10.1001/jama.2020.4756
21. Marr LC, Tang JW, Van Mullekom J, Lakdawala SS. Mechanistic insights into the effect of humidity on airborne influenza virus survival, transmission and incidence. *J R Soc Interface.* (2019) 16:20180298. doi: 10.1098/rsif.2018.0298
22. Anfinrud P, Stadnytskyi V, Bax CE, Bax A. Visualizing speech-generated oral fluid droplets with laser light scattering. *N Engl J Med.* (2020) 382:2061–3. doi: 10.1056/NEJMc2007800
23. Ong SWX, Tan YK, Chia PY, Lee TH, Ng OT, Wong MSY, et al. Air, surface environmental, and personal protective equipment contamination by severe acute respiratory syndrome coronavirus 2 (SARS-CoV-2) from a symptomatic patient. *JAMA.* (2020) 323:1610–2. doi: 10.1001/jama.2020.3227
24. Lu J, Gu J, Li K, Xu C, Su W, Lai Z, et al. COVID-19 outbreak associated with air conditioning in restaurant, Guangzhou, China, 2020. *Emerg Infect Dis.* (2020) 26:1628–31. doi: 10.3201/eid2607.200764
25. Shen Y, Li C, Dong H, Wang Z, Martinez L, Sun Z, et al. Community outbreak investigation of SARS-CoV-2 transmission among bus riders in Eastern China. *JAMA Intern Med.* (2020). doi: 10.1001/jamainternmed.2020.5225
26. Liu Y, Ning Z, Chen Y, Guo M, Liu Y, Gali NK, et al. Aerodynamic analysis of SARS-CoV-2 in two Wuhan hospitals. *Nature.* (2020) 582:557–60. doi: 10.1038/s41586-020-2271-3
27. van Doremalen N, Bushmaker T, Morris DH, Holbrook MG, Gamble A, Williamson BN, et al. Aerosol and surface stability of SARS-CoV-2 as compared with SARS-CoV-1. *N Engl J Med.* (2020) 382:1564–7. doi: 10.1056/NEJMc2004973
28. Guo ZD, Wang ZY, Zhang SF, Li X, Li L, Li C, et al. Aerosol and surface distribution of severe acute respiratory syndrome coronavirus 2 in hospital wards, Wuhan, China, 2020. *Emerg Infect Dis.* (2020) 26:1583–91. doi: 10.3201/eid2607.200885
29. Hui KPY, Cheung M-C, Perera RAPM, Ng K-C, Bui CHT, Ho JCW, et al. Tropism, replication competence, and innate immune responses of the coronavirus SARS-CoV-2 in human respiratory tract and conjunctiva: an analysis in *ex-vivo* and *in-vitro* cultures. *Lancet Respir Med.* (2020) 8:687–95. doi: 10.1016/S2213-2600(20)30193-4
30. Kampf G, Todt D, Pfaender S, Steinmann E. Persistence of coronaviruses on inanimate surfaces and their inactivation with biocidal agents. *J Hosp Infect.* (2020) 104:246–51. doi: 10.1016/j.jhin.2020.01.022
31. Public Health England. *COVID-19: Infection Prevention and Control (IPC).* (2020). Available online at: https://www.gov.uk/government/publications/wuhan-novel-coronavirus-infection-prevention-and-control (accessed April 16, 2020).
32. Chin AWH, Chu JTS, Perera MRA, Hui KPY, Yen H-L, Chan MCW, et al. Stability of SARS-CoV-2 in different environmental conditions. *Lancet Microbe.* (2020) 1:e10. doi: 10.1101/2020.03.15.20036673
33. Goldman E. Exaggerated risk of transmission of COVID-19 by fomites. *Lancet Infect Dis.* (2020) 20:892–3. doi: 10.1016/S1473-3099(20)30561-2
34. Pan L, Mu M, Yang P, Sun Y, Wang R, Yan J, et al. Clinical characteristics of COVID-19 patients with digestive symptoms in Hubei, China: a descriptive, cross-sectional, multicenter study. *Am J Gastroenterol.* (2020) 115:766–73. doi: 10.14309/ajg.0000000000000620
35. Xiao F, Tang M, Zheng X, Liu Y, Li X, Shan H. Evidence for gastrointestinal infection of SARS-CoV-2. *Gastroenterology.* (2020) 158:1831–3.e3. doi: 10.1053/j.gastro.2020.02.055
36. Young BE, Ong SWX, Kalimuddin S, Low JG, Tan SY, Loh J, et al. Epidemiologic features and clinical course of patients infected with SARS-CoV-2 in Singapore. *JAMA.* (2020) 323:1488–94. doi: 10.1001/jama.2020.3204
37. Wei WE, Li Z, Chiew CJ, Yong SE, Toh MP, Lee VJ. Presymptomatic transmission of SARS-CoV-2 - Singapore, January 23-March 16, 2020. *MMWR Morb Mortal Wkly Rep.* (2020) 69:411–5. doi: 10.15585/mmwr.mm6914e1
38. Bai Y, Yao L, Wei T, Tian F, Jin D-Y, Chen L, et al. Presumed asymptomatic carrier transmission of COVID-19. *JAMA.* (2020) 323:1406–7. doi: 10.1001/jama.2020.2565
39. Chan JF, Yuan S, Kok KH, To KK, Chu H, Yang J, et al. A familial cluster of pneumonia associated with the 2019 novel coronavirus indicating person-to-person transmission: a study of a family cluster. *Lancet.* (2020) 395:514–23. doi: 10.1016/S0140-6736(20)30154-9
40. Pan X, Chen D, Xia Y, Wu X, Li T, Ou X, et al. Asymptomatic cases in a family cluster with SARS-CoV-2 infection. *Lancet Infect Dis.* (2020) 20:410–1. doi: 10.1016/S1473-3099(20)30114-6
41. Buitrago-Garcia D, Egli-Gany D, Counotte MJ, Hossmann S, Imeri H, Ipekci AM, et al. Occurrence and transmission potential of asymptomatic and presymptomatic SARS-CoV-2 infections: a living systematic review and meta-analysis. *PLOS Med.* (2020) 17:e1003346. doi: 10.1371/journal.pmed.1003346
42. Guan WJ, Ni ZY, Hu Y, Liang WH, Ou CQ, He JX, et al. Clinical characteristics of coronavirus disease 2019 in China. *N Engl J Med.* (2020) 382:1708–20. doi: 10.1056/NEJMoa2002032
43. Li Q, Guan X, Wu P, Wang X, Zhou L, Tong Y, et al. Early transmission dynamics in Wuhan, China, of novel coronavirus-infected pneumonia. *N Engl J Med.* (2020) 382:1199–207. doi: 10.1056/NEJMoa2001316
44. Lauer SA, Grantz KH, Bi Q, Jones FK, Zheng Q, Meredith HR, et al. The incubation period of coronavirus disease 2019 (COVID-19) from publicly reported confirmed cases: estimation and application. *Anna Intern Med.* (2020) 172:577–82. doi: 10.7326/M20-0504
45. World Health Organisation. *Report of the WHO-China Joint Commission on Coronavirus disease 2019.* (2020). Available online at: https://www.who.int/docs/default-source/coronaviruse/who-china-joint-mission-on-covid-19-final-report.pdf (accessed April 16, 2020).
46. Poon CH. *Public Healthcare Sector to be Reorganised Into 3 Integrated Clusters, New Polyclinic Group to be Formed.* The Straits Times (2017). Available online at: https://www.straitstimes.com/singapore/health/public-healthcare-sector-to-be-reorganised-into-3-integrated-clusters-new (accessed April 24, 2020).
47. Lee S, Kim T, Lee E, Lee C, Kim H, Rhee H, et al. Clinical course and molecular viral shedding among asymptomatic and symptomatic patients with SARS-CoV-2 infection in a community treatment center in the Republic of Korea. *JAMA Intern Med.* (2020) 180:1447–52. doi: 10.1001/jamainternmed.2020.3862
48. Rothe C, Schunk M, Sothmann P, Bretzel G, Froeschl G, Wallrauch C, et al. Transmission of 2019-nCoV infection from an asymptomatic contact in Germany. *N Engl J Med.* (2020) 382:970–1. doi: 10.1056/NEJMc2001468
49. Centers for Disesase Control and Prevention. *Recommended Guidance for Extended. Use and Limited Reuse of N95 Filtering Facepiece Respirators in Healthcare Settings.* (2020). Available online at: https://www.cdc.gov/niosh/topics/hcwcontrols/recommendedguidanceextuse.html#respextended (accessed April 29, 2020).
50. Centers for Disesase Control and Prevention. *Interim Infection Prevention and Control Recommendations for Patients With Suspected or Confirmed Coronavirus Disease 2019 (COVID-19) in Healthcare Settings.* (2020). Available online at: https://www.cdc.gov/coronavirus/2019-ncov/hcp/infection-control-recommendations.html?CDC_AA_refVal=https%3A%2F%2Fwww.cdc.gov%2Fcoronavirus%2F2019-ncov%2Finfection-control%2Fcontrol-recommendations.html (accessed April 16, 2020).
51. Bowdle A, Munoz-Price LS. Preventing infection of patients and healthcare workers should be the new normal in the Era of novel coronavirus epidemics. *Anesthesiology.* (2020) 132:1292–5. doi: 10.1097/ALN.0000000000003295
52. Luo M, Cao S, Wei L, Tang R, Hong S, Liu R, et al. Precautions for Intubating Patients with COVID-19. *Anesthesiology.* (2020) 132:1616–8. doi: 10.1097/ALN.0000000000003288

53. World Health Organisation. *The COVID-19 Risk Communication Package for Healthcare Facilities*. (2020). Available online at: https://iris.wpro.who.int/handle/10665.1/14482 (accessed April 16, 2020).
54. Ministry of Health. *Stricter Safe Distancing Measures to Prevent Further Spread of COVID-19 Cases*. (2020). Available online at: https://www.moh.gov.sg/news-highlights/details/stricter-safe-distancing-measures-to-prevent-further-spread-of-covid-19-cases (accessed April 16, 2020).
55. Ang HM, Phua R. *COVID-19: Compulsory to Wear Mask When Leaving the House, Says Lawrence Wong*. Channel News Asia (2020). Available online at: https://www.channelnewsasia.com/news/singapore/covid19-wearing-masks-compulsory-lawrence-wong-12640828 (accessed April 24, 2020).
56. Dave M, Seoudi N, Coulthard P. Urgent dental care for patients during the COVID-19 pandemic. *Lancet*. (2020) 395:1257. doi: 10.1016/S0140-6736(20)30806-0
57. Oh T. *Dorscon Orange: NUS, NTU, SMU Move Large Lectures Online, Suspend Mass Events*. (2020). Available online at: https://www.todayonline.com/singapore/wuhan-coronavirus-dorscon-orange-nus-ntu-smu-move-large-lectures-online-suspend-mass-events (accessed April 26, 2020).
58. Lim EC, Oh VM, Koh DR, Seet RC. The challenges of "continuing medical education" in a pandemic era. *Ann Acad Med Singapore*. (2009) 38:724–6. Retrieved from: https://www.annals.edu.sg/pdf/38VolNo8Aug2009/V38N8p724.pdf
59. Wong ML, Koh D, Phua KH, Lee HP. Teaching community, occupational and family medicine at the National University of Singapore: past, present and future. *Ann Acad Med Singapore*. (2005) 34:102C–7C. Retrieved from: https://www.annals.edu.sg/pdf/34VolNo6200506/V34N6p102C.pdf
60. Dickens BL, Koo JR, Lim JT, Park M, Quaye S, Sun H, et al. Modelling lockdown and exit strategies for COVID-19 in Singapore. *Lancet Regional Health Western Pacific*. (2020) 1:100004. doi: 10.1016/j.lanwpc.2020.100004
61. Kissler SM, Tedijanto C, Goldstein E, Grad YH, Lipsitch M. Projecting the transmission dynamics of SARS-CoV-2 through the postpandemic period. *Science*. (2020) 368:860–8. doi: 10.1126/science.abb5793

16

Dentistry Amidst the COVID-19 Pandemic: Knowledge, Attitude and Practices Among the Saudi Arabian Dental Students

*Basim Almulhim[1], Abdullah Alassaf[1], Sara Alghamdi[1], Riyadh Alroomy[2], Sami Aldhuwayhi[3], Abdullah Aljabr[4] and Sreekanth Kumar Mallineni[1]**

[1] *Department of Preventive Dental Science, College of Dentistry, Majmaah University, Al-Majmaah, Saudi Arabia,* [2] *Department of Restorative Dental Sciences, College of Dentistry, Majmaah University, Al-Majmaah, Saudi Arabia,* [3] *Department of Prosthodontics, College of Dentistry, Majmaah University, Al-Majmaah, Saudi Arabia,* [4] *Department of Medical Education, College of Dentistry, Majmaah University, Al-Majmaah, Saudi Arabia*

Correspondence:
Sreekanth Kumar Mallineni
s.mallineni@mu.edu.sa;
drmallineni@gmail.com

Background: The recent pandemic outbreak has created a huge impact on dentistry. Dental students and dental professionals are at a higher risk because dental practice comprises close communication and widespread exposure to blood, saliva, and other body fluids. It is imperative to evaluate the knowledge and perceptions regarding Coronavirus (COVID-19) among budding dentists.

Aim: To assess the knowledge, attitude, and practices of dental students regarding dental practices during COVID-19.

Materials and methods: A cross-sectional questionnaire-based study was conducted among undergraduate students in Riyadh, Saudi Arabia. An online questionnaire consisting of demographic, knowledge, and attitude-based questions were circulated among the study population, and the responses for the knowledge and attitude were scored. Their mean scores were then calculated. Chi-square test and nonparametric tests were computed using SPSS version 21 software, and p-values < 0.05 were considered statistically significant.

Results: 388 undergraduate dental students have participated in the study from Saudi Arabia. 68% of the respondents believed that they had sufficient knowledge regarding COVID-19. The mean score for knowledge was 5.84 out of 7. Females (6.24) scored statistically significantly higher than males (5.55, $p < = 0.001$). The mean attitude score was 6.34 out of 9. 93% were using PPE models, while 95% maintained social distancing. Out of all the participating dental students, only 16% were willing to treat patients during the pandemic, and 28% did not want to treat patients, 28% preferred teledentistry. The majority (44%) of dental undergraduates were willing to handle only emergency cases.

Conclusion: Accurate knowledge and attitude regarding COVID-19 and diversified opinion on preventive practices during the pandemic period among budding dental professionals evident from Saudi Arabia. Mixed opinions were witnessed among them in seeking help from professional societies. The majority of dental undergraduates were willing to handle only emergency cases.

Keywords: coronavirus, dentistry, dental students, practice, Saudi Arabia

INTRODUCTION

Shutters of dental offices were pulled down with dentistry flagged as a high-risk profession on the unforeseen advent of the highly contagious viral infection of severe acute respiratory syndrome coronavirus 2 (SARS-CoV-2), also known as COVID-19, in early 2020. The pandemic was declared by the World Health Organization (WHO) on Mar 11, 2020, following which, overnight, curfews and lockdowns had been implemented worldwide (1). It was identified that this highly infective virus is transmitted through direct and indirect modes. The natural mode of transmission took place via aerosols generated during surgical and dental procedures, in the form of respiratory droplet nuclei or other bodily secretions and fluids or mother-to-child. This increased the chances of a person getting infected if present in the proximity of 1m of the host. Indirectly, the transmission occurred on touching surfaces in the infected people's immediate environment or objects used by them (2).

The first dentist reported to have fallen prey to this virus was on January 23rd, 2020 the hospital at Wuhan University in China, a country where the infection is said to be originated from, and eventually other health professionals were tested COVID posted (3, 4). In context with this, the civic authorities urged delay of dental sittings unless there being an emergency, and thus, dentistry as a profession came to a standstill (5). The dental profession demands the patients violate the recommended one-meter safe distance and dental procedures generating aerosols. it was no surprise that all non-essential dental procedures were suspended as a part of the interim guidance (6). The oral health providers may accidentally provide direct care for infected or suspected yet not diagnosed COVID-19 patients. There have also been cases of asymptomatic infections wherein transmission may occur even before symptoms appeared (7, 8).

The pandemic took a toll on dental practices. A recent study by Wang et al. (9) reported that 138 hospitals admitted COVID positive patients in Wuhan and identified 29% of these hospitalized patients as healthcare workers. In contrast, Meng et al. reported nine COVID positive cases among dentists and students at Wuhan University, raising the alarm regarding healthcare professionals' safety, especially dentists (5). As much as 38% reduction in patients seeking dental treatment was observed by Guo et al. (10) during the Wuhan outbreak. Consequently, the authorities across the globe were jolted into formulating an action plan for dental services to be carried out post the initial interim suspension.

Several protocols have been set up to ensure minimum human-to-human contact during the pandemic. There is an overall consensus of screening patients prior to initiation of any dental procedures and triage. The dentists are advised to don personal protective equipment (PPE) kits, facemasks, preferably N-95, and face shields. Minimization of aerosol generation, adequately ventilated operatory, and strict compliance with infection control measures and bio-waste management are reinforced (11). Practices of "teledentistry" or web/ telephonic consultation are also being encouraged (12). The face of dentistry is changing, with COVID-19 presenting an unprecedented challenge to the dental industry. The future and sustenance of practicing and emerging dental professionals depend on their adherence to these new norms and protocols and adapting to post-COVID dentistry 2.0. Dentistry has been forced to evolve right from how dental education is imparted to how dental procedures are carried out. Upon identifying the scarcity of such studies conducted to date, this study aims at evaluating the knowledge, attitudes, and practices of undergraduate students in Saudi Arabia to assist in preparing the dental workforce in responding better to such pandemics.

METHODS

This cross-sectional questionnaire-based study has been carried out following the STROBE guidelines (13) specified for this type of study upon approval was obtained from the Institution Ethical Committee, Majmaah University under IRB No. MUREC-June,03/COM-202-/31-2. The study was conducted in Saudi Arabia among undergraduate dental students to investigate their knowledge, attitude, and preventive practices toward COVID-19 from 01-06-2020 to 25-09-2020. Only dental undergraduate students and included both genders. Only those who were willing to sign a written informed consent participated in the study. Postgraduates, Faculty, Private practitioners, those working outside Saudi Arabia, and other health care professionals were excluded from the study. The sample size was calculated using the Raosoft online sample size calculator (14). Based on the survey by Althomairy et al. (15) in an assumption of 3,000 active Saudi dental society members, a response distribution of 50%, while the margin of error and confidence intervals of 5 and 95%, respectively, were made to reach a sample size of 341 dental students (15).

A structured online self-administered questionnaire was administered for this cross-sectional survey to evaluate knowledge, attitudes, and practices regarding COVID-19 among dental undergraduate students. The questionnaire was divided into five main parts. The first constituted the study participants' demographic information (age and gender). The second part explored (i) Information about Coronavirus in your professional society sufficient, (ii) Government institutions able to control the pandemic, and (iii) Obtaining sufficient knowledge regarding COVID-19 information. The third part elicited knowledge of oral health professionals toward COVID-19 by giving correct or incorrect options for every question. The fourth part assessed attitudes toward COVID-19 infection. The fifth part was considered for preventive practice. Each response was scored as "1" (correct) and "0" (wrong), with knowledge scores ranging from 0 to 7 and attitude scores ranging from 0 to 9. Comparisons of knowledge and attitude scores based on gender and practice questions were evaluated. The correlation of knowledge and attitude scores was established based on practice questions. The questionnaire was circulated among the target population in the form of an online Google form, and the recruitment was done through various social media platforms and contact information obtained from the database. The data assimilated was analyzed using Statistical Package for Social Sciences (SPSS) version 21.0 software NY, USA (16). One-way-ANOVA with Bonferroni corrections was used to analyze more than three groups. A Chi-square test was computed to determine the association between study variables. All the tests were assessed at a 5% level of significance.

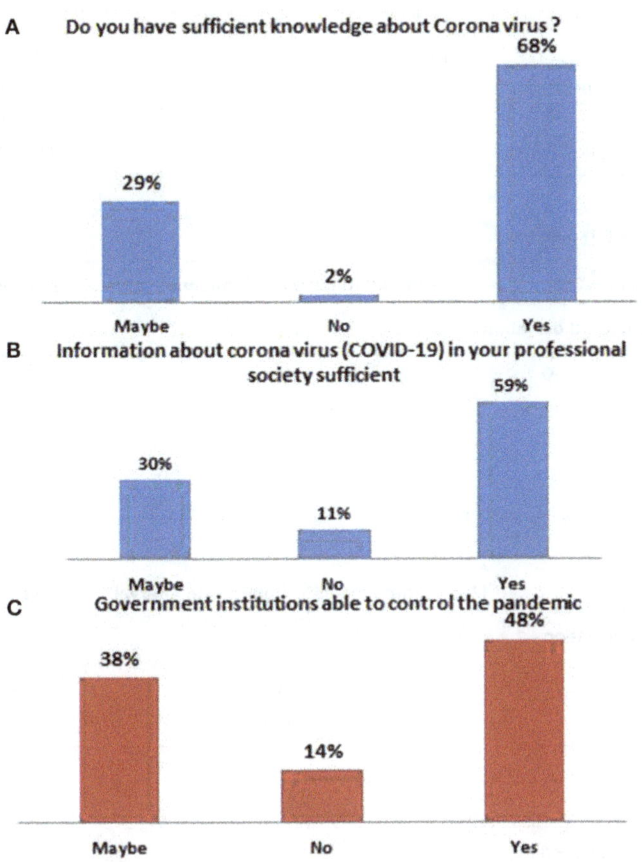

FIGURE 1 | Arabian undergraduate dental students opinions **(A)** sufficient knowledge about Corona virus (COVID-19) **(B)** available information about COVID-19 in your professional society sufficient and **(C)** the role government societies during COVID-19.

RESULTS

A total of 388 responses were received from undergraduate dental students, out of which 223 respondents were male while the remaining 165 were females with a mean age of 22 years. Amongst the participants, Saudis were 91%, and non-Saudis were 9%. When questioned about the knowledge regarding COVID-19, most of the participants (68%) believed that they had sufficient knowledge, while 29% were unsure, only 2% felt they didn't have the required knowledge (**Figure 1**). 48% thought that adequate information was available in their professional society, 38% were unsure, and 14% found the available information insufficient. Government institutions' ability to control the on-going pandemic was found satisfactory by the majority (59%) of the students, but 30% and 11% were unsure and found it insufficient, respectively (**Figure 1**). The mean score for knowledge was observed to be 5.84, where the maximum score was 7 (**Table 1**). Females (6.24) scored statistically significantly higher than males (5.55, $p < 0.001$). The mean attitude score was 6.34, where the maximum score was 9, and here too, females (6.53) managed to secure a higher mean score than males (6.19) (**Table 2**). Surprisingly, only 16% were treating patients during the pandemic, and 28% did not want to treat patients; 28% preferred teledentistry while a majority of 44% were willing to handle only emergency cases (**Table 3**). A 93% of the dental

TABLE 1 | Overall knowledge and attitude scores on COVID-19 among Arabian undergraduate dental students.

Overall total score	Mean	Standard deviation	Median	Mode	Percentile 25	Percentile 75
Knowledge (max = 7)	5.84	1.31	6.00	7.00	5.00	7.00
Attitude score (max = 9)	6.34	1.83	7.00	7.00	5.00	8.00

TABLE 2 | Comparison of knowledge and attitude scores on COVID-19 among Arabian undergraduate students based on gender.

Details	Female (n = 165)		Male (n = 223)		Mean Difference 95% Confidence Interval	p-value
	Mean	Standard deviation	Mean	Standard deviation		
Knowledge	6.24	0.83	5.54	1.50	0.69 (0.44 to 0.95)	0.00*
Attitude	6.52	1.47	6.19	2.038	0.33 (−0.03 to 0.70)	0.07

*$p < 0.05$ is considered statistically significant.

TABLE 3 | Responses of undergraduate students on practice-based questions during COVID-19.

Question	Response	N (%)
Are you using the personal protection equipment for safety?	No	29 (7)
	Yes	359 (93)
Are you maintaining social distancing?	No	20 (5)
	Yes	368 (95)
Are you treating your patients now?	No	327 (84)
	Yes	61 (16)
Do you want to treat patients during this lockdown?	I prefer online (tele dentistry) consultation	109 (28)
	No	108 (28)
	Only Emergency patients	171 (44)

TABLE 4 | Comparison of knowledge and attitudes scores based on use of personal protection equipment.

Using personal protection equipment	No ($n = 29$)		Yes ($n = 359$)		Mean Difference 95% Confidence Interval	p-value
	Mean	Standard deviation	Mean	Standard deviation		
Knowledge	5.34	1.31	5.88	1.30	−0.53 (−1.03 to −0.04)	0.03*
Attitude	5.72	1.19	6.38	1.86	−0.66 (−1.3 to 0.03)	0.06

$p < 0.05$ is considered statistically significant.

TABLE 5 | Comparison of knowledge and attitudes scores based on social distancing.

Social distancing	No ($n = 20$)		Yes ($n = 368$)		Mean Difference 95% Confidence Interval	p-value
	Mean	Standard deviation	Mean	Standard deviation		
Knowledge	5.8	0.89	5.84	1.32	−0.04 (−0.63 to 0.54)	0.88
Attitude	4.3	1.62	6.44	1.77	−2.14 (−2.94 to −1.34)	0.00*

$p < 0.05$ is considered statistically significant.

TABLE 6 | Comparison of knowledge and attitudes scores based on their practice in the dental operatory.

Treating patients	No ($n = 327$)		Yes ($n = 61$)		Mean Difference 95% Confidence Interval	p-value
	Mean	Standard Deviation	Mean	Standard Deviation		
Knowledge	5.87	1.28	5.65	1.43	0.22 (−0.130.58)	0.22
Attitude	6.15	1.83	7.31	1.42	−1.15 (−1.64 to −0.67)	0.00*

$p < 0.05$ is considered statistically significant.

TABLE 7 | Comparison of practice-based responses of Arabian undergraduate dental students.

Dependent Variable	Do you want treat patients during this lock down?		Mean Difference (95% Confidence Interval)	P-value
Knowledge	I prefer online (tele dentistry) consultation	No	−0.01(−0.43 to 0.42)	1.000
		Only Emergency patients	−0.054 (−0.44 to 0.33)	1.000
	No	Only Emergency patients	−0.05 (−0.43 to 0.34)	1.000
Attitude	I prefer online (tele dentistry) consultation	No	0.22 (−0.37 to 0.81)	1.000
		Only Emergency patients	−0.15 (−0.68 to 0.38)	1.000
	No	Only Emergency patients	−0.36 (−0.90 to 0.17)	0.304

$p < 0.05$ is considered statistically significant.

students revealed the use of PPE models when asked questions concerning prevailing practices and following protocols. They also had better knowledge, and attitude mean scores (5.88, 6.38) than those who didn't use PPE models (5.34, 5.72), summarized in **Table 4**. Social distancing was maintained by 95% of the undergraduates who had also scored statistically significantly higher than their peers on the attitude questions (6.44 > 4.3, $p < 0.001$) (**Table 5**). The 16% treating patient had statistically significantly higher mean attitude scores than those who did not treat patients (7.31 > 6.15, $p < 0.001$) but had lower knowledge mean scores (5.65 < 5.87, $p = 0.225$) (**Table 6**). No statistically significant difference was found in the mean knowledge and attitude scores when comparisons were made between those undergraduate dental students who preferred to teledentistry, who did not want to treat patients during the lockdown, and who only treated emergency patients using Bonferroni comparison (**Table 7**).

DISCUSSION

During the period of complete pandemonium across the globe, Saudi Arabia announced its first COVID-19 positive case on 2nd March 2020, and by 7th June, 2020, the total for confirmed cases had surpassed 1,00,000(17, 18). This unexpected outbreak put a strain on health systems of several countries and demanded that the health professionals step-up and accept the role of "Corona Warriors." Amidst the waves of rapidly transmitting infections was a wave of "mis-infodemic," which spread incorrect information, resulting in panic among the general population. The governments implemented varied guidelines, restrictions, bans, and curfews worldwide based on their healthcare systems, economies, and political ideologies. COVID-19 epidemics, etiology, clinical findings, epidemics, and treatment options necessitate widespread data from clinical trials (6, 19, 20). It has also been suggested that rapid discoveries can control the spread and further outbreaks of COVID-19. This disease spreads person-to-person, either through direct transmission by cough, sneeze, or droplet inhalation, or mucous membranes, or ocular contact of the eyes and saliva (8, 9, 19, 21). As a result of this hullabaloo, dental professionals had to face several challenges in the form of initial suspension of practice and later safe treatment of patients abiding by the prescribed infection control protocols (19). This study makes an effort to understand undergraduate dental student's knowledge, attitudes, and practices- training about COVID-19 and the transformed post- pandemic dentistry.

The current study evaluated the participating dental undergraduate students' knowledge by scoring them based on seven knowledge-based questions. The study demonstrated adequate knowledge about COVID-19 with a mean score of approximately six. This was in agreement with a previous study conducted by Srivastava et al. among dental health care professionals (22). Similarly, in a survey by Quadri et al. (23), dental interns, auxiliaries, and specialists scored above average scores when their knowledge was tested. However, in contrast to these findings, a prior study conducted in Georgia among the dental health care workers reported that more than half of the dental students, residents, and specialists did not have enough knowledge of viral infections (24). No prior studies have identified the correlation between gender and knowledge about COVID-19, whereas the current study reports a statistically significant difference in males' and females' knowledge, with females scoring better ($p \leq 0.001$).

In situations of public health crises like this, one's belief in government institutions' efforts shapes their morale, feeling of safety while also motivating them to effectively carry out duties assigned to them and ultimately be reflective in the nation's fight against the pandemic. 59% of the current study participants found government institutions' efforts satisfactory, others being unsure or finding it lacking. A similar study by Rabbani et al. (25) had found 75% of the Saudi Arabian healthcare workers unsatisfied with their institution's preparedness for the pandemic. These professionals' attitudes are associated with their practices, as noticed in this study wherein those with higher mean attitude scores were observed to practice social distancing. This difference was found to be statistically significant ($p \leq 0.001$).

After the interim suspension of non-essential dental treatments, new protocols have been imposed to resumption safe treatment of all cases. 84% of the participants have started treating patients. The respondents were questions about their adherence to safety protocols, and it was noted that 93% wore PPE models and 95% maintained social distancing guidelines. These numbers indicate awareness of required measures and implementation of set standards for infection control (26). However, despite relaxation regarding dental procedures that are allowed and precautionary measures, the majority (44%) still preferred to handle only emergency cases.

In the present study, accurate scores were obtained for knowledge and attitude by undergraduate students regarding COVID-19. Diverse scores were evident regarding preventive practice during COVID-19.especilly for the question on dental practice. Similarly, a recent Arabian study (27) found adequate knowledge and attitude scores and low practice scores, and the authors conducted the study with postgraduate and undergraduate students. Hence, the findings were not compared with the present study. COVID-19 plays a vital role in its control and prevention and would help formulate appropriate protocols and reform the prevailing practices to combat such pandemics in the future. The knowledge and attitudes scores of Arabian dental undergraduates were evaluated based on practices. Amongst these, overall knowledge mean scores showed correlation with the use of PPE, while social distancing and treating patients during pandemic showed correlation with attitude mean scores. Almost similar scores on knowledge among dental healthcare professionals regarding COVID-19 were reported (28, 29). The present study was conducted with dental undergraduate students; However, these findings with previous studies were not comparable. An interesting finding was the preference of teledentistry by 28% of the dental students. Teledentistry is an innovative way of rising against the challenge of social distancing by utilizing available information and technologies using smartphones, tablets, and computers for live video or phone consultation recorded videos, etc. (11, 30). It comprises remote assessment of patients with teleconsultation or telediagnosis, triage of patients, telemonitoring, and dental care provision remotely when possible and appropriate to the patients (9, 11, 31, 32). This pandemic has left many challenges to the dental profession, and it became mandatory to evaluate the knowledge and perception of oral healthcare professionals (9, 21). Prior surveys have shown this form of remote consultation gaining popularity for treatment for disabled, elderly, and patients who do not have access to health services and during the COVID-19 crises (31–33). COVID-19 plays a vital role in its control and prevention and would help formulate appropriate protocols and reform the prevailing practices to combat such pandemics in the future.

According to the best of our knowledge, this study is first conducted among undergraduate dental students in the Riyadh region, Saudi Arabia. However, while interpreting this study's results, certain limitations that this study had encountered need to be kept in mind. Firstly, due to the strict lockdowns imposed, face-to-face interviews were infeasible, resulting in this survey being conducted online, indicating the respondents' not having understood the questions accurately. The data assimilated has been self-reported by the respondents; thus reporting bias cannot be completely ruled out. In the present study dental undergraduate from Saudi Arabia was involved, and the authors tried to establish their perception of practicing dentistry during the pandemic period. It is a fact that dental undergraduate cannot do their own dental practices. Another limitation was using self-reported measures, convenience sampling, and a cross-sectional design, which cannot be generalized to the study findings. College and their province in Saudi Arabia of the dental undergraduate students did not take for evaluation. This might also make a difference that could be considered a potential limitation of the study. The questionnaire was sent to participants via social media, and we received only 388 responses; hence, the response rate was not sought. The present study looked into overall mean scores. The individual scores were not taken into consideration for the analysis. This also could be a potential limitation of the present study. Even though the dental undergraduates were not allowed to practice independently, the present study determines their knowledge and attitudes, and practices in the Arabian region. This study opens the arena to carry out nation-wide studies targeting a larger population from various regions of Saudi Arabia as well as in other counties to have a global comparison. Healthcare professionals form the backbone of any country's public health, and dentists play a vital role in this, with dental health being an integral part of general health. Correct knowledge about any disease plays an essential role in its control and prevention, especially in cases where the population is susceptible.

CONCLUSIONS

Accurate knowledge and attitude regarding COVID-19 and diversified opinions on dental practice during pandemic were evident among budding dental professionals from Saudi Arabia. The study observed mixed opinions among them in seeking help from professional societies. The majority of dental undergraduates were willing to handle only emergency cases.

AUTHOR CONTRIBUTIONS

BA: study conception. AAla and SAlg: study design. AAlj, BA, and SM: data collection. RA, SAlg, and SAld: data analysis and manuscript drafting. AAla and SM: data interpretation. RA, SAld and SM: critical revision of the manuscript. All authors approval of the final version. All authors contributed to the article and approved the submitted version.

ACKNOWLEDGMENTS

The authors would like to thank all the participants involve d in the study. The author would like to thank the Deanship of Scientific Research at Majmaah University for supporting this work under project number No. R-2021-55.

REFERENCES

1. WHO. *Coronavirus Disease (COVID-19) Situation Report 51*. (2020). Available online at: www.who.int/emergencies/diseases/novel-coronavirus-2019 (accessed March 11, 2020).
2. Karia R, Gupta I, Khandait H, Yadav A, Yadav A. COVID-19 and its modes of transmission. *SN Compr Clin Med.* (2020) 2:1798–801. doi: 10.1007/s42399-020-00498-4
3. Peng X, Xu X, Li Y, Cheng L, Zhou X, Ren B. Transmission routes of 2019-nCoV and controls in dental practice. *Int J Oral Sci.* (2020) 12:9. doi: 10.1038/s41368-020-0075-9
4. Smales FC SL. Maintaining dental education and specialist dental care during an outbreak of a new coronavirus infection. Part 1: a deadly viral epidemic begins. *Br Dent J.* (2003) 22:557–61. doi: 10.1038/sj.bdj.4810723
5. Meng L, Hua FBZ. Coronavirus disease 2019 (COVID-19): emerging and future challenges for dental and oral medicine. *J Dent Res.* (2020) 99:481–7. doi: 10.1177/0022034520914246
6. Wang C, Horby PW, Hayden FG GG. Concern, a novel coronavirus outbreak of global health. *Lancet.* (2020) 395:470–3. doi: 10.1016/S0140-6736(20)30185-9
7. Sabino-Silva R, Jardim ACG, Siqueira WL. Coronavirus COVID-19 impacts to dentistry and potential salivary diagnosis. *Clin Oral Investig.* (2020) 24:1619–21. doi: 10.1007/s00784-020-03248-x
8. Khurshid Z, Warsi I, Moin SF, Slowey PD, Latif M, Zohaib S, et al. Biochemical analysis of oral fluids for disease detection. *Adv Clin Chem.* (2021) 100:205–53 doi: 10.1016/bs.acc.2020.04.005
9. Wang D, Hu B, Hu C, Zhu F, Liu X, Zhang J, et al. Clinical characteristics of 138 hospitalized patients with 2019 novel coronavirus–infected pneumonia in Wuhan, China. *JAMA.* (2020) 323:1061–9. doi: 10.1001/jama.2020.1585
10. Guo H, Zhou Y, Liu X TJ. The impact of the COVID-19 epidemic on the utilization of emergency dental services. *J Dent Sci.* (2020) 15:564–56. doi: 10.1016/j.jds.2020.02.002
11. Turkistani K, Turkistani K. Dental risks and precautions during COVID-19 pandemic: a systematic review. *J Int Soc Prev Community Dent.* (2020) 10:540–8. doi: 10.4103/jispcd.JISPCD_295_20
12. Jampani ND, Nutalapati R, Dontula BSK BR. Applications of teledentistry: a literature review and update. *J Int Soc Prev Community Dent.* (2011) 1:37–44. doi: 10.4103/2231-0762.97695
13. Von Elm E, Altman DG, Egger M, Pocock SJ, Gøtzsche PC, Vandenbroucke JP. The strengthening the reporting of observational studies in epidemiology (STROBE) statement: guidelines for reporting observational studies. *J Clin Epidemiol.* (2008) 61:344–9. doi: 10.1016/j.jclinepi.2007.11.008
14. Available online at: http://www.raosoft.com/samplesize.html (accessed May 25, 2020).
15. Althomairy SA, Baseer MA, Assery M, Alsaffan AD. Knowledge and attitude of dental health professionals about middle east respiratory

syndrome in Saudi Arabia. *J Int Soc Prev Community Dent.* (2018) 8:137–44. doi: 10.4103/jispcd.JISPCD_9_18

16. IBM Corp. *IBM SPSS Statistics for Windows, Version 21.0.* Armonk, NY: IBM Corp (2012).
17. Arab News. *Saudi Arabia Announces First Case Of Coronavirus.* Arab News (2020). Available online at: https://arab.news/6xyan (accessed December 12, 2020).
18. Hilton T. *Coronavirus: Saudi Arabia now has over 100,000 COVID-19 Cases.* Al Arabiya English (2020). Available online at: https://english.alarabiya.net/en/coronavirus/2020/06/07/Coronavirus-Saudi-Arabia-now-has-more-than-100-000-COVID-19-cases-.html4 (accessed Junuary 7, 2020).
19. Seneviratne CJ, Lau MWJ, Goh BT. The role of dentists in COVID-19 is beyond dentistry: voluntary medical engagements and future preparedness. *Front Med.* (2020) 7:566. doi: 10.3389/fmed.2020.00566
20. Khurshid Z, Asiri FYI, Al Wadaani H. Human saliva: non-Invasive fluid for detecting novel coronavirus (2019-nCoV). *Int J Environ Res Public Health.* (2020) 17:2225. doi: 10.3390/ijerph17072225
21. Bhumireddy J, Mallineni SK, Nuvvula S. Challenges and possible solutions in dental practice during and post COVID-19. *Environ Sci Pollut Res Int.* (2021) 28:1275–7. doi: 10.1007/s11356-020-10983-x
22. Srivastava KC, Shrivastava D, Sghaireen MG, Alsharari AF, Alduraywish AA, Al-Johani K, et al. Knowledge, attitudes and practices regarding COVID-19 among dental health care professionals: a cross-sectional study in Saudi Arabia. *J Int Med Res.* (2020) 48:300060520977593. 48. doi: 10.1177/0300060520977593
23. Quadri MFA, Jafer MA, Alqahtani AS, Al Mutahar SAB, Odabi NI, Daghriri AA, et al. Novel corona virus disease (COVID-19) awareness among the dental interns, dental auxiliaries and dental specialists in Saudi Arabia: a nationwide study. *J Infect Public Health.* (2020) 13:856–64. doi: 10.1016/j.jiph.2020.05.010
24. Kochlamazashvili M, Kamkamidze G, McNutt LA, DeHovitz J, Chubinishvili O BM. Knowledge, attitudes and practice survey on blood-borne diseases among dental health care workers in Georgia. *J Infect Dev Ctr.* (2018) 12:864–70. doi: 10.3855/jidc.9911
25. Rabbani U, Al Saigul AM. Knowledge, attitude and practices of health care workers about Corona virus disease 2019 in Saudi Arabia. *J Epidemiol Glob Health.* (2020) 11:60–8. doi: 10.2991/jegh.k.200819.002
26. Al Jasser R, Al Sarhan M, Al Otaibi D, Al Oraini S. Awareness toward COVID-19 precautions among different levels of dental students in king saud university, riyadh, Saudi Arabia. *J Multidiscip Healthc.* (2020) 13:1317–24. doi: 10.2147/JMDH.S267956
27. Sezgin GP, Sirinoglu Çapan B. Assessment of dentists' awareness and knowledge levels on the Novel coronavirus (COVID-19). *Braz Oral Res.* (2020) 34:1–12. doi: 10.1590/1807-3107bor-2020.vol34.0112
28. Arora S, Saquib SA, Attar N, Pimpale S, Zafar KS, Saluja P, et al. Evaluation of knowledge and preparedness among indian dentists during the current COVID-19 pandemic: a cross-sectional study. *J Multidiscip Healthc.* (2020) 13:841–54. doi: 10.2147/JMDH.S268891
29. Mallineni SK, Bhumireddy JC, Nuvvula S. Dentistry for children during and post COVID-19 pandemic outbreak. *Child Youth Serv Rev.* (2020) 120:105734. doi: 10.1016/j.childyouth.2020.105734
30. Estai M, Kanagasingam Y, Xiao D, Vignarajan J, Bunt S, Kruger E TM. End-user acceptance of a cloud-based teledentistry system and android phone app for remote screening for oral diseases. *J Telemed Telecare.* (2017) 23:44–52. doi: 10.1177/1357633X15621847
31. Petcu R, Kimble C, Ologeanu-Taddei R, Bourdon I GN. Assessing patient's perception of oral teleconsultation. *Int J Technol Assess Heal Care.* (2017) 33:147–54. doi: 10.1017/S0266462317000319
32. Sa Y, Lin WS, Morton D, Huang C. Coronavirus disease 2019 (COVID-19): experiences and protocols from the department of prosthodontics at the Wuhan University. *J Prosthet Dent.* (2020) S0022-3913:30374-7. doi: 10.1016/j.prosdent.2020.06.004
33. McEachan R, Taylor N, Harrison R, Lawton R, Gardner P CM. Meta-analysis of the reasoned action approach (RAA) to understanding health behaviors. *Ann Behav Med.* (2016) 50:592–612. doi: 10.1007/s12160-016-9798-4

17

Knowledge, Attitudes and Social Responsiveness Toward Corona Virus Disease 2019 (COVID-19) Among Chinese Medical Students—Thoughts on Medical Education

*Haojun Yang [1,2], Yue Zheng [3], Fang Yu [1], Bohao Cheng [1], Ziqing Zhu [1], Sheng Liao [1], Yu Chen [1], Jianzhen Wu [4] and Fang Wang [1]**

[1] Department of Endocrinology, The Third Xiangya Hospital of Central South University, Changsha, China, [2] Department of Neurology, Xiangya Hospital of Central South University, Changsha, China, [3] West China School of Medicine, Sichuan University, Chengdu, China, [4] The Third Xiangya Hospital of Central South University, Changsha, China

***Correspondence:**
Fang Wang
285154425@qq.com

Purpose: To assess knowledge, attitudes, and social responsiveness toward COVID-19 among Chinese medical students.

Methods: Self-administered questionnaires were used to collect data from 889 medical students in three well-known Chinese medical universities. The questionnaire was comprised of three domains which consisted of demographic characteristic collection, seven items for knowledge, and eight items for attitudes and social responsiveness toward COVID-19. Data from different universities were lumped together and were divided into different groups to compare the differences, including (1) students at the clinical learning stage (Group A) or those at the basic-medicine stage (Group B) and (2) students who have graduated and worked (Group C) or those newly enrolled (Group D).

Results: Medical students at group B had a weaker knowledge toward COVID-19 than did students at group A, especially in the question of clinical manifestations ($p < 0.001$). The percentage of totally correct answers of COVID-19 knowledge in group C was higher than that in Group D ($p < 0.001$). There were significant differences between groups C and D in the attitudes and social responsiveness toward COVID-19. Surprisingly, we found that the idea of newly enrolled medical students could be easily affected by interventions.

Conclusions: In light of this information, medical education should pay attention not only to the cultivation of professional knowledge and clinical skills but also to the positive interventions to better the comprehensive qualities including communicative abilities and empathy.

Keywords: knowledge, attitude, COVID-19, Chinese medical students, social responsiveness

INTRODUCTION

Widespread interruptions of medical education have been seen throughout history by major conflicts or infectious pandemic (1). The structure, delivery, and future of both undergraduate and graduate medical education suffered as a result, requiring educators and learners to adapt to learning from a distance while aiming for normalization (2, 3). The suboptimal replication of patient encounters and gauging audience understanding and identifying knowledge gaps seemed to be the direct challenges faced by educators during the pandemic (3, 4). Importantly, the pandemic sounded a wake-up call for us and posed new challenges to medical education, such as insufficient emphasis on public health emergency preparedness, unsophisticated interdisciplinary cooperation mechanism, and insufficient guidance in medical ethics (5). In other words, it put forward higher and stricter requirements for disease prevention and control in the future, especially for public health security and emergency response capacity of infectious diseases (5, 6).

In late December 2019, a novel coronavirus pneumonia (NCP) epidemic occurred in Wuhan, Hubei Province, China. The World Health Organization (WHO) named the pneumonia caused by new coronavirus as Corona Virus Disease 2019 (COVID-19), and the International Committee on Taxonomy of Viruses (ICTV) named this pathogen as Severe Acute Respiratory Syndrome Coronavirus 2 (SARS-COV-2) (7). Compared with SARS, COVID-19 has the characteristics of a long incubation period, strong infectivity, and no obvious upper respiratory symptoms (8, 9). COVID-19 has been declared as a pandemic disease by the WHO on March 11, 2020, with approximately 81,000 confirmed cases in China and over 40,000 confirmed cases in other countries cumulatively (10, 11). Therefore, the Chinese government has implemented strict public health measures against the spread of COVID-19 and dispatched medical personnel from all over the country to support the first line of Hubei epidemic situation (5, 12).

At the same time, conflicts between doctors and patients in China are still difficult to resolve in recent years, mainly caused by the contradictions in the accumulation and distribution of medical resources, the defects of the medical system itself, and the low social trust between doctors and patients (13, 14). The total number of medical damage liability disputes was around 18,112 during 2019, almost 1.7 times of 2018 (15, 16). As The Lancet reported (17–19), Chinese doctors are under threat, which may explain the reason of the low professional happiness of Chinese doctors and the low conversion rate of Chinese medical students choosing to continue medical practice after graduation (13, 20–23). However, the relationship between doctors and patients seems to be more harmonious during this pandemic (24). Medical students in China, who cannot start their new term and are isolated at home, may be responding strongly to the COVID-19 pandemic, but no data are available to describe their perception and behaviors related to this infectious disease.

Generally, Chinese medical undergraduate education contains about 1-year public fundamental courses, nearly 2-year basic-medicine courses (physiology, pathology, anatomy, etc.), and 2-year clinical-medicine learning, including theoretical study (neurology, epidemiology, pediatrics, etc.) and clinical practice. The present study investigated the attitudes, knowledge, and social responsiveness of Chinese medical students in response to the pandemic for the first time, with the aim to compare the differences between medical students of different stages and better the phased cultivation of clinical medical students in the context of Chinese excellent doctor education program reform. Importantly, it is wise for us to put insight into public health and disease prevention, thus cultivating medical teams with enough public health knowledge in face of such major infectious events.

METHODS

Development of the Questionnaire

The modified questionnaire, which was conducted in Chinese and derived from the seventh edition of diagnosis and treatment plan for pneumonia infected by novel coronavirus (25), was composed of three blocks as follows: (1) demographic characteristic of medical students, (2) attitudes and social responsiveness toward COVID-19 and the profession of doctors, and (3) knowledge related to COVID-19 including epidemiology and clinical manifestations.

The first section collected demographic data including age, gender, enrollment year, specialty choice, and whether he/she was the only child in his/her family. The second section reflecting the attitudes and social responsiveness contained eight questions, including five open-ended questions and three single-choice questions as follows: (1) "The main reasons for choosing medicine"; (2) "Supposing you were at work, your first choice during the pandemic would be"; (3) "Supposing your family is against you supporting Hubei, your choice would be"; (4) "The reasons for your choice of being a front-line worker in Wuhan"; (5) "Things I can do as a medical student during the pandemic"; (6) "Do you agree that doctors are full of happiness"; (7) "What is your future plan after COVID-19"; and (8) "Which clinical department will you work in". Knowledge related to COVID-19 (the third section) was assessed by seven items, consisting of one single-choice question, and six multiple-choice questions where the respondent may only choose a single answer or may choose multiple answers.

Sample Recruitment

This was the first study of clinical medical students' knowledge, attitudes, and social responsiveness toward COVID-19 in China. All participants were required to be medical students, whose specialty choice was Eight-year MD program or Five-year Undergraduate program in some Chinese well-known medical colleges, such as Xiangya Medical College of Central South University, West China School of Medicine of Sichuan University, and Peking University Health Science Center. The enrollment year of the participants was not used as an exclusion criterion in this study. Informed consents were obtained, and all questionnaires were administered anonymously between January 2020 and March 2020. All the participants in our study were enrolled *via* convenience sampling and were required to answer the questionnaire without any intervention by the external factors through an online platform named Wenjuanxing.

Students with SARS-COV-2 infection were excluded from this study, which may affect the mental status of them. A total of 889 clinical medical students were enrolled in this study, including 428 students in Xiangya Medical College of Central South University, 244 students in West China School of Medicine of Sichuan University, and 217 students in Peking University Health Science Center.

Statistical Analysis

Data from different universities were lumped together and were divided into different groups to compare the differences, including (1) students at the stage of learning clinical courses (Group A) or students at the basic-medicine stage (Group B) and (2) students who have graduated and worked (Group C) or newly enrolled (Group D). Data were expressed as the means and standard deviations (SDs) in the case of normally distributed data. Pearson's or Spearman's correlation tests were conducted to determine the correlations between variables. The associations between the independent variables and the dependent variables related to medical education were assessed by using univariate odds ratios (ORs) and their 95% confidence intervals (CIs). Statistical Product and Service Solutions version 26.0 (SPSS 26.0) was used for data analyses, with $p < 0.05$ as the level of statistical significance.

Ethics

All participants signed an informed consent document as required by the institutional ethics committee. This study was approved by the ethics committees of the 3rd Xiangya Hospital of Central South University.

TABLE 1 | Demographic characteristics of Chinese clinical medical students.

Demographic characteristics	*n*	Percentage	Population (%)
Gender			
Male	387	43.5	36–47
Female	502	56.5	
Enrollment year			
2019	234	26.3	–
2018	146	16.4	–
2017	140	15.7	–
2016	122	13.7	–
2015	126	14.2	–
2014 and before	121	13.7	–
Specialty choice			
Eight-year MD program	543	61.1	–
Five-year Undergraduate program	346	38.9	–
The only child or not			
Yes	556	62.5	45–50
No	333	37.5	

The demography of the population was collected from the researches published in recent years, whose participants were clinical medical students in China (26–29).

RESULTS

Attitudes and Social Responsiveness Toward COVID-19 Among Chinese Clinical Medical Students

Table 1 shows the demographic characteristics of the participants, which matched the demography of the population to some extent (26–29). The proportion of students at different stages was balanced relatively (freshman, 26.3%; sophomore, 16.4%; junior student, 15.7%; senior student, 13.7%; fifth grade, 14.2%; senior 6 and above, 13.7%). It was found that 47.2% of the participants chose to volunteer to support Hubei Province and 46.9% chose to stick to their own hospitals if they had worked now (**Table 2**). Despite family opposition, 88.3% of the medical students surveyed were still willing to support the front-line in Wuhan, Hubei Province. Responsibilities of doctors were the main reason (92.7%) for those who wanted to work in the front-line (The vanguard and exemplary role of Communist Party members, 15.6%; Many doctors around me sign up for support, 8.2%; Be curious and want to experience, 11.4%; Others, 12.8%). As for the things medical students can do during the pandemic, the vast majority of participants said they would obey the arrangement of the government and the school (89.4%), encourage people around me to take active protective measures (86.3%), pay attention to the pandemic situation and learn efficiently (85.3%), and publish medical science articles and short videos (64.9%). When it came to the professional happiness of doctors, only 53% of the participants agreed or extraordinarily agreed Chinese doctors were full of happiness, 23.1% remained neutral, and 23.9% of the medical students were against the idea. In terms of target department, 12.5% of the participants preferred several departments with the heaviest workload during the outbreak (Department of infectious disease, 1.2%; Department of respiration, 3.6%; ICU or emergency, 7.7%), 87.5% preferred departments except abovementioned. The whole socio-demographic characteristics of the participants are presented in **Table 2**.

Knowledge, Attitudes, and Social Responsiveness Toward COVID-19 in Medical Students at Different Learning Stages

Comparison of Knowledge of COVID-19 Between Students in Basic-Medicine and Clinical-Medicine Stages

A total of 302 students at the stage of learning clinical courses (Group A) and 426 students during the basic-medicine courses (Group B) were approached. **Table 3** shows a similar percentage of gender, residence, and whether he/she was the only child in his/her family.

Table 4 shows medical students at the basic-medicine learning stage had a weaker knowledge toward COVID-19 than the clinical-medicine group, especially in clinical manifestations ($p < 0.001$). Less than 30% of the participants knew SARS-COV-2 is the correct name of the virus first-occurred in Wuhan, and nearly 70% confused the concepts of COVID-19 and SARS-COV-2. The significant differences in epidemiology between

TABLE 2 | Attitudes and social responsiveness toward COVID-19 among Chinese clinical medical students.

Questions	*n*	Percentage
The main reasons for choosing medicine		
Dream and hobby	652	73.4
Medical family	78	8.8
Family recommendation	356	40.1
Stable job	340	38.3
High social status	158	17.8
Others	127	14.3
Supposing you were at work, your first choice during the epidemic would be		
Volunteer to support Hubei	410	47.2
Stick to your hospital	417	46.9
Ask for leave	12	1.3
Resign and change profession	4	0.4
Others	46	3.9
Supposing your family is against you supporting Hubei, your choice would be		
I will try my best to persuade my family and support Hubei	694	78.1
I will support Hubei without telling my family	91	10.2
I will follow my family's advice and not go to Hubei for support	104	11.7
The reasons for your choice of being a front-line worker in Wuhan		
Responsibilities of doctors	824	92.7
The vanguard and exemplary role of Communist Party members	139	15.6
Many doctors around me sign up for support	73	8.2
Be curious and want to experience	101	11.4
Others	114	12.8
Things I can do as a medical student during the pandemic		
Obey the arrangement of the government and the school	795	89.4
Encourage people around me to take active protective measures	767	86.3
Publish Medical science articles and short videos	577	64.9
Pay attention to the pandemic situation and learn efficiently	758	85.3
Do you agree that doctors are full of happiness		
Agree extraordinarily	101	11.4
Agree	370	41.6
Neutral	205	23.1
Disagree	167	18.8
Disagree extraordinarily	46	5.1
What is your future plan after COVID-19		
Clinical work in China	549	61.8
Clinical work abroad	29	3.3
Become a full-time scientific research personnel	24	2.7
Engaged in medical related profession	41	4.6
Not decided yet	231	26.0
Separated from the medical profession completely	2	0.2
Others	13	1.4
Which clinical department will you work in		
Department of infectious disease	11	1.2
Department of respiration	32	3.6
ICU or emergency	68	7.7
Departments except abovementioned	778	87.5

two groups were mainly reflected in the choices of chlorine-containing disinfectant (Group A: 73.1%, Group B: 61.5%, $p < 0.01$, OR: 1.71) and ultraviolet radiation (Group A: 66.5%, Group B: 55.2%, $p < 0.01$, OR: 1.62). Higher frequencies of right answer were found in group A among all the three questions related with clinical manifestations than group B. Besides, the bold OR

TABLE 3 | Demographic characteristics of medical students in different groups.

C	Group A *n* (%)	Group B *n* (%)	*P*-value	Group C *n* (%)	Group D *n* (%)	*P*-value
N	302 (41.5)	426 (58.5)		75 (16.5)	380 (83.5)	
Gender						
Male	130 (43.1)	187 (43.8)	0.82	26 (34.7)	170 (44.7)	0.108
Female	172 (56.9)	239 (56.1)		49 (65.3)	210 (55.3)	
Residence						
Urban	236 (78.1)	325 (76.3)	0.558	52 (69.3)	298 (78.4)	0.088
Rural	66 (21.9)	101 (23.7)		23 (30.7)	82 (21.5)	
The only child or not						
Yes	191 (63.2)	264 (62.0)	0.727	36 (48.0)	256 (67.4)	**0.001**
No	111 (36.8)	162 (38.0)		39 (52.0)	124 (32.6)	

$p < 0.001$ is indicated in bold.

indicated a significant association between better knowledge of COVID-19 and the clinical-medicine learning stage students.

Comparison of Knowledge, Attitudes, and Social Responsiveness Toward COVID-19 Between Graduated and Newly Enrolled Clinical Medical Students

In this study, participants were grouped by whether they have graduated and worked or just entered school. Group C: Doctors enrolled in 2008 or 2009 when he/she was an undergraduate. Group D: Clinical medical students enrolled in 2018 or 2019. A total of 455 samples (Group C: 75; Group D: 380) were obtained, using the same questionnaire (**Table 3**). The percentage of totally correct answers in Group C was higher than that in Group D in most of the questions of epidemiology and clinical manifestations of COVID-19 ($p < 0.001$, **Table 5**). Interestingly, there were significant differences between the two groups in the attitudes of becoming a front-line doctor in Wuhan and the professional happiness of doctors. Further sub-analysis about the items above showed that Group D seemed more active than Group C (**Figure 1**). Surprisingly, the idea of supporting Wuhan diminished significantly after the objections of their family among newly enrolled medical students (**Figures 1A,B**).

DISCUSSION

Medical education under the context of prevention and control of COVID-19 has been pushed to the forefront. It has gone beyond the scope of maintaining health and disease diagnosis and treatment and is increasingly linked to social responsiveness and national security, which we should attach vital importance to. In the face of new challenges and requirements to the pandemic, it is necessary to comprehensively analyze all kinds of problems that may occur in medical education reform and take precautions. Our study was one of the first hospital-based attempts to obtain an initial estimate of Chinese medical students' attitudes, knowledge, and social responsiveness toward COVID-19, especially under the impact of different learning stages of medical students, so as to provide effective suggestions on medical students' education.

Medical students during the clinical learning stage showed more solid knowledge toward COVID-19 than those of the basic-medicine stage, which was plausible by their deepening clinical knowledge and intellectual curiosity about disease (30). Intellectual curiosity, the core of the humanistic practice of medicine, is a desire for knowledge that leads to exploratory behavior, including an inherent and stable baseline trait (trait curiosity) and a variable context-dependent state (state curiosity) (31, 32). Studies in educational psychology suggested that trait curiosity is positively associated with academic achievement, and the educational process itself may influence the state curiosity of medical students (30, 33). What is more, for a long time, medical education in China has emphasized "treatment" more than "prevention." Specifically, in the curriculum system of clinical, basic, and other majors in medical education, the proportion of public health courses is relatively small and the structure is unreasonable (34). There are few intersections between clinical and prevention teaching and few opportunities for students from clinical backgrounds to participate in public health practice. In addition, the curriculum setting of proofreading public health emergencies in most medical schools in China is far from enough, and the proportion of professional knowledge related to public health emergencies and psychological crisis management is seriously unbalanced, or even missing, and the contents are relatively outdated and lagging behind. The majority of medical personnel are obviously deficient in the knowledge and skills of responding to emergencies. They can only temporarily train and learn protective skills in the face of an outbreak, which increases the risk of infection (6, 35). In the early stage of the response to the epidemic, we had to reflect on the unexpected casualties caused by the insufficient public health literacy of front-line medical personnel. So we should strengthen the teaching management of public health and preventive medicine in medical majors. Moreover, the training of public health and epidemic prevention talents must be expanded in scale and improved in quality. Medical colleges must set up schools of public health and strengthen the construction of schools of public health. Only in this way can a team of professionals who not only know public health but also know systematic epidemic prevention and emergency response be trained quickly (36).

TABLE 4 | Knowledge related to COVID-19 including epidemiology and clinical manifestations.

Question	Frequency of YES answer (%)		OR
	Group A *n* (%)	Group B *n* (%)	
Which one do you think is the name of the virus occurred first in Wuhan?			
SARS-COV-2	84 (27.9)	112 (26.3)	1.08
COVID-19	203 (67.2)	279 (65.5)	1.08
MERSr-COV	14 (4.6)	25 (5.8)	0.78
Ebola virus*	1 (0.3)	10 (2.2)	**0.14**
Which ways do you think are the distribution of SARS-COV-2?§			
Droplet transmission	298 (98.7)	421 (98.8)	0.88
Air-borne transmission	166 (55.0)	236 (55.4)	0.98
Contagion**	247 (81.8)	306 (71.8)	1.76
Fecal–oral transmission	161 (53.3)	244 (57.3)	0.85
Mother–baby transmission	43 (14.2)	60 (14.1)	1.01
Which masks do you think can obstruct SARS-COV-2?§			
N95	302 (100.0)	424 (99.5)	/
PM2.5 respirator	30 (9.9)	37 (8.7)	1.16
Sponge mask	5 (1.6)	8 (1.9)	0.88
Active carbon mask	8 (2.6)	11 (2.6)	1.03
Surgical mask	290 (96.0)	412 (96.7)	0.82
Which ways do you think can inactivate SARS-COV-2 effectively?§			
Heating at 56°C for 30 min	270 (89.4)	383 (89.9)	0.95
75% ethyl alcohol	293 (97.0)	403 (94.6)	1.86
Chlorine-containing disinfectant**	221 (73.1)	262 (61.5)	1.71
Chlorhexidine	81 (26.8)	111 (26.1)	1.04
Ultraviolet radiation**	201 (66.5)	235 (55.2)	1.62
What are the initial manifestations of COVID-19?§			
Fever, weakness, and dry cough	301 (99.7)	424 (94.8)	1.42
Digestive symptoms, like nausea, vomiting, and diarrhea***	280 (92.7)	345 (81.0)	2.99
Neurological symptoms, such as headache***	187 (61.9)	201 (47.2)	1.82
Cardiovascular system symptoms, such as palpitation and chest tightness**	173 (57.3)	193 (45.3)	1.62
Ophthalmic symptoms, such as conjunctivitis***	220 (72.8)	193 (45.3)	**3.24**
Only mild limb or back muscle pain***	222 (72.9)	151 (35.4)	**5.05**
Which of the following specimens can detect nucleic acids of SARS-COV-2?§			
Nasopharyngeal swab***	290 (96.0)	343 (80.5)	**5.85**
Sputum***	279 (92.4)	311 (73.0)	**4.49**
Secretion of lower respiratory tract***	264 (87.4)	320 (75.1)	2.30
Blood	176 (58.3)	242 (56.8)	1.06
Feces***	253 (83.8)	291 (68.3)	2.40
What are the criteria for the release of isolation and discharge of patients?§			
Temperature returns to normal for more than 3 days***	252 (83.4)	298 (69.9)	2.16
Respiratory symptoms improved significantly***	223 (73.8)	248 (58.2)	2.03
Pulmonary imaging shows obvious absorption of inflammation*	245 (81.1)	318 (74.6)	1.46
The detection of respiratory pathogenic nucleic acid shows negative consecutive times (Sampling interval shall be at least 1 day)	300 (99.3)	411 (96.5)	**5.47**

*OR: odds ratio [(Medical students at clinical-learning stage confirmed/Medical students at clinical-learning stage not confirmed)/(Medical students at basic-medical learning stage confirmed/Medical students at basic-medical learning stage not confirmed)] OR>3 or OR<1/3 is indicated in bold. §Multiple responses possible. *$p < 0.05$. **$p < 0.01$. ***$p < 0.001$.*

When it came to the attitudes and social responsiveness toward COVID-19, almost all participants chose to do a favor to the society as medical students or as doctors supposing they were at work, revealing great social cohesion and adaptability. However, opinions seemed to differ greatly when talking about the professional happiness of doctors, which was definitely related to the high ratio of medical disputes in China (37–39). Occupational well-being is the key to maintaining the quantity and quality of new entrants (40–42), which may explain the low transformation rate from medical students

TABLE 5 | Percentage of totally correct answers to questions of COVID-19 between group C and group D.

General knowledge of NPC section items	Totally correct answer (%)		*P*-value
	Group C *n* (%)	Group D *n* (%)	
Which one do you think is the name of the virus in Wuhan?*	22 (28.8)	72 (18.9)	**0.042***
Which ways do you think are the distribution of SARS-COV-2?***	18 (24.0)	35 (9.1)	**<0.001*****
Which masks do you think can obstruct SARS-COV-2?	67 (89.3)	335 (88.2)	0.772
Which ways do you think can inactivate SARS-COV-2 effectively?***	44 (58.7)	67 (17.6)	**<0.001*****
What are the initial manifestations of COVID-19?***	35 (46.7)	52 (13.7)	**<0.001*****
Which of the following specimens can detect nucleic acids of SARS-COV-2?***	38 (50.7)	92 (24.1)	**<0.001*****
What are the criteria for the release of isolation and discharge of patients?***	55 (73.3)	166 (43.7)	**<0.001*****

*p < 0.05 is indicated in bold. *p < 0.05, **p < 0.01, ***p < 0.001.*

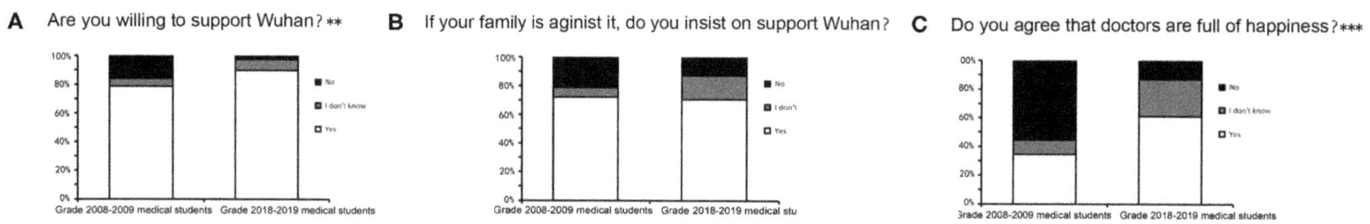

FIGURE 1 | Questions that were considered to be reflected attitudes and social responsiveness. **(A)** Are you willing to support Wuhan? **(B)** If your family is against it, do you insist on supporting Wuhan? **(C)** Do you agree that doctors are full of happiness? ** *p*-value is < 0.01. ****p*-value is < 0.001.

to doctors in China. Our results showed that newly enrolled medical students expected too much for professional happiness, which was much higher than that in the graduated group. Surprisingly, we found that the idea of newly enrolled medical students could be easily affected by interventions. In light of this information, more positive intervention such as policy guidance and communicative skills should be paid to medical students to maintain the high level of professional happiness, especially those newly enrolled. It is not only beneficial to medical students and doctors themselves but also conducive to ensuring the smooth and effective development of medical services and the stability and harmony of the entire society.

Being aware of the high conflict rate between doctors and patients in China, systemic managements and normalized media coverage and volunteerism have been performed to improve this situation (43–45). How to protect doctors from injuries in the process of practicing has always been the attention of the whole society. The Basic Health Care and Health Promotion Law is the first basic and comprehensive law in Chinese health field (45). The public have gradually realized the limitations of medicine during this pandemic, which will be helpful to build a stable foundation between the doctors and patients in China. Medical education is also constantly being reformed to cultivate modern high-quality doctors (46). Nowadays, medical education pays attention not only to the cultivation of professional knowledge and clinical skills but also to the comprehensive qualities including communicative abilities and empathy (47, 48). Surprisingly, a significant decline in empathy during medical school and residency was found in a systematic review, which was associated with gender, ethnicity, and specialty choice (49, 50). However, previous studies showed that well-received educational interventions could successfully cultivate empathy in undergraduate medical students, such as interventions of patient narrative and creative arts, writing, drama, communication skills training, and interpersonal skills training (51–53). It also emphasized the need for multicenter, randomized controlled trials, reporting long-term data to assess the longevity of intervention effects (51).

In addition, we further analyzed whether there were differences in knowledge and social responsiveness toward COVID-19 among participants of different demographic characteristics, because of the association of decreasing empathy and gender, ethnicity, and specialty choice (50). However, there were no significant differences in knowledge and social responsiveness toward COVID-19 among students in different gender (Male & Female), specialty choice (Eight-year MD program & Five-year Undergraduate program), and family (He/She is the only child & He/She is not the only child) (p both > 0.05).

However, there are some limitations in our study that must be acknowledged. (1) The participants may be worried about the confidentiality of this study since it was conducted by their peers, which may have impact on their responses. (2) We only focused on students in some well-known Chinese medical universities, which is a good attempt, but further research will need to be carried out to expand the context covering medical colleges at different levels so as to better match the demographic characteristics of the target population. Despite these limitations, our work provides a basis for international comparisons of medical students' knowledge, attitudes, and social responsiveness facing great public emergency health and safety problems.

CONCLUSIONS

This is the first study to evaluate the knowledge, attitudes, and social responsiveness toward COVID-19 among Chinese medical students and found some differences between students at different stages to better the phased cultivation of clinical medical students during the medical education reform. Medical students during the clinical learning stage showed more solid knowledge toward COVID-19 than those of basic-medicine stage, probably due to the deepening clinical knowledge and intellectual curiosity about disease. When it came to the attitudes and social responsiveness toward COVID-19, almost all participants chose to do a favor to the society revealing great social cohesion and adaptability. Surprisingly, we found the idea of newly enrolled medical students could be easily affected by interventions. In light of this information, medical education should pay attention not only to the cultivation of professional knowledge and clinical skills but also to the positive interventions to cultivate the comprehensive qualities including communicative abilities and empathy.

AUTHOR CONTRIBUTIONS

The study idea was conceived by FW and HY. HY, YZ, and FW were responsible for the writing and revising manuscript. All authors were involved in the data collecting and statistics.

ACKNOWLEDGMENTS

We would like to express our deepest gratitude to the medical students who completed the questionnaires. We are also grateful to the team members, as well as the volunteers and coordinators who assisted in this data collection.

REFERENCES

1. Yuen J, Xie F. Medical education during the COVID-19 pandemic: perspectives from UK trainees. *Postgrad Med J.* (2020) 96:432–3. doi: 10.1136/postgradmedj-2020-137970
2. Hilburg R, Patel N, Ambruso S, Biewald MA, Farouk SS. Medical education during the coronavirus disease-2019 pandemic: learning from a distance. *Adv Chronic Kidney Dis.* (2020) 27:412–7. doi: 10.1053/j.ackd.2020.05.017
3. Wijesooriya NR, Mishra V, Brand PLP, Rubin BK. COVID-19 and telehealth, education, and research adaptations. *Paediatr Respir Rev.* (2020) 35:38–42. doi: 10.1016/j.prrv.2020.06.009
4. Newman NA, Lattouf OM. Coalition for medical education-A call to action: a proposition to adapt clinical medical education to meet the needs of students and other healthcare learners during COVID-19. *J Card Surg.* (2020) 35:1174–5. doi: 10.1111/jocs.14590
5. Yang DY, Cheng SY, Wang SZ, Wang JS, Kuang M, Wang TH, et al. Preparedness of medical education in China: lessons from the COVID-19 outbreak. *Med Teach.* (2020). 42:787–90. doi: 10.1080/0142159X.2020.1770713
6. Rao R, Hawkins M, Ulrich T, Gatlin G, Mabry G, Mishra C. The evolving role of public health in medical education. *Front Public Health.* (2020) 8:251. doi: 10.3389/fpubh.2020.00251
7. Yang H, Chen Z, Fan Y, Xiang L, Hu X, Wu T, et al. Difficulties and countermeasures in hospital emergency management for fast-lane treatment of acute stroke during the COVID-19 epidemic prevention and control. *Front Neurol.* (2020) 11:604907. doi: 10.3389/fneur.2020.604907
8. Li Q, Guan X, Wu P, Wang X, Zhou L, Tong Y, et al. Early transmission dynamics in Wuhan, China, of novel coronavirus-infected pneumonia. *N Engl J Med.* (2020) 382:1199–207. doi: 10.1056/NEJMoa2001316
9. Yu N, Li W, Kang Q, Xiong Z, Wang S, Lin X, et al. Clinical features and obstetric and neonatal outcomes of pregnant patients with COVID-19 in Wuhan, China: a retrospective, single-centre, descriptive study. *Lancet Infect Dis.* (2020) 20:559–64. doi: 10.1016/S1473-3099(20)30176-6
10. Al-Balas M, Al-Balas HI, Jaber HM, Obeidat K, Al-Balas H, Aborajooh EA, et al. Distance learning in clinical medical education amid COVID-19 pandemic in Jordan: current situation, challenges, and perspectives. *BMC Med Educ.* (2020) 20:341. doi: 10.1186/s12909-020-02257-4
11. World Health Organisation. *WHO Coronavirus Disease (COVID-19) Dashboard.* World Health Organisation (2020). Available online at: https://covid19.who.int
12. Special Expert Group for Control of the pandemic of Novel Coronavirus Pneumonia of the Chinese Preventive Medicine Association, The Chinese Preventive Medicine Association. An update on the epidemiological characteristics of novel coronavirus pneumonia (COVID-19). *Chin J Viral Dis.* (2020) 10:81–7. doi: 10.3760/cma.j.issn.0254-6450.2020.02.002
13. Wang M, Tao H. How does patient safety culture in the surgical departments compare to the rest of the County Hospitals in Xiaogan City of China? *Int J Environ Res Public Health.* (2017) 14:1123. doi: 10.3390/ijerph14101123
14. Akologo A, Abuosi AA, Anaba EA. A cross-sectional survey on patient safety culture among healthcare providers in the Upper East region of Ghana. *PLoS ONE.* (2019) 14:e0221208. doi: 10.1371/journal.pone.0221208
15. Yang SZ, Wu D, Wang N, Hesketh T, Sun KS, Li L, et al. Workplace violence and its aftermath in China's health sector: implications from a cross-sectional survey across three tiers of the health system. *BMJ Open.* (2019) 9:e031513. doi: 10.1136/bmjopen-2019-031513
16. Lu L, Lok KI, Zhang L, Hu A, Ungvari GS, Bressington DT, et al. Prevalence of verbal and physical workplace violence against nurses in psychiatric hospitals in China. *Arch Psychiatr Nurs.* (2019) 33:68–72. doi: 10.1016/j.apnu.2019.07.002
17. Chinese doctors are under threat. *Lancet.* (2010). 376:657. doi: 10.1016/S0140-6736(10)61315-3
18. Huang J, Yan L, Zeng Y. Facing up to the threat in China. *Lancet.* (2010) 376:1823. doi: 10.1016/S0140-6736(10)62159-9
19. Yu D, Li T. Doctor stabbed to death two days after warning in The Lancet. *Lancet.* (2011) 377:639. doi: 10.1016/S0140-6736(11)60231-6
20. Liu C, Liu W, Wang Y, Zhang Z, Wang P. Patient safety culture in China: a case study in an outpatient setting in Beijing. *BMJ Qual Saf.* (2014) 23:556–64. doi: 10.1136/bmjqs-2013-002172
21. Tang N1, Thomson LE. Workplace violence in Chinese hospitals: the effects of healthcare disturbance on the psychological well-being of chinese healthcare workers. *Int J Environ Res Public Health.* (2019) 16:3687. doi: 10.3390/ijerph16193687
22. Cheung T, Yip PS. Workplace violence towards nurses in Hong Kong: prevalence and correlates. *BMC Public Health.* (2017) 17:196. doi: 10.1186/s12889-017-4112-3
23. Zhang L, Stone TE, Zhang J. Understanding the rise of Yinao in China: a commentary on the little known phenomenon of healthcare violence. *Nurs Health Sci.* (2017) 19:183–7. doi: 10.1111/nhs.12311
24. Gao B, Dong J. Does the impact of COVID-19 improve the doctor-patient relationship in China? *Am J Med Sci.* (2020).

360:305–6. doi: 10.1016/j.amjms.2020.05.039

25. Zhang S, Li L, Shen A, Chen Y, Qi Z. Rational use of tocilizumab in the treatment of novel coronavirus pneumonia. *Clin Drug Investig.* (2020) 40:511–8. doi: 10.1007/s40261-020-00917-3
26. Yin K, Yang L, Zhang R, Zheng D, Wilkes MS, Lai Y. Gender differences and influencing factors in specialty choices: findings from one medical school in China. *Front Public Health.* (2021) 9:648612. doi: 10.3389/fpubh.2021.648612
27. Chen J, Zhang Y, Zhou X. Effects of gender, medical school class year, and majors on sleep quality in Chinese medical students: a systematic review and meta-analysis. *Sleep Breath.* (2020) 24:259–66. doi: 10.1007/s11325-019-01905-4
28. Liu W, Hao Y, Zhao X, Peng T, Song W, Xue Y, et al. Gender differences on medical students' attitudes toward patient-centred care: a cross-sectional survey conducted in Heilongjiang, China. *PeerJ.* (2019) 7:e7896. doi: 10.7717/peerj.7896
29. Wen D, Ma X, Li H, Liu Z, Xian B, Liu Y. Empathy in Chinese medical students: psychometric characteristics and differences by gender and year of medical education. *BMC Med Educ.* (2013) 13:130. doi: 10.1186/1472-6920-13-130
30. Sternszus R, Saroyan A, Steinert Y. Describing medical student curiosity across a four year curriculum: an exploratory study. *Med Teach.* (2017) 39:377–82. doi: 10.1080/0142159X.2017.1290793
31. Reio TG Jr., Petrosko JM, Wiswell AK, Thongsukmag J. The measurement and conceptualization of curiosity. *J Genet Psychol.* (2006) 167:117–35. doi: 10.3200/GNTP.167.2.117-135
32. von Stumm S, Hell B, Chamorro-Premuzic T. The hungry mind: intellectual curiosity is the third pillar of academic performance. *Perspect Psychol Sci.* (2011) 6:574–88. doi: 10.1177/1745691611421204
33. Chamorro-Premuzic T, Furnham A, Ackerman PL. Incremental validity of the typical intellectual engagement scale as predictor of different academic performance measures. *J Pers Assess.* (2006) 87:261–8. doi: 10.1207/s15327752jpa8703_07
34. Mian SM, Lazorick S, Simeonsson KL, Afanador HF, Stowe CL, Novick LF. Prevention screening and counseling: strategy for integration into medical education and practice. *Am J Prev Med.* (2013) 44:666–71. doi: 10.1016/j.amepre.2013.01.034
35. Jin H, Dong G, Zou L, Shen X, Li D. History and status quo of higher public health education in China. *Public Health Rev.* (2020) 41:12. doi: 10.1186/s40985-020-00120-x
36. Maeshiro R, Carney JK. Public health is essential: COVID-19's learnable moment for medical education. *Acad Med.* (2020) 95:1799–801. doi: 10.1097/ACM.0000000000003517
37. Chen S, Pan Y, Yao Q, Yao L, Liu Z, Xiang L, et al. Publication pressure on Chinese doctors–another view. *Lancet.* (2014). 384:956. doi: 10.1016/S0140-6736(14)61630-5
38. Yuan HF, Xu WD, Hu HY. Young Chinese doctors and the pressure of publication. *Lancet.* (2013) 381:e4. doi: 10.1016/S0140-6736(13)60174-9
39. Ye B, Liu AH. Inadequate evaluation of medical doctors in China. *Lancet.* (2013) 381:1984. doi: 10.1016/S0140-6736(13)61200-3
40. Ortiz M, Teut M, Ben-Arye E, Reshef A, Kaffman M, Arnon Z, et al. Can complementary medicine enhance doctor-patient communication skills? Insights from an international medical student project. *Complement Ther Med.* (2018) 41:283–6. doi: 10.1016/j.ctim.2018.10.012
41. Thomas JS, Koo M, Shakib S, Wu J, Khanal S. Impact of a compulsory final year medical student curriculum on junior doctor prescribing. *Intern Med J.* (2014) 44:156–60. doi: 10.1111/imj.12316
42. Kadambari S. How a medical student taught me to become a better doctor. *Med Teach.* (2008) 30:544–5. doi: 10.1016/j.jsurg.2007.11.016
43. Hu DY. Play the key role in medical reform and take action to lead the "Healthy China 2020". *Zhonghua Xin Xue Guan Bing Za Zhi.* (2011) 39:1–2.
44. Zhou Y, Li LJ. New medical reform and the sustainable development of the pharmaceutical industry in China. *Chin Med J.* (2013) 126:775–82.
45. Cao X, Bai G, Cao C, Zhou Y, Xiong X, Huang X, et al. Comparing Regional Distribution Equity among Doctors in China before and after the 2009. Medical Reform Policy: a data analysis from 2002 to 2017. *Int J Environ Res Public Health.* (2020) 17:E1520. doi: 10.3390/ijerph17051520
46. Sanaee L. Medical education reform: a catalyst for strengthening the health system. Are we ready, Canada? *Can Med Educ J.* (2019) 10:e57–61. doi: 10.36834/cmej.61619
47. Rees CE, Garrud P. Identifying undergraduate medical students' attitudes towards communication skills learning: a pilot study. *Med Teach.* (2001) 23:400–6. doi: 10.1080/01421590120057067
48. Sulzer SH, Feinstein NW, Wendland CL. Assessing empathy development in medical education: a systematic review. *Med Educ.* (2016) 50:300–10. doi: 10.1111/medu.12806
49. Neumann M, Edelhäuser F, Tauschel D, Fischer MR, Wirtz M, Woopen C, et al. Empathy decline and its reasons: a systematic review of studies with medical students and residents. *Acad Med.* (2011) 86:996–1009. doi: 10.1097/ACM.0b013e318221e615
50. Rosenthal S, Howard B, Schlussel YR, Herrigel D, Smolarz BG, Gable B, et al. Humanism at heart: preserving empathy in third-year medical students. *Acad Med.* (2011) 86:350–8. doi: 10.1097/ACM.0b013e318209897f
51. Batt-Rawden SA, Chisolm MS, Anton B, Flickinger TE. Teaching empathy to medical students: an updated, systematic review. *Acad Med.* (2013) 88:1171–7. doi: 10.1097/ACM.0b013e318299f3e3
52. Bombeke K, Van Roosbroeck S, De Winter B, Debaene L, Schol S, Van Hal G, et al. Medical students trained in communication skills show a decline in patient-centred attitudes: an observational study comparing two cohorts during clinical clerkships. *Patient Educ Couns.* (2011) 84:310–8. doi: 10.1016/j.pec.2011.03.007
53. Mullen K, Nicolson M, Cotton P. Improving medical students' attitudes towards the chronic sick: a role for social science research. *BMC Med Educ.* (2010). 10:84. doi: 10.1186/1472-6920-10-84

18

A Dental Response to the COVID-19 Pandemic—Safer Aerosol-Free Emergent (SAFER) Dentistry

Habib Benzian [*†] ***and Richard Niederman*** [†]

WHO Collaborating Center Quality Improvement & Evidence-Based Dentistry, Department Epidemiology & Health Promotion, College of Dentistry, New York University, New York, NY, United States

***Correspondence:**
Habib Benzian
habib.benzian@nyu.edu

[†] *These authors have contributed equally to this work*

Dental services are significantly impacted by the COVID-19 pandemic. Almost all dental procedures carry a high infection risk for providers and patients due to the spread of aerosols. As a consequence, public health agencies and professional associations have issued guidelines for enhanced infection control and personal protection equipment and have also limited care to urgent or emergency services. However, there is no dental service concept for pandemic disaster preparedness or response that might be applied. Moreover, pathways to dental care provision in a post-pandemic future with persisting risks are needed. We propose *Safer Aerosol-Free Emergent Dentistry* (SAFER Dentistry) as one approach to dental services during and emerging from the pandemic. The concept's starting point is the identification of the most common patient needs. The next step is to replace common treatments addressing the most frequent needs with alternative interventions involving a lower infection risk because they do not generate aerosols. SAFER Dentistry is innovative, avoids risk, and responds to the requirements of a pandemic and post-pandemic emergency where the risk of airborne disease transmission remains high. SAFER Dentistry thereby ensures continuity of dental services while protecting providers and patients from infectious pathogens. Moreover, SAFER Dentistry allows dental service providers to remain operational and generate income even under pandemic conditions. Potential implementation and policy options for SAFER Dentistry include universal availability without co-payments by patients and a uniform bundled payment scheme for providers to simplify budgeting, reimbursement, and administration during a pandemic. Adaptations and adjustments of the concept are possible and encouraged as long as the principle of avoiding aerosol-generating procedures is maintained.

Keywords: COVID-19, infection control, pandemic preparedness and response, infectious dental aerosols, airborne transmission of diseases, dental care, emergency dental service

SARS-CoV-2 DISRUPTS HEALTH CARE AND DENTISTRY WORLDWIDE

In a crisis, be aware of the danger, but recognize the opportunity. John F. Kennedy.

Healthcare services are adapting to the COVID-19 pandemic, yet oral health care and dentistry are particularly affected due to the proximity to the patient and the generation of aerosols through common treatment procedures. The SARS-CoV-2 virus seriously disrupts routine dental procedures around the world. The reports, analyses, and recommendations emerging alongside first-hand experience from dental settings in China are alarming (1, 2). The risks of infection for oral health personnel as well as cross-infection between patients and anyone in a dental care setting are high.

The toll of the COVID-19 pandemic on health systems and availability of dental care has been unprecedented. At the height of the pandemic in the U.S., about 80% of practices offered only limited emergency services, and 17% did not see patients at all (3). This impacts heavily on service availability and patient access to essential services. At the same time, such service limitations result in significant economic losses for the entire dental sector, leading to layoffs of dental teams and growing unemployment. In addition, the prospect of re-starting services remains bleak and uncertain and will be so for months to come (4). Little is known so far about the impact on dental services in low- and middle-income countries, though recommendations for service limitations to emergency care and increased precautions were issued in many countries (5).

THE INFECTION RISK FROM AEROSOLS IN DENTISTRY

Dental teams are generally used to high standards of infection control and personal protection measures owing to the fact that dental personnel are among the most at risk for any kind of infection transmitted via contaminated aerosols and saliva, bodily fluids, blood, or tissue particles (6, 7).

Current evidence suggests three main pathways for virus transmission in dental settings: (1) direct transmission through inhalation of cough, sneeze, or droplets containing the virus; (2) transmission via eye, nasal, or oral mucous membranes; and (3) contact transmission through contaminated surfaces (2). All these transmission pathways are facilitated and possibly amplified by aerosols that are generated by most dental procedures (7, 8).

In reaction to the COVID-19 pandemic, international and U.S. federal public health agencies, as well as dental professional associations, have issued specific guidance for the control of SARS-CoV-2 in dental practice (5, 9–13).

These recommendations focus on three main areas where adaptation to the pandemic context is required to break potential transmission chains: patient management and teledentistry to prevent sick or possibly infected patients from coming to the practice, enhanced infection-control measures that include strict protocols for personal protective equipment (PPE), and limitation of dental care to urgent and emergency procedures. Some authorities demand that for patients with COVID-19 symptoms, emergency oral health care should be performed in a negative-pressure operatory with maximum PPE to reduce infectious health hazards (14, 15). Countries like the UK have therefore established special dental care centers to ensure appropriate protection (16).

In the U.S., the Occupational Safety and Health Administration (OSHA) considers work environments where aerosols may occur to be of high or very high infection risk for COVID-19 (14). In a specific update for dentistry, the OSHA requires telephone triage, office engineering controls that include air circulation and patient isolation, universal precautions for airborne pathogens, the use of PPE appropriate for the pandemic, limiting care to urgent and emergency procedures that do not generate aerosols, and environmental cleaning post-care. The recommendation for airborne infection isolation rooms (AIIR) with negative pressure is in line with the U.S. Centers for Disease Control and Prevention's (CDC) existing guidance (17).

Such measures beyond the standard dental infection-control procedures are challenging due to limited or costly supplies of PPE, and they would require significant infrastructure investments. Many of the requirements are unrealistic to achieve even in sophisticated university dental college settings, at least in the short term. For many dental care contexts, such as mobile dental services for schools, remote communities, nursing homes, prisons, homeless shelters, or refugee camps, as well as dental services in low-resource settings where the shortage of supplies is a constant challenge, such enhanced protective measures are near impossible.

The risks from infectious aerosols are central to all recommended alterations of current dental practice, yet uncertainties and open questions related to transmission details remain and oblige dental practitioners to assume they are operating under the highest possible infection risk and to act accordingly with appropriate precautions (18).

Dentistry as we know it is seriously disrupted and may not be able to return to the clinical routines of a pre-COVID-19 time. At this point of the pandemic, dentistry needs a concept for continued dental services that avoids procedures generating infectious aerosols while being able to address the most frequent patient oral health needs.

SAFER AEROSOL-FREE EMERGENT (SAFER) DENTISTRY

With aerosol-generating procedures being at the core of the current challenge for dental services, interventions that avoid aerosol generation should be the interventions of choice. Such procedures exist and may replace possibly hazardous "standard" therapies in an emergency context with airborne pathogens such as SARS-CoV-2. We propose the concept of *Safer Aerosol-Free Emergent Dentistry* (SAFER Dentistry). SAFER Dentistry builds on a prioritization of the most common patient needs, and systematically selects bundles of effective,

TABLE 1 | SAFER Dentistry Packages and intervention options.

	Package	Intervention options without aerosol risk	Conventional options with aerosol risk	References
1	Examination	• Teledentistry–remote triage, examination and counseling • Pre-examination antiseptic mouthrinse • Visual examination • Examination with instruments ○ Probing, percussion test ○ Pulp vitality testing (ice-pellet/heated gutta-percha/electric testing) • Extraoral X-ray if available and required (OPG)	• Intraoral x-ray (risk of avulsion & coughing) • Temperature test with cold air blow (saliva splatter) • Tactile examination/palpation	(19) (2) (20) (21) (1) (22)
2	Pain: Swelling & infection	• Local anesthesia • Incision of abscess & drainage • Or/and antibiotic therapy • Or tooth extraction (avoiding surgical separation or drilling)		(23) (1)
	Pain: Toothache & pulpitis	• Local anesthesia • Trepanation/opening of pulp chamber with hand instrument (excavator), extirpation & disinfection of root canal, temporary filling • Or tooth extraction (avoiding surgical separation or drilling)	• Trepanation with drill & spray • Machine preparation and cleaning of root canals	(22) (23) (24) (1)
3	Pain: Toothache & caries Caries prevention	• Silver diamine fluoride (SDF) • Glass ionomer sealants • Atraumatic Restorative Treatment (ART) with glass ionomer • Fluoride varnish • Fluoride gel/5,000 ppm F toothpaste	• Caries excavation & traditional restorative care (drilling & filling)	(25) (26) (27) (28) (29)
4	Acute periodontitis/pericoronitis	• Cleaning and scaling with hand instruments • Antibiotic therapy (if indicated) • Antiseptic mouthrinse/gel (i.e., CHX)	• Ultrasonic scaling and machine polishing	(22) (1) (30)
5	Broken denture Orthodontic emergency & post-surgery care	• Direct reline/rebase • Removal/adjustment of broken orthodontic wire causing serious irritation • Removal of stitches from previous surgery	• Indirect repair with impression/laboratory technician (risk of avulsion & coughing)	(31) (22)

evidence-based, and value-based care that do not require aerosol-generating procedures.

Focusing on emergency and urgent dental services, SAFER Dentistry addresses common care scenarios with a set of bundled interventions. **Table 1** details the treatment options with significantly lower risk of generating aerosols, including scientific references for the respective non-aerosol options. They comprise the following.

1. Examination/diagnosis via in-person teledentistry: when performed in person, this includes antiseptic mouthrinse and visual and/or tactile inspection without intraoral radiography for diagnosis.
2. Acute pain, swelling, or infection: depending on the diagnosis, pulp devitalization/temporary filling (pulpitis), antibiotic therapy (acute inflammation), and/or local anesthesia and tooth extraction.
3. Toothache due to caries without pulpal involvement: silver-diamine-fluoride application (SDF), glass-ionomer sealants/Atraumatic Restorative Treatment (ART), fluoride varnish/gel, and/or toothbrushing with high fluoride-containing toothpaste (HFT, 5,000 ppm fluoride).
4. Acute periodontitis: hand scaling and metronidazole/amoxicillin combination for 1 week.
5. Denture repair/reline, lost crown or orthodontic bracket, or orthodontic wire: denture repair with soft re-line, crown and bracket re-cementation, and wire adjustment, repair, or removal as well as removal of stiches from previous surgery.

The interventions of SAFER Dentistry are effective and realistic, even for resource-poor settings. Individually, they have been used for decades and have been promoted widely (30). The systematic bundling and prioritization, however, is new and innovative and responds to a pandemic and post-pandemic context where the risk of disease transmission remains high or might be intermittently increasing or decreasing. This approach ensures that dental services can continue during a pandemic by providing oral health care for the most frequent patient needs, while protecting providers and patients from pathogens. Dental teams will require little to no additional training to perform the interventions of SAFER Dentistry, since none of the procedures are new or unknown.

There is no clinical dental care situation without any infectious risk. The alternative interventions suggested are not completely risk-free, but carry a significantly lower and more manageable risk. We therefore use the acronym SAFER Dentistry in analogy to the HIV pandemic's response concept of *Safer Sex*, which also significantly reduces the risk of transmission of HIV and other sexually transmitted diseases (32).

HEALTHY SYSTEM OPTIONS FOR IMPLEMENTING SAFER DENTISTRY

Pandemics are a constant challenge to public health and reveal with relentless clarity the shortcomings of health systems in terms of capacity, coverage, quality, and financing. The same applies to inequalities and differential impact of the pandemic on different population groups. Oral health status and access to dental care has long been recognized as a prime example for such challenges (33). With millions of people unemployed due to the COVID-19 pandemic, many are losing their health insurance benefits at a time when most needed. There is growing recognition that basic health (and oral health) services are a public good that should be universally available for everyone, irrespective of their employment status (34). SAFER Dentistry, covering the most frequent oral health needs, is one starting point for a basic oral health benefit package. Further adaptations and evolving implementation may also include aerosol-free cavity prevention (dental sealants and the like) and other preventive measures to reduce the need for dental care as pandemics continue to emerge. In order to ensure maximum population coverage, we propose that SAFER Dentistry be universally available with no co-payments. Initial economic modeling for children shows that SAFER Dentistry is cost-saving and cost-effective compared to conventional aerosol-generating interventions (35).

Providers could be reimbursed through a single, uniform payment for any combination of examination and additional procedure, thereby simplifying documentation, billing, and reimbursement, which is of particular importance in an emergency context. Such an approach would work for health systems relying on a fee-for-service approach as well as for capitation-based systems. However, the details of the required changes in guidelines, service directives or other adaptations need to be determined nationally/locally depending on existing conditions, resources, local guidelines, and political support. Aspects of teledentistry should be included in the benefit package since they will become a more frequent practice and specific reimbursement positions are often not yet in place (19).

As the pandemic and related limitations of clinical practice endure, more and more patients will have to use emergency hospital services for relief of their dental problems. In the US, even without a pandemic, every 15 s a patient visits a hospital emergency service for dental care due to millions lacking dental insurance coverage (36). Universally available SAFER Dentistry would reduce such hospital visits for common dental ailments and unburden hospital personnel, infrastructure, and resources; it would instead offer an opportunity for dental service providers to remain operational and generate income. At the same time, SAFER Dentistry allows providers to offer a safe and hygienic service environment as a key component to regaining patient trust in the period of pandemic recovery.

CONCLUSIONS

The early experiences in dentistry from China during this COVID-19 pandemic are instructive and telling: They implemented rapid and bold actions to contain the pandemic, including limited emergency dental services in a tertiary care center with maximum precautions (1). The UK and other countries also established specialized emergency care centers for dentistry (37, 38). Yet, the level of infrastructure and service provisions possible in such centers are not realistic for general dental practices or oral health training programs in the U.S. or globally.

SAFER Dentistry, together with general measures to mitigate risk in dental settings, is an adaptation to a pandemic emergency and a pandemic recovery process by avoiding hazardous infectious aerosols. It is also a first step toward oral health care that does not require complex technology, as envisaged in the landmark Lancet Series on Oral Health (39). If continued and institutionalized as a universally available benefit and coverage feature, substantial gains in oral health status and significant reductions in oral health care expenditure could be achieved in the long run.

The dangers of the crisis are clear. Continuation of dentistry as usual during the COVID-19 pandemic will result in incalculable risks for patients and providers. For U.S. governmental agencies and professional organizations, oral healthcare training institutions, clinicians, and patients not willing to accept a complete shutdown of oral healthcare, including deterioration of health and well-being, there is no alternative to SAFER Dentistry.

AUTHOR CONTRIBUTIONS

All authors listed have made a substantial, direct and intellectual contribution to the work, and approved it for publication.

REFERENCES

1. Meng L, Hua F, Bian Z. Coronavirus Disease 2019 (COVID-19): emerging and future challenges for dental and oral medicine. *J Dent Res.* (2020) 99:481–7. doi: 10.1177/0022034520914246
2. Peng X, Xu X, Li Y, Cheng L, Zhou X, Ren B. Transmission routes of 2019-nCoV and controls in dental practice. *Int J Oral Sci.* (2020) 12:9. doi: 10.1038/s41368-020-0075-9
3. Health Policy Institute (HPI), American Dental Association (ADA). *COVID-19: Economic Impact on Dental Practices (week of April 20 results).* Available online at: https://bit.ly/2z9tLcY (accessed May 25, 2020).
4. Nasseh K, Vujicic M. *Modeling the Impact of COVID-19 on U.S. Dental Spending.* Chicago: Health Policy Institute/American Dental Association (2020).
5. COVID-19 Dental Services Evidence Review (CoDER) Working Group. *Recommendations for the Re-Opening of Dental Services: A Rapid Review of International Sources* (Version 1.3). Available at: https://oralhealth.cochrane.org/sites/oralhealth.cochrane.org/files/public/uploads/covid19_dental_reopening_rapid_review_07052020.pdf (accessed May 13, 2020)
6. Gamio L. *The Workers Who Face the Highest Coronavirus Risk.* New York Times. 15 March (2020).
7. Harrel SK, Molinari J. Aerosols and splatter in dentistry: a brief review of the literature and infection control implications. *J Am Dent Assoc.* (2004) 135:429–37. doi: 10.14219/jada.archive.2004.0207
8. Ge Z-y, Yang L-m, Xia J-j, Fu X-h, Zhang Y-z. Possible aerosol transmission of COVID-19 and special precautions in dentistry. *J Zhejiang Univ Sci B.* (2020) 21:361–8. doi: 10.1631/jzus.B2010010
9. Centers for Disease Control and Prevention (CDC). *Guidance for Dental Settings: Interim Infection Prevention and Control Guidance for Dental Settings During the COVID-19 Response.* Available online at: https://www.cdc.gov/coronavirus/2019-ncov/hcp/dental-settings.html (accessed May 19, 2020).
10. Indian Dental Association. *COVID-19 Advisory.* Available online at: https://www.ida.org.in/pdf/20200317_Advisory_on_Corona.pdf (accessed March 17, 2020).
11. Lazzerini M, Putoto G. COVID-19 in Italy: momentous decisions and many uncertainties. *Lancet Glob Health.* (2020) 8:e641–2. doi: 10.1016/S2214-109X(20)30110-8
12. Ordre National des Chirugiens-Dentistes [French National Dental Council]. *Recommandations d'experts pour la prise ne charge des patients en cabinet dentaire de ville au stade 3 de l'epidemie de COVID-19 [Expert recommendations for patient care in urban dental clinics during phase 3 of the COVID-19 epidemic.* Available online at: https://lescdf.fr/sites/default/files/inline-files/Recommandations%20COVID%2019%20v1%2024%20mars%202020_0.pdf (accessed March 24, 2020).
13. Shan S. *Study Highlights Cancer Risks From Betel-Nut Chewing.* Taipei Times 20062.
14. Occupational Safety and Health Administration (OSHA), Department of Labor. *Guidance on Preparing Workplaces for COVID-19 (OSHA 3990-02 2020).* Available online at: www.osha.gov/Publications/OSHA3990.pdf (accessed May 25, 2020).
15. Ather A, Patel B, Ruparel N, Diogenes A, Heargreaves K. Coronavirus Disease 19 (COVID-19): implications for clincial dental care. *J Endod.* (2020) 46:584–95. doi: 10.1016/j.joen.2020.03.008
16. Carter E, Currie C, Asuni A, Goldsmith R, Toon G, Horridge C, et al. The first 6 weeks: setting up a UK urgent dental care centre during the COVID-19 pandemic. *Br Dent J.* (2020) 228:842–8. doi: 10.1038/s41415-020-1708-2
17. Cleveland JL, Robison VA, Panlilio AL. Tuberculosis epidemiology, diagnosis and infection control recommendations for dental settings: an update on the Centers for Disease Control and Prevention guidelines. *J Am Dent Assoc.* (2009) 140:1092–9. doi: 10.14219/jada.archive.2009.0335
18. Beltrán-Aguilar E, Benzian H, Niederman R. Rational perspectives on risk and certainty for dentistry during the COVID-19 pandemic. *Am J Infect Control.* (2020). doi: 10.1590/SciELOPreprints.537
19. Alabdullah JH, Daniel SJ. A systematic review on the validity of teledentistry. *Telemed e-Health.* (2018) 24:639–48. doi: 10.1089/tmj.2017.0132
20. Chen E, Abbott PV. Dental pulp testing: a review. *Int J Dent.* (2009) 2009:365785. doi: 10.1155/2009/365785
21. Bartoloni J, Basquill L. Infection control and dental radiography. *Infection Control Pract.* (2003) 2:1–8.
22. Alharbi A, Alharbi S, Alqaidi S. Guidelines for dental care provision during the COVID-19 pandemic. *Saudi Dental J.* (2020) 32:181–6. doi: 10.1016/j.sdentj.2020.04.001
23. Dave M, Seoudi N, Coulthard P. The oral surgery response to urgent dental care for patients during the COVID-19 pandemic. *Lancet.* (2020) 395:1257. doi: 10.1016/S0140-6736(20)30806-0
24. Yu J, Zhang T, Zhao D, Haapasalo M, Shen Y. Characteristics of endodontic emergencies during COVID-19 outbreak in Wuhan. *J Endodontics.* (2020).
25. Seifo N, Robertson M, MacLean J, Blain K, Grosse S, Milne R, et al. The use of silver diamine fluoride (SDF) in dental practice. *British Dental J.* (2020) 228:75–81. doi: 10.1038/s41415-020-1203-9
26. Marinho VC, Worthington HV, Walsh T, Chong LY. Fluoride gels for preventing dental caries in children and adolescents. *Cochrane Database Syst Rev.* (2015) 6:CD002280. doi: 10.1002/14651858.CD002280.pub2
27. Frencken JE. Atraumatic restorative treatment and minimal intervention dentistry. *Br Dent J.* (2017) 223:183–9. doi: 10.1038/sj.bdj.2017.664
28. Slayton RL, Urquhart O, Araujo MWB, Fontana M, Guzmán-Armstrong S, Nascimento MM, et al. Evidence-based clinical practice guideline on nonrestorative treatments for carious lesions: a report from the American Dental Association. *J Am Dent Assoc.* (2018) 149:837–49.e19. doi: 10.1016/j.adaj.2018.07.002
29. Douglas GV, Ramsdale MP, Vinall-Collier K, Csikar JI. Using high fluoride concentration products in public policy: a rapid review of current guidelines for high fluoride concentration products. *Caries Res.* (2016) 50(Suppl. 1):50–60. doi: 10.1159/000443409
30. Niederman R, Feres M, Ogunbodede E. *Chapter 10: Dentistry.* In: Debas H, Donkor P, Gawande A, J amison D, Kruk M, Mock C, Washington DC: World Bank (2015). p. 173–195. doi: 10.1596/978-1-4648-0346-8_ch10
31. Felton D, Cooper L, Duqum I, Minsley G, Guckes A, Haug S, et al. Evidence-based guidelines for the care and maintenance of complete dentures: a publication of the American College of Prosthodontists. *J Prosthodontics.* (2011) 20:S1–S12. doi: 10.1111/j.1532-849X.2010.00683.x
32. Merson MH, O'Malley J, Serwadda D, Apisuk C. The history and challenge of HIV prevention. *Lancet.* (2008) 372:475–88. doi: 10.1016/S0140-6736(08)60884-3
33. Peres MA, Daly B, Guarnizo-Herreno C, Benzian H, Watt R. Oral diseases: a global public health challenge - Author's Reply. *Lancet.* (2020) 395:186–7. doi: 10.1016/S0140-6736(19)32997-6
34. Chakrabarti M. COVID-19: *Make Health Systems a Global Public Good (27 April 2020); OECD Development Matters (Blog).* Available at: https://oecd-development-matters.org/2020/04/29/covid-19-make-health-systems-a-global-public-good/ (accessed April 27, 2020).
35. Huang SS, Ruff RR, Niederman R. An economic evaluation of a comprehensive school-based caries prevention program. *JDR Clin Trans Res.* (2019) 4:378–87. doi: 10.1177/2380084419837587
36. Health Policy Institute (HPI), American Dental Association (ADA). *Emergency Departments Visits for Dental Conditions - A Snapshot.* (2020). Available online at: https://www.ada.org/media/ADA/Science%20and%20Research/HPI/Files/HPIgraphic_0420_1.pdf?la=en (accessed May 25, 2020).
37. NHS England, NHS Improvement. *COVID-19 Guidance and Standard Operating Procedure. Urgent Dental Care Systems in the Context of the Coronavirus.* Available at: https://bit.ly/3b4BAhw (accessed April 15, 2020).
38. Bundeszahnärztekammer [German Federal Dental Council]. Position zur Ausbreitung von Sars-CoV-2/COVID 19. *Risikomanagement in Zahnarztpraxen [Position on the Sars-CoV-2/COVID 19 epidemic. Risk management in dental clinics].* available at https://www.bzaek.de/fileadmin/PDFs/b/2020_Position_Sars-CoV-2.pdf (accessed March 27, 2020).
39. Watt RG, Daly B, Allison P, Macpherson LMD, Venturelli R, Listl S, et al. Ending the neglect of global oral health – time for radical action. *Lancet.* (2019) 394:261–72. doi: 10.1016/S0140-6736(19)31133-X

19

The Impact of Periodontal Disease on Hospital Admission and Mortality During COVID-19 Pandemic

*Harriet Larvin[1], Sheryl Wilmott[2], Jianhua Wu[1,3] and Jing Kang[4]**

[1] School of Dentistry, University of Leeds, Leeds, United Kingdom, [2] Leeds Dental Institute, Leeds Teaching Hospitals Trust, Leeds, United Kingdom, [3] Leeds Institute for Data Analytics, University of Leeds, Leeds, United Kingdom, [4] Oral Biology, School of Dentistry, University of Leeds, Leeds, United Kingdom

***Correspondence:**
Jing Kang
j.kang@leeds.ac.uk

Introduction: COVID-19 has had a huge impact on society and healthcare and it has been suggested that people with periodontal disease are at risk of having worse outcomes from the disease. The aim of this study was to quantify the impact of periodontal disease on hospital admission and mortality during the COVID-19 pandemic.

Materials and Methods: The study extracted UK Biobank participants who had taken a COVID-19 test between March and June 2020 (n = 13,253), of which 1,616 were COVID-19 positive (12%) and 11,637 were COVID-19 negative (88%). Self-reported oral health indicators of painful or bleeding gums and loose teeth were used as surrogates for periodontal disease, participants who did not report any of the aforementioned indicators were used as controls. Multivariable logistic regressions were used to obtain crude and adjusted odds ratios of COVID-19 infection, subsequent hospital admission and mortality adjusted for demographics, BMI, biomarkers, lifestyle and co-morbidities.

Results: Painful gums, bleeding gums and loose teeth were reported in 2.7, 11.2 and 3.3% of participants with COVID-19 infection, respectively. Risk of COVID-19 infection in participants with painful or bleeding gums and loose teeth compared to controls was not increased (odds ratio [OR]: 1.10, 95% CI: 0.72–1.69; OR: 1.15, 95% CI: 0.84–1.59). COVID-19 positive participants with painful or bleeding gums had a higher risk of mortality (OR: 1.71, 95% CI: 1.05–2.72) but not hospital admission (OR: 0.90, 95% CI: 0.59–1.37). Participants with loose teeth did not show higher risk of hospital admission or mortality compared to the control group (OR = 1.55, 95% CI: 0.87–2.77; OR: 1.85; 95% CI: 0.92–2.72).

Conclusion: There was insufficient evidence to link periodontal disease with an increased risk of COVID-19 infection. However, amongst the COVID-19 positive, there was significantly higher mortality for participants with periodontal disease. Utilization of linked dental and hospital patient records would improve the understanding of the impact of periodontal disease on COVID-19 related outcomes.

Keywords: COVID-19, oral health, periodontal disease, hospital admission, mortality, UK Biobank

INTRODUCTION

The COVID-19 pandemic has resulted in a huge burden on society and healthcare. Studies have shown that sex, older age and co-morbidities including diabetes, hypertension, cardiovascular disease and cancer may increase risk of COVID-19 associated deaths (1, 2). There are also suggestions that COVID-19 related deaths may be associated with deprivation and ethnicity (3). As yet no study has examined the impact of periodontal disease on COVID-19 infection and associated outcomes.

Over a lifetime, ~90% of adults will experience oral disease. Periodontal disease is a main cause of tooth loss in adults and the sixth most prevalent disease globally (4), affecting between 10 and 50% of adults (5, 6). Existing evidence suggests that people with periodontitis may have an increased risk in developing subsequent systemic diseases including cardiovascular disease, hypertension, respiratory disease, diabetes and cancer (7–12). It has been suggested that COVID-19 could be linked to periodontal disease given their shared risk factors, which include obesity, age and hypertension (13, 14). Additionally, there is growing evidence of bacterial co-infection in COVID-19 hospitalizations (15), while ventilator associated pneumonia is also a reported complication of patients hospitalized with COVID-19 (16). Oral dysbiosis as a result of increased dental plaque in periodontitis may provide an environment for oral carriage of respiratory pathogens and cause COVID-19 complications. As yet there is insufficient evidence to provide robust conclusions on how periodontal disease may be associated to COVID-19 infection and outcomes.

During the COVID-19 pandemic UK Biobank has provided live-feed information of its participants on COVID-19 testing, subsequent hospital admission and mortality. The UK Biobank dataset provides an extensive resource to aid in understanding the impact of various factors including periodontal disease during the pandemic. The aim of this study was to quantify the impact of periodontal disease on COVID-19 infection and related outcomes utilizing the UK Biobank data.

MATERIALS AND METHODS

Database

Data from the UK Biobank cohort was used in this analysis. UK Biobank is a national, longitudinal cohort study of over 500,000 participants. The dataset includes information from UK Biobank assessment centers; self-reported responses *via* online questionnaires, linked HES data including ICD-10 diagnoses and hospital admissions provided by NHS Digital, and death records extracted from the death register. Since 16th March 2020 COVID-19 test results provided by Public Health England have been linked to UK Biobank core data as a live-feed for the purposes of COVID-19 related research during the pandemic. The COVID-19 test result data reflects the change in national testing capacity, which has moved from mostly inpatient to more community testing. The data is accessible by researchers with an approved UK Biobank application (reference no: 54633) for a prior study and may carry out additional COVID-19 related research without further approval according to UK Biobank guidelines.

Study recruitment was between 2006 and 2010. Linked follow-up information from HES and death records were available until May and June 2020, respectively. COVID-19 test results were available until the date of data extraction (August 2020). All participant information was fully anonymised prior to data acquisition. HES data, death records and COVID-19 test results were linked to the core UK Biobank dataset by a unique study ID therefore we do not anticipate any missing outcome data. Participants are free to remove themselves from the UK Biobank study cohort at any point (17).

Study Sample

For this study we included participants who were tested for COVID-19 (n = 13,502) with their results linked to the core UK Biobank dataset. The final dataset included information on participant demographics, biomarkers, co-morbidities, COVID-19 test results, hospital admissions and mortality.

Study Outcomes

Hospital admission and mortality following positive COVID-19 test result.

Exposures

The self-reported oral health indicators of bleeding gums, painful gums and loose teeth were utilized as surrogates for periodontal disease as they have demonstrated their validity in the absence of a clinical diagnosis (18). Painful and bleeding gums were associated with mild to moderate periodontal disease, while loose teeth indicated severe periodontal disease. Periodontal disease status was determined by the presence of any of the aforementioned indicators, while no mention of the indicators identified the control group, comprising participants with no self-reported history of periodontal disease.

Covariates

Information on participant demographics (age, sex, ethnicity, household income) and BMI was collated during attendance to UK Biobank assessment centers. Periodontal disease status was also determined from self-reported responses taken from UK Biobank assessment centers. Age at COVID-19 test was derived from age at assessment center attendance and date of test. Information on biomarkers such as blood pressure (systolic and diastolic) and resting heart rate was also acquired from attending UK Biobank assessment centers. Where there were multiple entries for biomarkers the most recent report was extracted. History of smoking was derived according to self-reported current or ex-smoking status. The following conditions were also considered as covariates: cancer, hypertension, angina, cardiac arrest, diabetes, myocardial infarction (MI), stroke, peripheral artery disease (PAD), heart failure, atrial fibrillation and respiratory conditions. Validated ICD-10 code lists within the Cardiovascular Research Using Linked Bespoke Studies and Electronic Health Records (CALIBER) resource were used to classify the aforementioned conditions (19), and the presence of the appropriate ICD-10 code in a participants health records denoted history of the disease. The code list meanings were also adapted to identify relevant self-reported conditions that were not coded with ICD-10 classification. Participants were considered to have disease history if relevant ICD-10 codes were found in their health records, or if the condition was self-reported at the assessment center. No participants had history of heart failure therefore it was excluded from further analysis. A history of hypertension was determined if ICD-10 code was present in health record data, or if the blood pressure reading from the assessment center exceeded 140/90 mmHg.

Data Analysis

Descriptive statistics for baseline characteristics were presented using frequency (percentage) for categorical data and mean [standard deviation (SD)] or median [interquartile range (IQR)] for continuous variables depending on their distribution. Among participants who had COVID 19 test results available, the risk of COVID-19 infection was investigated for those with periodontal disease (self-reported painful gums, bleeding gums or loose teeth) using logistic regression, and further adjusted for covariates including demographics, BMI,

TABLE 1 | Summary table of UK Biobank participants stratified by oral health indicator and COVID-19 test result.

		No self-reported history of periodontal disease		Painful gums		Bleeding gums		Loose teeth	
		COVID-19 test result		COVID-19 test result		COVID-19 test result		COVID-19 test result	
	Overall	–	+	–	+	–	+	–	+
n	13,253	9,815	1,338	321	44	1,148	181	353	53
Age at test, mean (SD)	68.55 (8.38)	69.10 (8.20)	67.15 (9.19)	67.88 (8.71)	69.27 (9.20)	66.10 (8.22)	63.24 (8.50)	69.82 (7.27)	68.13 (8.28)
Sex, female (%)	6,802 (51.3)	5,026 (51.2)	627 (46.9)	174 (54.2)	18 (40.9)	677 (59.0)	98 (54.1)	150 (42.5)	32 (60.4)
Ethnicity, white (%)	12,268 (92.9)	9,231 (94.3)	1,180 (88.5)	276 (86.5)	34 (77.3)	1,047 (91.4)	148 (82.2)	307 (87.2)	45 (84.9)
Average Total Household Income, £ (%)	3,349 (28.3)	411 (4.7)	34 (2.9)	114 (43.3)	11 (29.7)	263 (27.0)	40 (26.0)	126 (43.4)	21 (51.2)
<18,000									
18,000–30,999	2,836 (24.0)	2,108 (24.1)	279 (23.5)	59 (22.4)	13 (35.1)	256 (26.3)	43 (27.9)	73 (25.2)	5 (12.2)
31,000–51,999	2,578 (21.8)	1,925 (22.0)	258 (21.8)	47 (17.9)	6 (16.2)	235 (24.2)	42 (27.3)	54 (18.6)	11 (26.8)
52,000–100,000	1,871 (15.8)	1,424 (16.3)	180 (15.2)	36 (13.7)	5 (13.5)	171 (17.6)	21 (13.6)	30 (0.3)	4 (9.8)
>100,000	517 (4.4)	481 (5.5)	73 (6.2)	7 (2.7)	2 (5.4)	48 (4.9)	8 (5.2)	7 (2.4)	NA
BMI, mean (SD)	28.24 (5.18)	28.08 (5.06)	28.68 (5.28)	28.83 (6.18)	30.55 (5.13)	28.61 (5.52)	28.27 (4.94)	28.76 (5.42)	30.81 (7.21)
Systolic blood pressure/mmHg, mean (SD)	140.69 (20.11)	141.03 (20.01)	140.78 (20.65)	138.43 (19.33)	143.28 (20.34)	138.44 (20.11)	138.06 (19.09)	141.88 (21.25)	136.21 (19.39)
Diastolic blood pressure/mmHg, mean (SD)	82.27 (10.79)	82.16 (10.74)	82.73 (11.16)	81.42 (9.86)	83.49 (10.76)	82.55 (10.92)	82.65 (10.99)	83.18 (10.77)	81.08 (11.95)
Resting heart rate/BPM, mean (SD)	63.85 (9.87)	64.12 (10.29)	57.67 (5.20)	58.00 (NA)	NA	67.14 (8.91)	65.00 (NA)	74.50 (7.78)	NA
History of smoking (%)	6,731 (51.0)	4,937 (50.5)	677 (51.0)	186 (58.7)	25 (56.8)	538 (47.0)	82 (45.6)	256 (73.1)	30 (56.6)
Cancer (%)	2,334 (17.6)	1,813 (18.50)	179 (13.4)	53 (16.5)	2 (4.5)	190 (16.6)	23 (12.7)	66 (18.7)	8 (15.1)
Hypertension (%)	7,781 (58.7)	5,776 (58.8)	793 (59.3)	197 (61.4)	31 (70.5)	636 (55.4)	90 (49.7)	229 (64.9)	29 (54.7)
Angina (%)	1,711 (12.9)	1,251 (12.7)	159 (11.9)	64 (19.9)	13 (29.5)	135 (11.8)	20 (11.0)	61 (17.3)	8 (15.1)
Cardiac arrest (%)	204 (1.5)	160 (1.6)	20 (1.5)	6 (1.9)	NA	11 (1.0)	1 (0.6)	5 (1.4)	1 (1.9)
Diabetes (%)	551 (4.2)	376 (3.8)	62 (4.6)	26 (8.1)	3 (6.8)	36 (3.1)	10 (5.5)	31 (8.8)	7 (13.2)
Myocardial infarction (%)	1,133 (8.5)	830 (8.5)	114 (8.5)	56 (17.4)	5 (11.4)	74 (6.4)	14 (7.7)	37 (10.5)	3 (5.7)
Stroke (%)	769 (5.8)	547 (5.6)	92 (6.9)	35 (10.9)	5 (11.4)	55 (4.8)	8 (4.4)	22 (6.2)	5 (9.4)
Peripheral artery disease (%)	963 (7.3)	695 (7.1)	110 (8.2)	36 (11.2)	2 (4.5)	67 (5.8)	12 (6.6)	36 (10.2)	5 (9.4)
Atrial fibrillation (%)	1,100 (8.3)	826 (8.4)	116 (8.7)	34 (10.6)	5 (11.4)	74 (6.4)	16 (8.8)	30 (8.5)	1 (1.9)
Respiratory disease (%)	3,056 (23.1)	2,213 (22.5)	335 (25.0)	88 (27.4)	9 (20.5)	255 (22.2)	49 (27.1)	96 (27.2)	11 (20.8)
Hospital admission	4,083 (30.2%)	2,723 (27.7)	665 (49.7)	89 (27.7)	18. (40.9)	297 (25.9)	81 (44.8)	101 (28.6)	26 (49.1)
Mortality	644 (4.8%)	292 (3.0)	247 (18.5)	12 (3.7)	7 (15.9)	25 (2.2)	21 (11.6)	11 (3.1)	16 (30.2)

BMI, body mass index; n, number of participants; SD, standard deviation; NA, not applicable as not enough data; –, negative COVID-19 test result; +, positive COVID-19 test result. Means and percentages are calculated for variables excluding missing data. There was missing data in the following variables: oral health (1.88%), ethnicity (0.3%), household income (15.9%), BMI (3.0%), systolic and diastolic blood pressure readings (3.4%), heart rate (99.4%), history of smoking (0.4%).

biomarkers, lifestyles and comorbidities. Among participants with a positive COVID-19 test result, the risks of hospital admission and mortality were investigated for those with periodontal disease using logistic regression and further adjusted for the relevant covariates mentioned above. Crude and adjusted odds ratios (OR) with 95% confidence interval were reported.

Multiple imputations were used for missing data, and Rubin's rule was used to combine the coefficients (20). To assess the impact of missing data, sensitivity analyses were performed using only the complete cases. Data processing and analyses were performed using R version 4.0.0 (21). Statistical significance level was set as 0.05.

RESULTS

Of the 13,253 participants involved in the final analysis cohort, there were 365 (2.4%) participants with painful gums, 1,329 (8.7%) with bleeding gums, 406 (2.7%) with loose teeth and 11,153 (84.1%) with no self-reported history of periodontal disease. Overall there were 1,616 (10.5%) confirmed COVID-19 cases and 11,637 negative test results in the study sample.

The mean age of all participants was 68.55 ± 8.38 years. There were 51.3% females in the final cohort. 92.9% of participants were of white ethnicity. On average participants were considered overweight with a mean BMI of 28.24 ± 5.18.Mean BMI was higher in COVID-19 positive participants when compared to negative participants across all periodontal disease indicator groups. 58.7% of all participants had a history of hypertension and 23.1% had respiratory disease (**Table 1**).

COVID-19 infection risk was not higher in participants with painful/bleeding gums or loose teeth compared to controls (OR = 1.10, 95% CI = 0.72–1.69; OR = 1.15, 95% CI = 0.84–1.59) (**Table 2**).

Though participants with painful/bleeding gums did not have a higher risk of hospital admission (OR = 0.90, 95% CI = 0.59–1.37), their mortality was almost doubled (OR = 1.71, 95% CI = 1.05–2.72) compared to the control group. Participants with loose teeth did not have significantly increased risk of hospital admission or mortality (OR = 1.55, 95% CI = 0.87–2.77; OR = 1.85; 95% CI = 0.92–2.72) (**Table 3**).

Sensitivity analysis on complete cases showed similar effects of periodontal disease on COVID-19 infection risk, hospital admission and mortality rate, but the effects were not significant due to a smaller sample size.

TABLE 2 | Association between oral health indicators and risk of COVID-19 infection.

	Oral health status, OR (95% CI)		
	Control	**Bleeding or painful gums**	**Loose teeth**
Crude OR (95% CI)	**1 (ref)**	1.07 (0.70-1.63)	0.99 (0.73-1.38)
Adjusted* OR (95% CI)	**1 (ref)**	1.10 (0.72-1.69)	1.15 (0.84-1.59)

CI, confidence interval; OR, odds ratio; ref, reference value.
**Adjusted by age at test, sex, ethnicity, average total household income, BMI, systolic and diastolic blood pressure, history of smoking, history of previous conditions including: cancer, hypertension, angina, cardiac arrest, diabetes, myocardial infarction, stroke, peripheral artery disease, atrial fibrillation, and respiratory disease.*

DISCUSSION

Our study did not find a difference in the risk of COVID-19 infection between participants with periodontal disease and those with no self-reported history of periodontal disease. However, logistic regression showed that participants with painful or bleeding gums were at much higher risk of mortality following COVID-19 infection after adjusting for covariates, though hospital admission risk was not higher in these participants. Loose teeth did not affect COVID-19 infection risk, or hospital admission and mortality following COVID-19 infection.

In this study, risk of mortality was significantly increased in participants with painful or bleeding gums following COVID-19 infection. A recent retrospective study of COVID-19 patients found dominant bacterial, viral and fungi co-infections in ~94% of cases (22). These pathogens have also been identified in the oral biofilms associated with periodontal disease (23). Our results suggest oral bacterial load in people with periodontal disease may influence prognosis following COVID-19 infection, and supports the suggestion that the oral microbiome could be associated with severe COVID-19 complications (13). Conversely, risk of hospital admission following COVID-19 infection in participants with painful or bleeding gums did not significantly increase. This could be due to a reduction in the number of people attending hospital for acute disease during the social containment mandate ("lockdown") period of the pandemic (24). People with severe COVID-19 may have chosen to avoid hospital which may have impacted the risk estimates for this outcome. The follow up time for mortality outcomes from the UK Biobank cohort was longer than for the HES data available in determining hospital admission (June 2020 and May 2020, respectively). This may also influence the accuracy of estimates for risk of hospital admission.

Risk of hospital admission and mortality was not higher in participants with self-reported loose teeth, due to smaller sample size in this subgroup. Loose teeth is an indicator of severe periodontal disease (25). Participants with this response in the UK Biobank cohort could have since undergone periodontal treatment, had the affected teeth extracted, or in severe cases, the affected teeth may have self-exfoliated. This could result in a change in participant oral health status between the time of self-report and the COVID-19 infection as most of the self-reported information was collected at baseline. A study of a larger sample size with up-to-date dental measures is required to understand this phenomenon.

The results of this study have clinical implications for the management of COVID-19 infections in the general population, and in hospitalized patients. In England, routine dental services were suspended in March 2020 (26) and, at the time of writing, two-thirds of dental practices were operating at or below 25% of

TABLE 3 | Association between oral health indicators and hospital admission and mortality for participants with COVID-19 infection.

	Crude OR (95% CI) for oral health status			Adjusted* OR (95% CI) for oral health status		
	Control	**Painful or bleeding gums**	**Loose teeth**	**Control**	**Painful or bleeding gums**	**Loose teeth**
Hospital admission	**1 (ref)**	0.99 (0.13–3.02)	0.88 (0.16–10.04)	**1 (ref)**	0.91 (0.12–2.94)	0.90 (0.16–10.63)
Mortality	**1 (ref)**	1.60 (1.03–2.42)	1.34 (0.71–2.76)	**1 (ref)**	1.71 (1.05–2.72)	1.85 (0.92–2.72)

CI, confidence interval; OR, odds ratio; ref, reference value.

**Adjusted by age at test, sex, ethnicity, average total household income, BMI, systolic and diastolic blood pressure, history of smoking, history of previous conditions including: cancer, hypertension, angina, cardiac arrest, diabetes, myocardial infarction, stroke, peripheral artery disease, atrial fibrillation, and respiratory disease.*

their pre-COVID-19 activity levels (27). Dental practices are also having difficulties sourcing Personal Protective Equipment (PPE) (28). In the absence of routine dental care, remote consultations are an opportunity to emphasize self-care methods such as thorough brushing and interdental cleaning, both to prevent oral disease and to reduce the risk of COVID-19 mortality. UK government strategy has focused on tackling obesity to reduce the risk of serious illness or death from COVID-19 (29). Our results show that periodontal disease may be another preventable risk factor that the government could target to improve population outcomes before and after COVID-19 infection. The oral health of patients who have been hospitalized with COVID-19 should not be neglected. There is a wealth of evidence establishing an association between good hospital mouth-care and a reduced risk of pneumonia and acute viral respiratory infections (13). Furthermore, simple measures such as chlorhexidine mouth rinses have been shown to reduce the risk of ventilator associated pneumonia in critically ill patients from 24 to 18% (30). Improving the mouth care provided to COVID-19 patients in hospital could be a straightforward method for improving their outcomes, and Public Health England have supported this by publishing mouth care guidance for patients with COVID-19 (31).

This is the first study to quantify the effect of periodontal disease on risk of COVID-19 infection and related outcomes. As such, there are several strengths to our study. First of all, this is the largest study to date to quantify the association between periodontal disease and COVID-19. Secondly, the utilization of UK Biobank, a national resource with high quality measures linked to COVID-19 test results enabled our quantitative analysis of association between periodontal disease and COVID-19 outcomes. Finally, our study demonstrates robust results using both imputed and complete cases.

Our study also has some limitations. Delayed information of hospital admission and mortality (updated until June 2020) limited the number of study cases, and has been recognized as an avenue for further investigation. The use of self-reported oral health indicators as a surrogate for signs of periodontal disease could introduce bias, as research suggests self-reported periodontal disease prevalence is underestimated in populations (32, 33). We are also aware that loose teeth, and painful or bleeding gums could result from trauma or endodontic diseases, however, there is evidence that the validity of a periodontal disease diagnosis is not compromised when self-reported responses of bleeding gums and loose teeth are utilized (18). In addition, the dataset held no information regarding any periodontal treatment that the participants had received in the time between reporting the oral measures and receiving the results of the COVID-19 test. Given that periodontal therapy can reverse or prevent disease activity, participants may have experienced changes to periodontal disease status between self-report at UK Biobank assessment center and undertaking a COVID-19 test. Furthermore, the oral measures (painful gum, bleeding gum and loose teeth) in this study may be due to oral dysbiosis but this causal association was not measurable within the UK Biobank dataset. Lastly, as the pandemic continues to take hold, the study follow up time for hospital admission and mortality was relatively short (until May and June 2020); the numbers of COVID-19 positive cases may have been underreported during the early stages of the pandemic.

Suggestions for future research include: (1) Using updated information of additional COVID-19 test results with longer follow up in order to acquire more precise estimates of the effect of periodontal disease on risk of COVID-19 infection and associated outcomes. (2) Utilization of linked dental and hospital records in future analyses. This could provide more accurate and recent information on oral health status in comparison to the self-reported periodontal disease responses at UK Biobank assessment centers and account for any change in oral health status following dental treatment.

CONCLUSIONS

Our study demonstrated an increased risk of mortality following COVID-19 infection in people with periodontal disease. The findings suggest that while periodontal disease might not increase risk of COVID-19 infection directly, it may be associated with COVID-19 pathology and increase the risk of death. This indicates the importance of good oral hygiene and periodontal disease management, particularly while dental services are working below their pre-COVID-19 capacity levels.

AUTHOR CONTRIBUTIONS

JW and JK contributed to study design and data acquisition and interpretation of the results. HL contributed to data analysis and interpretation and drafted the manuscript. SW contributed to interpretation of the results. All authors critically revised the manuscript. All authors contributed to the article and approved the submitted version.

ACKNOWLEDGMENTS

This research has been conducted using the UK Biobank Resource under Application Number 54633.

REFERENCES

1. Zandkarimi E, Moradi G, Mohsenpour B. The prognostic factors affecting the survival of Kurdistan Province COVID-19 patients: a cross-sectional study from February to May 2020. *Int J Health Policy Manag.* (2020). doi: 10.34172/ijhpm.2020.155. [Epub ahead of print].
2. Boulle A, Davies MA, Hussey H, Ismail M, Morden E, Vundle Z, et al. Risk factors for COVID-19 death in a population cohort study from the Western Cape Province, South Africa. *Clin Infect Dis.* (2020). doi: 10.1093/cid/ciaa1198. [Epub ahead of print].
3. Williamson EJ, Walker AJ, Bhaskaran K, Bacon S, Bates C, Morton CE, et al. Factors associated with COVID-19-related death using OpenSAFELY. *Nature.* (2020) 584:430–6. doi: 10.1038/s41586-020-2521-4
4. Jin LJ, Lamster IB, Greenspan JS, Pitts NB, Scully C, Warnakulasuriya S. Global burden of oral diseases: emerging concepts, management and interplay with systemic health. *Oral Dis.* (2016) 22:609–19. doi: 10.1111/odi.12428
5. Eke PI, Thornton-Evans GO, Wei L, Borgnakke WS, Dye BA, Genco RJ. Periodontitis in US adults: National Health and Nutrition Examination Survey 2009–2014. *J Am Dent Assoc.* (2018) 149:576–88.e6. doi: 10.1016/j.adaj.2018.04.023
6. Petersen PE, Bourgeois D, Ogawa H, Estupinan-Day S, Ndiaye C. The global burden of oral diseases and risks to oral health. *Bull World Health Organ.* (2005) 83:661–9.
7. Batty GD, Jung KJ, Mok Y, Lee SJ, Back JH, Lee S, et al. Oral health and later coronary heart disease: cohort study of one million people. *Eur J Prev Cardiol.* (2018) 25:598–605. doi: 10.1177/2047487318759112
8. Ide R, Hoshuyama T, Wilson D, Takahashi K, Higashi T. Periodontal disease and incident diabetes: a seven-year study. *J Dent Res.* (2011) 90:41–6. doi: 10.1177/0022034510381902
9. Joshipura KJ, Wand HC, Merchant AT, Rimm EB. Periodontal disease and biomarkers related to cardiovascular disease. *J Dent Res.* (2004) 83:151–5. doi: 10.1177/154405910408300213
10. Lee J-H, Kweon HH-I, Choi J-K, Kim Y-T, Choi S-H. Association between periodontal disease and prostate cancer: results of a 12-year longitudinal cohort study in South Korea. *J Cancer.* (2017) 8:2959–65. doi: 10.7150/jca.20532
11. Rivas-Tumanyan S, Spiegelman D, Curhan GC, Forman JP, Joshipura KJ. Periodontal disease and incidence of hypertension in the health professionals follow-up study. *Am J Hypertens.* (2012) 25:770–6. doi: 10.1038/ajh.2012.32
12. Scannapieco FA, Ho AW. Potential associations between chronic respiratory disease and periodontal disease: analysis of National Health and Nutrition Examination Survey III. *J Periodontol.* (2001) 72:50–6. doi: 10.1902/jop.2001.72.1.50
13. Sampson V, Kamona N, Sampson A. Could there be a link between oral hygiene and the severity of SARS-CoV-2 infections? *Br Dent J.* (2020) 228:971–5. doi: 10.1038/s41415-020-1747-8
14. Pitones-Rubio V, Chávez-Cortez EG, Hurtado-Camarena A, González-Rascón A, Serafín-Higuera N. Is periodontal disease a risk factor for severe COVID-19 illness? *Med Hypotheses.* (2020) 144:109969. doi: 10.1016/j.mehy.2020.109969
15. Chen N, Zhou M, Dong X, Qu J, Gong F, Han Y, et al. Epidemiological and clinical characteristics of 99 cases of 2019 novel coronavirus pneumonia in Wuhan, China: a descriptive study. *Lancet.* (2020) 395:507–13. doi: 10.1016/S0140-6736(20)30211-7
16. Yang X, Yu Y, Xu J, Shu H, Xia J, Liu H, et al. Clinical course and outcomes of critically ill patients with SARS-CoV-2 pneumonia in Wuhan, China: a single-centered, retrospective, observational study. *Lancet Respir Med.* (2020) 8:475–81. doi: 10.1016/S2213-2600(20)30079-5
17. UK Biobank. *Protocol for a Large-Scale Prospective Epidemiological Resource.* (2006). Available online at: www.ukbiobank.ac.uk/resources/ (accessed September 01, 2020).
18. Abbood HM, Hinz J, Cherukara G, Macfarlane TV. Validity of self-reported periodontal disease: a systematic review and meta-analysis. *J Periodontol.* (2016) 87:1474–83. doi: 10.1902/jop.2016.160196
19. Denaxas SC, George J, Herrett E, Shah AD, Kalra D, Hingorani AD, et al. Data resource profile: cardiovascular disease research using linked bespoke studies and electronic health records (CALIBER). *Int J Epidemiol.* (2012) 41:1625–38. doi: 10.1093/ije/dys188
20. Rubin DB. *Multiple Imputation for Nonresponse in Surveys.* New York, NY: John Wiley & Sons (2004).
21. R Core Team. *R: A Language and Environment for Statistical Computing.* Vienna, Austria: R Foundation for Statistical Computing (2017).
22. Zhu X, Ge Y, Wu T, Zhao K, Chen Y, Wu B, et al. Co-infection with respiratory pathogens among COVID-2019 cases. *Virus Res.* (2020) 285:198005. doi: 10.1016/j.virusres.2020.198005
23. Vieira Colombo AP, Magalhães CB, Hartenbach FA, Martins do Souto R, Maciel da Silva-Boghossian C. Periodontal-disease-associated biofilm: a reservoir for pathogens of medical importance. *Microb Pathog.* (2016) 94:27–34. doi: 10.1016/j.micpath.2015.09.009
24. Wu J, Mamas M, Rashid M, Weston C, Hains J, Luescher T, et al. Patient response, treatments and mortality for acute myocardial infarction during the COVID-19 pandemic. *Eur Heart J Qual Care Clin Outcomes.* (2020). doi: 10.1093/ehjqcco/qcaa062
25. Petersen PE, Ogawa H. Strengthening the prevention of periodontal disease: the WHO approach. *J Periodontol.* (2005) 76:2187–93. doi: 10.1902/jop.2005.76.12.2187
26. Hurley S. *Preparedness Letter for Primary Dental Care.* London: NHS England (2020).
27. British Dental Association. *Investigation into the Resilience of Mixed NHS/Private Dental Practices Following the First Wave of the COVID-19 Pandemic 2020.* (2020). Available online at: https://bda.org/advice/Coronavirus/Documents/Investigation-into-the-resilience-of-mixed-dental-practices-following-the-first-wave-of-the-COVID-19-pandemic.pdf (accessed September 01, 2020).
28. Public Health England. *Considerations for Acute Personal Protective Equipment (PPE) Shortages.* London: Public Health England (2020).
29. *New Obesity Strategy Unveiled as Country Urged to Lose Weight to Beat Coronavirus (COVID-19) and Protect the NHS* [press release] (2020).
30. Hua F, Xie H, Worthington HV, Furness S, Zhang Q, Li C. Oral hygiene care for critically ill patients to prevent ventilator-associated pneumonia. *Cochrane Database Syst Rev.* (2016) 10:Cd008367. doi: 10.1002/14651858.CD008367.pub3
31. Public Health England. *Mouth Care for Hospitalized Patients With Confirmed or Suspected COVID-19.* London: Public Health England (2020).
32. Heloe LA. Comparison of dental health data obtained from questionnaires, interviews and clinical examination. *Scand J Dent Res.* (1972) 80:495–9. doi: 10.1111/j.1600-0722.1972.tb00318.x
33. Pitiphat W, Garcia RI, Douglass CW, Joshipura KJ. Validation of self-reported oral health measures. *J Public Health Dent.* (2002) 62:122–8. doi: 10.1111/j.1752-7325.2002.tb03432.x

20

The Impact of Coronavirus Disease 2019 on the Disease Pattern of Oral and Maxillofacial Surgery Inpatients

*Jingya Jane Pu[1], Colman Patrick McGrath[2], Yiu Yan Leung[1], Wing Shan Choi[1], Wei-fa Yang[1], Kar Yan Li[1] and Yu-xiong Su[1]**

[1] Division of Oral and Maxillofacial Surgery, Faculty of Dentistry, The University of Hong Kong, Pokfulam, Hong Kong,
[2] Division of Applied Oral Sciences and Community Dental Care, Faculty of Dentistry, The University of Hong Kong, Pokfulam, Hong Kong

***Correspondence:**
Yu-xiong Su
richsu@hku.hk

Objective: Oral and maxillofacial surgery (OMFS) is a high-risk specialty involving airway and aerosol-generating procedures, which is potentially of more risk in the era of coronavirus disease 2019 (COVID-19). We aimed to identify the impact of COVID-19 on the disease pattern of OMFS inpatients and surgeries under general anesthesia in a comparative study.

Materials and Methods: We reviewed the admission and operating theater records of OMFS patients from Jan 1 to Aug 31 in 2020 and 2019. The total number of cases, presenting disease patterns, and proportion of essential and non-essential medical services were compared between 2020 and 2019.

Results: There were 664 admissions and 356 general anesthesia surgical procedures included in this study. Both admission and surgery numbers were significantly reduced in 2020, compared with 2019 ($p = 0.012$ and 0.007, respectively). The proportion of malignancy cases increased significantly, whereas that of cleft lip and palate and temporomandibular disorder (TMD) decreased. There was a significant increase in the proportion of essential services compared with non-essential services in 2020 compared with 2019.

Conclusion: Our results first reported the epidemiological data of the impact of COVID-19 on OMFS disease pattern in a comparative study. The change of disease pattern and caseload will have a long-term impact on OMFS patient care, education, and training during the pandemic. Our paper provides evidence for health policy makers to consider the relocation of medical resources and optimization of medical education and services.

Keywords: COVID-19, coronavirus, oral and maxillofacial surgery, oral cancer, essential services, healthcare, pandemic, disease pattern

INTRODUCTION

The pandemic outbreak of severe acute respiratory syndrome coronavirus-2 (SARS-CoV-2), which is also known as coronavirus disease 2019 (COVID-19), has been posing major impacts on health care (1). Since the declaration of the World Health Organization (WHO) of COVID-19 outbreak as an international public health emergency, different health-care policies have been adopted by countries worldwide. In general, there is a reduction in the number of elective procedures due to the risk of COVID infection and limited medical resources (2).

During the pandemic, prioritizing medical services is crucial to avoid collapse of medical systems. The health-care system failures during the outbreak of Ebola virus in 2014–2015 contributed to the increased number of deaths caused by measles, malaria, HIV/AIDS, and tuberculosis (3). Therefore, maintaining the essential medical services during an outbreak is of premier importance to avoid increased morbidity and mortality contributed indirectly by the insufficiency or inappropriate distribution of medical resources. According to the guidance by the WHO, priorities of elective surgeries change over time and vary from country to country. The main factors to consider while scheduling the elective treatments including the level of outbreak, availability of the health-care service in the area, and estimated length of the shortage of services (4).

Despite the high population mobility and density in Hong Kong, the citizens, government, and medical professionals have been striving for a reasonable control of the pandemic. From January 1, 2020, to September 19, 2020, there were a total of 5,010 cases of COVID-19 documented by the Department of Health of Hong Kong. Most of the cases were discharged after full recovery (4,708/5,010), while 103 (2.1%) were fatal. The number of patients hospitalized or pending admission was kept below 1,000 most of the time (**Figure 1**), which was within the isolation ward capacity in Hong Kong (5).

Oral and maxillofacial surgery (OMFS) is considered as one of the high-risk specialties due to the involvement of airway and aerosol-generating procedures. However, the impact of COVID-19 on the disease pattern of inpatients and operations in OMFS has yet to be studied. Globally, OMFS services were severely affected during the pandemic, while we have been keeping a certain level of OMFS services including elective cases in Hong Kong. This provides an ideal model to study the service pattern changes of OMFS during the COVID-19 era. Although WHO suggested health conditions and acute presentations that require time-sensitive intervention to be considered as essential medical services, the context-relevant definition in OMFS field is still lacking (4). The aim of this study is to investigate the impact of COVID-19 on the disease pattern in OMFS inpatients and surgeries under general anesthesia and to identify the context-relevant essential services in OMFS field for future reference when it comes to policy making and resource distribution.

MATERIALS AND METHODS

The study was approved by the Institutional Review Board of the University of Hong Kong (IRB Reference Number: UW 20-684), with the patient informed consent waived. We performed a comparative study in the Department of Oral and Maxillofacial Surgery, University of Hong Kong, Queen Mary Hospital, a tertiary hospital in Hong Kong. The study consisted of two parts. The first part focused on the distribution of inpatients admitted to the OMFS ward, Queen Mary Hospital; while the second part analyzed the cases operated in the operating theater (OT) under general anesthesia by the OMFS team. Records from January 1 to August 31 in 2019 and 2020 were reviewed and divided into eight groups below, with dental extraction cases excluded.

1. Dentofacial deformities
2. Benign pathologies
3. Malignancy
4. Dentoalveolar diseases
5. Infections
6. Cleft lip and palate
7. Temporomandibular joint diseases
8. Others (sleep endoscopy, trauma, nerve repair, etc.).

The total number of cases and proportions of different categories of cases were documented and compared so as to illustrate the difference in disease pattern between 2019 and 2020. Cases of malignancy, infection, and trauma were considered as in need of time-sensitive management, thus proposed as "essential medical services" according to the WHO guideline (4).

Polymerase chain reaction screening test for SARS-CoV-2 infection was conducted within 24 h before the operation or admission. Patients would be operated only if they had no travel history within 14 days, had not been in close contact with confirmed cases, were showing no symptom suggesting possible COVID-19 infection, and had negative PCR results. Patients in close contact with confirmed cases were observed for at least 14 days before presenting to the hospital unless they require a life-saving emergency surgery.

All statistical analyses were performed using IBM SPSS Statistics Version 26. Binomial test was performed to compare the difference in total number of cases, while chi square test was used to compare the proportions of essential medical services as well as different groups of cases. Bonferroni adjustment was applied for multiple group comparisons. All tests and reported p-values were two-sided. A $p < 0.05$ was considered statistically significant.

RESULTS

Comparison of Disease Distribution of Inpatients

A total of 664 patients were admitted in the designated periods. Significantly fewer patients were admitted to the hospital in 2020 compared with 2019 ($p = 0.012$) (**Figure 2**). None of the patients tested positive for COVID-19 upon admission or developed COVID-19 infection during their inpatient stay. No health-care professional in our team developed symptoms or tested positive for COVID-19 during the studied period.

The numbers and percentages of different groups of admissions are shown in **Table 1** and **Figure 3**. A significantly larger proportion of patients with malignancies were admitted in 2020 compared with 2019. In contrast, significantly fewer patients were admitted for dentoalveolar diseases,

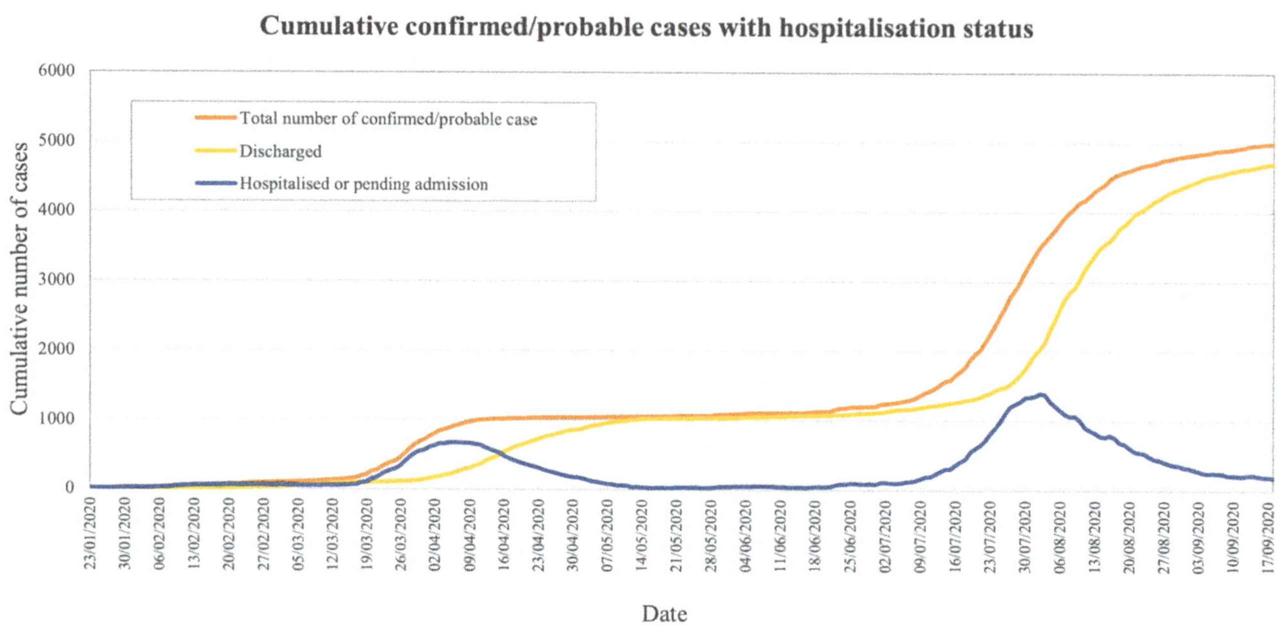

FIGURE 1 | Cumulative confirmed/probable cases with hospitalization status (5).

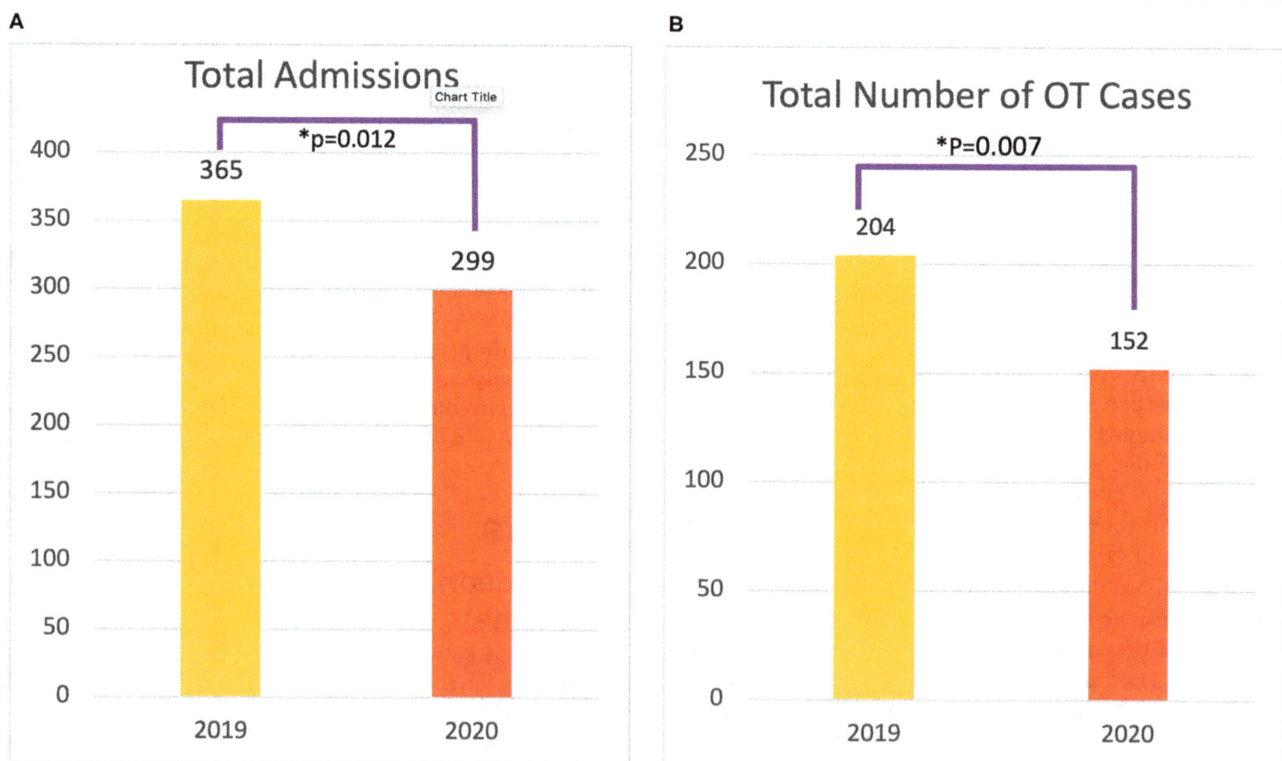

FIGURE 2 | Total number of admissions **(A)** and operating theater (OT) operations **(B)** from Jan 1 to Aug 31 in 2019 and 2020.

cleft lip and palate, and temporomandibular joint diseases. The admissions for the category of "others" also showed significant difference probably due to the decreased number of admissions for obstructive sleep apnea patients in 2020. The proportion of patients admitted for dentofacial deformity, benign pathology, and infections were similar

TABLE 1 | Number of admissions and OT cases in from Jan 1 to Aug 31 in 2019 and 2020.

	Admissions					**OT**				
	2019		**2020**		***p*-value**	**2019**		**2020**		***p*-value**
Dentofacial deformities	78	21.4%	58	19.4%	<0.001	63	30.9%	40	26.3%	0.001
Benign pathology	114	31.2%	91	30.4%		70	34.3%	52	34.2%	
Malignancy	39	10.7%	80	26.8%		16	7.8%	29	19.1%	
Dentoalveolar diseases	46	12.6%	21	7.0%		19	9.3%	11	7.2%	
Infections	33	9.0%	34	11.4%		8	3.9%	14	9.2%	
Cleft	13	3.6%	3	1.0%		8	3.9%	0	0.0%	
TMJ diseases	19	5.2%	4	1.3%		11	5.4%	1	0.7%	
Others (OSA, trauma, etc.)	23	6.3%	8	2.7%		9	4.4%	5	3.3%	
Total	365	100.0%	299	100.0%	0.012	204	100.0%	152	100.0%	0.007

NS, not significant; OT, operating theater; TMJ, temporomandibular joint; OSA, obstructive sleep apnea.

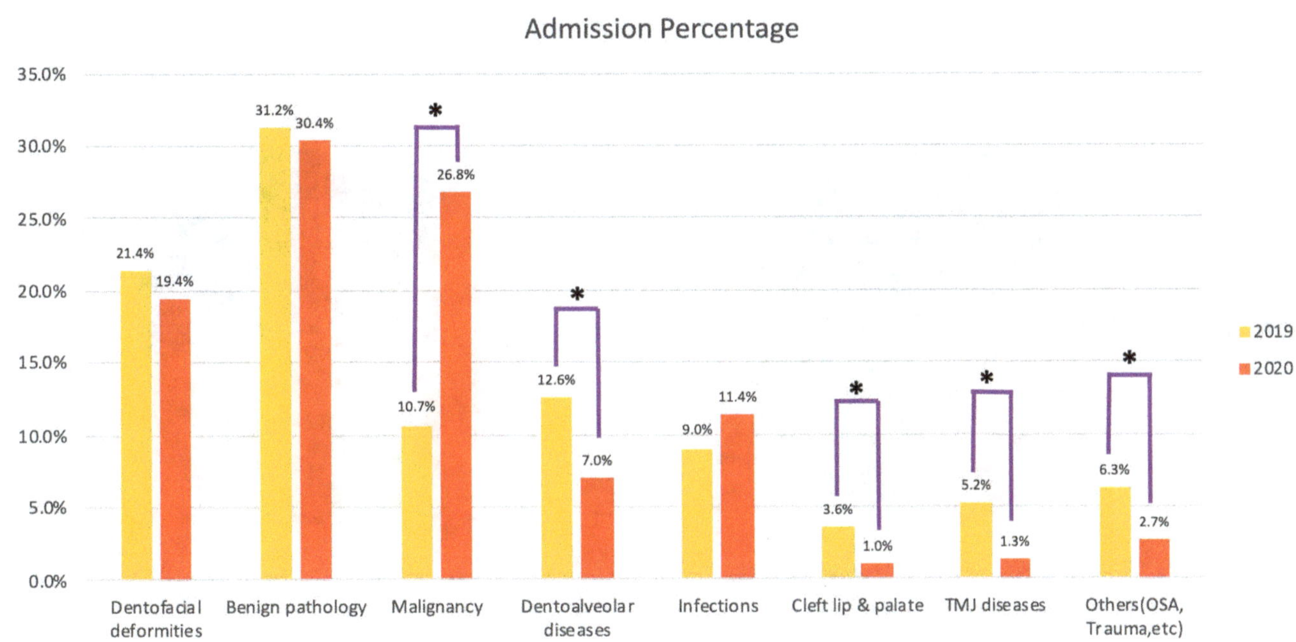

FIGURE 3 | Percentage of different categories of admissions. *Groups with significant difference between 2019 and 2020 after Bonferroni adjustment.

in 2019 and 2020. Percentage distributions of different groups of admissions in 2019 and 2020 are shown in **Figure 4**.

Comparison of Surgery Under General Anesthesia

A total of 356 patients were operated in the theater under general anesthesia. Compared with that in 2019, there was a decrease in total number of cases ($p = 0.007$) (**Figure 2**). None of the patients operated tested positive for COVID-19.

The number of percentage of cases in different categories is shown in **Table 1** and **Figure 5**. Significant increases in the percentage of malignancy and infection cases were observed in 2020. Priorities were given to the malignant cases with no limitation imposed. Different than most other hospitals during pandemic, we performed microvascular free flap reconstruction for oral malignancy cases as usual. No cleft lip or palate repair surgery was performed in 2020. The difference was significant between 2019 and 2020. Significantly less operations for temporomandibular joint dysfunction were performed in 2020. The proportions of surgeries for dentofacial deformity,

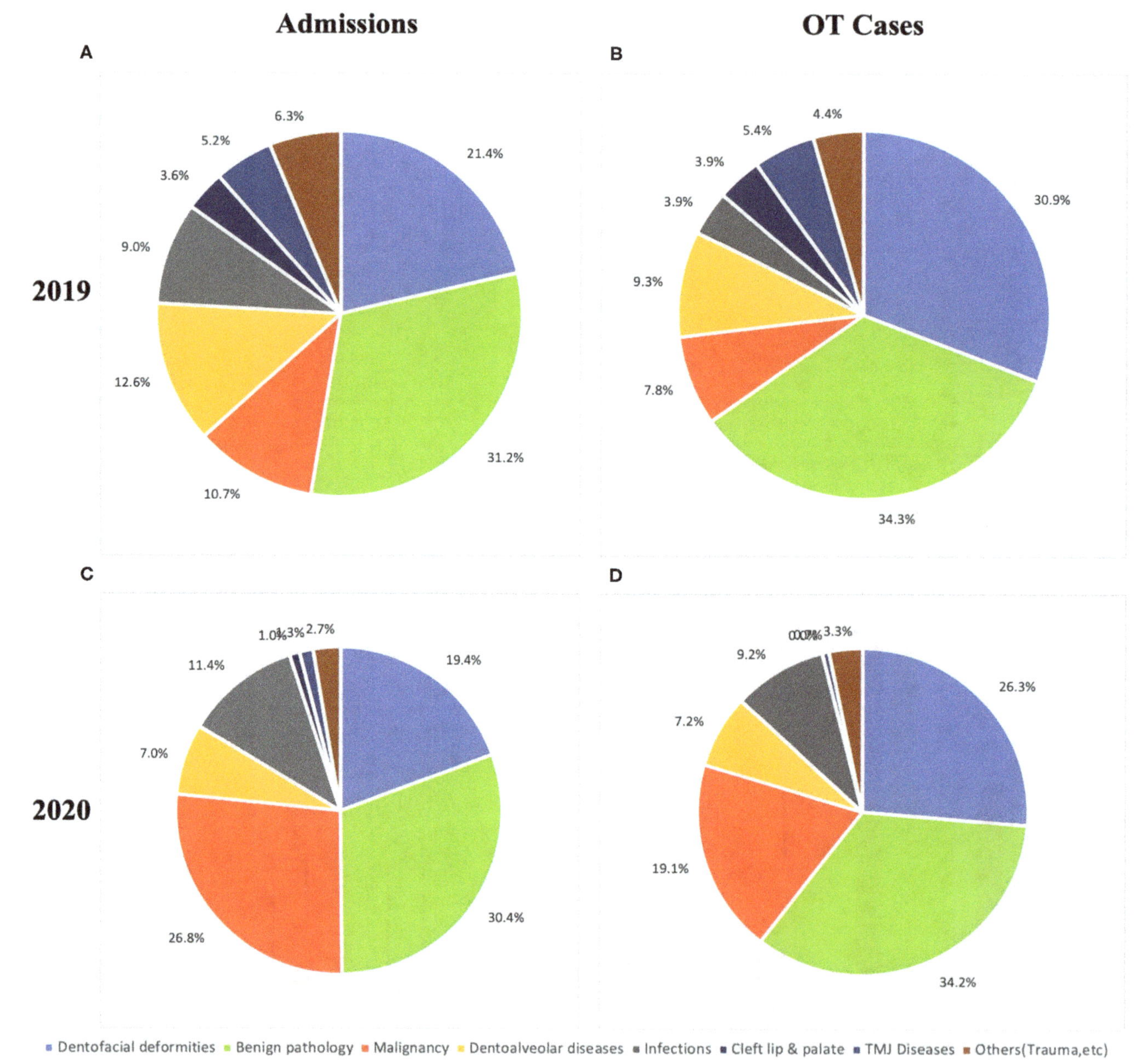

FIGURE 4 | Distribution of admissions and operating theater (OT) cases. **(A)** Admissions in 2019. **(B)** OT cases in 2019. **(C)** Admissions in 2020. **(D)** OT cases in 2020.

benign pathology, dentoalveolar diseases, and others (trauma, nerve repair, etc.) were kept at a similar level. The distribution of cases in 2019 and 2020 is shown in **Figure 4**.

Essential Medical Services

When malignancy, infection, and trauma were considered as time-sensitive essential medical services, the proportion of essential services increased significantly in both inpatient admissions and surgeries, with the $p < 0.001$. The decrease in the proportion of non-essential cases was also significant in both groups (**Figure 6**).

DISCUSSION

Since the outbreak of COVID-19, there have been numerous guidelines on the management of patients during the pandemic (6–8). However, to the best of our knowledge, the current study is the first comparative study to objectively report the significant decrease in total number of patients, the increase in malignancy cases, and essential medical services in OMFS under the influence of COVID-19 pandemic.

Compared with that pre-COVID-19, the total number of cases operated in the OT decreased mainly due to the limited supply of personal protection equipment and the reduction in OT sessions

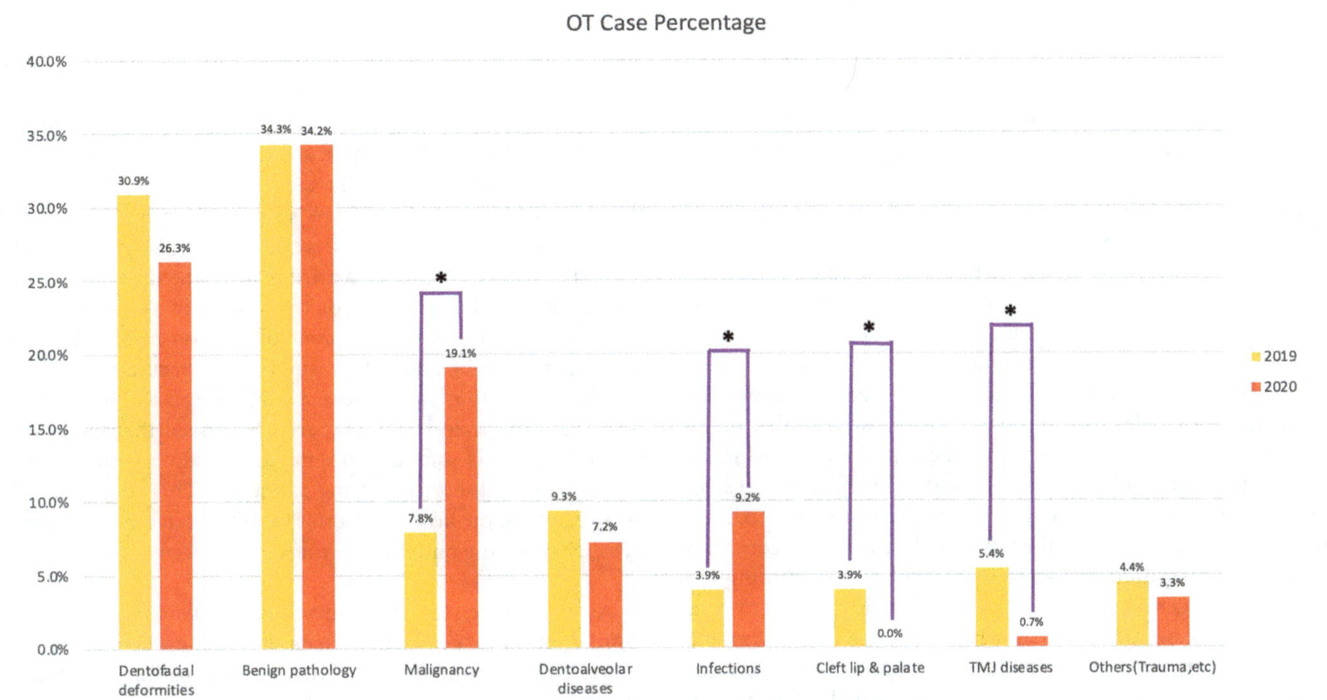

FIGURE 5 | Percentage of different categories of operating theater (OT) cases. *Groups with significant difference between 2019 and 2020 after Bonferroni adjustment.

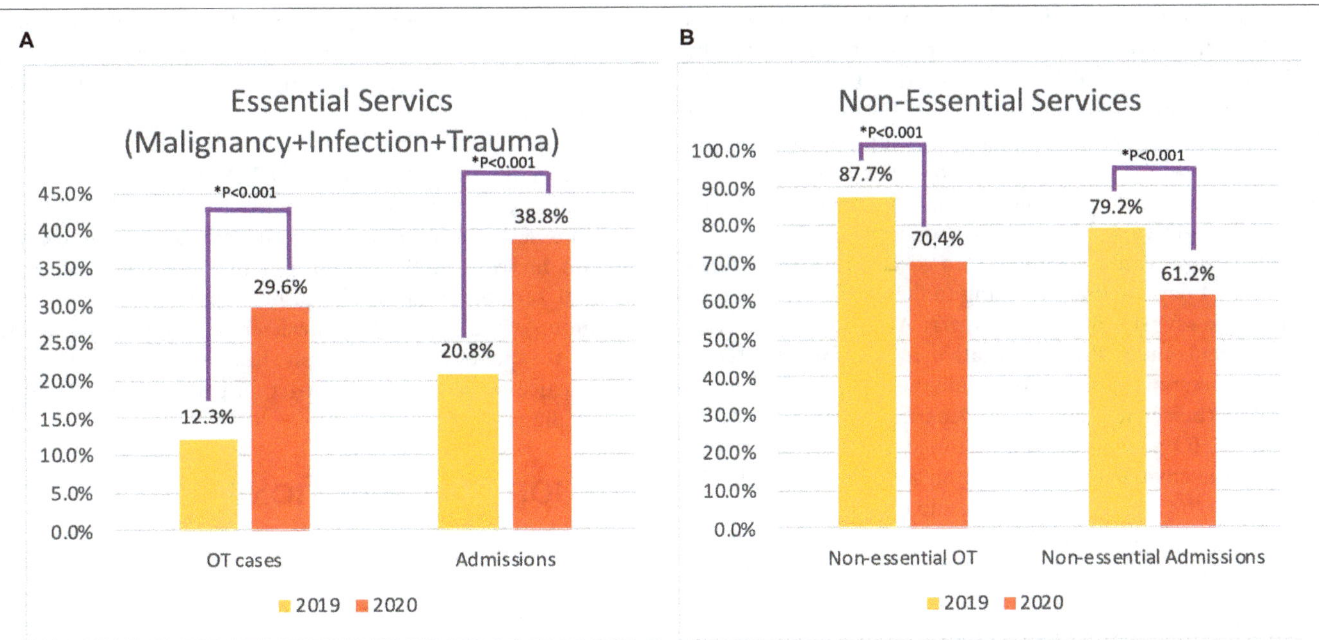

FIGURE 6 | Proportion of essential medical services **(A)** and non-essential services **(B)**.

assigned to OMFS. The reduction in the number of admissions could be attributed to reduction in operations as well as decrease of elective inpatient and outpatient services during the outbreak of COVID-19.

The proportion of essential medical services, especially the percentage of malignancy cases, increased significantly under the influence of COVID-19. Although there were no supportive scientific data available so far, various subjective recommendations have been proposed to determine the priority of surgical treatments. From the country with the earliest outbreak, Yang et al. from China defined four categories of OMFS patients according to severity. The critically ill patients include those who require emergency interventions due to life-threatening conditions such as hemorrhage and obstruction of the upper respiratory tract following trauma, tumors, and infections. Subacute patients include those with stable vital signs but requiring urgent interventions such as closed fractures. This is followed by the patients who require expedited interventions including patients diagnosed with malignant tumors, chronic infections, osteomyelitis, etc., while the last group of patients are those who require elective procedures such as those with cleft lip and palate, dentofacial deformities, and benign tumors (9). The malignancy, infection, and trauma cases we included in the "essential medical service" belong to the first three categories in this classification, while the "non-essential medical services" in our study agreed with the last category of elective procedures. Others suggested balancing the risk of delaying the surgery with the resources required for the treatment when determining the priority of surgeries (10, 11). In most situations, priority was given to the essential services when resources were limited. However, when the current pandemic is expected to persist for a relatively long period of time, the changed disease pattern in OMFS might become the new norm. This will have long-term effects in patient care as well as education and training of surgeons. Our data provide reference for policy making and resource distribution in the future.

The precautions we adopted for managing patients in COVID-19 era were similar as the joint recommendations by OMFS in Spain (12). PCR screening test for SARS-CoV-2 infection was conducted within 24 h before the operation or admission. Patients would be operated on only if they had no travel history within 14 days, had not been in close contact with confirmed cases, were showing no symptoms suggesting possible COVID-19 infection, and had negative PCR results. Patients in close contact with confirmed cases were observed for at least 14 days before presenting to the hospital unless they require a life-saving emergency surgery. All cases documented in the current study showed negative results for COVID-19 tests. The operations were performed in the designated COVID-19-negative theater for the OMFS Department in Queen Mary Hospital. WHO guidelines were followed in terms of level of personal protective equipment (PPE) in ward and OT (13, 14). Regardless of the negative results, oral and maxillofacial surgeons were required to wear surgical masks at all time. Aerosol-generating procedures in ward such as changing or removing of tracheostomy tubes and irrigation of intra-oral wound were performed with whole body protection including surgical mask with facial shield, gown, gloves, surgical cap, and eye protection. The same recommendation of protection was applied in the OT. During the period studied, all of our patients and health-care professionals were kept safe from COVID-19 infection, which proved the effectiveness of the precautions we adopted.

In Hong Kong, although the proportion of non-essential services significantly decreased in 2020, we were able to maintain a certain level of service on orthognathic surgery, benign pathology, and dentoalveolar surgeries during the pandemic. This contrasts with the report by Barca et al. about the practice in Italy where all cases treated from Feb 29 to April 16, 2020, were due to either malignancy or trauma (15). A similar situation was observed in the UK where all non-urgent elective surgeries were suspended for 3 months starting April 15, 2020 (16). In the worldwide survey of OMFS surgeons conducted by Maffia et al., only 5.8% of surgeons were still performing orthognathic surgeries (17). This could be attributed to the different levels of pandemic in different parts of the world. In the future, when the pandemic is reasonably controlled, non-essential medical services need to be gradually resumed. The accumulated load of elective procedures might pose a challenge in the recovery and post-recovery periods. Our experience proved that with proper precautions, it is safe and pragmatic to keep a certain level of elective medical services during pandemic. This could also serve as a reference on how to resume OMFS service in a controlled manner when the outbreak is winding down.

As a single-center study, there are intrinsic limitations. The number of trauma cases in our center and the whole Hong Kong is limited, which made the statistical analysis for traumatology as an independent category difficult. There was no COVID-19-positive patient in our cohort. If a multicenter study could be conducted in the future, more comprehensive and widely applicable experience in OMFS patient management in COVID-19 era will be more valuable. Our study only investigated hospital admissions and operations. When the outbreak period is prolonged, data on outpatient management will be needed to guide the outpatient services, which could be time-dependent and lifesaving.

Compared with that pre-COVID-19, the number of admissions and surgeries decreased in the COVID-19 era. There was a significant difference in the disease pattern of OMFS with an increase in the proportion of malignancy cases and essential services. Our results also support that with proper precautions, non-essential medical services can be maintained during the pandemic. Our study has implication for policy and practice for OMFS with impact on patient care, education, and training.

AUTHOR CONTRIBUTIONS

JJP: conceptualization, methodology, data curation, formal analysis, writing—original draft, and writing—review and editing. CPM: conceptualization, formal analysis, project administration, validation, and writing—review and editing. YYL, WSC, and WFY: project administration, supervision, validation, and writing—review and editing. YXS: conceptualization, formal analysis, funding acquisition, supervision, validation, and writing—review and editing. KYL: statistical analysis and validation. All authors approved the final manuscript for publication.

REFERENCES

1. Tao ZY, Chu G, McGrath C, Hua F, Leung YY, Yang WF, et al. Nature and diffusion of COVID-19-related oral health information on Chinese Social Media: analysis of tweets on Weibo. *J Med Internet Res.* (2020) 22:e19981. doi: 10.2196/19981
2. Ralli M, Greco A, de Vincentiis M. The effects of the COVID-19/SARS-CoV-2 pandemic outbreak on otolaryngology activity in Italy. *Ear Nose Throat J.* (2020) 99:565–6. doi: 10.1177/0145561320923893
3. Parpia AS, Ndeffo-Mbah ML, Wenzel NS, Galvani AP. Effects of response to 2014-2015 ebola outbreak on deaths from malaria, HIV/AIDS, and tuberculosis, West Africa. *Emerg Infect Dis.* (2016) 22:433–41. doi: 10.3201/eid2203.150977
4. World Health Organization. *COVID-19: Operational Guidance for Maintaining Essential Health Services During an Outbreak: Interim Guidance.* WHO (2020). Available online at: https://apps.who.int/iris/handle/10665/331561 (accessed June 1, 2020).
5. Centre for Health Protection of the Department of Health, Hong Kong SAR. *Latest Situation of Cases of COVID-19.* Available online at: https://www.chp.gov.hk/files/pdf/local_situation_covid19_en.pdf (accessed September 19, 2020).
6. Federation of Surgical Specialty Associations. *Clinical Guide to Surgical Prioritisation During the Coronavirus Pandemic.* FSSA (2020). Available online at: https://fssa.org.uk/_userfiles/pages/files/covid19/prioritisation_master_240820.pdf (accessed September 27, 2020).
7. Givi B, Schiff BA, Chinn SB, Clayburgh D, Iyer NG, Jalisi S, et al. Safety recommendations for evaluation and surgery of the head and neck during the COVID-19 pandemic. *JAMA Otolaryngol Head Neck Surg.* (2020) 146:579–584. doi: 10.1001/jamaoto.2020.0780
8. Chigurupati R, Panchal N, Henry AM, Batal H, Sethi A, D'innocenzo R, et al. Considerations for oral and maxillofacial surgeons in COVID-19 era: can we sustain the solutions to keep our patients and healthcare personnel safe? *J Oral Maxillofac Surg.* (2020) 78:1241–56. doi: 10.1016/j.joms.2020.05.027
9. Yang Y, Soh HY, Cai ZG, Peng X, Zhang Y, Guo CB. Experience of diagnosing and managing patients in oral maxillofacial surgery during the prevention and control period of the new coronavirus pneumonia. *Chin J Dent Res.* (2020) 23:57–62. doi: 10.3290/j.cjdr.a44339
10. Caplan AL, Thomas SA. A better way to prioritize "essential" vs. "elective" care during COVID-19. *Perspective Medscape.* (2020). Available online at: https://www.medscape.com/viewarticle/928537 (accessed April 17, 2021).
11. Stahel PF. How to risk-stratify elective surgery during the COVID-19 pandemic? *Patient Saf Surg.* (2020) 14:8. doi: 10.1186/s13037-020-00235-9
12. Gil FM, Carretero JLC, Cembranos JLL, Alamillos MR, Beltrán AV, Parra FA, et al. Management of patients in oral and maxillofacial surgery during the stage of crisis and subsequent control of COVID-19 pandemic. *Rev Esp Cir Oral Maxilofac.* (2020) 42:51–9. doi: 10.20986/recom.2020.1162/2020
13. World Health Organization. *Infection Prevention and Control During Health Care When COVID-19 Is Suspected: Interim Guidance, 19 March 2020.* Geneva: World Health Organization (2020).
14. World Health Organization. *Rational Use of Personal Protective Equipment (PPE) for Coronavirus Disease (COVID-19): Interim Guidance, 19 March 2020.* Geneva: World Health Organization (2020).
15. Barca I, Cordaro R, Kallaverja E, Ferragina F, Cristofaro MG. Management in oral and maxillofacial surgery during the COVID-19 pandemic: Our experience. *Br J Oral Maxillofac Surg.* (2020) 58:687–91. doi: 10.1016/j.bjoms.2020.04.025
16. Iacobucci G. Covid-19: all non-urgent elective surgery is suspended for at least three months in England. *BMJ.* (2020) 368:m1106. doi: 10.1136/bmj.m1106
17. Maffia F, Fontanari M, Vellone V, Cascone P, Mercuri LG. Impact of COVID-19 on maxillofacial surgery practice: a worldwide survey. *Int J Oral Maxillofac Surg.* (2020) 49:827–35. doi: 10.1016/j.ijom.2020.04.015

21

Anxiety, Practice Modification and Economic Impact Among Iraqi Dentists During the COVID-19 Outbreak

Anas F. Mahdee[1], Sarhang S. Gul[2], Ali A. Abdulkareem[3] and Syed Saad B. Qasim[4]*

[1] Department of Restorative and Aesthetic Dentistry, College of Dentistry, University of Baghdad, Baghdad, Iraq, [2] Department of Periodontics, College of Dentistry, University of Sulaimani, Sulaimani, Iraq, [3] Department of Periodontics, College of Dentistry, University of Baghdad, Baghdad, Iraq, [4] Department of Bioclinical Sciences, Faculty of Dentistry, Kuwait University, Safat, Kuwait

***Correspondence:**
Sarhang S. Gul
sarhang.hama@univsul.edu.iq
orcid.org/0000-0003-1413-4934

Objectives: As health care workers on the front line during the coronavirus (COVID-19) pandemic, dental practitioners are amongst those at risk due to their close contact with potentially infected individuals. The aim of the current study was to assess the anxiety, awareness practice modification, and economic impact amongst Iraqi dentists whilst working during the outbreak.

Methods: This study was performed using an online survey questionnaire with aid of Google forms from 2nd to 23rd July 2020. A total of 484 clinicians responded. The questionnaire was composed of open end, closed end, and Likert five-point scale questions to assess anxiety, awareness and financial impact of COVID-19 on dentists. Mann–Whitney test was used to compare two groups, whilst Kruskal–Wallis was performed by *post-hoc* test for multigroup comparisons.

Results: The mean age of participants was 36.51 ± 9.164 years and the majority (75.2%) of these were graduate dentists only. More than 80% of participants reported anxiety of catching COVID-19. The recorded anxiety level was higher amongst younger dentists and females. Awareness and practice levels among these dentists of precautions and infection-control measures associated with COVID-19 (94%) was found to be high and to be statistically significantly affected by age, qualification and designation (except GP vs. Specialist). With respect to the economic impact, about 75% of practitioners, regardless of demographical variables, reported that their income had declined by about 50%.

Conclusions: The investigation provides clear insights into the anxiety, practice modifications and economic impact on dentists working in Iraq. Although there is a high level of knowledge and awareness of required practice regarding the COVID-19 outbreak among Iraqi dentists, they also reported a high level of anxiety.

Keywords: anxiety, coronavirus, Iraqi dentists, economic, practice management

INTRODUCTION

Since the emergence of the novel coronavirus disease (COVID-19) in Wuhan, China, all aspects of life have been influenced worldwide. The COVID-19 pandemic has spread in an exponential manner (1, 2), affecting millions of people worldwide and causing hundreds of thousands of deaths (3). Many countries have shut down their teaching institutes, industries, sport activities, social gatherings, public events, and airports. Drastic measures such as individual self-quarantine and social distancing rules have been introduced in an attempt to control the spread of the infection (4). The condition in Iraq has been no better than in many other countries. Since the first registered case of COVID-19 was recorded on the 24th of February 2020 in an Iranian student attending the city of Najaf in the south of Iraq, the spread of the virus has been escalating and as of 1st of July there were 51,524 confirmed cases and 2,050 deaths.

COVID-19 belongs to the Coronaviridae virus family, which is characterized by a single strand RNA structure (5). This virus has potential to cause severe respiratory tract infection and pneumonia among infected individuals, and can be easily transmitted via hand contact, saliva, nasal droplets and contaminated surfaces (2, 6). Health care workers and dentists in particular are categorized as at high risk of catching this infection (7). This could be because their close contact with patients during routine dental procedures increases the possibility of infection transmission (8, 9). Droplets and aerosols that are generated during dental procedures by such as high speed handpieces, air-water syringes, and ultrasonic scaling could produce a contaminated pathogenic environment within the dental working field during treatment of an infected person (6, 9, 10). Therefore, the risk of infection transmission within the dental team cannot be controlled through the standard protective measures of daily dental practice (8). This categorization as high-risk professionals could increase fear within the dental community (11, 12).

Regarding the rapid spread of the infection, the World Health Organization (WHO) and American Dental Association (ADA) published specific precaution guidelines to be implemented by dentists during treatment of urgent and emergency cases only. Otherwise, they stipulated that dental offices should be kept closed during the outbreak (13, 14). These guidelines emphasized the use of the appropriate precautions including wearing personal protective equipment (PPE) during dental procedures (13, 14). In addition, the use of antibacterial mouth washes, rubber dam, and high-volume section during treatment procedures with frequent cleaning and disinfecting of surfaces of chairs, door handles and floors was highly recommended (8, 15). Providing a secure environment is of paramount importance for dentists and dental staff to conduct dental work in a safe working environment. The high infection rate of COVID-19 and lack of PPE might affect the anxiety of the dentist. The levels anxiety of dentists have shown a negative impact on decision making, quality of work, and burnout (16).

On the other hand, in dental practice the demand arose for more expensive aerosol controlling equipment such as the high efficiency particulate arrestor (HEPA) during the outbreak period (10). The expense of these precautionary measures and limitations in the treatment of patients may have had serious economic impact on the dentistry field. Hence, the future careers of dentists could be affected if the outbreak continues for an indefinite period.

Meanwhile, no study has assessed the levels of anxiety among Iraqi dentists in the wake of the COVID-19 outbreak, their awareness about this illness and the infection control guidelines to prevent its spread, or the financial impact on their current practice. Therefore, the aim of this study was to use a specially designed online-based questionnaire to assess the impact of the COVID-19 outbreak on Iraqi dentists in terms of their anxiety, awareness and practice modification, and the financial implications for their dental practice.

METHODS

Survey Administration

A cross-sectional survey was conducted using an online questionnaire that was electronically sent to Iraqi dentists by Iraqi Dental Association (IDA). Administration of the questionnaire started on 02/07/2020 for a period of 2 weeks, which was extended for another week after a reminder was sent, and ended on 23/07/2020. The study was approved by the ethics committee of the College of Dentistry, University of Baghdad in compliance with the Helsinki declaration (Ref No. 579/06/2020).

Study Population and Sample Size

The survey was exclusively sent to registered Iraqi dentists and only completed forms were included in the final analysis. All incomplete forms and those returned outside the required timeframe were excluded.

The total number of registered Iraqi dentists, as officially provided by the IDA, was 6,463. Sample size was determined according to the following formulas (17, 18):

$$\begin{aligned}\text{Sample size} &= (\text{distribution of } 50\%)/[(\text{margin of error}\%/\\ &\quad \text{confidence level score})^2]\\ \text{Confidence level} &= 1.96 \text{ (for confidence level of } 95\%),\\ &\quad \text{margin of error} = 0.05.\\ \text{True sample} &= (\text{sample size} \times \text{population})/\\ &\quad (\text{sample size} + \text{population} - 1)\end{aligned}$$

The calculated sample size was equal to 363 which was further adjusted to take account of the dropout risk, previously estimated from a pilot study, by using the following formula:

$$N = n/[1 - (z/100)]$$

Where N is the adjusted sample size, n is the calculated sample size, z represents the hypothesized attrition rate (25%). The final sample size was equal to 484 dentists. Accordingly, the questionnaire link was distributed via emails to corresponding number of randomly selected dentists.

TABLE 1 | The study questionnaire.

Age					
Country					
Sex	A-Male	B-Female			
Qualification	A-Graduate	B-Postgraduate			
Designation	A-General practitioner	B-Specialist	C-Consultant		
Working place	A-Clinic	B-Hospital	C-Both		
Working type	A-Private	B-Government	C-Both		
1- Do you have a anxiety of being infected with COVID-19 by a patient or co-worker?				Yes	No
2- Are you afraid of providing treatment for any patient?				Yes	No
3- If a patient is coughing or suspected to be infected with COVID-19, are you afraid to provide treatment for him/her?				Yes	No
4- Do you anxious talking to the patients in close proximity?				Yes	No
5- Are you afraid that you could carry the infection from your practice back to your family?				Yes	No
6- Do you feel anxious when you hear that one of your co-workers or colleagues has been infected with COVID-19?				Yes	No
7- Do you know the illness problems associated with COVID-19 virus?				Yes	No
8- Do you know the mode of transmission of COVID-19 virus?				Yes	No
9- Are you updated with the current WHO guidelines for cross-infection control for COVID-19 virus?				Yes	No
10- Are you currently asking every patient if he/she has recently been in contact with an infected COVID-19 person?				Yes	No
11- Are you or your staff members taking every patient's body temperature before performing dental treatment?				Yes	No
12- Are you deferring dental treatment for patients with suspicious symptoms?				Yes	No
13- Do you think the routine surgical mask is effective to prevent COVID-19 cross infection?				Yes	No
14- Do you think that N-95 masks should be used routinely in dental practice because of the current COVID-19 outbreak?				Yes	No
15- Do you routinely follow universal infection control protocol for every patient?				Yes	No
16- Do you currently use rubber dam isolation for every patient as a part of your infection control?				Yes	No
17- Do you routinely use high volume section for every patient as part of droplets and airborne isolation precautions?				Yes	No
18- Do you routinely prepare antimicrobial mouth rinse for every patient to be used before starting treatment?				Yes	No
19- Have you changed or increased the procedure of infection control during the COVID-19 pandemic?				Yes	No
20- Has the schedule of your practice been changed to make it safer for you and the patient?				Yes	No
21- Do you routinely wash your hands with soap and water/ use sanitizer before and after treatment of every patient?				Yes	No
22- Do you and your staff members get tested for COVID-19 as a precautionary measure?				Yes	No
23- Do you know which authority to contact if you come across a patient with suspected COVID-19 infection?				Yes	No
25- What is the average drop in the number of patients visiting your practice as compared to the period before the COVID-19 pandemic?					
A- N/A	B- <25%	C- 25–50%	D- 50–75%	E- >75%	
26- How many appointments for non-urgent cases have you canceled recently as a part of COVID-19 precaution protocol?					
A- N/A	B- <25%	C- 25–50%	D- 50–75%	E- >75%	
27- Because of the COVID-19 pandemic, how much have the prices for your dental services been reduced, if at all?					
A- N/A	B- <25%	C- 25–50%	D- 50–75%	E- >75%	
28- If any, how much financial compensation (governmental and non-governmental) are you receiving for your losses in your practice?					
A- N/A	B- <25%	C- 25–50%	D- 50–75%	E- >75%	
29- To what extent have you reduced the staff numbers in your clinic?					
A- N/A	B- <25%	C- 25–50%	D- 50–75%	E- >75%	
30- By how much has the practice's income been reduced due to the COVID 19 pandemic?					
A- N/A	B- <25%	C- 25–50%	D- 50–75%	E- >75%	
31- What percentage of your stored dental materials have expired during the COVID-19 pandemic?					
A- N/A	B- <25%	C- 25–50%	D- 50–75%	E- >75%	
32- If applicable, what has been the average reduction of working days during the COVID-19 outbreak?					
A- N/A	B- <25%	C- 25–50%	D- 50–75%	E- >75%	

Questionnaire Design

Google forms was used to create the link for the questionnaire (illustrated in **Table 1**) that was distributed to the targeted population electronically via IDA to ensure uniform and validated distribution across all groups of dentists, including general practitioners, specialists, and consultants, throughout the country. Before distributing the questionnaire, a pilot study was conducted which included 36 dentists (about 10% of the sample size). Then data were entered on spreadsheet and double-checked by two authors which was followed pre-launch analysis was performed to check the internal consistency of all questionnaire's components.

The questionnaire was adapted and modified from previously published surveys (19, 20). The questionnaire used for this study was composed of demographic/practice-related, closed end, and Likert five-point scale questions. These questions were divided into four sections:

Section 1 was designed to collect demographic/practice-related variables of the respondents.
Section 2, questions #1 to #6, was intended to assess the anxiety among dentists deriving from the COVID-19 infection.
Section 3, questions #7 to #23, was designed to evaluate the dentists' awareness and practice modification about the precautions and infection-control measures for COVID-19 infection.
Section 4, questions #24 to #32, consisted of questions that explored the economic impact of COVID-19 on dental practice.

For closed end questions, each positive response "Yes" was marked as "1" while "No" was marked with "0." The frequency of the positive/negative responses was used to assess the dentists' anxiety (section 2) and awareness (section 3) regarding the COVID-19 infection. For section 4, the responses "N/A," "<25%," "25–50%," "50–75%," ">75%" received sequential scores of "1," "2," "3," "4," "5," respectively. The scores for each section were summed together to calculate the mean of the answers to evaluate the response according to the different independent variables.

Statistical Analysis

Demographic data and total responses for each question were analyzed by descriptive statistics expressed by mean, standard deviation, and frequency/percentage. Inferential analysis for sections 2, 3, and 4 was performed by using Mann–Whitney test for comparing two groups while Kruskal–Wallis followed by *post-hoc* test was used for multiple groups comparisons. The statistically significant value was set at $p < 0.05$. All analyses were performed by using GraphPad Prism (Version 8.4.3, GraphPad Software, San Diego, CA, USA).

RESULTS

A total of 435 dentists (218 male and 217 female) with mean age of 36.51 ± 9.164 years (ranging from 23 to 70 years) participated in the study (**Table 2**). The number of respondents represented 89.9% of the calculated sample size (484) after excluding 49 dentists who did not response to the questionnaire within the specified time. The number of the respondents (435) was considered as a satisfactory response rate (89.8%). The majority of respondents (327, 75.2%) were graduate dentists, in comparison to 108 (24.8%) who had postgraduate degrees. The proportions of general practitioners, specialists and consultants were 47.8% (208), 47.4% (206), and 4.8% (20), respectively. Furthermore, 202 (46%) of respondents working in clinics worked in both the private and governmental sector (**Table 2**).

Responses to section 2 questions relating to dentists' feelings about the COVID-19 pandemic indicated that the majority of respondents (386, > 80%) (**Figure 1A**) were anxious of catching the COVID-19 infection (Q1). Over 60% (274) of the dentists were afraid of treating any patients (Q2). This anxiety was further aggravated (397, 91%) if a patient was showing a sign of suspected infection such as coughing (Q3). Moreover, about 72% (316) of the respondents were not comfortable with being in close contact with their patients (Q4). The highest scoring response among the participants (413, 94%) was associated with the anxiety of carrying infection home to their family (Q5), whilst the second highest response (395, 90%) related to hearing that a co-worker had been infected with COVID-19 (Q6).

TABLE 2 | Demographic characteristics of the study population.

AGE (YEARS)	
(mean± SD)	36.51 ± 9.16
Age range	23–70
AGE GROUPS (YEARS)	
≤35	222 (51)[§]
>35	213 (49)[§]
Gender	
Male	218 (50.1) [§]
Female	217 (49.9)[§]
QUALIFICATION	
Graduate	327 (75.2)[§]
Postgraduate	108 (24.8)[§]
DESIGNATION	
General practitioner	208 (47.8)[§]
Specialist	206 (47.4)[§]
Consultant	21 (4.8)[§]
WORKPLACE	
Clinic	202 (46.4)[§]
Hospital	70 (16.1)[§]
Both	163 (37.5)[§]
EMPLOYMENT TYPE	
Private	135 (31.1)[§]
Governmental	98 (22.5)[§]
Both	202 (46.4)[§]
Total	435 (100)[§]

[§] *Frequency, percentage.*

Regarding responses to section 3 questions, the dentists' highest scores related to their knowledge about the COVID-19 illness (Q7, 413, 94%) (**Figure 1B**) and its modes of transmission (Q8, 424, 97%), modification in infection control procedure (Q19, 410, 94%) re-scheduling patients' appointments (Q20, 404, 93%), and washing hands before and after treatment (Q21, 416, 95%). Additionally, three questions achieved (>80%) positive responses including: the dentist had updated information about the current WHO guidelines for infection control (Q9), deferring treatment of patients with suspicious symptoms (12), and following universal infection control protocol (Q15). Whereas, the lowest awareness score (138, 31.7%) related to the effectiveness of surgical masks to prevent cross infection (Q13), in comparison to nearly 80% of respondents who thought that N95 masks should be used routinely in dental practice (Q14). The response to (Q16) about the use of rubber dam as an infection control measure was equally low at 31.7% (138), but a higher

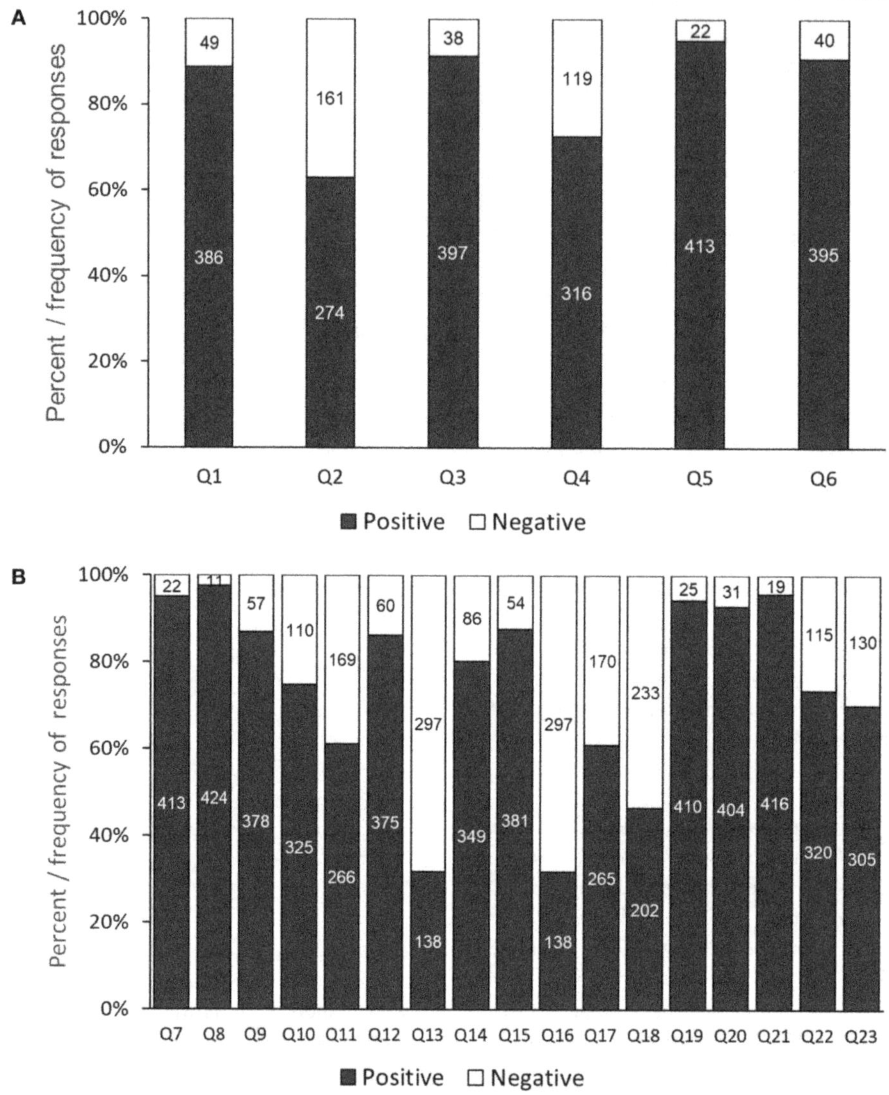

FIGURE 1 | Dentists' responses to anxiety and awareness questions: **(A)** responses to individual questions on anxiety of COVID-19 and **(B)** awareness of precaution and infection control-measures.

percentage of respondents (265, >60%) confirmed that they used high volume section as a droplets precaution measure (Q17).

The economic impact of COVID-19 was investigated in this study via the section 4 questions (**Figure 2**). About 27% of the respondents suggested that the price of personal protection equipment had increased by >75% of the original price (Q24). Meanwhile, 32% of the dentists indicated that the number of patients had declined by 25–50% (Q25). The influence of COVID-19 on income was very apparent as >75% of the dentists reported that their income had dropped by 25–50% (Q30), with a similar response regarding the reduction in their working days (Q32). The level of financial compensation received by the dentists was unsatisfactory as more than half of the respondents were not eligible for any support programmes (Q28). However, the majority of the respondent dentists had not decreased their staff numbers (Q29) (**Figure 2**).

Inferential analysis of the questionnaire sections showed that older (>35 years old) and male respondents exhibited a statistically significant lower degree of anxiety of COVID-19 compared to younger ($\leq$35 years old, $p = 0.018$) and female ($p = 0.003$) respondents, respectively (**Table 3**). Furthermore, the respondents who worked only in a hospital or in a clinic and hospital showed a statistically significantly higher anxiety than those working only in a clinic. Similarly, those working only in the government sector or in the government and private sector showed statistically significantly higher anxiety from COVID-19 than those working only in private clinics. However, respondents' qualifications and designation did not show a statistically significant impact on anxiety of COVID-19 (**Table 3**). Generally, the mean of responses showed a high level of anxiety of COVID-19 infection (5.01 ± 1.37; **Table 3**).

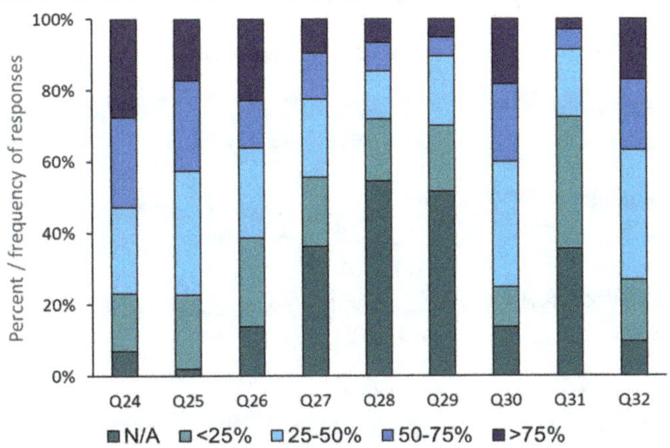

FIGURE 2 | Dentists' responses on the economic impact of COVID-19 outbreak on their practice.

TABLE 3 | Respondents' anxiety of the COVID-19 infection.

Variables	Mean ± SD	Comparison	*p*-value
AGE			
≤35	5.14 ± 1.27	≤ 35 vs. > 35	0.018*
>35	4.87 ± 1.45		
GENDER			
Male	4.78 ± 1.57	Male vs. female	0.003*
Female	5.24 ± 1.08		
QUALIFICATION			
Graduate	4.9 ± 1.39	Postgraduate vs. Graduate	0.363*
Postgraduate	5.04 ± 1.36		
DESIGNATION			
General practitioner (GP)	4.89 ± 1.43	GP vs. Specialist	0.377†
Specialist	5.11 ± 1.34	GP vs. Consultant	>0.999†
Consultant	5.23 ± 0.88	Consultant vs. Specialist	>0.999†
WORKPLACE			
Clinic	4.76 ± 1.45	Clinic vs. Both	0.003†
Hospital	5.31 ± 1.08	Clinic vs. Hospital	0.015†
Both	5.19 ± 1.33	Hospital vs. Both	>0.999†
EMPLOYMENT TYPE			
Private	4.71 ± 1.51	Private vs. Governmental	0.046†
Governmental	5.12 ± 1.09	Private vs. Both	0.015†
Both	5.2 ± 1.36	Governmental vs. Both	0.064†
Total	5.01 ± 1.37		

**Mann–Whitney test, †Kruskal–Wallis test.*

The mean awareness of respondents (section 3) was 12.65 ± 2.36 (**Table 4**). Age of the study participants have shown a statistically significant impact on respondents' awareness, whereas, this is not the case when male and female compared. Furthermore, qualification and designation (except for GP vs. Specialist) were found to have a statistically significant effect on respondents' awareness ($P < 0.05$, **Table 4**). Meanwhile, no statistically significant differences in respondents' awareness were identified according to workplace and employment type (**Table 4**).

Regarding the economic impact, no demographic variables emerged as having a statistically significant economic effect (**Table 5**). However, the mean economic effect was recorded as equal to 2.72 ± 0.71 out of 5 (**Table 5**), i.e., the economic losses incurred by the dental community amounted to more than 50%.

DISCUSSION

The present cross-sectional study reported a high level of anxiety among Iraqi dentists as a result of the COVID-19 outbreak and high awareness about preventing its transmission and avoiding infection; in addition, they and their practices have been economically affected due to this pandemic situation. These findings are understandable because dentists fall within the highest risk category, since their practice is associated with generation of droplets and aerosols which is considered as a main route of virus transmission (6). The high levels of anxiety recorded among these Iraqi dentists can be considered as natural human feelings during the pandemic situation, especially in light of the increasing infection and mortality rates. In Iraq the mortality rate is considered to be higher (about 3.9%) in comparison to other regional countries, such as the UAE with only a (0.5%) mortality rate (3). This could possibly be due to differences in available health resources between these two countries (21). The general weakness in the medical foundations and care system in Iraq after four decades of military conflicts (22), and the exaggerated pressure on the health care system due to the quick spread of the virus, general feelings of stress and fear among healthcare workers for their own safety and that of their families (23). Additionally, the nature of this disease, with its prolonged incubation period (as long as 14 days), its spectrum that ranged from asymptomatic to death, and the absence of a vaccine or treatment, are all factors potentially exacerbating stressful feelings among healthcare workers, especially dentists. This confirms findings from studies about COVID-19 (11), or previous outbreaks of similar infectious respiratory diseases such as SARS, which demonstrated severe and sustained psychological trauma, especially among the front line healthcare workers (24, 25).

Another interesting finding within the present study was that the recorded anxiety level was higher among younger than older dentists and females than males. This goes against the reports that among infected individuals there are higher risk groups, including older and male adults, who are more likely to develop severe respiratory symptoms and die than younger individuals and females (26). It may be that older dentists are more experienced than younger dentists in dealing with similar pandemic situations. This may make them more confident and less prone to anxiety. This was also reflected in the finding by this study of a statistically significant higher level of awareness about the virus and its mode of transmission among dentists aged above 35 years in comparison to those aged below 35 years. Moreover, since females, as mothers, tend to have closer contact with their

TABLE 4 | Respondents' awareness of COVID-19 infection-control measures.

Variables	Mean ± SD	Comparison	p-value
AGE			
≤35	11.14 ± 2.41	≤35 vs. >35	<0.001*
>35	12.99 ± 2.24		
GENDER			
Male	12.32 ± 2.58	Male vs. female	0.121*
Female	12.8 ± 2.09		
QUALIFICATION			
Graduate	11.98 ± 2.49	Postgraduate vs. Graduate	0.003*
Postgraduate	12.75 ± 2.28		
DESIGNATION			
General practitioner (GP)	12.48 ± 2.24	GP vs. Specialist	>0.999†
Specialist	12.53 ± 2.48	GP vs. Consultant	0.016†
Consultant	13.91 ± 1.92	Consultant vs. Specialist	0.027†
WORKPLACE			
Clinic	12.76 ± 2.07	Clinic vs. Both	0.569†
Hospital	12.44 ± 2.58	Clinic vs. Hospital	0.963†
Both	12.36 ± 2.58	Hospital vs. Both	>0.999†
EMPLOYMENT TYPE			
Private	12.82 ± 2.09	Private vs. Governmental	0.196†
Governmental	12.26 ± 2.38	Private vs. Both	>0.999†
Both	12.53 ± 2.52	Governmental vs. Both	0.674†
Total	12.65 ± 2.36		

Mann–Whitney test, †Kruskal–Wallis test.

TABLE 5 | Economic impact of the COVID-19 outbreak.

Variables	Mean ± SD	Comparison	*p*-value
AGE			
≤35	2.71 ± 0.69	≤ 35 vs. > 35	0.955*
>35	2.72 ± 0.72		
GENDER			
Male	2.67 ± 0.72	Male vs. female	0.109*
Female	2.77 ± 0.69		
QUALIFICATION			
Graduate	2.66 ± 0.8	Postgraduate vs. Graduate	0.468*
Postgraduate	2.73 ± 0.67		
DESIGNATION			
General practitioner (GP)	2.71 ± 0.73	GP vs. Specialist	0.463†
Specialist	2.74 ± 0.65	GP vs. Consultant	0.463†
Consultant	2.54 ± 0.94	Consultant vs. Specialist	0.353†
WORKPLACE			
Clinic	2.73 ± 0.73	Clinic vs. Both	>0.999†
Hospital	2.68 ± 0.67	Clinic vs. Hospital	>0.999†
Both	2.71 ± 0.69	Hospital vs. Both	>0.999†
EMPLOYMENT TYPE			
Private	2.63 ± 0.74	Private vs. Governmental	>0.999†
Governmental	2.69 ± 0.67	Private vs. Both	0.077†
Both	2.79 ± 0.69	Governmental vs. Both	0.877†
Total	2.72 ± 0.71		

Mann–Whitney test, †Kruskal–Wallis test.

children than other family members, the anxiety of transferring infection to family members, especially their children, could increase feelings of stress among female in comparison to male dentists. In the same way, dentists who were working in the public sector, in clinics or hospitals, reported higher anxiety levels than others. This could be attributed to the large number of dental patients visiting the public centers per day in comparison to private clinics (27). Consequently, this may increase dentists' concerns and anxiety of being infected compared to those working only in private clinics, who have more control over their appointments, case selection and cancellation of non-emergency cases. Finally, consultant dentists and those with postgraduate degree have higher levels awareness than their counterparts and this can be explained by the fact the majority of these dentists work in academic field, thus more update about the new developments in their field including the COVID-19 outbreak.

Almost all of the responding dentists were aware of the nature of the COVID-19 illness and its mode of transmission. This information is considered to be crucial in terms of applying infection control measures while carrying out dental treatment. In the same way, over 80% of the dentists responded that they were up to date about the current WHO guidelines for cross-infection control measures within dental practice (14). This was reflected through over 70% of the respondents asking their patients if they had been in contact with an infected COVID-19 individual, and above 60% recording patients' body temperature. Logically, this is basic information required during the routine examination to identify potentially infectious conditions among patients and the necessary precautionary management. Indeed, under such pandemic circumstances, the conventional precautions already recommended by WHO and any other infectious control authority worldwide should be rigorously applied to prevent cross-infection within dental practice. But unfortunately, more than 60% of the respondents were not using rubber dam for every patient as a cross-infection control. Rubber dam effectively limits the spread of aerosols during use of rotary instruments, decreases the hazard of fine instrument swallowing, gives excellent isolation of the working field and increases patients' acceptance of dental procedures (28). Therefore, training courses and workshops are suggested for Iraqi dentists, especially new graduates, to increase their awareness about the effectiveness of rubber dam in controlling the spread of infection. This could improve their hand skills and increase their willingness to consider rubber dam as part of their routine practice. The usage of high volume suction should also be considered as an essential method during routine dental practice to control aerosols and droplets evacuation (10).

The use of antimicrobial mouth washes before starting dental procedure is also recommended in the WHO guidelines for the current pandemic. Interestingly, over 40% of the respondents were complying with this recommendation. Mouthwashes such as chlorhexidine (29), 1% hydrogen peroxide (6), or povidone iodine (30) can be employed to decrease microbial loading inside the oral cavity. The latter has virucidal activity against SARS-CoV and MERS-CoV coronaviruses and is recommended to be used at 0.5% concentration as a mouthwash for patients before initiating a clinical procedure. Additionally, the operator is also advised to use povidone iodine as a nasal spray (0.4%) and mouthwash (0.5%) before and after suspected patient contact (31).

A positive finding by the current study was that the majority of Iraqi dentists were routinely focusing on hand hygiene before and after treating each patient, which is considered as an essential infection control measure for dental practitioners. Frequent hand washing with water and soap or using alcohol containing sanitizer is included in the WHO infection control guidelines for the current pandemic (14). The spread of respiratory viruses can be effectively avoided by proper hand washing and cleaning with alcohol-based sanitizers (8, 32). Furthermore, the majority of the study respondents agreed with the routine use of N-95 respirators rather than surgical masks in dental practice during the COVID-19 outbreak. The use of such personal protection equipment (PPE) is also recommended by the WHO and ADA guidelines when performing aerosols generating procedures (33).

Carefulness in selecting cases, controlling appointments, and receiving only emergency cases were also recommended by the ADA and WHO guidelines (13, 14). Almost all of the respondents in the current study stated that they had altered their appointment schedules to control the spread of the virus. This process could be started by initially calling patients or having video conferences to identify their need and decide if their condition requires clinical intervention (34). This could help in limiting face-to-face contact, making diagnoses through remote dental screening, deterring any COVID-19 susceptible patients, delaying nonemergency work, and planning effectively for the emergency cases (8, 34).

According to the findings of the present study, the economic losses caused by the COVID-19 outbreak to the dental community in Iraq amounted to about 50%. This is understandable during such a pandemic situation. The whole country has been affected by quarantines and lockdowns in an attempt to control the spread of the infection. The lockdowns consisted of intermittent periods of complete closure for all sectors followed by partial lockdown for specific sectors including schools, universities, tourism, and others. This has had severe economic impact on almost all activities, including dentistry (4). Additionally, the majority of respondents in the current study reported reduction of their working days, rescheduling of their appointments to see emergency cases only, absence of governmental support, and reduction in their total income. On the other hand, as some of the study participants received financial compensation, the degree of economic impact has shown to be varied from one to another dentist. However, none of demographical variables have shown an impact on income. This can be explained by the fact that during the national lockdown, working in private dental clinics was stopped by government and the only source of income were their monthly salary by the government. According to a recent investigation conducted in the U.S., this economic impact on dental services could be extended to 2022 because of financial hardship among dental patients (35). These financial impacts on dentistry as a profession may have serious implications for the future of this career.

The limitations of this study that should be considered is the rapid changes in respondents' psychology and practice in accordance with the progression of the current outbreak, the attitudes and awareness of dentists will certainly be altered by future alteration in the scientific knowledge about COVID-19. Additionally, although the distribution of the questionnaire for the present study was done through the IDA, fewer responses were obtained from consultants in comparison to the other designations. This possibly because of the general panic situation during the COVID-19 outbreak altered the priorities for potential respondents. Thus, the findings of the current study should be carefully interpreted to avoid generalization of the data.

CONCLUSIONS

The emergence of the novel coronavirus has increased concern among healthcare workers, especially dentists, regarding aerosols borne microbes rather than the conventional blood borne microbes. This has dramatically increased the anxiety among dentists about getting the infection and has altered their awareness toward a new era. Although, Iraqi dentists have gained a high level of knowledge and practice to address the COVID-19 outbreak, their anxiety was high. It is important in the current scenario to modify the conventional dental practice to deal with emergencies only or close down practices until the outbreak recedes. However, this situation may last for an indefinite period, which would have a dramatic impact not only on the economy which have shown to affect the majority of responders by reducing their income by 50% but also on the future of the dental profession such as increasing levels of anxiety amongst dentist and adapting to practice modification.

AUTHOR CONTRIBUTIONS

AM: study conception. AA and SG: study design. AM, AA, SG, and SQ: data collection. AA and SG: data analysis and manuscript drafting. AA and SG: data interpretation. SG and SQ: critical revision of the manuscript. All authors: approval of the final version. All authors contributed to the article and approved the submitted version.

ACKNOWLEDGMENTS

The authors would like to thank all the dentists who responded to this survey.

REFERENCES

1. Neher RA, Dyrdak R, Druelle V, Hodcroft EB, Albert J. Potential impact of seasonal forcing on a SARS-CoV-2 pandemic. *Swiss Med Wkly.* (2020) 150:w20224. doi: 10.4414/smw.2020.20224
2. Khurshid Z, Asiri FYI, Al Wadaani H. Human saliva: Non-invasive fluid for detecting novel coronavirus (2019-nCoV). *Int J Environ Res Public Health.* (2020) 17:2225. doi: 10.3390/ijerph17072225
3. WHO. *World Health Organization Coronavirus Disease (COVID-19) Dashboard.* (2020). Available online at: https://covid19.who.int/?gclid=

EAIaIQobChMItvnC1ej16gIVxYjVCh0YUwNkEAAYASAAEgJRDfD_BwE.
4. Nicola M, Alsafi Z, Sohrabi C, Kerwan A, Al-Jabir A, Iosifidis C, et al. The socio-economic implications of the coronavirus pandemic (COVID-19): areview. *Int J Surg.* (2020) 78:185–93. doi: 10.1016/j.ijsu.2020.04.018
5. Chen Y, Liu Q, Guo D. Emerging coronaviruses: genome structure, replication, and pathogenesis. *J Med Virol.* (2020) 92:418–23. doi: 10.1002/jmv.25681
6. Peng X, Xu X, Li Y, Cheng L, Zhou X, Ren B. Transmission routes of 2019-nCoV and controls in dental practice. *Int J Oral Sci.* (2020) 12:1–6. doi: 10.1038/s41368-020-0075-9
7. Administration OSaH. *COVID-19 Control and Prevention/ Dentisrty Worker and Employers.* United States Deparment of Labor (2020).
8. Ather A, Patel B, Ruparel NB, Diogenes A, Hargreaves KM. Coronavirus disease 19 (COVID-19): implications for clinical dental care. *J Endod.* (2020) 46:584–95. doi: 10.1016/j.joen.2020.08.005
9. Meng L, Hua F, Bian Z. Coronavirus disease 2019 (COVID-19): emerging and future challenges for dental and oral medicine. *J Dent Res.* (2020) 99:481–7. doi: 10.1177/0022034520914246
10. Ge Z-y, Yang L-m, Xia J-j, Fu X-h, Zhang Y-z. Possible aerosol transmission of COVID-19 and special precautions in dentistry. *J Zhejiang Univ Sci B.* (2020) 21:361–8. doi: 10.1631/jzus.B2010010
11. Ahmed MA, Jouhar R, Ahmed N, Adnan S, Aftab M, Zafar MS, et al. Fear and practice modifications among dentists to combat Novel Coronavirus Disease (COVID-19) outbreak. *Int J Environ Res Public Health.* (2020) 17:2821. doi: 10.3390/ijerph17082821
12. Ng K, Poon BH, Kiat Puar TH, Shan Quah JL, Loh WJ, Wong YJ, et al. COVID-19 and the risk to health care workers: a case report. *Ann Intern Med.* (2020) 172:766–7. doi: 10.7326/L20-0175
13. ADA. *Summary of ADA Guidance During the COVID-19 Crisis.* American Dental Association (2020). Available online at: https://www.ada.org/en/press-room/news-releases/2020-archives/april/summary-of-ada-guidance-during-the-covid-19-crisis (cited September 16, 2020).
14. WHO. *Considerations for the Provision of Essential Oral Health Services in the Context of COVID-19.* Interim Guidance: World Health Organization (2020). Available online at: https://apps.who.int/iris/bitstream/handle/10665/333625/WHO-2019-nCoV-Oral_health-2020.1-eng.pdf (cited September 16, 2020).
15. CDC. *Interim Infection Prevention and Control Recommendations for Healthcare Personnel During the Coronavirus Disease 2019 (COVID-19) Pandemic.* Centers for Disease Control and Prevention (2020). Available online at: https://www.cdc.gov/coronavirus/2019-ncov/hcp/infection-control-recommendations.html?CDC_AA_refVal=https%3A%2F%2Fcdc.gov%2Fcoronavirus%2F2019-ncov%2Finfection-control%2Fcontrol-recommendations.html (cited September 16, 2020).
16. Chipchase SY, Chapman HR, Bretherton R. A study to explore if dentists' anxiety affects their clinical decision-making. *Br Dent J.* (2017) 222:277–90. doi: 10.1038/sj.bdj.2017.173
17. Taherdoost H. Determining sample size; how to calculate survey sample size. *Int J Econ Manag.* (2017) 2:237–9. Avialable online at: https://papers.ssrn.com/sol3/papers.cfm?abstract_id=3224205
18. Charan J, Biswas T. How to calculate sample size for different study designs in medical research? *Indian J Psychol Med.* (2013) 35:121–6. doi: 10.4103/0253-7176.116232
19. Tysiac-Miśta M, Dziedzic A. The attitudes and professional approaches of dental practitioners during the COVID-19 outbreak in Poland: a cross-sectional survey. *Int J Environ Res Public Health.* (2020) 17:4703. doi: 10.3390/ijerph17134703
20. Kamate SK, Sharma S, Thakar S, Srivastava D, Sengupta K, Hadi AJ, et al. Assessing Knowledge, Attitudes and Practices of dental practitioners regarding the COVID-19 pandemic: a multinational study. *Dent Med Probl.* (2020) 57:11–7. doi: 10.17219/dmp/119743
21. Ji Y, Ma Z, Peppelenbosch MP, Pan Q. Potential association between COVID-19 mortality and health-care resource availability. *Lancet Glob Health.* (2020) 8:e480. doi: 10.1016/S2214-109X(20)30068-1
22. Al Hilfi TK, Lafta R, Burnham G. Health services in Iraq. *Lancet.* (2013) 381:939–48. doi: 10.1016/S0140-6736(13)60320-7
23. Xie J, Tong Z, Guan X, Du B, Qiu H, Slutsky AS. Critical care crisis and some recommendations during the COVID-19 epidemic in China. *Intens Care Med.* (2020) 46:837–40. doi: 10.1007/s00134-020-05979-7
24. Tam CW, Pang EP, Lam LC, Chiu HF. Severe acute respiratory syndrome (SARS) in Hong Kong in 2003: stress and psychological impact among frontline healthcare workers. *Psychol Med.* (2004) 34:1197. doi: 10.1017/S0033291704002247
25. McAlonan GM, Lee AM, Cheung V, Cheung C, Tsang KW, Sham PC, et al. Immediate and sustained psychological impact of an emerging infectious disease outbreak on health care workers. *Can J Psychiatry.* (2007) 52:241–7. doi: 10.1177/070674370705200406
26. Jordan RE, Adab P, Cheng K. Covid-19: risk factors for severe disease and death. *BMJ.* (2020) 368:m1198. doi: 10.1136/bmj.m1198
27. Fernández-Feijoo J, Garea-Gorís R, Fernández-Varela M, Tomás-Carmona I, Diniz-Freitas M, Limeres-Posse J. Prevalence of systemic diseases among patients requesting dental consultation in the public and private systems. *Med Oral Patol Oral Cir Bucal.* (2012) 17:e89. doi: 10.4317/medoral.17313
28. Madarati A, Abid S, Tamimi F, Ezzi A, Sammani A, Shaar MBAA, et al. Dental-dam for infection control and patient safety during clinical endodontic treatment: preferences of dental patients. *Int J Environ Res Public Health.* (2018) 15:2012. doi: 10.3390/ijerph15092012
29. Nayak SU, Kumari A, Rajendran V, Singh VP, Hegde A, Pai KK. Comparative evaluation of efficacy of chlorhexidine and herbal mouthwash as a preprocedural rinse in reducing dental aerosols: a microbiological study. *Int J Dent.* (2020) 2020:2021082. doi: 10.1155/2020/2021082
30. Eggers M, Koburger-Janssen T, Eickmann M, Zorn J. *In vitro* bactericidal and virucidal efficacy of povidone-iodine gargle/mouthwash against respiratory and oral tract pathogens. *Infect Dis Ther.* (2018) 7:249–59. doi: 10.1007/s40121-018-0200-7
31. Mady LJ, Kubik MW, Baddour K, Snyderman CH, Rowan NR. Consideration of povidone-iodine as a public health intervention for COVID-19: Utilization as "Personal Protective Equipment" for frontline providers exposed in high-risk head and neck and skull base oncology care. *Oral Oncol.* (2020) 105:104724. doi: 10.1016/j.oraloncology.2020.104724
32. Fung ICH, Cairncross S. Effectiveness of handwashing in preventing SARS: a review. *Trop Med Int Health.* (2006) 11:1749–58. doi: 10.1111/j.1365-3156.2006.01734.x
33. Coulthard P. Dentistry and coronavirus (COVID-19)-moral decision-making. *Br Dent J.* (2020) 228:503–5. doi: 10.1038/s41415-020-1482-1
34. Ghai S. Teledentistry during COVID-19 pandemic. *Diabetes Metab Syndr.* (2020) 14:933–5. doi: 10.1016/j.dsx.2020.06.029
35. Nasseh K, Vujicic M. *Modeling the Impact of COVID-19 on U.S. Dental Spending: Health Policy Institute Research Brief.* American Dental Association (2020). Available online at: https://www.ada.org/$\sim$/media/ADA/Science%20and%20Research/HPI/Files/HPIBrief_0420_1.pdf?la=en.~

22

COVID-19 Awareness Among Dental Professionals in Indonesia

Armelia Sari Widyarman [1], Endang W. Bachtiar [2], Citra Fragrantia Theodorea [2], M. Ihsan Rizal [3], M. Orliando Roeslan [3], Melanie S. Djamil [3], Didi N. Santosa [3] and Boy M. Bachtiar [2]*

[1] Department of Microbiology, Faculty of Dentistry, Trisakti University, Jakarta, Indonesia, [2] Department of Oral Biology, Faculty of Dentistry, Universitas Indonesia, Depok, Indonesia, [3] Department of Oral Biology, Faculty of Dentistry, Trisakti University, Jakarta, Indonesia

***Correspondence:**
Armelia Sari Widyarman
armeliasari@trisakti.ac.id

Background: The COVID-19 pandemic caused by SARS-CoV-2 has claimed thousands of lives worldwide. To enhance knowledge and awareness of COVID-19, considerable online resources have been made available, including aspects related to the dental profession. The study aim was to examine the knowledge, perception, and attitude of dental professionals in Indonesia toward COVID-19. We conducted a survey via a questionnaire created using Google docs and distributed to 632 members of the Indonesian Dental Association in the context of a webinar hosted by the Indonesian Oral Biology Association on first June, 2020.

Materials and Methods: The questionnaire consisted of 17 items pertaining to demographic data, knowledge and virus identification, awareness regarding drugs commonly used in dentistry during pandemic and research opportunities. Participants were asked to complete the questionnaire after the webinar by choosing one answer to each question. For the analysis, participants were divided into three groups according to their professional background i.e., employment at national hospital, private hospital, or academic faculty. Data were analyzed using descriptive statistics and expressed as frequencies and percentages. The chi-square test was used to investigate the association between professional activity and the level of knowledge, perceptions, and attitudes about COVID-19.

Results: Sixty percent of the participants correctly identified the pathogenesis of the disease. This knowledge was not associated with their professional affiliation ($p = 0.95$). Sixty-seven percentage had comprehensive knowledge about virus detection methods. This knowledge was not associated with their affiliation either ($p = 0.54$). Questions regarding drugs of choice, prevention, and the spread of COVID-19 were correctly answered by 89, 96, and 82% of the participants, respectively. Knowledge of these aspects were significantly associated with the professional affiliation ($p < 0.05$). All respondents were optimistic regarding research opportunities ($p < 0.01$). Respondents from academics were more interested in joining COVID-19-related research projects with governmental institutions ($p < 0.01$).

Conclusion: Knowledge and awareness of COVID-19 among Indonesian dentists are reasonably good. However, further improvement would be beneficial to manage patients during this pandemic. As the number of COVID-19 cases continue to rise in Indonesia, it is important that dentists keep abreast of the updated knowledge on this moving field. Dentist knowledge on infection control should be strengthened through continuous educational programs.

Keywords: SARS-COV-2, knowledge, dentist, COVID-19, awareness

INTRODUCTION

Since it was first reported in Wuhan City, Hubei Province, Central China in December 2019, coronavirus disease 2019 (COVID-19) has become a major health concern worldwide (1). COVID-19 is caused by a novel coronavirus called severe acute respiratory syndrome coronavirus 2 (SARS-CoV-2) which causes pneumonia, with symptoms ranging from mild to deadly. SARS-CoV-2 infection can cause an acute inflammatory response (cytokine storm) and respiratory failure (2, 3). The World Health Organization (WHO) declared COVID-19 a pandemic on March 11, 2020 (4). As of July 6, 2020, COVID-19 had spread to 216 countries, causing 11,496,926 confirmed cases and over 535,390 deaths (5). Indonesia reported its first two cases on March 2, 2020. By July 6, it had reported 63,749 cases and 3,171 deaths (6). Indonesia currently has the highest COVID-19-related mortality rate in Southeast Asia.

Dental schools and their affiliated hospitals, as well as research laboratories have also been significantly affected by the pandemic. As a consequence, most research work has been stopped or undergone radical changes with severe limitations. These difficulties have been compounded by the absence of technical support as some experienced laboratory personnel belong to high-risk groups. However, this challenging situation has offered an opportunity to re-evaluate the our knowledge and understanding of the infection control measures related to dentistry and formulate new strategies in the post-COVID era (7).

The risk of viral transmission is higher for those who are close to or work near patients, such as relatives and health workers. To evaluate the preparedness of dentists to cope with the pandemic, many researchers around the globe are trying to assess their knowledge of COVID-19. In this study, we included the knowledge of characterization and method identification of SARS-CoV-2.

Due to the involvement of aerosol generating procedures, the dental profession is regarded as one of the occupations at the highest risk of SARS-CoV-2 infection. Therefore, it is critical that the risk of transmission through dental procedures is minimized through proper understanding and actions. Dentists should be well-aware of the characteristics of SARS-CoV-2 and new infection control standards. In the Indonesian context, many dentists, particularly in the private practice has opted to perform only emergency procedures during the pandemic. Hence, dental pain of the patients has been commonly managed with prescription of analgesics. In order to enhance knowledge on COVID-19 and the management of dental patients during the pandemic, Indonesian Oral Biology Association organized a series of webinars through Zoom platform. However, there

TABLE 1 | Demographic characterisatic of participants.

Characteristic		*n*	%
Sex	Woman	524	82.9
	Man	108	17.1
Age	20–30 years	139	22.0
	31–40 years	188	29.7
	41–50 years	146	23.1
	51–65 years	159	25.2
Occupation	Academic	175	27.7
	Government hospital	158	25
	Private hospital/private practice	299	47.3
Province	Riau	10	1.6
	Riau Islands	7	1.1
	Bangka-Belitung Islands	5	0.8
	Aceh	6	1.0
	North Sumatra	10	1.6
	West Sumatra	12	1.9
	South Sumatera	14	2.2
	Bengkulu	3	0.5
	Jambi	2	0.3
	Lampung	3	0.5
	Banten	42	6.7
	Jakarta	155	24.6
	West Java	109	17.3
	Central Java	54	8.6
	Yogyakarta	25	4.0
	East Java	88	13.9
	Bali	18	2.9
	East Nusa Tenggara	2	0.3
	West Nusa Tenggara	4	0.6
	Central Kalimantan	4	0.6
	North Kalimantan	4	0.6
	South Kalimantan	1	0.2
	West Kalimantan	3	0.5
	East Kalimantan	10	1.6
	South Sulawesi	29	4.6
	North Sulawesi	3	0.5
	North Maluku	1	0.2
	Papua	7	1.1

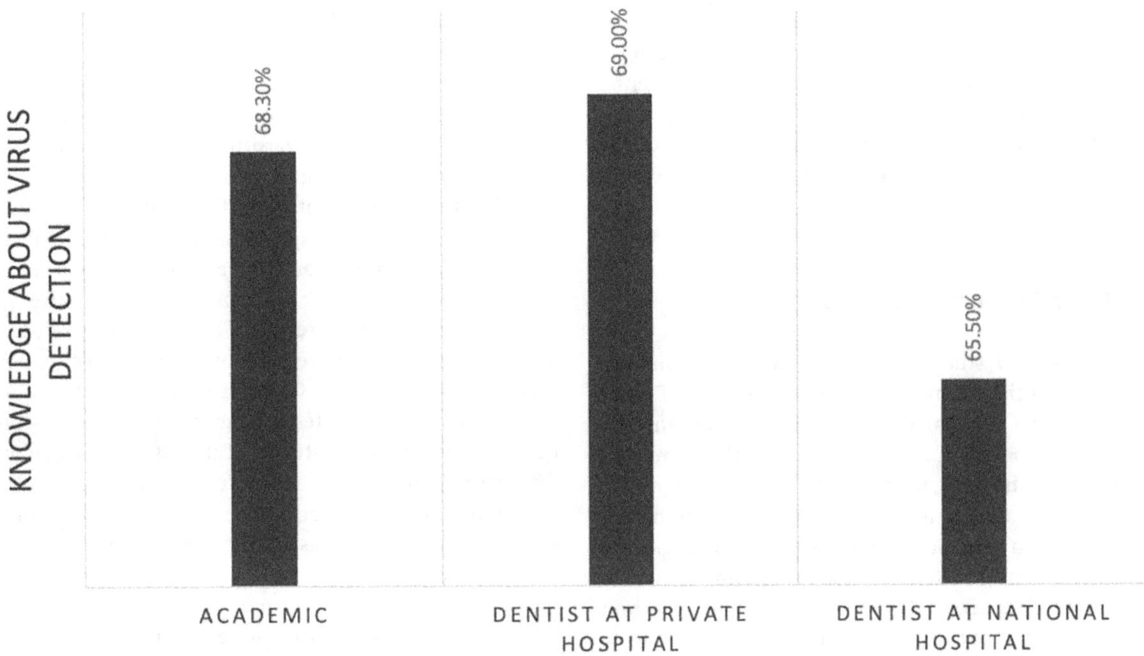

FIGURE 1 | Sixty percent of the participants correctly identified the pathogenesis of COVID-19. This knowledge was not associated with the professional affiliation ($p = 0.95$).

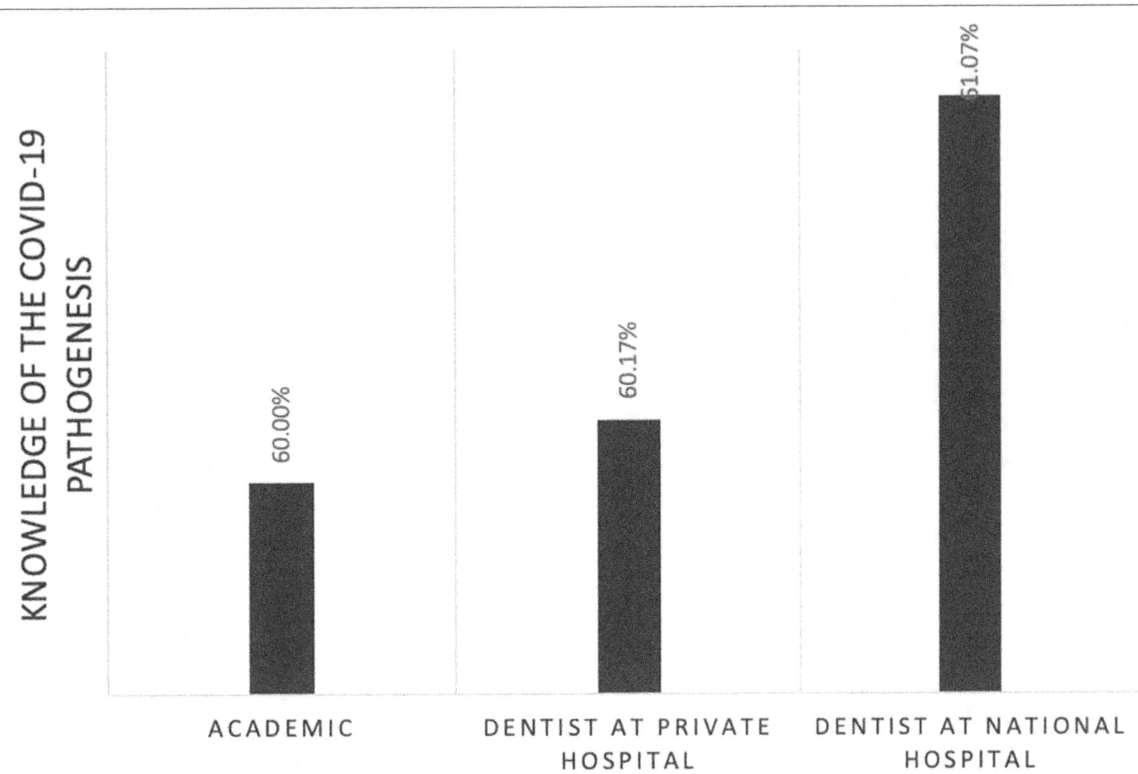

FIGURE 2 | Sixty-seven percent of the participants had comprehensive knowledge about virus detection. This knowledge was not associated with the professional affiliation ($p = 0.54$).

are no studies which has assessed the knowledge, perception, and attitude of Indonesian dentists on COVID-19. Considering this research gap, in the present study we evaluated the level of knowledge on SARS-CoV-2 and COVID-19 among dental professionals in Indonesia. In this study, we highlighted the most important research questions concerning the knowledge of the virus, the pathogenesis as well as the virus detection and infection prevention of COVID-19.

MATERIALS AND METHODS

This was a survey-based study conducted via a questionnaire distributed to all dentist members of the Indonesian Dental Association attending a webinar hosted by the Indonesian Oral Biology Association on first June, 2020 on COVID-19 related topic. The questionnaire was prepared in Indonesian native language. The original and translated version the questionnaire to English is given in the **Supplementary Material**. Google docs were used as a platform to create the questionnaire, which was then distributed online. Participants from any region of Indonesia were granted password-protected access to a URL hosting the questionnaire. A unique study ID ensured confidentiality of all self-reported data. The participants' responses were stored in a cloud database, where the data were automatically sorted, scaled, and scored using custom Microsoft Office Excel formulas. This study was approved by the Institutional Review Board of Faculty of Dentistry, Trisakti University (Jakarta, Indonesia) with approval number: 360/s3/KEPK/FKG/2020.

The questionnaire consisted of 17 items, including four pertaining to demographic information (age, gender, and residence and work locations), three regarding knowledge about the virus, two regarding the method identification of COVID-19, two regarding knowledge about its pathogenesis, two about infection control and precautions, two pertaining to awareness regarding drugs commonly used in dentistry during the pandemic, one regarding research opportunities, and one regarding research collaborations (Questionnaire is given in the **Supplementary Material**). The questionnaire was developed and confirmed after review by a panel of experts (EWB, BMB, MSD, and DNS). Construct validity of this questionnaire was done through intense discussion. The reliability of the questionnaire was statistically scaled as alpha Cronbach = 0.66. The participants were asked to choose one answer to each question. The level of optimism regarding research opportunities during the pandemic was assessed with a question that had three possible answers: "optimistic," "doubtful," and "pessimistic." Participants' willingness to cooperate with the government in COVID-19-related research projects was assessed with a question that had three possible answers: "yes," "maybe," and "no."

For the statistical analysis, the participants were divided into three groups according to their professional affiliation i.e., dentists employed at national hospital consist of dentist who work in the health center and government hospital. Dentists employed at private hospital consist of dentist who

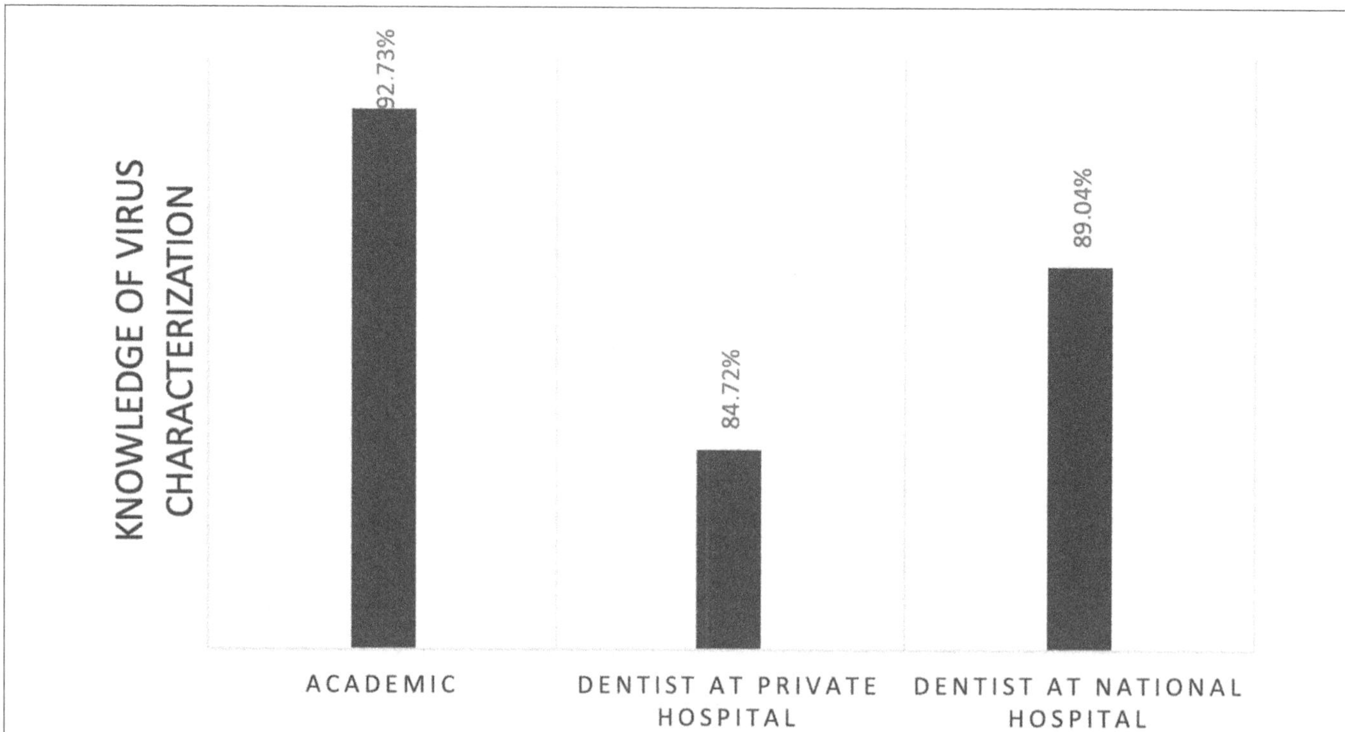

FIGURE 3 | Eighty-nine percent of the participants correctly identified the characterization of the virus. This knowledge was associated with the professional affiliation ($p < 0.05$).

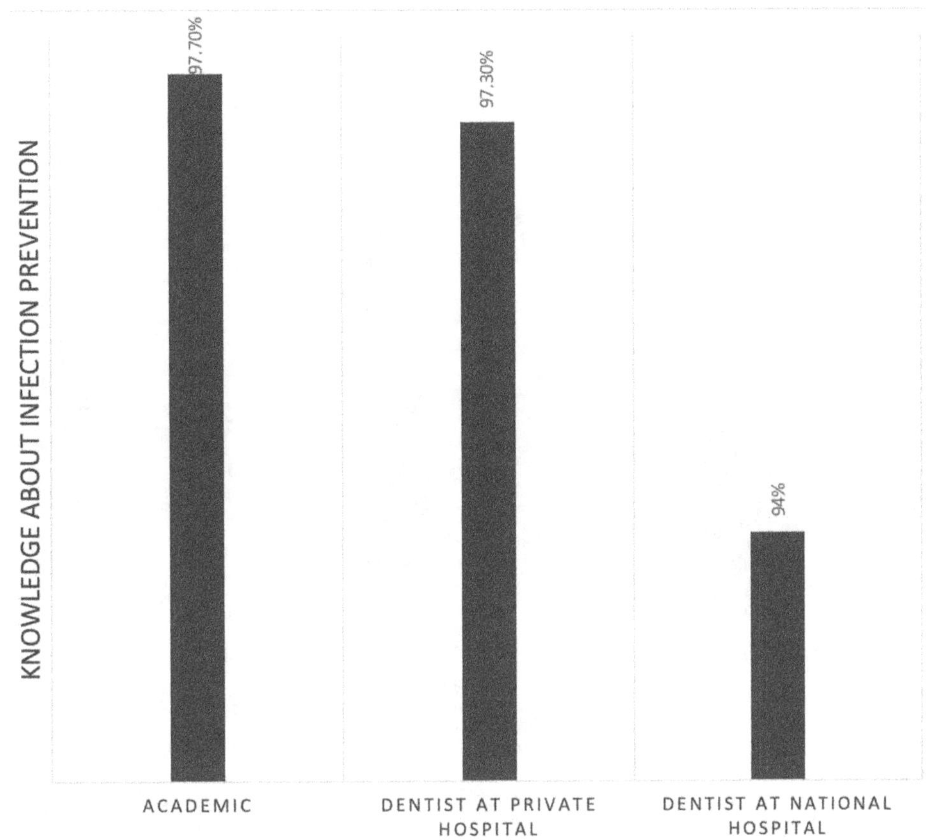

FIGURE 4 | Ninety-six percent of the participants were knowledgeable about infection prevention methods. The distribution showed a significant association between professional affiliation and knowledge ($p < 0.05$).

work in private hospital, private dental practice or dental clinic and employment as an academic in a dental school. Researchers downloaded questionnaire responses in multiple formats (Microsoft Office Excel), which were then analyzed using descriptive statistics and expressed as frequencies and percentages. The response rate to the study was 100%. We exclude participants who did not answer all the questions. We analyzed the correctness rate by calculating the average percentage of correct answer for all related questions in each topic. The chi-square test was used to investigate associations between professional background and knowledge, perceptions, attitudes about COVID-19 and to compare the levels of optimism regarding research opportunities and willingness to collaborate with the government between the three groups. IBM SPSS Statistics version 25 (IBM, Armonk, NY, USA) was used for the statistical analyses. The $p < 0.05$ was considered statistically significant.

RESULTS

The study cohort consisted of a total of 632 dentists who participated in the survey. Demographic features include 524 (82.9%) female and 108 (17.1%) male, age range from 20 to 65 years old, and from 28 provinces in Indonesia. The distribution of the professional affiliation includes 175 (27.7%) academics, 158 (25%) national hospital practitioners, and 299 (47.3%) private hospital/private practice practitioners as shown in **Table 1**.

Of those, 60% correctly identified the pathogenesis of COVID-19 (**Figure 1**). However, this knowledge was not significantly associated with their professional affiliation ($p = 0.95$). Sixty-seven percent had comprehensive knowledge about virus detection methods (**Figure 2**). This knowledge was not associated with their professional affiliation either ($p = 0.54$). Questions regarding virus characterization, prevention and drugs of choice for the dental treatment during COVID-19 pandemic were correctly answered by 89, 96, and 82% of the participants, respectively (**Figures 3–5**). Knowledge related to these aspects was significantly associated with the professional affiliation ($p < 0.05$). All respondents were optimistic regarding research opportunities ($p < 0.01$) (**Figure 6**). Respondents with an academic background from the dental schools were more interested in participating in collaborative research with governmental institutions ($p < 0.01$) (**Figure 7**).

DISCUSSION

This is the first study to assess the knowledge of COVID-19 among the dental professional in Indonesia. The most of

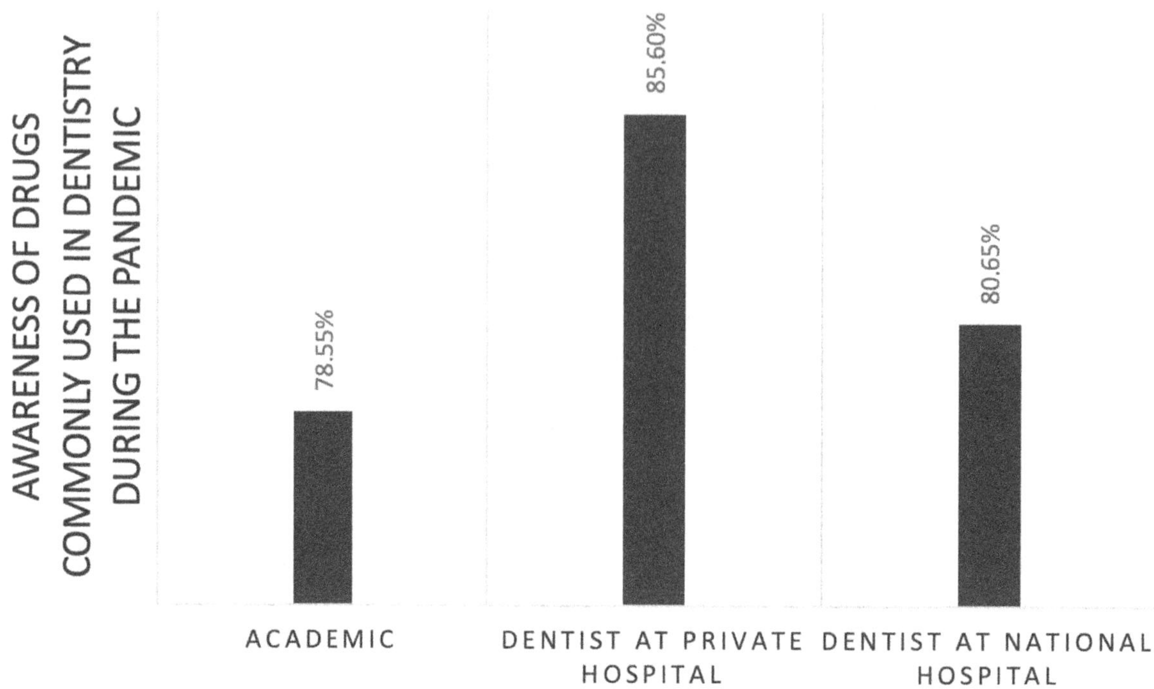

FIGURE 5 | Eighty-two percent of the participants correctly identified the drugs of choice. The distribution showed a significant association between professional affiliation and knowledge ($p < 0.05$).

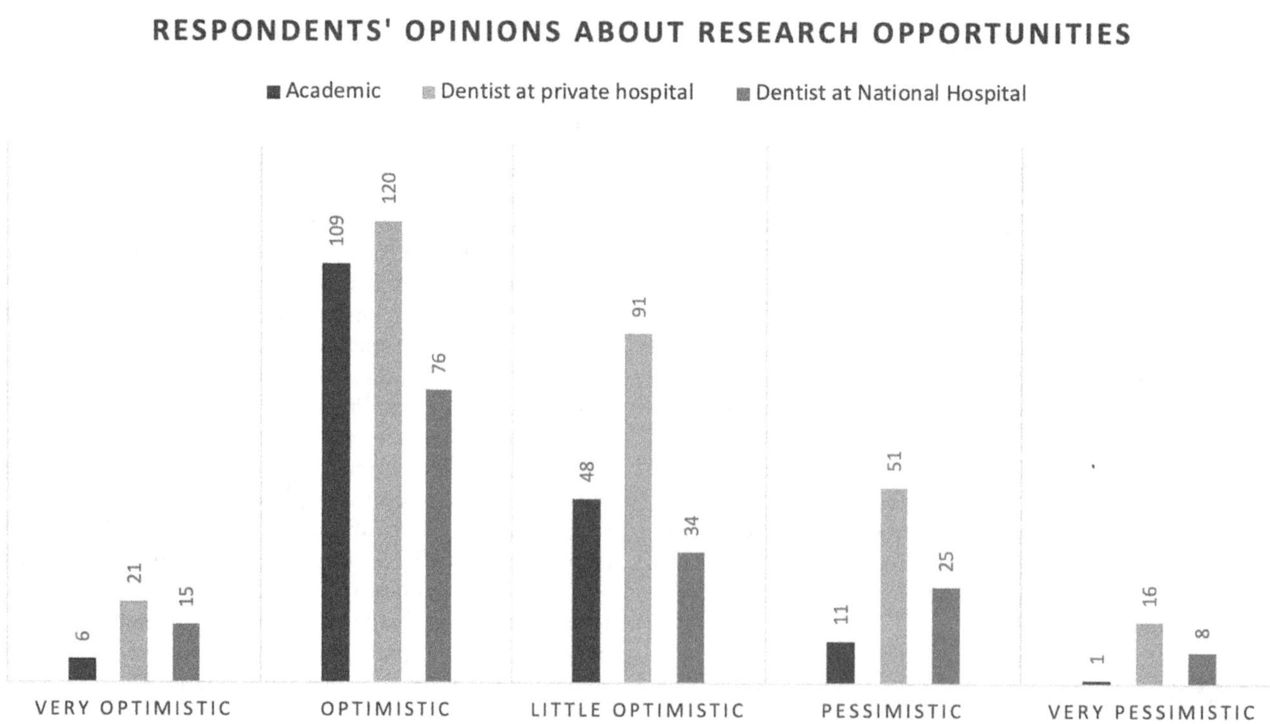

FIGURE 6 | All respondents were optimistic regarding research opportunities ($p < 0.01$).

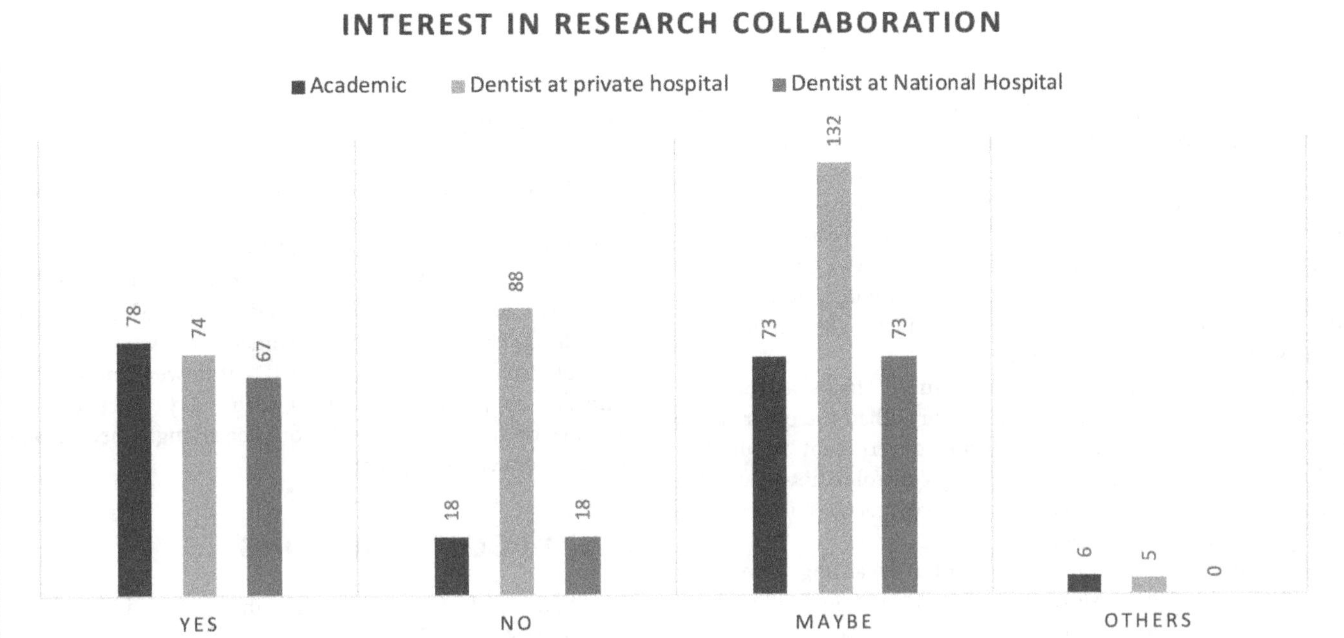

FIGURE 7 | Respondents from dental faculties were more interested in research collaboration with governmental institutions ($p < 0.01$).

the participants (47.3%) were dentists practicing in private hospitals or private practitioners. This result may be attributed to the fact that the recent increase of number of private dental hospitals in Indonesia. Although the government has launched an infrastructure development strategy in the recent years, with a target of 54 government dental hospitals in 2018 and 64 hospitals in 2019, much of this growth were seen in the private healthcare sector (8). Hence, it is important to educate the private dental practitioners in Indonesia on the post-COVID infection control measures.

The role of dental professionals in preventing the transmission of COVID-19 is critically important. In this study, 96% of the participants were knowledgeable about infection prevention methods. The distribution showed a significant association between professional affiliation and knowledge. In a similar study in Jordan which conducted among practicing dentists, it was found that 71.7% were aware of mode of transmission of COVID-19, and infection controls measures in dental clinics, and has the perspective that COVID-19 is a dangerous disease (9).

Our results showed that the knowledge regarding the general information and transmission, of COVID-19 among the dentist in Indonesia is sufficient, since most of dentists answer the survey questions correctly. Not only that, they also acknowledge their profession as a high-risk zone for virus transmission. This knowledge was associated with the professional affiliation, as dentists affiliated in private hospital and academics had a better knowledge compared to dentists in national hospital ($p < 0.05$). However, the majority of dentist who participated in this study was not able to differentiate the clinical symptom between common cold and COVID-19, as both of them share the same symptoms, such as fever, cough, sore throat, headache, and fatigue. Moreover, COVID-19 patients could be asymptomatic or even without fever. Therefore, suspected cases should be tested positive with specific molecular tests to confirm (10). Similar observations have been reported by researchers in United Arab Emirates, Iran and India in a study led by Bhagavathula et al. involving health care workers globally showed that factors such as age and profession were associated with inadequate knowledge and a poor perception of COVID-19 (11). Another study conducted in Saudi Arabia showed that the basic knowledge on COVID-19 among the dental health care workers in Saudi Arabia is acceptable (12).

Herein we also assessed how professional background and affiliation affect the knowledge of COVID-19 among Indonesian dentists. In general, dentists irrespective of their professional background i.e., in private practice or academics in dental school had a good understanding regarding SARS CoV-2, COVID-19 and its relationship with their professional affiliation, and the differences between the virus and the disease. However, our data showed that academics were more knowledgeable about the characterization of SARS-CoV-2, whereas private hospital dentists tended to know more about the identification method of SARS-CoV-2. This may be due to specific professional interests. Dentists in an academic background especially affiliated to basic sciences are likely to be more interested in biomolecular and technological approaches, while practicing dentists are more interested in applied sciences (13).

Private hospital dentists showed a better understanding of medicines used in dentistry than the other two groups. Academics exhibited the lowest level of understanding. The academics teaching basic science subjects in the dental schools may not engage in clinical practice which may have contributed to their relatively lower understanding of the medicine. On the contrary, private hospital dentists who engage in patient care on daily basis continuously learn about developments in medicines to uphold their professional care (14).

At the beginning of the COVID-19 pandemic, a study claimed that taking ibuprofen could increase the risk factor of severe with SARS-CoV-2 because it could increase the levels of angiotensin-converting enzyme 2, to which the virus binds to infect the host (15). Subsequently, studies reported that ibuprofen was not found to increase risk of severe consequences from SARS CoV-2 (16–18). This is an example of why practicing dentists follow the latest developments about safe analgesics during the pandemic, as shown by the results of this study.

Dentists with academic background had a better understanding of infection control measures than the other two groups. Comparatively dentists serving government hospitals had a lowest understanding of infection control. Knowledge of infection prevention and daily preventive practices is critical during the COVID-19 pandemic.

Academics were the most optimistic regarding research opportunities (65.7%). Moreover, they were more willing to collaborate with governmental institutions (41.1%) in COVID-19 research. This is in line with the increasing number of studies on COVID-19. As of the time of writing this manuscript, according to the WHO, 39,608 COVID-19-related studies were published globally (19). Despite this exponential growth of research on COVID-19, further studies are needed to address many remaining research questions.

CONCLUSION

Although knowledge and awareness of COVID-19 among Indonesian dentists are reasonably good, further improvement would be beneficial to manage patients during this pandemic. As the number of COVID-19 cases continue to rise, it is important that dentists keep abreast of the updated knowledge on this moving field. The Indonesian government has assumed a major role in containing the spread of COVID-19, however more efforts are needed to protect dentists in their daily practice. Their knowledge on infection control should be strengthened through continuous educational programs.

AUTHOR CONTRIBUTIONS

ASW, EWB, and BMB contributed to the concept and design of the study. ASW and CFT collected and analyzed the data. ASW, MSD, and DNS interpreted the results. CFT, MIR, ASW, and MOR wrote sections of the manuscript. All authors contributed to the article and approved the submitted version.

REFERENCES

1. Huang C, Wang Y, Li X, Ren L, Zhao J, Hu Y, et al. Clinical features of patients infected with 2019 novel coronavirus in Wuhan, China. *Lancet.* (2020) 395:497–506. doi: 10.1016/S0140-6736(20)30183-5
2. Giovanetti M, Benvenuto D, Angeletti S, Ciccozzi M. The first two cases of 2019-nCoV in Italy: where they come from? *J Med Virol.* (2020) 92:518–21. doi: 10.1002/jmv.25699
3. Chen Y, Liu Q, Guo D. Emerging coronaviruses: genome structure, replication, and pathogenesis. *J Med Virol.* (2020) 92:418–23. doi: 10.1002/jmv.25681
4. *Naming the Coronavirus Disease (COVID-19) and the Virus That Causes It.* Available online at: https://www.who.int/emergencies/diseases/novel-coronavirus-2019/technical-guidance/naming-the-coronavirus-disease-(covid-2019)-and-the-virus-that-causes-it (accessed July 10, 2020).
5. *Coronavirus Update (Live): 11,496,926 Cases and 535,390 Deaths From COVID-19 Virus Pandemic - Worldometer.* Available online at: https://www.worldometers.info/coronavirus/?utm_campaign=homeAdvegas1? (accessed July 6, 2020).
6. COVID-19 GTPP. *Gugus Tugas Percepatan Penanganan COVID-19.* Available online at: https://covid19.go.id/ (accessed July 6, 2020).
7. Rosales-Mendoza S, Comas-García M, Korban SS. Challenges and opportunities for the biotechnology research community during the coronavirus pandemic. *Trends Biotechnol.* (2020) 38:823–4. doi: 10.1016/j.tibtech.2020.04.016
8. Hp+ P. *Expanding Markets While Improving Health in Indonesia: The Private Health Sector Market in the JKN Era.69.* Washington, DC: Health Policy Plus (2018).
9. Khader Y, Al Nsour M, Al-Batayneh OB, Saadeh R, Bashier H, Alfaqih M, et al. Dentists' awareness, perception, and attitude regarding COVID-19 and infection control: cross-sectional study among Jordanian dentists. *JMIR Public Health Surveill.* (2020) 6:e18798. doi: 10.2196/preprints.18798
10. Singhal T. A review of coronavirus disease-2019 (COVID-19). *Indian J Pediatr.* (2020) 87:281–6. doi: 10.1007/s12098-020-03263-6
11. Bhagavathula AS, Aldhaleei WA, Rahmani J, Mahabadi MA, Bandari DK. Knowledge and perceptions of COVID-19 among health care workers: cross-sectional study. *JMIR Public Health Surveill.* (2020) 6:e19160. doi: 10.2196/19160
12. Quadri MFA, Jafer MA, Alqahtani AS, Al mutahar SAB, Odabi NI, Daghriri AA, et al. Novel corona virus disease (COVID-19) awareness among the dental interns, dental auxiliaries and dental specialists in Saudi Arabia: a nationwide study. *J Infect Public Health.* (2020) 13:856–64. doi: 10.1016/j.jiph.2020.05.010
13. Guven Y. Scientific basis of dentistry. *J Istanb Univ Fac Dent.* (2017) 51:64–71. doi: 10.17096/jiufd.04646
14. Mosadeghrad AM. Factors affecting medical service quality. *Iran J Public Health.* (2014) 43:210–20. doi: 10.15171/ijhpm.2014.65
15. Fang L, Karakiulakis G, Roth M. Are patients with hypertension and diabetes mellitus at increased risk for COVID-19 infection? *Lancet Respir Med.* (2020) 8:e21. doi: 10.1016/S2213-2600(20)30116-8
16. Mancia G, Rea F, Ludergnani M, Apolone G, Corrao G. Renin–angiotensin–aldosterone system blockers and the risk of Covid-19. *N Engl J Med.* (2020) 382:2431–40. doi: 10.1056/NEJMoa2006923
17. Reynolds HR, Adhikari S, Pulgarin C, Troxel AB, Iturrate E, Johnson SB, et al. Renin–angiotensin–aldosterone system inhibitors and risk of Covid-19. *N Engl J Med.* (2020) 382:2441–8. doi: 10.1056/NEJMoa2008975
18. Vaduganathan M, Vardeny O, Michel T, McMurray JJV, Pfeffer MA, Solomon SD. Renin–angiotensin–aldosterone system inhibitors in patients with Covid-19. *N Engl J Med.* (2020) 382:1653–9. doi: 10.1056/NEJMsr2005760
19. *Global Research on Coronavirus Disease (COVID-19).* Available online at: https://www.who.int/emergencies/diseases/novel-coronavirus-2019/global-research-on-novel-coronavirus-2019-ncov (accessed July 10, 2020).

Dental Education in the Time of COVID-19 Pandemic: Challenges and Recommendations

Mohamed G. Hassan [1,2]* *and Hala Amer* [3]

[1] Department of Orthodontics, Faculty of Oral and Dental Medicine, South Valley University, Qena, Egypt, [2] Department of Orthodontics, Faculty of Dentistry, October 6 University, Giza, Egypt, [3] Department of Pediatric Dentistry and Dental Public Health, Faculty of Dentistry, Alexandria University, Alexandria, Egypt

***Correspondence:**
Mohamed G. Hassan
mgamal@dent.svu.edu.eg

Moving within the second wave of the coronavirus (COVID-19) pandemic, dental education delivery has been profoundly affected by this crisis, so has the structure, evaluation, and future of dental education. Both pre-clinical and clinical dental education have experienced challenges ranging from fully online educational content to limited dental training for senior dental students. This crisis appears to be a tipping point that produced confusion in dental teaching especially clinical sciences. Although medical institutions immediately started to adapt to the unexpected COVID-19 crisis, dental and oral health educational services are profoundly impaired due to the dental team's propinquity to the patient and the aerosols generated during routine dental therapeutic procedures. Dental students unlike other medical students are considered to be at the highest risk due to the nature of their clinical training that includes working in the oral cavity of patients using aerosol-generating equipment. Some dental schools have taken the leadership and documented their modifications during this pandemic; however, there is a serious need for further investigation and wide range screening of the situation in the dental schools during the COVID-19 crisis. The aim of this mini-review is to present these challenges and how academic dental institutions have implemented strategies to overcome them.

Keywords: dental school, dental students, dental education, COVID-19, pandemic

INTRODUCTION

December 2019, Coronavirus disease 2019 (COVID-19) was firstly spotted in Wuhan, China, as pneumonia of unknown origin (1). COVID-19 flare-up spread rapidly not only in China, but also worldwide, therefore, on 11 March 2020, the World Health Organization (WHO) affirmed the SARS-CoV-2 virus, more commonly known as COVID-19 as a pandemic (2). The overall number of confirmed cases and mortalities are 78,194,105 and 1,754,369, respectively, in 216 countries as of December 25, 2020 (3). Human-to-human contact via droplets and aerosol has been linked to the transmission of the SARS-CoV-2 virus (4). On the 15 March 2020, the majority of countries all over the world started to impose a lockdown of their population and dental practices were asked to close temporarily. Not to mention, dentists were reported to be among the highest professional risk groups of being infected and a possible vector of the transmission of the SARS-CoV-2 virus (5).

Academic dental schools are considered as competitive and demanding learning communities. Although there have been many outstanding innovations in teaching methodologies during the last few years in higher education, the COVID-19 pandemic highlighted the structural difference between dental and medical schools in the methods of instruction, and the practical and clinical educational daily activities. In the academic dental schools, students have a 2-year preclinical and a 2-year clinical dental course curriculum designed to prepare them for licensure and practice upon graduation (6). Dental chairside teaching is far more complex than most higher education, as senior dental students take the responsibility for the management of the patient's oral health under guidance from clinical specialists (7). Moreover, clinical dental interventions demand the integration of both intellectual and technical skills, including a sensitivity to the patients' needs as well as technical ability, and most critical, risk consideration. In other words, dental students learn what should be done, when to intervene effectively, and finally how to critically appraise treatment outcomes.

All levels of the educational system in Egypt and worldwide have been affected by COVID-19 (8). The worldwide temporary closure of the academic institutions affected around 931,345,922 students in 94 countries representing 54% of total enrolled learners (9). Egyptian private and public universities either canceled or postponed all campus in-person events in order to minimize gatherings and hence control the routes of the virus transmission (10). However, these actions elevated the medical, economical, and social burden on both undergraduate and graduate communities (11). The experiences of oro-dental health education in clinical settings varied remarkably based on the national spread of the virus. Due to the rapid second wave spread of COVID-19, it is imperative for dental schools to apply dynamic adjustments to the delivery of educational clinical services and community services, in order to protect students, patients, and educators meanwhile sustaining continued student academic and research progress.

Some medical academic institutions have taken the action and documented their adjustments during the pandemic; yet; there is an urgent demand for further analysis and wide range screening of the condition in the Egyptian dental schools during the COVID-19 crisis. Thus, the current review aims to illustrate how one of public dental schools in Egypt acted in response to the COVID-19 pandemic and to present the ongoing challenges, and how academic and clinical educators have worked to overcome them.

SOUTH VALLEY UNIVERSITY DENTAL SCHOOL EXPERIENCE

On March 25, South Valley University undergraduate dental students were not allowed to perform in-person activities within the dental school and clinics based on the Egyptian prime minister decree for holding all the educational activities. Administrative and secretarial activities were only part-time accessible (2 days/week). Lectures and examinations moved on the web. The professors started recording video lectures to be available online on the e-learning platform of the University (*http://app.svu.edu.eg/ecourses/faculties3.aspx*). Moreover, intermediate and summative examinations have been performed online, except for final year students, who performed their written examination at the university halls following social distancing rules and strict protective infection control measures.

Early July, the university council regulated the process of carrying out clinical training for healthcare professionals. There were many specific challenges for educators which required rigorous attention in balancing the safety of dental students and staff and the adoption of effective protective measures whilst maintaining high quality educational services. The dental clinics remained available only for the management of dental emergencies. Restorative, esthetic, prophylactic, and all non-essential treatments were canceled. Mid October, the start of fall semester witnessed the restart of education activities on patients. Part of the clinical training activities of dental students was performed through case presentation, reading and critical appraisal of scientific literature, interactive discussions based on clinical scenarios, and update training in cross-infection control. The dental faculty administration placed strict rules to regulate the dental clinics including the limitation of patients' daily numbers, limitations of the accompanying person (one person allowed), temperature checking at the entrance of the clinics.

NON-CLINICAL EDUCATION CHALLENGES

According to the Egyptian Supreme Council of Universities regulations, the majority of Egyptian dental programs adopted the Hybrid Learning Model, in which lectures (theoretical part) were introduced via e-learning platforms, while in-person learning was limited to preclinical (laboratory), and practical (clinical) courses that cannot be delivered remotely. This strategy was implemented to minimize the physical interaction between students, in order to control the outspread of the infection. Meanwhile it allowed dental students to acquire their practical competencies essential for dental education and important for students' satisfaction, in spite of the compromised educational environment.

Teaching practical courses remotely requires resources and unhurried critical planning. For example, the presence of a stable internet connection is mandatory to provide online educational services, which might be a challenge to some of the developing countries. Besides, this new system requires a fundamental change in the mentality of both the faculty and students to perform differently in the educational process (10). Learning a new skill (preclinical or clinical) requires the integration of both; verbal and non-verbal educational methods (12). Dental students gain many practical skills without meaningful verbal expressions, such tacit knowledge usually provides a strong base to much of our dental skills (13). COVID-19 pandemic highlighted the need for educators and clinical teachers to understand the importance of tacit knowledge and how to provide alternative teaching modalities. Internationally, some dental programs started to monitor the students preclinical performance via novel methods like ZOOM, Microsoft Teams, and Whatsapp. The use of distant video illustrations, and the evaluation of the students' practical performance online might be a practical solution, although more studies are essential to evaluate their effectiveness. Some methods like the five-step method (14) can be modified for preclinical dental teaching. Before the students perform the procedure, the students visualize the procedure without any verbal explanation in order to help them to imagine the procedure before applying it. Then, the procedure demonstrated by the educator is repeated with verbal narration and detailed explanation of steps. Later, the students are asked to repeat the steps so that they can be internalized. And finally, the students perform the procedure with the educator observing and providing feedback as needed.

With the gradual breakthrough that has taken place in the lockdown procedures done in Egypt as well as many other countries, the majority of dental students have resumed their in-person practical classes since October 2020. The return to the practice had to deal with new challenges such as social distancing in classes, management of modified schedules, and the new mandatory public health guidelines (15). The Association for Dental Education, Asia Pacific (ADEAP) developed and published detailed guidelines for safe provision of dental education (including pre-clinical and clinical settings) during the COVID-19 pandemic (16). Although we serendipitously followed many of these items (like the majority of dental programs) during the pandemic (17), it's important to exchange these guidelines and distribute them globally in order to facilitate providing dental education in a safe environment. Regarding the in-person classes, dental academics need to emphasize strict infection control measures (protective face masks and shields, social distancing, and hand hygiene) among students, educators, and staff. The application of these measures is crucial for the safety of the work environment. Students, faculty, and staff should be only allowed to participate in limited, in-person classes, activities, and events that permit attendees to remain spaced at least six feet apart (e.g., lecture hall with seating spaced six feet apart). Besides, dental school should completely avoid out-of-class social activities and events and communications. It's important to continuously remind students, faculty, and staff not to share objects (e.g., laboratory and/or clinical supplies). Routinely scheduled cleaning and disinfection of frequently touched areas should be applied and monitored (e.g., on-time and consistently).

Despite these challenges, it may be a great opportunity to share experiences and information between dental schools, and to implement novel strategies in dental education, especially there are few hindrances to traditional dental learning scenarios. The main aim is to offer the dental students a new alternative that is satisfactory for their training. Although this might look enthusiastic, future studies are important to evaluate the impact of these guidelines and techniques on the learning outcomes, due to the unique demands of dental education (18).

PRACTICE-BASED CLINICAL CHALLENGES

The resumption of routine clinical dental activities was a difficult decision and should be guided by the virus updated status and national health guidelines to manage it. Dental academics had to plan for a safe recovery of clinical teaching for students, patients, educators, and staff with contingency plans. This is very crucial as SARS-CoV-2 is known to be highly contagious and the status of virus transmission in the Egyptian community remains unclear. Certain clinical training (like journal club and case presentation) were well-suited for teledentistry (19). In these cases, case presentation, and discussions could be done using online platforms (ZOOM, Webex, Microsoft Teams) (20). This approach can aid in conducting problem-focused interactions with students without the need of their physical presence (21, 22). On the other side, the therapeutic clinical training in the university clinics represented the main challenge for clinical dental education, specially the management of bio-aerosol, the insurance of the dental team compliance with the obligatory additional infection control measures, the application of social distancing policies to reduce overcrowding in the clinic, and thus reduce the exposure to others as well as the bio-aerosol generated during the clinical procedures (23).

Dental Bio-Aerosols

Almost all dental procedures include a set of mechanical preparation, this includes the use of air turbines, air-water syringe, ultrasonic scalers, rotary handpieces, and air abrasion which generate bio-aerosols. Interestingly, these procedures include routine dental examination and hand-scaling which many dentists would consider safe to perform (24). Bio-aerosol generated during dental procedures contains a spectrum of microorganisms within tiny particles called droplet nuclei (1–5 μm) or droplets (>5 μm) (25). Large droplets tend to fall quickly due to the gravity, while droplet nuclei are airborne for hours due to their low settling velocity with the ability to propagate further before being inhaled inside the respiratory system or contaminate the clinic exposed surfaces (26).

Recent evidence demonstrated three main routes for the transmission of SARS-CoV-2 in dental settings: (1) direct transmission via inhalation of the virus via cough droplets; (2) transmission via oral, nasal, or eye membranes; and (3) direct contact transmission (27). All these three transmission routes are facilitated by dental procedures generated aerosols (28). It's important to highlight here that the majority of previous studies quantifying bio-aerosol generation during dental instrumentations have a range of differences in between them. Nevertheless, their findings should be taken into consideration when operating in this pandemic.

The reduction of bio-aerosol generation can be accomplished by using many protocols (26, 29). In our experience, we followed two different approaches to control bio-aerosol generation: (1) the use of pre-operative mouthwash; and (2) the regulation of daily dental procedures (30, 31). The use of pre-operative mouthwash (1% hydrogen peroxide, 0.2% povidone iodine, or alcohol free options such as 0.2% chlorhexidine rinse) has been shown to control the bacterial burden (23). In order to regulate the daily clinical practice, it was logical to prioritize senior dental students in the clinic as the most skillful clinical cohort with more structured clinical skills (32). Less experienced dental students have been found taking significantly longer time (2–3 h) than those of experienced dentists for doing the same clinical intervention, which exposes patients, students, educators, and staff to bio-aerosol for an extended period of time. Besides, it's preferable to prioritize patients with dental emergencies or acute dental pain, and mandate the use of the rubber dam (with aerosol generating procedures) until the situation becomes clearer or with the mass distribution of the vaccine.

Infection Control

Infection control continues to be one of the most critical issues in healthcare service worldwide including dental schools. Infection control and prevention is crucial in providing a safe environment for students, patients, educators, and healthcare workers within clinical settings in dental schools (33–35). Since its establishment, the Faculty of Oral and Dental Medicine at South Valley University has followed the infection control regulations published in the Summary of Infection Prevention Practices in Dental Settings published by the Center for Disease Control and Prevention (CDC) as the standard infection control measures (36). The transmission of SARS-CoV-19 virus from human to human through the respiratory droplets of the patients (37) requires new regulations in order to control the infection outbreak.

Recently, multiple guidelines and recommendations have been published in order to share the modification in the infection control measures between dental professionals (26, 38). Although we applied many of these measures serendipitously, it is crucial to establish rational evidence-based protocols for all clinical settings to make sure that students, educators, and staff are understanding and applying these protocols properly, and thus do not compromise infection control measures especially at this crisis.

During the pandemic, we strictly applied the social-distancing regulation in the operating as well as patients' waiting rooms. Moreover, the clinic administrative board effectively monitored the hygiene levels in the clinic and patients waiting areas between appointments. This was achieved by using a hospital grade disinfectant that is effective against other viruses such as norovirus or 0.1% sodium hypochlorite or >60% alcohol based wipes (23). These applied measures are closely matching these applied in other countries like France, China, and Iran (15, 26, 38).

According to recent evidence, dental schools should perform primary screening when scheduling an appointment online or over the phone (26, 38). As we don't have online or phone scheduling at the dental clinics in South Valley University, screening of students, patients, faculty, and staff was applied including temperature checking and a questionnaire of any recent respiratory problems or fever at the entrance of the dental hospital. Inside the clinics, dental students, assistants, clinicians, and educators followed strictly the standard precautions for the airborne, as well as contact infections, which include but not limited the use of PPE and the hand hygiene protocols (39). Dental schools need to oblige students and assistants to use disposable surgical caps and long-sleeved polyethylene gowns with elasticized wrists which are cautiously disposed of after every patient. In some high-risk facilities, faculties, and/or clinical educators may be forced to change gowns between each student/patient, and patients are asked to wear disposable gowns. Furthermore, students, staff, and educators are required to wear a surgical mask or N95/P2 respirators inside the dental clinic. The N95/P2 surgical respirators have been known to provide more effective protection from both: airborne particles (0.3–0.6 μm) and from liquid droplets (40). Moreover, protective eyewear is an important protective gadget as the virus has been isolated from conjunctival samples from COVID-19 positive patients (41). Recent studies (42–45) showed that whilst dental students have a positive attitude toward infection control, their compliance is poor, specifically regarding eye protection, with 28% of senior students in some schools admitting to only use eyewear protection sometimes. Finally, all academic dental institutions should clinically assess the compliance of their students periodically to the infection control in the dental settings to ensure their understanding of the infection control obligations.

QUESTIONS CONCERNING THE FUTURE OF DENTAL INSTITUTIONS AND EDUCATION

Although COVID-19 pandemic has a worldwide unlimited devastating impact, this pandemic should alarm the health professionals to be more prepared for any future emerging pandemic. Dental academic institutions must learn from this experience and remember the binding professional responsibility and sharing information. Regarding dental clinical education, it's crucial to answer many questions that may help in understanding what could be done in the future; what will be the basic infection control standards, after the COVID-19 vaccination? The design and infrastructure of educational clinics including patients waiting areas may also need to be reconsidered in the future regarding the positioning, spacing of dental units, and the central air ventilation. In the same context, it is important to know when dental students and educators will receive the vaccine? Are they considered among high risk groups or just educational institutions? Institutional support plans for students, educators, and staff will be vital to help them dealing with the negative consequences of this current crisis.

Regarding pre-clinical dental education, the main challenge that e-learning faces is how to teach efficiently practical pre-clinical lessons in a safe environment. Since most of the dental subjects require practical interaction; therefore, it is not feasible to teach them only online. We believe that dental students will face a difficulty to fulfill the dental practical skills only with an online-based education system. That's why it is suggested that e-learning can be improved by enhancing its interactivity, showing dental procedures in real situations, in addition to providing 3D simulations to mimic the real teaching experience. Finally, It will be important to evaluate in the future the pedagogical effects of the structural change in the dental educational techniques caused by the COVID-19 crisis.

CONCLUSION

The SARS-CoV-2 crisis has forced a paradigm shift on the performance of the dental academic institutions. Due to its uniqueness, clinical dental education faces special challenges compared to other medical specialties. Hybrid learning will probably be a cornerstone of future dental education. Educational clinical dental settings need to be re-adjusted as quickly as possible, according to the new infection control measures, to ensure high quality training for dental students, as well as continuation of community dental services, in a safe clinical environment. Finally, post-pandemic, dental academic institutions must consider documenting and sharing their guidelines and experiences in published research. This knowledge will help dental institutions to improve the overall educational process and to provide both pre-clinical and clinical dental education in a safe environment.

AUTHOR CONTRIBUTIONS

All authors have read and approved the final article. MGH conceived and designed the review. HA revised the manuscript. MGH and HA wrote and revised the final manuscript.

ACKNOWLEDGMENTS

The authors would like to thank all the workers in the Egyptian healthcare system that are saving lives each day. It is because of your dedication, commitment, and hard work that we are all here today. We are all proud to be working with all of you.

REFERENCES

1. Li Q, Guan X, Wu P, Wang X, Zhou L, Tong Y, et al. Early transmission dynamics in Wuhan, China, of novel coronavirus-infected pneumonia. *N Engl J Med.* (2020) 382:1199–207. doi: 10.1056/NEJMoa2001316
2. WHO/Europe. *WHO Announces COVID-19 Outbreak a Pandemic.* Available online at: https://www.euro.who.int/en/health-topics/health-emergencies/coronavirus-covid-19/news/news/2020/3/who-announces-covid-19-outbreak-a-pandemic (accessed December 25, 2020).
3. *WHO Coronavirus Disease (COVID-19) Dashboard.* Available online at: https://covid19.who.int (accessed December 25, 2020).
4. Huang C, Wang Y, Li X, Ren L, Zhao J, Hu Y, et al. Clinical features of patients infected with 2019 novel coronavirus in Wuhan, China. *Lancet.* (2020) 395:497–506. doi: 10.1016/S0140-6736(20)30183-5
5. Available online at: https://www.osha.gov/Publications/OSHA3990.pdf (accessed December 30, 2020).
6. Akinkugbe AA, Garcia DT, Smith CS, Brickhouse TH, Mosavel M. A descriptive pilot study of the immediate impacts of COVID-19 on dental and dental hygiene students' readiness and wellness. *J Dent Educ.* (2020) 85:401–10. doi: 10.1002/jdd.12456
7. Sweet J, Pugsley L, Wilson J. Stakeholder perceptions of chairside teaching and learning in one UK dental school. *Br Dent J.* (2008) 205:499–503. doi: 10.1038/sj.bdj.2008.934
8. Nicola M, Alsafi Z, Sohrabi C, Kerwan A, Al-Jabir A, Iosifidis C, et al. The socio-economic implications of the coronavirus pandemic (COVID-19): a review. *Int J Surg.* (2020) 78:185–93. doi: 10.1016/j.ijsu.2020.04.018
9. *School Closures Caused by Coronavirus (Covid-19).* Available online at: https://en.unesco.org/covid19/educationresponse (accessed December 26, 2020).
10. Shehata MH, Abouzeid E, Wasfy NF, Abdelaziz A, Wells RL, Ahmed SA. Medical education adaptations post COVID-19: an Egyptian reflection. *J. Med. Educ. Curic. Dev.* (2020) 7:2382120520951819. doi: 10.1177/2382120520951819
11. Esposito S, Principi N. School closure during the coronavirus disease 2019 (COVID-19) pandemic: an effective intervention at the global level? *JAMA Pediatr.* (2020) 174:921–2. doi: 10.1001/jamapediatrics.2020.1892
12. Maddox WT, Ashby FG. Dissociating explicit and procedural-learning based systems of perceptual category learning. *Behav Processes.* (2004) 66:309–32. doi: 10.1016/j.beproc.2004.03.011
13. Fugill M. Tacit knowledge in dental clinical teaching. *Eur J Dent Educ.* (2012) 16:2–5. doi: 10.1111/j.1600-0579.2011.00716.x
14. George JH, Doto FX. A simple five-step method for teaching clinical skills. *Fam Med.* (2001) 33:577–8.
15. Gaudin A, Arbab-Chirani R, Pérez F. Effect of COVID-19 on dental education and practice in France. *Front Dent Med.* (2020) 1:5. doi: 10.3389/fdmed.2020.00005
16. Hong G, Chang T-Y, Terry A, Chuenjitwongsa S, Park Y-S, Tsoi JK, et al. Guidelines for innovation in dental education during the coronavirus disease 2019 pandemic. *J Oral Sci.* (2020) 63:107–10. doi: 10.2334/josnusd.20-0399
17. Gurgel BCdV, Borges SB, Borges REA, Calderon PDS. COVID-19: perspectives for the management of dental care and education. *J Appl Oral Sci.* (2020) 28:e20200358. doi: 10.1590/1678-7757-2020-0358
18. Ahmed SA, Hegazy NN, Malak HWA, Kayser CW, Elrafie NM, Hassanien M, et al. Model for utilizing distance learning post COVID-19 using (PACT)™ a cross sectional qualitative study. *BMC Med Educ.* (2020) 20:400. doi: 10.1186/s12909-020-02311-1
19. Farooq I, Ali S, Moheet IA, AlHumaid J. COVID-19 outbreak, disruption of dental education, and the role of teledentistry. *Pak J Med Sci Q.* (2020) 36:1726–31. doi: 10.12669/pjms.36.7.3125
20. Chang T-Y, Hong G, Paganelli C, Phantumvanit P, Chang W-J, Shieh Y-S, et al. Innovation of dental education during COVID-19 pandemic. *J Dent Sci.* (2021) 16:15–20. doi: 10.1016/j.jds.2020.07.011
21. Abbas B, Wajahat M, Saleem Z, Imran E, Sajjad M, Khurshid Z. Role of teledentistry in COVID-19 pandemic: a nationwide comparative analysis among dental professionals. *Eur J Dent.* (2020) 14:S116–22. doi: 10.1055/s-0040-1722107
22. Yadav V, Kumar V, Sharma S, Chawla A, Logani A. Palliative dental care: ignored dimension of dentistry amidst COVID-19 pandemic. *Spec Care Dentist.* (2020) 40:613–5. doi: 10.1111/scd.12517
23. Sukumar S, Dracopoulos SA, Martin FE. Dental education in the time of SARS-CoV-2. *Eur J Dent Educ.* (2020) 25:325–31. doi: 10.1111/eje.12608
24. Huntley DE, Campbell J. Bacterial contamination of scrub jackets during dental hygiene procedures. *J Dent Hyg.* (1998) 72:19–23.
25. Zemouri C, de Soet H, Crielaard W, Laheij A. A scoping review on bio-aerosols in healthcare and the dental environment. *PLoS ONE.* (2017) 12:e0178007. doi: 10.1371/journal.pone.0178007
26. Ge Z-Y, Yang L-M, Xia J-J, Fu X-H, Zhang Y-Z. Possible aerosol transmission of COVID-19 and special precautions in dentistry. *J Zhejiang Univ Sci B.* (2020) 21:361–8. doi: 10.1631/jzus.B2010010
27. Pan Y, Liu H, Chu C, Li X, Liu S, Lu S. Transmission routes of SARS-CoV-2 and protective measures in dental clinics during the COVID-19 pandemic. *Am J Dent.* (2020) 33:129–34.
28. Innes N, Johnson IG, Al-Yaseen W, Harris R, Jones R, Kc S, et al. A systematic review of droplet and aerosol generation in dentistry. *J Dent.* (2021) 105:103556. doi: 10.1016/j.jdent.2020.103556
29. Gandolfi MG, Zamparini F, Spinelli A, Sambri V, Prati C. Risks of aerosol contamination in dental procedures during the second wave of COVID-19-experience and proposals of innovative IPC in dental practice. *Int J Environ Res Public Health.* (2020) 17:8954. doi: 10.3390/ijerph17238954
30. Bidra AS, Pelletier JS, Westover JB, Frank S, Brown SM, Tessema B. Comparison of *in vitro* inactivation of SARS CoV-2 with hydrogen peroxide and povidone-iodine oral antiseptic rinses. *J Prosthodont.* (2020) 29:599–603. doi: 10.1111/jopr.13220
31. Clementini M, Raspini M, Barbato L, Bernardelli F, Braga G, Di Gioia C, et al. Aerosol transmission for SARS-CoV-2 in the dental practice. A review by SIdP covid-19 task-force. *Oral Dis.* (2020). doi: 10.1111/odi.13649. [Epub ahead of print].

32. Quinn B, Field J, Gorter R, Akota I, Manzanares M-C, Paganelli C, et al. COVID-19: the immediate response of european academic dental institutions and future implications for dental education. *Eur J Dent Educ.* (2020) 24:811–4. doi: 10.1111/eje.12542
33. Bebermeyer RD, Dickinson SK, Thomas LP. Guidelines for infection control in dental health care settings–a review. *Tex Dent J.* (2005) 122:1022–6.
34. Cleveland JL, Bonito AJ, Corley TJ, Foster M, Barker L, Gordon Brown G, et al. Advancing infection control in dental care settings: factors associated with dentists' implementation of guidelines from the Centers for Disease Control and Prevention. *J Am Dent Assoc.* (2012) 143:1127–38. doi: 10.14219/jada.archive.2012.0044
35. Dagher J, Sfeir C, Abdallah A, Majzoub Z. Infection control measures in private dental clinics in Lebanon. *Int J Dent.* (2017) 2017:5057248. doi: 10.1155/2017/5057248
36. Centers for Disease Control and Prevention. *Summary of Infection Prevention Practices in Dental Settings* (2016).
37. Wu Z, Harrich D, Li Z, Hu D, Li D. The unique features of SARS-CoV-2 transmission: comparison with SARS-CoV, MERS-CoV and 2009 H1N1 pandemic influenza virus. *Rev Med Virol.* (2020) 31:e2171. doi: 10.1002/rmv.2171
38. Falahchai M, Babaee Hemmati Y, Hasanzade M. Dental care management during the COVID-19 outbreak. *Spec Care Dentist.* (2020) 40:539–48. doi: 10.1111/scd.12523
39. Jadhav GR, Mittal P. Coronavirus disease 2019: implications for clinical dental care. *J Endod.* (2020) 46:1341–2. doi: 10.1016/j.joen.2020.05.026
40. Available online at: http://www.cec.health.nsw.gov.au/__data/assets/pdf_file/0006/590307/Application-of-PPE-in-COVID-19.pdf (accessed December 26, 2020).
41. *Transmission of SARS-CoV-2: Implications for Infection Prevention Precautions.* Available online at: https://www.who.int/news-room/commentaries/detail/transmission-of-sars-cov-2-implications-for-infection-prevention-precautions (accessed December 26, 2020).
42. Ahmad IA, Rehan EA, Pani SC. Compliance of Saudi dental students with infection control guidelines. *Int Dent J.* (2013) 63:196–201. doi: 10.1111/idj.12030
43. de Abreu MHNG, Lopes-Terra MC, Braz LF, Rímulo AL, Paiva SM, Pordeus IA. Attitudes and behavior of dental students concerning infection control rules: a study with a10-year interval. *Braz Dent J.* (2009) 20:221–5. doi: 10.1590/s0103-64402009000300009
44. Acosta-Gío AE, Borges-Yáñez SA, Flores M, Herrera A, Jerónimo J, Martínez M, et al. Infection control attitudes and perceptions among dental students in Latin America: implications for dental education. *Int Dent J.* (2008) 58:187–93. doi: 10.1111/j.1875-595x.2008.tb00347.x
45. Hoover TE, Kirk J, Fredekind RE. Clinical quality assurance surveillance and targeted interventions: managing unfavorable trends in a dental school clinic. *J Dent Educ.* (2007) 71:746–58. doi: 10.1002/j.0022-0337.2007.71.6.tb04331.x

24

Modeling the Behavioral Response of Dentists to COVID-19 and Assessing the Perceived Impacts of Pandemic on Operative Dentistry Practices in Pakistan

Syeda Afshan Manzoor[1*] *and Abdul-Hakeem Alomari*[2]

[1] *Department of Operative Dentistry & Endodontics, Bakhtawar Amin Medical & Dental College, Multan, Pakistan,* [2] *Biomedical Engineering Department, College of Engineering, Imam Abdulrahman Bin Faisal University (IAU), Dammam, Saudi Arabia*

Correspondence:
Syeda Afshan Manzoor
drafshan205@gmail.com

COVID-19 pandemic has affected dentistry in unprecedented ways. This study investigates the perceived effects of the pandemic on operative dentistry procedures and dentistry profession in Pakistan and the factors that determine the behavioral changes among dentists to adapt to the "new normal." A Capability Opportunity Motivation-Behavioral model (COM-B) was utilized to investigate the factors that determine the behavior of dentists in Punjab, Pakistan to adhere to COVID-19 standard operating procedures (SOPs). Using social media, an online questionnaire was sent to operative dentistry professionals in Pakistan, and 312 responses were received. 81.4% of the respondents believed that the COVID-19 pandemic has severely affected the level of care provided to the patients, 66% were extremely worried about the risk of contagion during clinical practices, and more than 75% of the respondents opined that the pandemic has led to an increased emphasis on disinfection and oral hygiene instructions. The multiple regression model suggests that the behavior of Pakistani dentists to adhere to the COVID-19 SOPs is significantly affected by their Capabilities ($\beta = 0.358$) and Opportunities ($\beta = 0.494$). The study concluded that dentists in Punjab, Pakistan are concerned about the risk of contagion and report a serious concern about consequences such as financial loss and inappropriate care of patients. The current study results can feed the policymaking in Pakistan and other developing countries. Facilities and training to improve dentists' opportunities and capabilities can improve their ability to cope with the COVID-19 challenges.

Keywords: COVID-19, COM-B model, dentistry, operative dentistry, Pakistan

INTRODUCTION

Worldwide, healthcare professionals are on the first lines in fighting the COVID-19 pandemic. They have become highly vulnerable to COVID-19 transmission, constituting 9% of all the infected cases (1, 2). Dental practitioners are among high-risk healthcare professionals because of direct exposure to blood and saliva (3). The Occupational Safety and Health Administration (OSHA) devised an occupational risk pyramid which shows the vulnerability of healthcare professionals based on their exposure to COVID-19 virus (https://www.osha.gov/Publications/OSHA3990.pdf; United States, Department of Labor). According to the OSHA (Department of Labor, USA), dentists are at "very high risk." Earlier studies confirmed that aerosol transmission and respiratory droplets are potential pathways of COVID-19 transmission (4).

Dental professionals are especially vulnerable when carrying out aerosol-generating procedures (AGPs) on infectious patients (5). Evidence suggests that while a dentist is treating a patient on a dental chair, the highest levels of aerosol contaminants are within 50–60 cm of the face of the patient. Furthermore, aerosols are highest on face masks of patients, and around their nose and eyes (6). The aerosol contaminants generated by ultrasonic devices can remain in the air for half an hour after the procedure (7). Thus, dentists are highly vulnerable to infection because of close proximity to the patient, contact with patients' blood and saliva as well as due to the use of instruments that generate aerosols (8, 9).

Evidence suggests that returning to work after the COVID-19 outbreak requires dentists and healthcare professionals to adopt a behavioral change to adhere to COVID-19 SOPs during clinical practices (5). The main SOPs include the use of personal protective equipment (PPE) in line with government advice, use of robust infection prevention and control procedures and use of high-power rubber suction and rubber dam where an aerosol generating procedure is necessary (5, 8, 9). This is especially true for operative dentistry professionals since several operative dentistry procedures involve AGPs, which makes dentists critically exposed to infection risk (5, 10, 11). Furthermore, COVID-19 also led to increased anxiety and practice modification as well as had economic consequences for dentists (12). Thus, it is critical to identify and understand the factors driving behavioral change in operative dentistry professionals.

Capability Opportunity Motivation-Behavior model (COM-B) has been used to study and understand the behavioral change in dentistry (5). The COM-B consists of three components that drive behavioral change: Capability, Opportunity, and Motivation (13, 14). In the proposed COM-B model, Capability is defined as the internal factors that enable an individual to engage in a given behavior. Opportunity is defined as the external variables or factors that allow an individual to engage in a given behavior. Motivation consists of a "conscious motivation" (intentional plans to engage in a given behavior) and "automatic motivation" (defined as an individual's habitual or instinctive response) (13). In another study (4), COM-B is utilized as a framework to understand the factors underpinning behavioral change for intervention.

Due to a high exposure to infection, wearing of PPE was made mandatory for healthcare professionals all around the world. PPE includes protective eyewear, N-95 mask, full-length gowns covering body from head to toe, air-purifying respirators, and surgical gloves. Compared to the countries such as New Zealand (15), Canada (9), and Saudi Arabia (16), dentists in developing countries have shown far less knowledge and compliance to the COVID-19 infection control SOP's (10). Although there is evidence of positive attitude toward the use of PPE by dentists in some developing countries including Iraq (6), in most developing countries, attitude toward the use of PPE during COVID-19 outbreak has not been encouraging.

In developing countries including Pakistan, the usage of PPE and adherence to the COVID-19 infection control SOP's is still quite challenging (17). Limited evidence is available which suggests that one of the key factors influencing the attitude of dentists toward the use of PPE are financial constraints and poor knowledge about the use of PPE among dentists in Pakistan (17). Studies in dental hospital in Rawalpindi and Karachi suggest that as low as 20 percent of the dental students complied to COVID-19 SOPs (18). This is an alarming situation for a country like Pakistan as dentists' lack of compliance of COVID-19 SOPs could lead to increased burden on scarce resources of the country. Therefore, it is vital to investigate how the COVID-19 pandemic has affected the dentistry profession in Pakistan and what factors underpin the behavioral change in the dentists of Pakistan.

This study aims to understand the perceived impacts of the COVID-19 pandemic on the dental profession in the Punjab province of Pakistan and understand the factors that underpin the behavioral change in the dentists to adapt to the COVID-19 SOPs. Punjab is the most populous province of Pakistan, containing more than 110 million people. Also, Punjab is the most affected province of the country by COVID-19 pandemic. So far, 506,018 confirmed cases of COVID-19 have been reported in Punjab. Of these confirmed cases, 13,560 patients died (https://covid.gov.pk/stats/punjab). Dentists working in all departments are vulnerable to COVID-19 exposure. Current study focuses on dentists who specialize and work in operative dentistry departments. This study specifically concentrated on this group of dentists as these dentists are among the most affected professionals by the challenges and risks associated with treatments frequently requiring AGPs. Although this study could have involved other professionals such as periodontists and oral hygienists, limiting this study to operative dentists allowed a more comprehensive and in-depth survey of the perception of a specific department of dentistry.

The specific objectives of this study are (a) to identify the perceived effects of COVID-19 on dentistry practices in Pakistan, (b) to identify the perceived impacts of COVID-19 on operative dentistry procedures in Pakistan, and (c) to identify the drivers of behavioral change of adherence of COVID-19 SOPs among dentists of Pakistan using COM-B model.

METHODOLOGY

A survey-based cross-sectional study was conducted to collect data for this project. A structured questionnaire was prepared through review of literature and consultation with expert biostatisticians, operative dentists, and psychologists. The questionnaire was approved by the Institutional Research Board (IRB) of Bakhtawar Amin Dental College & Hospital Multan, Pakistan (reference BADC&H No. 300/21). The questionnaire was pre-tested once with a pilot survey of 25 respondents. The demographic profile of these 25 respondents was fairly similar to the profile of the respondents in the actual survey (i.e., of the 25 respondents, 18 were female and six were male. Eighteen respondents aged between 20 and 30 years, five respondents 30–40 years old and two respondents were above 60 years age. In terms of type of workplace, 19 respondents worked in Government hospitals, three worked in private hospitals and three respondents worked in both Government and private hospitals). Informed consent of all respondents was obtained.

Sample Selection

According to Pakistan Medical Dental Council Islamabad, total number of registered dentists in Pakistan are approximately 25,000 (https://www.pbs.gov.pk/sites/default/files//tables/rename-as-per-table-type/Registered%20Dental%20Doctor.pdf). Of these, 9,000 dentists are registered in Punjab (https://tribune.com.pk/story/1975950/pakistan-facing-acute-shortage-doctors). The sample size for this survey was determined by the total number of dentists in Punjab province of Pakistan (i.e., 9,000), using the sample size calculation formula proposed by Yamane (19). The confidence interval was set to 6% and a 95% confidence level was used. With these parameters, the sample size derived was 260.

Questionnaire Development

An online questionnaire was created using Google Forms and cascaded to registered operative dentistry professionals in Punjab, Pakistan, through social media (WhatsApp groups of dentists). The survey started on May 20th, 2021. The online survey was kept open for 10 weeks. Four reminders were sent to the respondents, each after 2 weeks (through messages in the WhatsApp groups) to record their responses during this time.

The questionnaire for this study consisted of 32 questions which were divided into eight sections. A complete draft of the questionnaire is provided in the **Table 1**.

The first section recorded the demographic details of the respondents. The respondents were asked about their age, gender, location, years in dentistry professions, dental education/training, type of workplace and nature of their jobs.

The second section enquires about respondents' perceived impacts of COVID-19 pandemic on dentistry profession. All answers were recorded on a Likert scale of 1–5 where 1 = "Not at all" and 5 = "Extremely."

The purpose of the third section was to explore the perceived impacts of pandemic situation on various dental procedures. The respondents were asked to record their answers on Likert scale, ranging from 1 to 5 (Completely disagree to Completely agree).

In the fourth section, the questionnaire inquired the participants about the perceived impacts of COVID-19 on various procedures in operative dentistry. Operative dentistry procedures include aesthetic (e.g., tooth whitening, veneers, crowns etc.), endodontics (e.g., root canal treatment), implant, and restorative procedures (e.g., tooth restoration.). The respondents were asked to record their responses on a Likert scale. The sections 2–4 were used to assess the perceived effects of the pandemic on dentistry practice and operative dentistry procedures.

Sections 5 to 8 in the survey was used to assess the behavior of respondents to adhere to COVID-19 SOPs. COM-B model is utilized to predict the "behavior to adhere to COVID-19 SOPs" using opportunities, motivation, and capabilities as independent variables. Behavior was measured using three items: (i) On a scale of 1–10, how regularly do you wear PPE during your clinical practices? (ii) On a scale of 1–10, how often do you ensure that your patients follow SOPs during your clinical practices? (iii) On a scale of 1–10, how often do you follow infection control measures during clinical practice? Opportunities were measured using three items: (i) On a scale of 1–10, how confident you are that you have the required physical resources available to follow COVID-19 SOPs at your workplace? (ii) On a scale of 1–10, how confident you are that your colleagues support you to follow COVID-19 SOPs at your workplace? (iii) On a scale of 1–10, how confident you are that you have the required time available to follow COVID-19 SOPs at your clinic/hospital/workplace? Motivation was measured using three items: (i) I feel that it is my moral obligation to follow the COVID SOPs during practice. (ii) I follow COVID SOPs automatically/unconsciously without reminding myself (has become a habit for me) (iii) If I implement COVID-19 SOPs correctly and regularly, I will be a role model for my colleagues. All questions of COM-B constructs were recorded on a Likert scale (1–10).

Data Analysis

Descriptive statistics is used to report the frequency and percentages of the respondents in each category of the demographic variables. Stacked bar charts were used to report the proportions of the respondents who chose various levels of agreements to the questions asked in section 2–4.

In order to establish a relationship between COVID-19 SOPs adherence behavior and the opportunities, capabilities, and motivations of the respondents, a multiple linear regression analysis is utilized. The significance level was set at $p \leq 0.05$.

Before running the regression model, Cronbach's alpha test was used to test the internal consistency in each of the four constructs (Behavior, Opportunities, Motivation and Capabilities). All data analysis were carried out in SPSS v. 21 and R statistical software. The results were then collected and performed using Statistical Package 21 for the Social Sciences SPSS® (IBM®, SPSS® Statistics, Armonk, NY, USA).

RESULTS

Demographics

A total of 312 valid survey responses were received. There were no missing data on responses. Among the respondents, 74.36 % ($n = 232$) were female. Most of the respondents aged between 20 and 30 years ($n = 210$). The details of the demographics of the respondents are given in **Table 2**.

Perceived Impacts of COVID-19 Pandemic on Your Profession

The results suggest that a large proportion of the respondents (66%) were "Extremely" worried about the risk of contagion during their clinical practices

TABLE 1 | List of sections and questions included in the questionnaire for this study.

Section	Questions	
Demographic information	Age (Years)	20–30. 30–40. 40–60. Above 60
	Type of workplace	Government. Private. Work in both Government and Private workplaces simultaneously
	Gender	Male. Female
	Nature of Job	Clinical. Teaching. Both clinical and teaching.
	Clinical experience (years)	Less than 1. 1–3. 3–5. 5–10. 10–15. More than 15.
	Dental education	BDS (Or equivalent). Post-graduation (In progress). Post-graduation (Completed)
Impacts of COVID-19 pandemic on your profession	To what extent has COVID-19 pandemic affected the ability of dentists to provide appropriate levels of care to the patients?	
	To what extent do you think COVID-19 pandemic is likely to cause loss of clinical skills in dentists?	
	To what extent do you think COVID-19 pandemic has financially affected dentists?	
	To what extent COVID-19 pandemic causes risk of contagion in dentists due to unavailability of appropriate PPE?	
Impacts of COVID-19 pandemic on dental practices	COVID-19 pandemic has positively impacted dental practice because it has allowed better spaced appointments	
	COVID-19 pandemic has positively impacted dental practice because it has led to more emphasis on disinfection procedures	
	COVID-19 pandemic has positively impacted dental practice because it has led to more emphasis on Oral Health Instructions (OHI)	
	COVID-19 pandemic has negatively impacted dental practices by causing reduced number of patients	
	COVID-19 pandemic has negatively impacted dental practices by causing reduced number of follow-up visits	
Impacts of COVID-19 pandemic on procedures in operative dentistry	COVID-19 pandemic has affected restorative procedures	
	COVID-19 pandemic has affected endodontic procedures	
	COVID-19 pandemic has affected aesthetic procedures (veneers, bleaching, etc)	
	COVID-19 pandemic has affected implants procedures	
Opportunities to follow COVID-19 SOPs	On a scale of 1–10, how regularly do you wear PPE during your clinical practices?	
	On a scale of 1–10, how often do you ensure that your patients follow SOPs during your clinical practices?	
	On a scale of 1–10, how often do you follow infection control measures (high volume suction, rubber dam isolation, etc) during clinical practice?	
	On a scale of 1–10, how confident you are that you have the required physical resources available to follow COVID-19 SOPs at your workplace?	
	On a scale of 1–10, how confident you are that your colleagues support you to follow COVID-19 SOPs at your workplace?	
	On a scale of 1–10, how confident you are that you have the required time available to follow COVID-19 SOPs at your clinic/hospital/workplace?	
Motivation to follow COVID-19 SOPs	I feel that it is my moral obligation to follow the COVID SOPs during practice.	
	I follow COVID SOPs automatically/unconsciously without reminding myself (has become a habit for me)	
	If I implement COVID-19 SOPs correctly and regularly, I will be a role model for my colleagues	
Capability to follow COVID-19 SOPs	I have enough physical strength to follow COVID SOPs during clinical practice	
	I have sufficient knowledge/information about how to follow COVID SOPs during clinical practice	
	Even if I commit an error, I feel confident to implement COVID-19 SOPs correctly again	

(**Figure 1**). More than two-third of the respondents recorded their perceived level of impact as "Quite a lot" (59%) and "Extreme" (22.4%) when asked if the COVID-19 pandemic has affected the level of care provided to the patients.

Perceived Impacts of COVID-19 Pandemic on Dental Practices

The results suggest that more than two-third of the respondents were either "Completely Agree" or "Somewhat Agree" that the pandemic situation has reduced the number of patients and reduced the number of follow-up visits (**Figure 2**). Almost two-third of the respondents opined that the pandemic has led to an increased emphasis on the disinfection procedures and OHI in dental practices in Pakistan.

Perceived Impacts of COVID-19 Pandemic on Procedures in Operative Dentistry

More than 75% of the respondents agreed that the pandemic has affected the aesthetic, endodontics, implants and restorative dentistry procedures (**Figure 3**). The highest agreement was found in response to the question about aesthetic procedures followed by restorative dentistry procedures.

Regression Modeling (COM-B)

Internal Consistency and Computation of Variables

Cronbach's alpha is used to assess the internal consistency of the items in each construct (i.e., capability, opportunity, motivation, and behavior). Results suggested an acceptable degree of internal consistency for all four constructs: Capability (0.825), Opportunity (0.801), Motivation (0.707), and Behavior (0.695). Then, "Compute Variable" function in SPSS version

TABLE 2 | Demographic profile of the respondents ($n = 312$).

	Frequency (*n*)	Percentage (%)		Frequency (*n*)	Percentage (%)
Age (Years)			**Type of workplace**		
20–30	210	67.31	Govt.	148	47.43
30–40	70	22.44	Private	90	28.84
40–60	22	7.05	Both Govt. & Private	74	23.71
Above 60 years	10	3.21			
Gender			**Nature of job**		
Male	80	25.64	Clinical	252	80.76
Female	232	74.36	Teaching	12	3.20
			Both Clinical & Teaching	48	15.38
Clinical experience (years)			**Dental education/training**		
Less than a1	26	8.33	BDS (or equivalent)	138	44.23
1–3	106	33.97	Post-graduation (in-progress)	22	7.05
3–5	106	33.97	Post-graduation (completed)	152	48.71
5–10	54	17.31			
10–15	10	3.21			
More than 15	10	3.21			

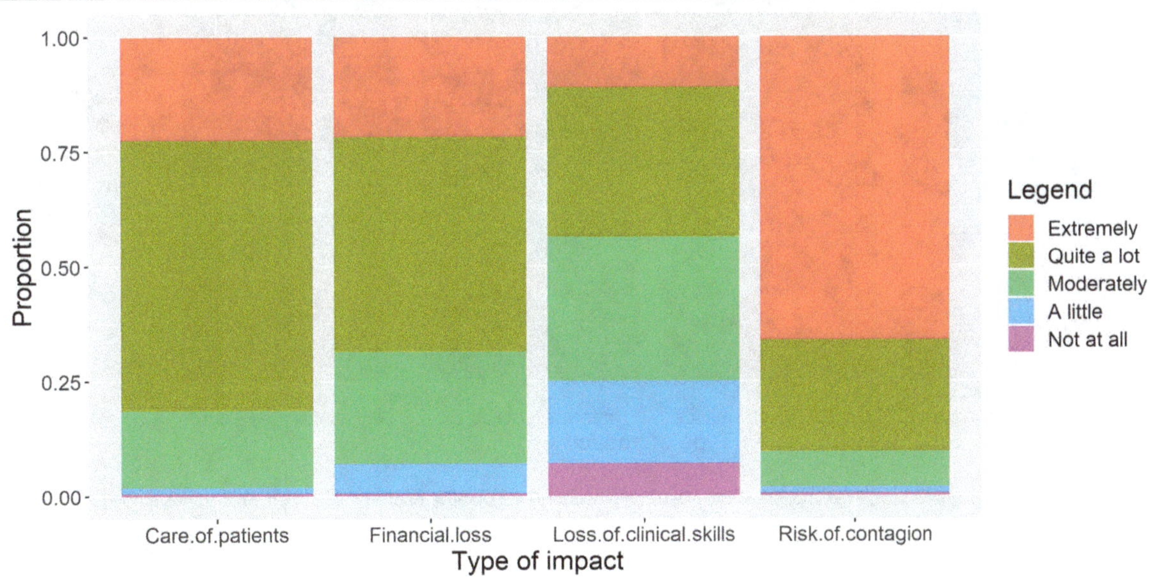

FIGURE 1 | Participant responses about "perceived impacts of COVID-19 on their profession" ($n = 312$). Proportions among respondents are reported.

21 (SPSS® (IBM®, SPSS® Statistics, Armonk, NY, USA) was used to compute four continuous variables from the items within each of the four constructs (i.e., the scores of all questions within a construct were averaged and the resulting score was used as a continuous variable). Thus, four continuous variables: Capability, Opportunity, Motivation, and Behavior were generated. **Figure 4** shows the response of participants.

Multiple Linear Regression Model

Table 3 shows that a significant regression equation was found ($F_{(3,303)} = 85.451$, $p < 0.0001$), with an adjusted R^2 of 0.453. The regression model shows that the dependent variable is significantly affected by the Opportunities and Capabilities of respondents. With increasing Opportunities, the respondents were significantly more likely to adhere to COVID-19 SOP's ($\beta = 0.494$). Similarly, with an increase in the Capabilities of the

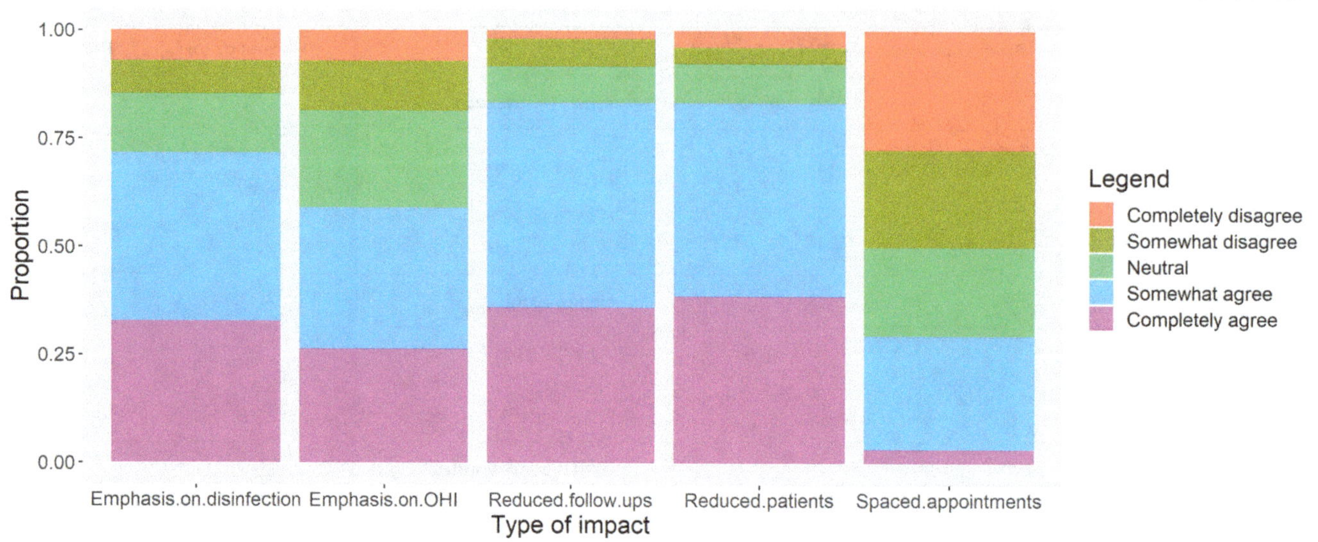

FIGURE 2 | Participant responses about "perceived impacts of COVID-19 on different practices in dentistry" ($n = 312$). Proportions among respondents are reported.

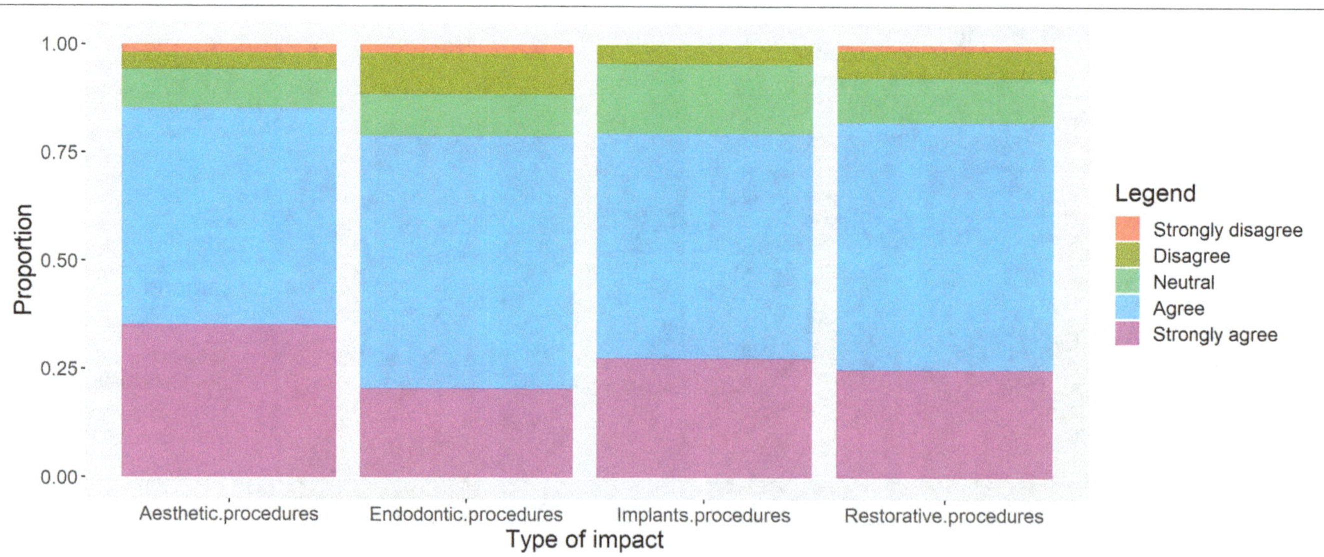

FIGURE 3 | Participant responses about "perceived impacts of COVID-19 on procedures in operative dentistry" ($n = 312$). Proportions among respondents are reported.

respondents, there was a significant increase in the Behavior to adhere to COVID-19 SOP's ($\beta = 0.358$).

DISCUSSION

Healthcare professionals around the world are the most vulnerable groups to COVID-19 exposure as they are most likely to be directly exposed to the infected patients. Healthcare professionals have reported mental stress and physical fatigue due to insufficient health care protection. This study was aimed to understand how the COVID-19 pandemic affected the dentistry professionals in Pakistan, taking a case study of Punjab province in the country. The study also aimed to understand the factors determining the dentists' behavior to adhere to the COVID-19 SOPs.

The results showed that the respondents are most concerned about the risk of contagion. This can be attributed to the fact that the contagious nature of COVID-19 has caused large-scale mortality among the healthcare professionals, especially in the developing countries of South Asia (20). A large number of operative dentistry procedures lead to generation of aerosols due to which dentists are at a high risk of infection (5, 9). Furthermore, scarcity of personal protective equipment also threatens safety of dentists, especially in the developing countries (21). Therefore, it is understandable why most of the respondents

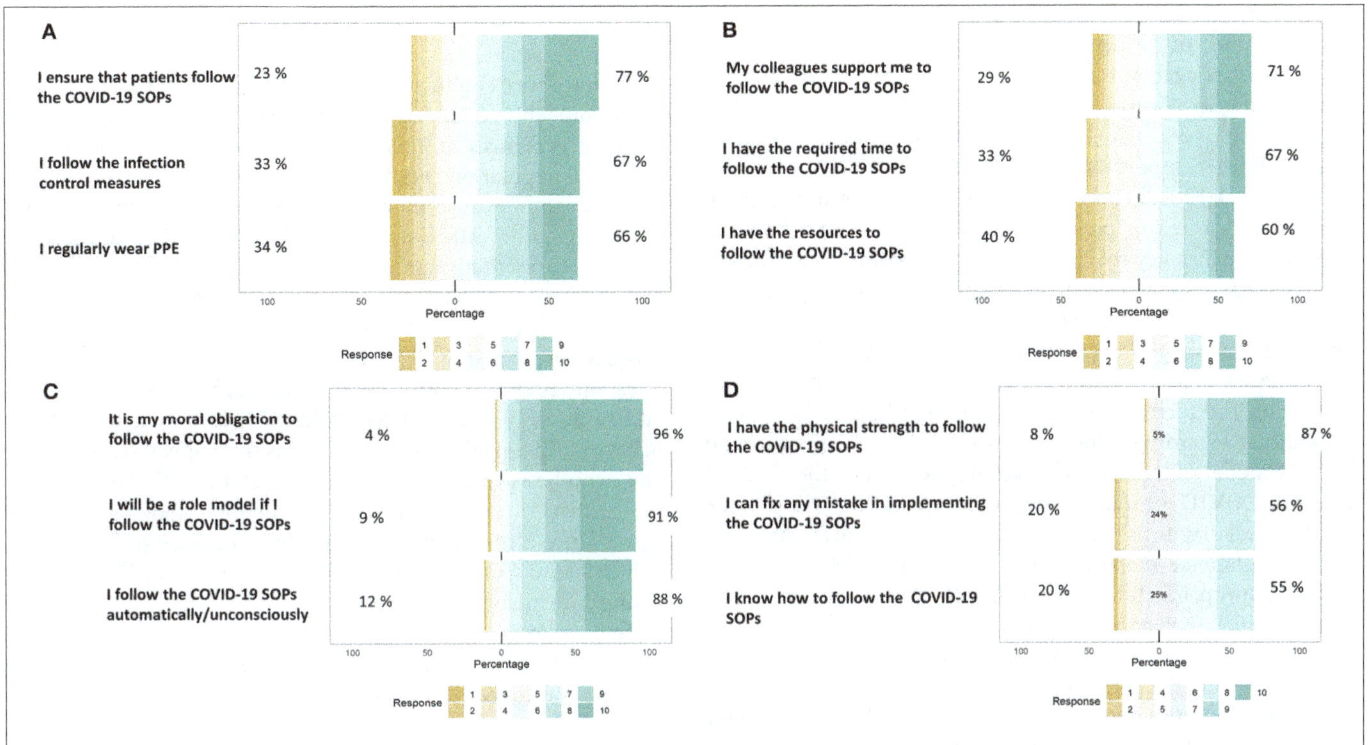

FIGURE 4 | Distribution of responses to the questions asked under the constructs: **(A)** Adherence to COVID-19 SOP's (Behavior), **(B)** Opportunities to follow COVID-19 SOP's, **(C)** Motivation to follow COVID-19 SOP's, and **(D)** Capabilities to follow COVID-19 SOP's. All responses were recorded on a Likert scale (0–10).

TABLE 3 | Multiple regression analysis results showing relationships between dependent variable (Behavior toward adherence to COVID-19 SOPs) and independent variables (Opportunities, Motivation and Capabilities to adhere to COVID-19 SOPs).

Model	Unstandardized coefficients		Standardized coefficients	*p*-Value
	B	Standard Error	*β*	
(Constant)	−0.977	0.674		0.148
Opportunities	0.516	0.047	0.494	0.000
Motivation	−0.091	0.087	−0.057	0.297
Capabilities	0.612	0.096	0.358	0.000

Constructs were created from questions in a survey administered to the dentists in Pakistan (n = 312).

in this survey showed highest concern about the risk of contagion.

After the risk of contagion, the respondents were most concerned about inappropriate levels of care provided to the patients. These results are in agreement with earlier reports where dentists in the UK reported a similar concern (5). This could be due to the fact that most of the operative dentistry treatments require a physical presence of the patients (22). However, due to the closure of clinics and dental hospitals, dentists were inaccessible for patients (23). Furthermore, most of the patients, especially those coming from remote rural areas do not have access to the internet for online appointments and follow-ups (24). Thus, it is expected that dentists would show concern about insufficient healthcare provision to their patients.

More than 60% of the respondents also showed high levels of concern about financial loss due to COVID-19 pandemic. The financial aspect of COVID-19 pandemic is not unheard of (25). Several studies have reported that the pandemic situations have caused financial insecurities among health professionals (26, 27). A study in the UK concluded that more than 75% of the dentists are worried about the financial losses caused by the pandemic (5). Similarly, in a large-scale survey of dentists in the Eastern Mediterranean, Europe, North America, and Western Pacific regions, 73.6% of the respondents strongly agreed that the pandemic situations has caused a substantial financial impact on their income (28). In Iraq, a study reported that 75% of dental practitioners believed their income had decreased by as much as 50% due to the pandemic situation (12). In case of developing countries like Pakistan where resources are limited, one could expect financial stress to be a major outcome of the pandemic.

About two-third of the respondents agreed that there has been an increased emphasis on the disinfection procedures and OHI. This could be attributed to the extraordinary awareness campaigns about disinfection procedures (29). Most people, including doctors and the patients, are extremely cautious about the risk of contagion and therefore an unusually high level of emphasis has been made on disinfection procedures in the dental hospitals (30–32). Similar results have been reported in several other studies. In Turkey, for example, dentists reported a significant decrease in the number of patient admitted to dental hospitals (33). The researchers attributed this decrease in the number of patients to the measures taken by dentists and authorities against the COVID-19 pandemic in view of the growing number of cases (33).

In this study, the COM-B model was used to demonstrate how capabilities, opportunities and motivation of dentists predict their COVID-19 adherence behavior. Understanding human behavior in the era of pandemic is critical because behavioral adaptations play a key role in the spread and control of infection (34). Evidence suggests that behavioral science is pivotal to understanding the factors that encourage stakeholders to adopt behaviors that shape the progression of the outbreak (35). The British Psychological Society Behavioral Science and Disease Prevention Taskforce recommends understanding the behavioral adaptations regarding adherence to COVID-19 SOPs through COM-B model of behavior change. Application of the COM-B model to COVID-19 transmission-related behavior will provide a "behavioral diagnosis" that can help us identify the factors most likely to influence the behavior of individuals (13) and, thus, identify appropriate targets for behavior change interventions. The identified behavioral change interventions can then be designed and implemented to improve adherence to preventive behaviors during the period of social isolation.

The results of the regression model showed that the behavior is significantly affected by capabilities and opportunities. Various studies on this subject have reported contrasting results. For example, a study in the UK reported that motivation is the strongest predictor of an individual's behavior to adhere to COVID-19 SOPs (34). In this study, however, motivation was not a significant determinant of behavior. Instead, opportunities and capabilities were the strongest predictors in the regression model. This can be attributed to the fact that in countries with scarce resources, opportunities and capabilities of individuals are often more important than their motivation. Due to lack of resources and feasible environment, people fail to adopt or avoid a behavior despite motivation. The COM-B model gives a theoretical insight of the drivers of COVID-19 SOPs adherence behavior. In the recent past, COM-B model has been extensively used by researchers to model behavior to adhere to different COVID-19 SOPs (5, 34, 36).

This study makes an argument that the policymakers must emphasize more on improving the facilities, infrastructures, and resources for dentists to adopt COVID-19 SOPs. This is because the regression model in the study highlighted the fact that even though the respondents reported high levels of motivation, their behavior was not significantly affected by their motivation. Instead, better capabilities and opportunities lead to a more promising behavior change. Therefore, the scarce financial resources must be spent on providing PPE and other essential equipment and trainings to enable dentists to counter a pandemic situation.

Limitations of the Study

The study was conducted in the Punjab province of Pakistan. Therefore, the results of this study should not be generalized to other provinces of Pakistan, especially where socioeconomic profile of population is different and where severity of pandemic was different. Furthermore, most of the respondents in this study are under 40 years of age. Under ideal circumstances, a more representative sample of Pakistani dentists in terms of age and years of work experience would have been desirable. However, this study was conducted during periods of lock-down where meeting dentists in-person was not possible. The questionnaires were disseminated through WhatsApp groups and response was completely voluntary. However, the authors believe it did not affect the outcomes as this study did not include any hypothesis regarding the age, gender, or work experience of the dentists. Moreover, most of the dentists above 50 years of age did not attend clinics and hospitals because of being most vulnerable to COVID. Therefore, it is understandable that only younger dentists responded to this questionnaire as they were the ones who practiced dentistry during epidemic and were able to respond to the questions about the impacts of COVID-19 on dentistry profession in Pakistan.

CONCLUSION

This study concludes that COVID-19 pandemic has caused considerable worry to operative dentistry professionals in Pakistan. Dentists in the Punjab province of Pakistan reported financial loss, increased focus on disinfections procedures as major outcomes of the pandemic. The study further concludes that there is a need to spend more resources on providing opportunities and improving capabilities of dentists to allow them to successfully follow the COVID-19 guidelines during their clinical practices.

AUTHOR CONTRIBUTIONS

SM: writing original draft, research, and analysis. A-HA: analysis, editing, review, and supervision. Both authors contributed to the article and approved the submitted version.

ACKNOWLEDGMENTS

The authors are thankful to Dr. Syed Amir Manzoor, Bahauddin Zakariya University Multan for his advice on the design of questionnaire and statistical analysis in this study.

REFERENCES

1. *sars-cov-2-sorveglianza-dati* @ www.epicentro.iss.it [Internet]. Available online at: https://www.epicentro.iss.it/coronavirus/sars-cov-2-sorveglianza-dati (acessed April 20, 2022).
2. Passarelli PC, Rella E, Manicone PF, Garcia-Godoy F, D'Addona A. The impact of the COVID-19 infection in dentistry. *Exp Biol Med.* (2020) 245:940–4. doi: 10.1177/1535370220928905
3. Spagnuolo G, De Vito D, Rengo S, Tatullo M. COVID-19 outbreak: an overview on dentistry. *Int J Environ Res Public Health.* (2020) 17:3–5. doi: 10.3390/ijerph17062094
4. Liu Y, Ning Z, Chen Y, Guo M, Liu Y, Gali NK, et al. Aerodynamic

analysis of SARS-CoV-2 in two Wuhan hospitals. *Nature.* (2020) 582:557–60. doi: 10.1038/s41586-020-2271-3

5. Nibali L, Ide M, Ng D, Buontempo Z, Clayton Y, Asimakopoulou K. The perceived impact of Covid-19 on periodontal practice in the United Kingdom: a questionnaire study. *J Dent.* (2020) 102:103481. doi: 10.1016/j.jdent.2020.103481
6. Chasib NH, Alshami ML, Gul SS, Abdulbaqi HR, Abdulkareem AA, Al-Khdairy SA. Dentists' practices and attitudes toward using personal protection equipment and associated drawbacks and cost implications during the COVID-19 pandemic. *Front Public Heal.* (2021) 9:1–7. doi: 10.3389/fpubh.2021.770164
7. Bescos R, Casas-Agustench P, Belfield L, Brookes Z, Gabaldón T. Coronavirus disease 2019 (COVID-19): emerging and future challenges for dental and oral medicine. *J Dent Res.* (2020) 99:1113. doi: 10.1177/0022034520932149
8. Veena HR, Mahantesha S, Joseph PA, Patil SR, Patil SH. Dissemination of aerosol and splatter during ultrasonic scaling: a pilot study. *J Infect Public Health.* (2015) 8:260–5. doi: 10.1016/j.jiph.2014.11.004
9. Madathil S, Siqueira WL, Marin LM, Sanaulla FB, Faraj N, Quiñonez CR, et al. The incidence of COVID-19 among dentists practicing in the community in Canada: a prospective cohort study over a six-month period. *J Am Dent Assoc.* (2021) 153:450–9.e1. doi: 10.1016/j.adaj.2021.10.006
10. Das G, Samejo I, Ahmed S, Jabeen B, Shaikh MI, Mushtaque K. Cross infection control in private dental practice in Karachi, Sindh. *Prof Med J.* (2019) 26:1354–8. doi: 10.29309/TPMJ/2019.26.08.17
11. NHS England, NHS Improvement. COVID-19 guidance and standard operating procedure urgent dental care systems in the context of coronavirus. *Delay Phase NHS Engl.* (2020) 2:2–35. Available online at: https://go.digitalsmiledesign.com/hubfs/BIOSAFETY/C0282-covid-19-urgent-dental-care-sop.pdf (accessed September 30, 2021).
12. Mahdee AF, Gul SS, Abdulkareem AA, Qasim SSB. Anxiety, practice modification, and economic impact among iraqi dentists during the COVID-19 outbreak. *Front Med.* (2020) 7:595028. doi: 10.3389/fmed.2020.595028
13. Michie S, Van Stralen MM, West R. The behaviour change wheel: a new method for characterising and designing behaviour change interventions. *Implement Sci.* (2011) 6:1–12. doi: 10.1186/1748-5908-6-42
14. Asimakopoulou K, Newton JT. The contributions of behaviour change science towards dental public health practice: a new paradigm. *Community Dent Oral Epidemiol.* (2015) 43:2–8. doi: 10.1111/cdoe.12131
15. Loch C, Kuan IBJ, Elsalem L, Schwass D, Brunton PA, Jum'ah A. COVID-19 and dental clinical practice: students and clinical staff perceptions of health risks and educational impact. *J Dent Educ.* (2021) 85:44–52. doi: 10.1002/jdd.12402
16. Al-Khalifa KS, AlSheikh R, Al-Swuailem AS, Alkhalifa MS, Al-Johani MH, Al-Moumen SA, et al. Pandemic preparedness of dentists against coronavirus disease: a Saudi Arabian experience. *PLoS ONE.* (2020) 15:e0237630. doi: 10.1371/journal.pone.0237630
17. Kamran R, Saba K, Azam S. Impact of COVID-19 on Pakistani dentists: a nationwide cross sectional study. *BMC Oral Health.* (2021) 21:59. doi: 10.1186/s12903-021-01413-6
18. Qamar MK, Shaikh BT, Afzal A. What do the dental students know about infection control? A cross-sectional study in a teaching hospital, Rawalpindi, Pakistan. *Biomed Res Int.* (2020) 2020:3413087. doi: 10.1155/2020/3413087
19. Yamane T. *Statistics, An Introductory Analysis.* 2nd ed. New York, NY: Harper and Row (1967).
20. Jatoi NN, Ahmad S, Sajid E ud din, Yasmin F, Asghar MS, Farhan SA, et al. Are doctors protected enough during COVID-19 in South Asia? *Glob Heal Res Policy.* (2021) 6:36. doi: 10.1186/s41256-021-00219-x
21. Spinazzè A, Cattaneo A, Cavallo DM. COVID-19 outbreak in Italy: protecting worker health and the response of the Italian Industrial Hygienists Association. *Ann Work Expo Health.* (2020) 64:559–64. doi: 10.1093/annweh/wxaa044
22. Gambarini E, Galli M, Di Nardo D, Miccoli G, Patil S, Bhandi S, et al. A survey on perceived COVID-19 risk in dentistry and the possible use of rapid tests. *J Contemp Dent Pract.* (2020) 21:718–22. doi: 10.5005/jp-journals-10024-2851
23. Welti R, D'Mello G, Ramalingam L, Silva M. COVID-19: implications for paediatric dental care in the hospital setting. *J Paediatr Child Health.* (2020) 56:1661–2. doi: 10.1111/jpc.15198
24. Nuvvula S, Mallineni SK. Remote management of dental problems in children during and post the COVID-19 pandemic outbreak: a teledentistry approach. *Dent Med Probl.* (2021) 58:237–41. doi: 10.17219/dmp/133182
25. Gasparro R, Scandurra C, Maldonato NM, Dolce P, Bochicchio V, Valletta A, et al. Perceived job insecurity and depressive symptoms among Italian dentists: the moderating role of fear of COVID-19. *Int J Environ Res Public Health.* (2020) 17:5338. doi: 10.3390/ijerph17155338
26. Amato A, Ciacci C, Martina S, Caggiano M, Amato M. COVID-19: the dentists' perceived impact on the dental practice. *Eur J Dent.* (2021) 15:469–74. doi: 10.1055/s-0041-1734470
27. Ahmadi H, Ebrahimi A, Ghorbani F. The impact of COVID-19 pandemic on dental practice in Iran: a questionnaire-based report. *BMC Oral Health.* (2020) 20:1–9. doi: 10.1186/s12903-020-01341-x
28. Bakaeen LG, Masri R, AlTarawneh S, Garcia LT, AlHadidi A, Khamis AH, et al. Dentists' knowledge, attitudes, and professional behavior toward the COVID-19 pandemic: a multisite survey of dentists' perspectives. *J Am Dent Assoc.* (2021) 152:16–24. doi: 10.1016/j.adaj.2020.09.022
29. Alzyood M, Jackson D, Aveyard H, Brooke J. COVID-19 reinforces the importance of handwashing. *J Clin Nurs.* (2020) 29:2760–1. doi: 10.1111/jocn.15313
30. Israel S, Harpaz K, Radvogin E, Schwartz C, Gross I, Mazeh H, et al. Dramatically improved hand hygiene performance rates at time of coronavirus pandemic. *Clin Microbiol Infect.* (2020) 26:1566. doi: 10.1016/j.cmi.2020.06.002
31. Li G, Chang B, Li H, Wang R, Li G. Precautions in dentistry against the outbreak of corona virus disease 2019. *J Infect Public Health.* (2020) 13:1805–10. doi: 10.1016/j.jiph.2020.09.013
32. Alomari AH, Aga O, El Sahmarany L, Hegazi M, Almulla L. Public perception towards medical waste generated in the environment during the COVID-19 pandemic in Eastern Province, Saudi Arabia. *Heliyon.* (2021) 7:e08363. doi: 10.1016/j.heliyon.2021.e08363
33. Duruk G, Gümüşboga ZS, Çolak C. Investigation of Turkish dentists' clinical attitudes and behaviors towards the COVID-19 pandemic: a survey study. *Braz Oral Res.* (2020) 34:e054. doi: 10.1590/1807-3107bor-2020.vol34.0054
34. Gibson Miller J, Hartman TK, Levita L, Martinez AP, Mason L, McBride O, et al. Capability, opportunity, and motivation to enact hygienic practices in the early stages of the COVID-19 outbreak in the United Kingdom. *Br J Health Psychol.* (2020) 25:856–64. doi: 10.1111/bjhp.12426
35. West R, Michie S, Rubin GJ, Amlôt R. Applying principles of behaviour change to reduce SARS-CoV-2 transmission. *Nat Hum Behav.* (2020) 4:451–9. doi: 10.1038/s41562-020-0887-9
36. Schmidtke KA, Drinkwater KG A cross-sectional survey assessing the influence of theoretically informed behavioural factors on hand hygiene across seven countries during the COVID-19 pandemic. *BMC Public Health.* (2021) 21:1–14. doi: 10.1186/s12889-021-11491-4

25

Practical Applicability of Teledentistry in Pediatric Patients Amidst Pandemic

Mousumi Goswami [1*], *Tanu Nangia* [1], *Aditya Saxena* [1], *Sakshi Chawla* [1], *Anam Mushtaq* [1], *Shrey R. Singh* [2] *and Palak Jain* [1]

[1] I.T.S Dental College, Hospital and Research Centre, Noida, India, [2] School of Medical Science and Research, Sharda University, Noida, India

***Correspondence:**
Mousumi Goswami
mousumi87goswami@gmail.com*

The coronavirus disease-2019 (COVID-19) pandemic has imposed a situation where all healthcare facilities except emergency services remain suspended. These times generated the necessity for the implementation of a healthcare delivery system that can be accessed digitally and, thus, benefit the majority of children as well as healthcare professionals. This review aims to propose a sound model of less technique sensitive, safe and handy strategies for dental traumatic injuries, endodontic and restorative concerns, and orthodontic urgencies until complete clinical help can be sought. Five hundred thirty articles were obtained from the PubMed, Google Scholar, Embase, Lilacs, and Cochrane databases published from 2011 to 2021. Nineteen articles that described teledentistry in the COVID-19 era were included. Teledentistry can serve as a vital patient management strategy that can aid in triaging urgent and elective patient treatment needs, ultimately easing the burden of clinics and at the same time providing a safer means of consultation.

Keywords: teledentistry, telehealth, teleconsultation, pediatric dentistry, COVID-19

INTRODUCTION

Dentistry has been considered as the most susceptible profession to get affected by the COVID-19 pandemic, as it involves close inspection, examination, diagnosis, and therapeutic interventions around the naso-oropharyngeal region (1). This enormously aggressive novel coronavirus SARS CoV-2, whose epicenter was Hubei province in China, was declared as a health emergency of global concern by the World Health Organization (WHO) on January 30, 2020 (2). Around the world, even after 1 year, people are still experiencing suspension of ongoing dental practices except for addressing emergent needs (3–5). A rising number of pediatric cases of COVID-19 infection with greater severity and higher risk of transmission have been seen in the second wave of the pandemic (6, 7). This has made it imperative for pediatric dentists to be vigilant in triaging, assessing, and managing patients.

During these difficult times, adapting a telehealth model has been the most sound approach practiced by all nations to manage patients presenting with health problems during lockdown and otherwise. Advisories also focus on managing the majority of patients affected by COVID-19 within the home under the supervision of a treating doctor *via* telehealth (8). In dentistry, this approach has been proven to be successful, as it satisfies social distancing norms and allows halting the transmission of the virus to contain its spread.

Teledentistry has been defined by Cook in 1997 as "the practice of using video-conferencing technologies to diagnose and advice about treatment over a distance" (9, 10). Teledentistry, a form of telehealth comprising of a synergism between telecommunications and dentistry that involves the exchange of clinical derived information and relevant images for consultation and treatment planning.

The concept has proven to be a boon for the continuous delivery of necessary healthcare services during difficult situations of the pandemic (11). Innovations in the form of mobile applications and other technical developments have eased the learning and referral protocol necessary to minimize direct contact between patients and doctors.

METHODOLOGY

An electronic search from databases of PubMed, Google Scholar, Embase, Lilacs, and Cochrane was conducted for articles published from 2011 to June 2021. The use of MeSH terms "teledentistry", "teledentistry" AND "COVID-19" yielded a total of 530 articles (Pubmed: 256, Google scholar: 270, and Embase *via* Cochrane: 2) out of which 211 duplicates and 5 non-English publications were removed. Screening of the remaining 314 articles was performed based on title and abstract, and the articles were sought for retrieval. Full texts of only 147 articles were retrieved and screened for further eligibility. Articles published as reviews, systematic reviews, meta-analysis, observational studies, and randomized clinical trials were included while those published as case reports, books or documents, and conference proceedings were excluded. The exclusion was also made after screening based on relevance to dentistry, pediatric or general dentistry, triaging of patients, guidelines, protocol, and reviews from clinical experience. Out of the 147 articles, 19 that described a practical implementation of teledentistry service in the COVID-19 era were selected for the review (3–5, 8, 11–25). Refer to the flowchart in **Supplementary Figure 1**.

Types of Teledentistry

1. **Two-Way Interactive or Real-Time Consultation/ Synchronous**
   Real-time consultation caters to video conferencing between a dentist and a patient with simultaneous exchange of information, medical history, and reports in order to reach a diagnosis within the same appointment. It also aids in the prompt exchange of information and reporting with a peer dentist or specialist. Two- way interactive technology allows procuring live images or sound occurring in an originating site to a person in a remote or distant site (26–31).
2. **Store and Forward Teledentistry/Asynchronous**
   Information is gathered from one location, stored, and transferred to the treating consultant in a different location. Relevant data in the form of x-rays, photographs, and scanned images are uploaded and forwarded to the consultant after screening or storing it in the system.
   This system is beneficial for consulting a specialist/team from a different place/city/country before referring or managing the patient. The data can be used to educate colleagues after obtaining a prior consent. A pattern of asynchronous consultation is also available on many webpages for fetching a potential diagnosis by entering serology or pathology reports (30, 31).
3. **Remote Monitoring of Patient**
   Information on health and other medical data are transmitted from one location to another *via* electronic media for healthcare and supportive management.
4. **Mobile Health (mHealth)**
   The use of mobile communication devices to support public health practice and education by using devices such as cell phones, tablets, computers, and personal digital assistants (PDAs).

Telehealthcare Model

Teletriaging

Categorizing patients based on the urgency of treatment can be managed by teletriage. The dental team or front office can characterize if the case of a patient is elective or emergent. Emergent cases can be prioritized, and elective cases can be scheduled at a convenient time for teleconsultation, and appointments can be postponed to a more appropriate time (12). "Forward triage" helps to reduce the workload of a caregiver by managing non-emergent patients before they visit a hospital (32, 33). It foresees any crisis that can occur and prevents unnecessary movements in times of pandemic.

Teleconsultation

Interactive consultation with a clinician by telephonic or video conferencing is the prime component of the telehealth model. Consultation with a specialist can also be included if the software allows multiple participants at a time. Exchange of chief complaint, medical history, recent and previous laboratory reports, extraoral photographs, intraoral photographs, dental cast photographs, and radiographs, and examination by virtual appointments comprises a teleconsultation.

Telediagnosis

Analysis of collected information in teleconsultation leads to formulation of a diagnosis. The appropriate diagnosis and devised treatment plan are projected to the patient. Efforts were made in the past by Haron et al. to develop "Mobile Mouth Screening Anywhere (MeMoSA®)" for detection of oral cancer (34). Limited access to specialist has also lead to the development of tablet based mobile microscope (Cellscope Device) as an adjust to oral cancer screening (35).

Telemonitoring

Follow-ups and routine checkups in dentistry have always been of less priority among patients. Monitoring of postoperative cases with the help of telecommunication can be effectively carried out. Taking the help from scheduled telephonic calls, video conferencing, or merely by filling e-forms about resolution of symptoms can pave the way for sound dental health and can anticipate any treatment failure to occur (36).

Applicability in Pediatric Dentistry

The American Academy of Pediatric Dentistry (AAPD) recognizes COVID-19 as an ongoing community and global problem with ever increasing number of cases among children and have, thereby, added a COVID-19 resource page in the recent reference manual, AAPD 2020–2021 namely "Re-emergence A Report on Pediatric Dental Practice Re-entry into Practice During the COVID-19 Pandemic" (13), also holds the statement for parent-FAQ (37). It also highlights the implementation of public health initiatives and the impact on oral healthcare delivery during the suspension of dental practice.

Adoption of teledentistry in daily practice:

1. Conduction of regular virtual continuous dental education programs and webinars for dentists to appraise various recent software and technological platforms as a medium for practicing teledentistry.
2. Dissemination of approaches for adequate management by dentists can be delivered by hospital-based software with stepwise triaging of patients. The hospital-based software can also be converted into a self-help application with which patients can direct themselves according to their chief complaint and acquire help from a specialist by scheduling a call or initiating a conversation. Another approach of providing management options can be applicable in private dental practices where patients can talk to their treating doctors directly for help.

Pediatric patients may have a variety of treatment needs that requires definitive operative, endodontic, orthodontic, or surgical intervention in a dental clinic/hospital. We propose a model of teledentistry-assisted management of pediatric dental problems during the COVID-19 pandemic that can be augmented with video-based and live teleconsultation demonstrations in order to minimize the need for dental clinic visits. It includes at-home recommendations for non-emergency concerns that can be disseminated *via* teleconsultation mode for parents and caregivers.

The main aim of this approach is to provide help during the pandemic when patients are unable to seek definitive treatment at the professional level because of the risk of infection, overburdened hospitals, and unavailability of functioning dental offices during lockdowns. The proposed specific problem-oriented management model is described in **Tables 1, 2.** These tables describe proposed advice and possible modified management based on established guidelines. It must not replace the definitive treatment required for a patient in a dental clinic that involves thorough clinical examination and adjunctive tests for accurate diagnosis and treatment plan (14, 38–47).

Recent Evidence of Teledentistry

As the dynamics of the pandemic are changing with time, the acquisition of updated knowledge of the usage and practical applications as well as challenges of teledentistry is important before designing any robust model of action. According to a survey by Dusseja et al. almost 70.7% of respondents were unwilling to visit dental clinics during the COVID-19 pandemic, and 80.5% of the participants were in favor of teledentistry to resolve their dental problems. Out of them, 58% of the responders received prescriptions *via* WhatsApp, 35% through telephone, 5% through video call, and 2% *via* e-mail and other means (17). Similarly, in a study by Davies et al. findings show that over 50% of photographic referrals resulted in either advice or antibiotics being prescribed, without the need for face-to-face contact. Over 70% of the images received during the study period were related to children aged 10 and under, and the majority related to swelling, pain, and dental trauma (18). Furthermore, a survey by Statista reports that 97% of those between the ages of 16 and 54 yr now own a smartphone with the capability to take photographs and send email (48).

In a survey by Rahman et al., patient satisfaction was evaluated along with ease of use, effectivity in accessing clinical services, and reliability of the teledentistry system; 94% of the respondents were satisfied with telephonic consultation and willing to utilize it in the future. Majority of the respondents were able to express themselves satisfactorily and clearly (19). A recent study from Google interest trends on self-medication during the COVID-19 pandemic depicted an increase in the number of searches regarding self-medication, which indicates the need to reach out to the population in different ways, one of which can be through teledentistry, as reported by Sen Tunc et al. (20).

A few more acceptance-oriented studies have achieved good responses with teledentistry consultation for pain as well as for monitoring and follow-ups. Teledentistry has been beneficial in various fields, such as orthodontics, maxillofacial surgery, and pediatric dentistry (21–23).

Barriers in the Use of Teledentistry

1. Technology: The complexity of technology might make it difficult for clinicians to accept teledentistry, as they may be hesitant to learn and adopt a new skill.
2. Practical implications: Inability to perform a tactile examination of lesion/oral cavity and two-dimensional pictures, and improper evaluation of interproximal contact and posterior-most teeth might offer a limitation in accurate diagnosis (24). Clinicians might get afraid of making a wrong diagnosis and inappropriate treatment plan.
3. Communication: Patient acceptance due to lack of in-person communication may hamper in adopting a devised treatment plan, although many surveys being conducted support the gaining popularity of teledentistry (17–20, 48).
4. Rural setting: Lack of infrastructure such as internet connectivity, computer or smartphone, x-ray machine and other advance armamentarium to help in diagnosing the tooth/lesion, providing it to the patient or transferring to a specialist at different location (25).
5. Privacy: The lack of privacy of transferred information may be a roadblock in gaining the confidence of patients, although the law for breach in privacy of a patient without his/her consent is strict. It is advised to all healthcare workers and portals working for telehealth to obey the Health Insurance Portability and Accountability Act (HIPAA)[1].

[1]Available online at: https://www.cdc.gov/phlp/publications/topic/hipaa.html. (accessed July 06, 2021).

TABLE 1 | Management of common pediatric dental problems.

Table 1: MANAGEMENT OF COMMON PEDIATRIC DENTAL PROBLEMS

COMMON PEDIATRIC DENTAL CONCERNS [26,27,28,29]

Teething problems

- Maintain oral hygiene.
- Clean gums regularly after each meal using clean moistened cotton guaze/cloth.
- Advise using cold -non sweetened teething rings/pacifiers to relieve discomfort .

Exfoliating/ Mobile tooth

- Assist in at home extraction/ removal of tooth .
- Apply topical anaesthetic gel (Available online) .
- Hold the tooth with clean guaze piece/sterile cotton, twist and pull out.
- Arrest bleeding by pressure gauze.
- Advise post-extraction instructions : Biting down on guaze for at least 30-40 mins, avoid hard or hot foods and avoid spitting for 24 hours.
- Prescribe analgesics (available online)
- Use of orthodontic elastic/elastic module (available online) around the tooth * may be considered to stimulate exfoliation in over - retained teeth.

Oral ulcers

- Identify the cause of ulcer. Virtual diagnosis by the dentist.
- Avoid spicy and hot foods
- Application of lignocaine based topical anaesthetic gel or glycerin over the area.
- Maintain oral hygiene by brushing twice daily and mouthrinsing after every meal.

Decementation/ Accidental swallowing of crown/restoration

- Do not attempt to fix the dislodged crown.
- If swallowed, usually crowns go into the gastrointestinal tract and pass out eventually.
- In case of choking : Induce coughing or attempt Heimlich Maneouver.*
- Visit Emergency service if choking persists.

*Video based consultation and assistance can be more effective.

CARIOUS LESION & LESION INVOLVING PULP [30,31,32,33,34]

Initial cavity/Blackspot/ Discoloration

- Non-restorative cavity control (NRCC) which involves:
- Proper brushing twice daily with fluoridated toothpaste.*
- Dietary modification.
- Flouride mouth rinse/ Self applied topical fluoride gels.(Available online)

Considerably deep cavitated lesion

Asymptomatic:

- Maintain oral hygiene with effective cleaning of cavitated tooth using intra-oral aids such as regular flossing and interdental brushes to avoid food lodgement.
- Follow NRCC protocol of topical fluoride use at home.
- Dietary modification

Symptomatic cavities (Pain/sensitivity) :

Dietary modification and maintenance of oral hygiene.

Mild-moderate and intermittent:

- Small cotton pellet soaked in clove oil may give temporary pain relief in cavities.
- Analgesic coverage as and when required till dental visit is feasible.

Severe and continous:

- Analgesics for immediate relief but schedule dental visit as soon as possible.

Dislodged restoration:

- Maintain oral hygiene.
- Pack teflon tape into the cavity or a clean cotton pellet soaked in clove oil (in case of pain or sensitivity) using a clean toothpick/ tweezer and change daily till dental visit is feasible.

Dental abscess :

- Teleconsultation for appropriate antibiotic and analgesic coverage.
- Advise warm saline rinses for swollen gums and soft tissue.
- Abstinence from any extraoral hot/cold fomentation.
- Maintain stringent oral hygiene.
- Follow up on teleconsultation and accordingly decide if emergency visit needs to be scheduled.
- Cellulitis/Facial swelling/ difficulty in swallowing: EMERGENCY DENTAL VISIT

Ongoing endodontic treatment

If intermediate restorative material is dislodged and root canals are exposed:

- Irrigate with chlorhexidine mouthwash / clean water using a syringe/ water flosser.
- Pack teflon tape or clean cotton pellet into the cavity and change daily till dental visit is feasible.

*Video based consultation, assistance and live demonstration for age appropriate tooth brushing can be more effective.

TABLE 2 | Management of common pediatric dental problems.

Table 2: MANAGEMENT OF COMMON PEDIATRIC DENTAL PROBLEMS

DENTAL TRAUMA [35,36]

Minor Soft Tissue Injury

Control Bleeding :

- Apply pressure with clean cotton/ guaze piece.
- If bleeding persists: Use moist tea bag to apply pressure.
- Analgesic for pain relief (Over the counter /Available online)

Tooth Fracture

Very small fractured segment- Non-painful:

- No emergency treatment required.

Considerable fracture of tooth crown:

- Use densensitizing paste.

In case of sharp tooth edges:

- Cover tooth w ith paraffin wax/ orthodontic wax (available online)*

OR

- Wrap tooth and cover edges with Teflon tape (PTFE) and change it regularly till the time dental visit is possible.*

Excessively Mobile tooth fragment:

- Apply topical anaesthetic gel (Available online)
- If possible; remove the mobile fragment with a clean gauze/cloth.

Displaced tooth / Luxation Injury :

- *Displacement without mobility:* Teleconsultation and regular follow-up required. Consider analgesics in case of pain and visit dental clinic when possible for a definitive treatment.
- *Displacement with mobility :*
  -Repositioning of permanent tooth can be attempted using finger pressure.*
  -Consider soft diet and analgesics till dental clinic visit is feasible (as soon as possible).

Knocked out tooth/ Avulsion:

- Assess whether tooth is milk tooth or permanent tooth via Teleconsultation.
- Attempt to reimplant permanent tooth only.
- Wash tooth under clean running water
- Try to put the tooth back in socket.*
- Ask the child to bite down on the clean cloth.
- Seek simultaneous Tele-help from dentist
- Store in cold milk/ coconut water if unable to replant tooth . Do not let it dry!
- **Visit dentist immediately.**

Jaw Fracture/ Bone fracture.

- Teleconsultation for immediate help.
- Try to control bleeding by pressure pack.
- **EMERGENCY DENTAL VISIT**

*Video based consultation, assistance and live demonstration for tooth repositioning and reimplantation can be provided. Advise maintenance of strict oral hygiene

PEDIATRIC ORTHODONTICS [37,38]

Broken space maintainers / appliances

- Attempt seating the orthodontic bands of appliances back on to the tooth. with finger pressure in case the appliance has de-cemented .
- Remove loose and completely broken appliances with sharp wire ends in order to avoid injury.
- In case of inability to remove damaged fixed appliance, cover sharp areas with orthodontic wax till help can be sought at dental clinic.
- Remove broken or debonded brackets .
- Stop usage of broken removable appliances.
- Elastic modules (available online) can be changed at home with the help of tweezer using video demonstrations during teleconsultation.*

Impinging wires and brackets

- Cover impinging bracket areas with orthodontic wax.
- Loose or debonded brackets to be removed.
- Attempt can be made at carefully clipping impinging wire ends using a nail clipper (cleaned and sterlized at home).*

Accidental swallowing

- Swallowing of small component that does not cause choking/breathing problem or irritation does not require any intervention as it will eventually pass out via digestive tract.
- In case of choking :
  Induce coughing or attempt Hemlich Maneouver.*:
- If it doesn/t help : It is an **EMERGENCY SITUATION. Visit a doctor.**

*Video based consultation, assistance and live demonstration for removal or adjusting appliance can be done.

SUMMARY

Telemedicine has been widely used in the COVID-19 pandemic. Dentistry in the newer times does not only rely on technological advancements in terms of armamentarium and instruments but also ways to reach out to patients using convenient and advanced modes of communication media that include teleconsultation support anytime and anywhere as well as internet-based social media platforms for creating health awareness and disseminating valuable information to patients during times of crisis. Teledentistry can, therefore, serve as a vital patient management strategy that aids in triaging urgent and elective patient treatment needs, ultimately easing the burden of clinics and at the same time providing a safer means of consultation.

AUTHOR CONTRIBUTIONS

MG, TN, AS, SC, AM, SS, and PJ organized database, wrote first draft, sections of the manuscript, conception, and design of the study. All authors contributed to the manuscript revision, read, and approved the submitted version.

REFERENCES

1. Peng X, Xu X, Li Y, Cheng L, Zhou X, Ren B. Transmission routes of 2019-nCoV and controls in dental practice. *Int J Oral Sci.* (2020) 12:9. doi: 10.1038/s41368-020-0075-9
2. World Health Organization. Statement on the second meeting of the International Health Regulations (2005). Emergency Committee regarding the outbreak of novel coronavirus (2019-nCoV). Available online at: https://www.who.int/news-room/detail/30-01-2020-statement-on-the-second-meeting-of-the-international-health-regulations-(2005)-emergency-committee-regarding-the-outbreak-of-novel-coronavirus-(2019-ncov) (accessed May 15, 2021).
3. Amato A, Caggiano M, Amato M, Moccia G, Capunzo M, De Caro F. Infection control in dental practice during the COVID-19 pandemic. *Int J Environ Res Public Health.* (2020) 17:4769. doi: 10.3390/ijerph17134769
4. Duruk G, Gumusboga ZS, Colak C. Investigation of Turkish dentists' clinical attitudes and behaviors towards the COVID-19 pandemic: a survey study. *Braz Oral Res.* (2020) 34:e054. doi: 10.1590/1807-3107bor-2020.vol34.0054
5. Guo H, Zhou Y, Liu X, Tan J. The impact of the COVID-19 epidemic on the utilization of emergency dental services. *J Dent Sci.* (2020) 15:564–67. doi: 10.1016/j.jds.2020.02.002
6. Iftimie S, López-Azcona AF, Vallverdú I, Hernández-Flix S, de Febrer G, Parra S, et al. First and second waves of coronavirus disease-19: a comparative study in hospitalized patients in Reus, Spain. *PLoS ONE.* (2021) 16:e0248029. doi: 10.1101/2020.12.10.20246959
7. Brookman S, Cook J, Zucherman M, Broughton S, Harman K, Gupta A. Effect of the new SARS-CoV-2 variant B117 on children and young people. *Lancet Child Adolesc Health.* (2021) 5:9–10. doi: 10.1016/S2352-4642(21)00030-4
8. Monaghesh, E., Hajizadeh, A. The role of telehealth during COVID-19 outbreak: a systematic review based on current evidence. *BMC Public Health.* (2020) 20:1193. doi: 10.1186/s12889-020-09301-4
9. Fricton J, Chen H. Using teledentistry to improve access to dental care for the underserved. *Dent Clin North Am.* (2009) 53:537–48. doi: 10.1016/j.cden.2009.03.005
10. Cook J, ISDN. video conferencing in postgraduate dental education and orthodontic diagnosis. Learning Technology in Medical Education Conference. *CTI Med.* (1997) 1997:111–6.
11. Ghai S. Teledentistry during COVID-19 pandemic. *Diabetes Metab Syndr.* (2020) 14:933–35. doi: 10.1016/j.dsx.2020.06.029
12. Goswami, M. Chawla S. Time to restart: a comparative compilation of triage recommendations in dentistry during the Covid-19 pandemic. *J Oral Biol Craniofac Res.* (2020) 10:374–84. doi: 10.1016/j.jobcr.2020.06.014
13. American Academy of Pediatric Dentistry. Re-emergence Pediatric Dentistry Practice Checklist: A guide for re-entry into practice for pediatric dentists during the COVID-19 pandemic. Available online at: https://www.aapd.org/link/8a3864bdb3684db19145486aca0d4bcc.aspx (accessed May 15, 2021).
14. Martignon S, Cortes A, Douglas GV, Newton JT, Pitts NB, Avila V, et al. CariesCare International adapted for the pandemic in children: Caries OUT multicentre single-group interventional study protocol. *BMC Oral Health.* (2021) 21:329. doi: 10.1186/s12903-021-01674-1
15. Aziz SB, Kapoor P. Customized orthodontic triage during COVID-19 pandemic. *J Indian Orthodontic Soc.* (2020) 54:391–3. doi: 10.1177/0301574220963495
16. Luzzi V, Ierardo G, Bossù M, Polimeni A. Paediatric Oral Health during and after the COVID-19 Pandemic. *Int J Paediatr Dent.* (2021) 31:20–6. doi: 10.1111/ipd.12737
17. Dusseja SH, Rao D, Panwar S, Ameen S. Patients' views regarding dental concerns and tele dentistry during COVID-19 pandemic *Int J Sci Healthc Res.* (2020) 5:423–9. Available online at: https://ijshr.com/IJSHR_Vol.5_Issue.4_Oct2020/IJSHR_Abstract.0056.html
18. Davies A, Howells R, Lee SMG, Sweet CJ, Dominguez-Gonzalez S. Implementation of photographic triage in a paediatric dental, orthodontic, and maxillofacial department during COVID-19. *Int J Paediatr Dent.* (2020) 31:547–53. doi: 10.1111/ipd.12773
19. Rahman N, Nathwani S, Kandiah T. Teledentistry from a patient perspective during the coronavirus pandemic. *Br Dent J.* (2020) 229:1–4. doi: 10.1038/s41415-020-1919-6
20. Sen Tunc E, Aksoy E, Arslan HN, Kaya Z. Evaluation of parents' knowledge, attitudes, and practices regarding self-medication for their children's dental problems during the COVID-19 pandemic: a cross-sectional survey. *BMC Oral Health.* (2021) 21:98. doi: 10.1186/s12903-021-01466-7
21. Saccomanno S, Quinzi V, Sarhan S, Laganà D, Marzo G. Perspectives of tele-orthodontics in the COVID-19 emergency and as a future tool in daily practice. *Eur J Paediatr Dent.* (2020) 21:157–62. doi: 10.23804/ejpd.2020.21.02.12
22. Menhadji P, Patel R, Asimakopoulou K, Quinn B, Khoshkhounejad G, Pasha P et al. Patients' and dentists' perceptions of Tele-Dentistry at the time of COVID-19. A questionnaire-based study: Tele-dentistry at the time of COVID-19. *J Dent.* (2021) 13:103782. doi: 10.1016/j.jdent.2021.103782
23. Machado RA, de Souza NL, Oliveira RM, Martelli Júnior H, Bonan PRF. Social media and telemedicine for oral diagnosis and counselling in the COVID-19 era. *Oral Oncol.* (2020) 105:104685. doi: 10.1016/j.oraloncology.2020.104685
24. Smith AC, Thomas E, Snoswell CL, Haydon H, Mehrotra A, Clemensen J, et al. Telehealth for global emergencies: implications for coronavirus disease 2019 (COVID-19). *J Telemed Telecare.* (2020) 26:309–13. doi: 10.1177/1357633X20916567
25. Nuvvula S, Mallineni SK. Remote management of dental problems in children during and post the COVID-19 pandemic outbreak: a teledentistry approach. *Dent Med Probl.* (2021) 58:237–41. doi: 10.17219/dmp/133182
26. Jampani ND, Nutalapati R, Dontula BS, Boyapati R. Applications of teledentistry: a literature review and update. *J Int Soc Prev Community Dent.* (2011) 1:37–44. doi: 10.4103/2231-0762.97695
27. Clark GT. Teledentistry: What is it now, and what will it be tomorrow? *J Calif Dent Assoc.* (2000) 28:121–7.
28. Folke LE. Teledentistry. An overview. *Tex Dent J.* (2001) 118:10–8.
29. Farman AG, Farag AA. Teleradiology for dentistry. *Dent Clin North Am.* (1993) 37:669–81.
30. Bhambal A, Saxena S, Balsaraf SV. Teledentistry: potentials unexplored. *J Int Oral Health.* (2010) 2:1–6. doi: 10.1177/2229411220110105
31. Golder DT, Brennan KA. Practicing dentistry in the age of telemedicine. *J Am Dent Assoc.* (2000) 131:734–44. doi: 10.14219/jada.archive.2000.0272
32. Daniel SJ, Wu L, Kumar S. Teledentistry: a systematic review of clinical outcomes, utilization and costs. *J Dent Hyg.* (2013) 87:345–52.
33. Estai M, Kanagasingam Y, Tennant M, Bunt S. A systematic review of the research evidence for the benefits of teledentistry. *J Telemed Telecare.* (2018) 24:147–56. doi: 10.1177/1357633X16689433

34. Haron N, Zain RB, Ramanathan A, Abraham MT, Liew CS, Ng KG. m-Health for early detection of oral cancer in low- and middle-income countries. *Telemed J e Health.* (2020) 26:278–85. doi: 10.1089/tmj.2018.0285
35. Skandarajah A, Sunny SP, Gurpur P, Reber CD, D'Ambrosio MV, Raghavan N, et al. Mobile microscopy as a screening tool for oral cancer in India: a pilot study. *PLoS ONE.* (2017) 12:e0188440. doi: 10.1371/journal.pone.0188440
36. Mariño R, Ghanim A. Teledentistry: a systematic review of the literature. *J Telemed Telecare.* (2013) 19:179–83. doi: 10.1177/1357633x13479704
37. American Academy of Pediatric Dentistry. Talking to Parents about the COVID-19 Pandemic. Available online at: https://www.aapd.org/globalassets/media/covid-19/aapdparentfaq.pdf (accessed May 1, 2021).
38. Owais AI, Zawaideh F, Bataineh O. Challenging parents' myths regarding their children's teething. *Int J Dent Hygiene.* (2010) 8:28–34. doi: 10.1111/j.1601-5037.2009.00412.x
39. Regev E, Lustmann J, Nashef R. Atraumatic teeth extraction in bisphosphonate-treated patients. *J Oral Maxillofac Surg.* (2008) 66:1157–61. doi: 10.1016/j.joms.2008.01.059
40. Tarakji B, Gazal G, Al-Maweri SA, Azzeghaiby SN, Alaizari N. Guideline for the diagnosis and treatment of recurrent aphthous stomatitis for dental practitioners. *J Int Oral Health.* (2015) 7:74–80.
41. Vranić DN, Jurković J, Jeličić J, Balenović A, Stipančić G, Cuković-Bagić I. Medical Emergencies in Pediatric Dentistry. *Acta Stomatol Croat.* (2016) 50:72–80. doi: 10.15644/asc50/1/10
42. Fontana M. Nonrestorative management of cavitated and noncavitated caries lesions. *Dental Clinics.* (2019) 63:695–703. doi: 10.1016/j.cden.2019.06.001
43. Olcay K, Steier L, Erdogan H. Polytetrafluoroetylene tape as temporary restorative material: a fluid filtration study. *J IstanbUnivFac Dent.* (2015) 49:17–22. doi: 10.17096/jiufd.08659
44. Azim AA, Shabbir J, Khurshid Z, Zafar MS, Ghabbani HM, Dummer PM. Clinical endodontic management during the COVID-19 pandemic: a literature review and clinical recommendations. *Int Endod J.* (2020) 53:1461–71. doi: 10.1111/iej.13406
45. Jyoti BB. Phytotherapeutics in conservative dentistry & endodontics -a review. *J Conserv Dent.* (2005) 8:31–9. doi: 10.4103/0972-0707.42602
46. Fouad AF, Abbott PV, Tsilingaridis G, Cohenca N, Lauridsen E, Bourguignon C, et al. International Association of Dental Traumatology guidelines for the management of traumatic dental injuries: 2 avulsion of permanent teeth. *Dent Traumatol.* (2020) 36:331–42. doi: 10.1111/edt.12573
47. Bourguignon C, Cohenca N, Lauridsen E, Flores MT, O'Connell A, Day PF, et al. International Association of Dental Traumatology guidelines for the management of traumatic dental injuries: 1 Fractures and luxations. *Dent Traumatol.* (2020) 36:314–30. doi: 10.1111/edt.12578
48. O'Dea S.Smartphone Ownership in the United Kingdom (UK). 2012–2020, by Age. 2020. Available online at: www.statista.com/statistics/271851/smartphone-owners-in-the-united-kingdom-uk-by-age/. (accessed July 25, 2020).

26

Impact on Utilization and Shift in Treatment Needs Post-COVID Lockdown of Pediatric Dentistry in a Tertiary Care Hospital

Bhojraj Nandlal[1]*, Birti Singh[1] and Arun Gopi[2]

[1] Department of Pediatric and Preventive Dentistry, Jagadguru Sri Shivarathreeshwara Dental College and Hospital, Jagadguru Sri Shivarathreeshwara Academy of Higher Education and Research, Mysuru, India, [2] Department of Community Medicine, Jagadguru Sri Shivarathreeshwara Medical College and Hospital, Jagadguru Sri Shivarathreeshwara Academy of Higher Education and Research, Mysuru, India

***Correspondence:**
Bhojraj Nandlal
dr_nandlal@yahoo.com

Background: The COVID-19 pandemic has brought all treatments other than emergencies to a halt. Dental disease, being a multifactorial microbial disease, is capable of progressing to pulpits and its sequelae. The purpose of this study is to predict the impact of utilization of dental services and the progression of treatment needs in children during the lockdown and partial lockdown.

Methods: Outpatient department data from the year 2017–2019 from the Department of Pediatric and Preventive Dentistry, JSS Dental College was collected. A table of treatments provided was prepared. Utilization of services as care-seeking rates at 10, 25, and 50% were assumed and modeled corresponding to each stage of the lockdown using linear regression analysis. Dental caries progression was calculated as shifts in treatment needs from permanent restorations to temporary restorations, pulpectomies, or extraction, assuming a 10% progress to each sequela.

Results: The *p*-values for 10, 25, and 50% care-seeking rates were 0.021, <0.001, and <0.001, respectively.

Conclusion: The number and severity of cases were predicted to have increased. However, after removal of lockdown, it was noted that the number of patients seeking care was significantly less. The advancement in progression of dental disease further adds to the burden of society and caregivers.

Keywords: disease accumulation, COVID-19, dental caries, epidemiology, pediatric dentistry, disease progression

INTRODUCTION

Dental caries is a multifactorial microbial disease process caused by the bacterial metabolism of acids diffusing into hard dental tissues and dissolving the mineral content. It is progressive in nature involving the pulp followed by the dissolution of enamel and dentin, which may further progress to pulpitis and its sequelae (1). Caries prevalence in the children of India is as high as 70–80%. Pediatric dentistry is a specialized branch of dentistry catering to the dental needs of children and adolescents as well as that of special patients.

The novel coronavirus disease-2019 (COVID-19) pandemic due to severe acute respiratory syndrome virus-2 (SARS-CoV-2) was declared by WHO as an international concerning public health emergency on January 30, 2020, with Chinese horshoe bat being the source of origin (2). Its transmission is through droplet spread and contact routes, thereby increasing the risk of cross infection between dental professionals and patients (3). India, having the second largest population in the world with a underdeveloped healthcare system and a majority of the population following an unhygienic lifestyle, managed to follow a strict and early social distancing protocol during the lockdown (4).

The timeline of lockdown in India can be divided into four phases. Phase one began on March 25, 2020 and lasted for 21 days, followed by phase two beginning on April 15, 2020, and ending on May 3, 2020. Phase three and four beginning on May 4, 2020 and May 18, 2020, respectively lasted for 2 weeks each (5). Lockdown restrictions were partially lifted from June 1, 2020 onwards, with services being resumed in a phased manner; this was termed as unlock. Unlock 1.0 lasted the month of June followed by unlock 2.0 announced for the period of July with more ease in restrictions. Unlock 3.0 was further extended for the month of August followed by unlock 4.0.

The Ministry of Health and Family Welfare (MoHFW), Indian Dental Association (IDA), and the Dental Council of India (DCI) issued several guidelines for dental professionals allowing only emergency dental procedures which increased the risk of a patient to death. In children, acute pulpitis and unavoidable dental extractions were treated as "very high" risk. Modifications of dental operatories were also mentioned as per WHO and CDC guidelines. These restrictions ensued during the lockdown and unlock phases in light of the novel COVID-19 pandemic, which caused most activities to halt. This included all elective medical and dental procedures (6). With this regard, many medical and dental institutions including JSS Dental College and Hospital had shut their out-patient department (OPD) as of March 19, 2020, with only emergency procedures being performed. The beginning of March itself had warranted screening of in-patients and preferable postponement of elective procedures of new OPD patients. The lockdown that began on March 25, 2020 has created a large gap in the demand and supply operations as well as an increasing attention toward optimal patient management and treatment with available resources due to acute shortage of provision of routine dental treatments (7, 8). Treatments began upon beginning of the unlock phase in India in June with added infection control measures including personal protective equipment (PPE) kits in dentistry, a field with preexisting high standards of infection control.

The objectives for this study were set to compare the assumed care-seeking rates at 10, 25, and 50% to the actual rates upon the beginning of unlock period in India commencing on June 1, 2020, as well as to predict the treatment needs due to progression and accumulation of dental caries using linear regression analysis. This was carried out utilizing the average outpatient data for treatments done between the years 2017 and 2019 at the Department of Pediatric and Preventive Dentistry, JSS Dental College and Hospital. Such a prediction model would enable the department to be better prepared for the future in terms of resources and manpower, as literature states that children reporting for treatment are to be considered as potential carriers of the disease unless otherwise proven (9–11). This would further enable health care providers to reduce overcrowding in the out-patient area and improve scheduling of appointments so as to provide better quality patient care services. The care-seeking rates upon the beginning of unlock were to be reviewed as the impact of utilization of services due to the lockdown.

MATERIALS AND METHODS

This study was done in the Department of Pediatric and Preventive Dentistry at JSS Dental College and Hospital, Mysuru. It was designed as a retrospective observational study. Data used as sample population was the outpatient data records of the years 2017–2020. This data was retrieved from the Medical Records Department of JSS Dental College and Hospital. Analysis has been done cumulatively from 2017 to 2019 as well as individually for each of the treatment procedures.

Data from the department were retrospectively collected from monthly records of the Medical Records Department of the years 2017–2019 and used as database. Average out-patient (OP) numbers of the years 2017 to 2019 were modeled at 10, 25, and 50% using linear regression analysis to predict the expected number of treatments for the year 2020. These were compared with the actual OP numbers of 2020 coming to a halt during the lockdown and inflow during the unlock phase post the lockdown. These numbers represent the care-seeking rates of the pediatric population.

Data of the various treatment procedures done in the Department of Pediatric and Preventive Dentistry were tabulated for the years 2017–2019 on Microsoft excel spreadsheet into nine categories including temporary restorations (TEMP), indirect pulp capping (IPC), direct pulp capping (DPC), glass ionomer cement restorations (GIC), light cure composite restorations (LC), pulpectomies (PULPEC), permanent teeth root canal treatments (RCT), extractions of deciduous teeth (EXT), and extractions of permanent teeth (EXT) from the database. Data on cleft lip and palate management, orthodontic treatments, and trauma have been excluded from this analysis. The average number of treatments done from 2017 to 1019 were used in calculating the predictions of this study (**Table 1**). A linear regression analysis has been done to predict the expected number of treatment procedures during the lockdown and postlockdown period.

This research was approved by the Institutional Ethics Committee of JSS Dental College and Hospital (JSSDCH IEC Research Protocol No: 27/2020).

CALCULATIONS

Calculations for acquiring expected OP numbers were made assuming a possible turn up of 10, 25, and 50% corresponding to the end of May (lockdown phases one and two), June

TABLE 1 | Average OP statistics of the Department of Pediatric and Preventive Dentistry, JSS Dental College and Hospital, Mysuru.

Treatment	January	February	March	April	May	June	July	August	September	October	November	December
New OP	201	138	152	320	341	178	200	153	147	226	162	184
Old OP	787	722	486	725	850	619	592	501	395	507	438	582
Total OP	985	860	638	1,046	1,191	797	791	661	543	731	601	767
Treated OP	809	687	690	840	1,068	806	774	638	471	608	592	628
Temporary Restorations (TEMP)	60	59	58	72	62	60	49	55	35	74	86	113
Indirect pulp capping (IPC)	38	29	26	30	52	32	22	27	19	23	23	36
Direct pulp capping (DPC)	3	3	1	7	4	5	3	2	3	1	1	4
Glass ionomer cement (GIC)	170	151	137	210	247	168	188	161	109	143	125	159
Light cure composite (LC)	44	33	41	28	42	33	32	20	18	13	17	26
Pulpectomies (PULPEC)	23	42	43	40	53	48	33	39	25	30	41	63
Root canal treatment (RCT)—Permanent teeth	36	33	30	30	29	29	37	29	20	29	26	36
Extractions—deciduous teeth (EXT)	105	75	80	122	138	93	90	73	55	76	67	82[a]

[a]*Average OP statistics, Department of Pediatric and Preventive Dentistry, JSSDCH, Mysuru.*

TABLE 2 | Initial baseline prediction and possible care-seeking rates.

Treatment	May (Lockdown phases 1 and 2)			June (Lockdown phases 3 and 4)			September (Unlock 1.0–3.0)		
Turn up	10%	25%	50%	10%	25%	50%	10%	25%	50%
New OP	81	203	407	99	248	496	149	373	745
Old OP	206	515	1,031	268	670	1,340	417	1,042	2,084
Total OP	287	719	1,437	367	918	1,836	567	1,417	2,833
Temporary Restorations (TEMP)	19	48	96	25	63	126	39	98	195
Indirect pulp capping (IPC)	11	27	54	14	35	70	21	52	104
Direct pulp capping (DPC)	1	3	6	2	4	8	2	6	12
Glass ionomer cement (GIC)	60	149	298	76	191	382	122	305	610
Light cure composite (LC)	11	28	56	14	36	72	21	54	107
Pulpectomies (PULPEC)	14	34	68	18	46	92	28	70	141
Root canal treatment (RCT)—Permanent teeth	9	22	45	12	30	59	21	51	102
Extractions—deciduous teeth (EXT)	34	85	170	43	108	217	65	163	326

The initial baseline prediction and possible care-seeking rates as observed as utilization of pediatric dental services by patients modeled at 10, 25, and 30% care-seeking rates.

(lockdown phases three and four), and September (unlock 1.0–3.0), respectively (**Table 2**).

Dental caries progression was calculated as shifts in treatment needs, modeled on the following criteria:

1) A 10% progression of the treatments took place every month. A 10% progression was assumed as per observations of previous data from the department revealing an 8–10% shift in treatment needs.
2) The disease progressed such that there was a 10% shift in progression of the disease to the next treatment need as per the flow chart in **Figure 2** with the following: 10% temporary restoration progressed to IPC; 10% IPC progressed to DPC; 10% DPC to PULPEC and RCT. Ten percent GIC and LC progressed to temporary restorations; 10% of which moved to IPC followed by DPC and further followed by PULPEC and RCT. Ten percent of PULPEC and RCT shifted to deciduous and permanent teeth extractions, respectively (**Figure 1**).
3) The elective procedures were restricted in March 2020 while undertaking only emergency treatment as per government interim advisories; hence calculations on progression were made from March onwards.
4) Treatments were resumed upon unlock beginning in June 2020 with additional personal protective equipment.

The progression of treatment needs was calculated using linear regression analysis for the months of May, June, and September which corresponded with the end of lockdown phases one and

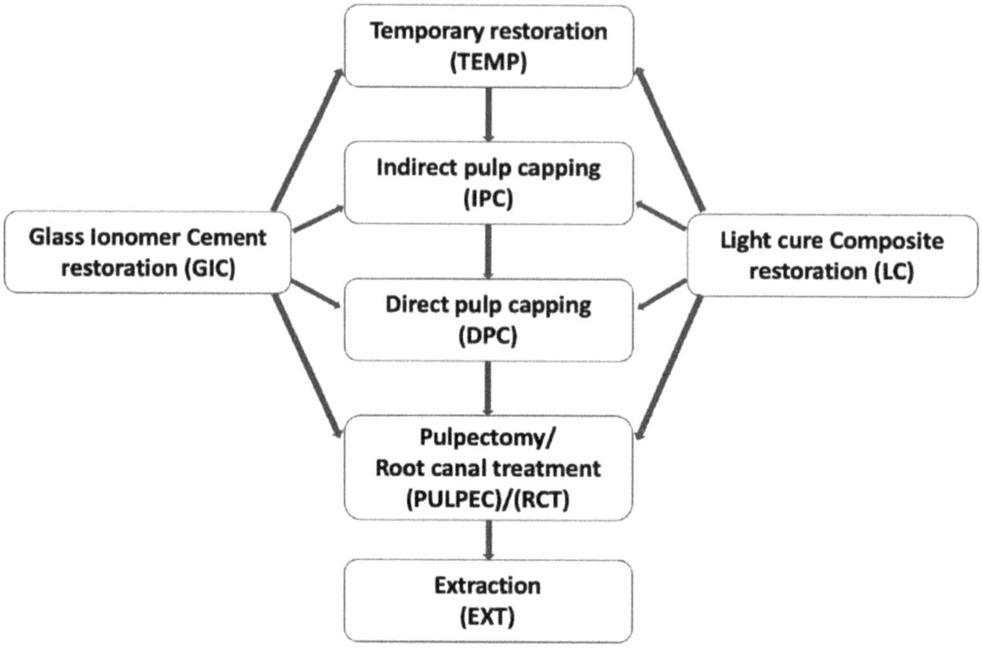

FIGURE 1 | Progression of Treatment Needs. The progression of dental caries as shift in treatment needs: 10% temporary restoration progressed to IPC; 10% IPC progressed to DPC; 10% DPC to PULPEC and RCT. 10% GIC and LC progressed to temporary restorations; 10% of which moved to IPC followed by DPC and further followed by PULPEC and RCT. Ten percent of PULPEC and RCT shifted to deciduous and permanent teeth extractions respectively.

TABLE 3 | Prediction of progression of treatment needs in pediatric dentistry.

Treatment	May average cases	Expected May 2020 cases	June average cases	Expected June 2020 cases	September average cases	Expected September 2020 cases
Temporary Restorations (TEMP)	62	249	60	303	35	597
Indirect pulp capping (IPC)	52	189	32	212	19	506
Direct pulp capping (DPC)	4	74	5	83	3	277
Glass ionomer cement (GIC)	247	390	168	559	109	425
Light cure composite (LC)	42	70	33	106	18	70
Pulpectomies (PULPEC)	53	157	48	223	25	372
Root canal treatment (RCT)—Permanent teeth	29	78	29	110	20	152
Extractions—deciduous teeth (EXT)	138	357	93	447	55	742
Extractions—permanent teeth (EXT)	0	12	0	9	0	52

Prediction of shift in treatment needs due to progression of dental disease modeled as per the assumptions taken in the study. The expected cases in progression of diseases as viewed due to accumulation and underutilization of services corresponding to various stages of the lockdown and unlock in India.

two; lockdown phases three and four; and unlock 1.0–3.0 in India, respectively. Further calculations were completed using Microsoft excel spreadsheet (**Table 3**). The calculations were then compared with the actual care-seeking rates upon beginning of unlock.

RESULTS

The average and expected care-seeking rates obtained on performing linear regression analysis of the Department of Pediatric and Preventive Dentistry are presented in **Table 2**, and comparison with the actual care-seeking rates upon the beginning of unlock period are presented in **Figure 2**, respectively. It can be noted that the expected care-seeking rates at 10, 25, and 50% for each month amount to a very high value that further increases as the number of untreated cases of previous months get accumulated. However, the actual care-seeking behavior can be observed to be lesser than the lowest assumed value of 10%, with slight improvement as the months progressed. Thus, it can be concluded that the number of patients seeking care and utilizing dental services are significantly lesser than those predicted to report to the pediatric department.

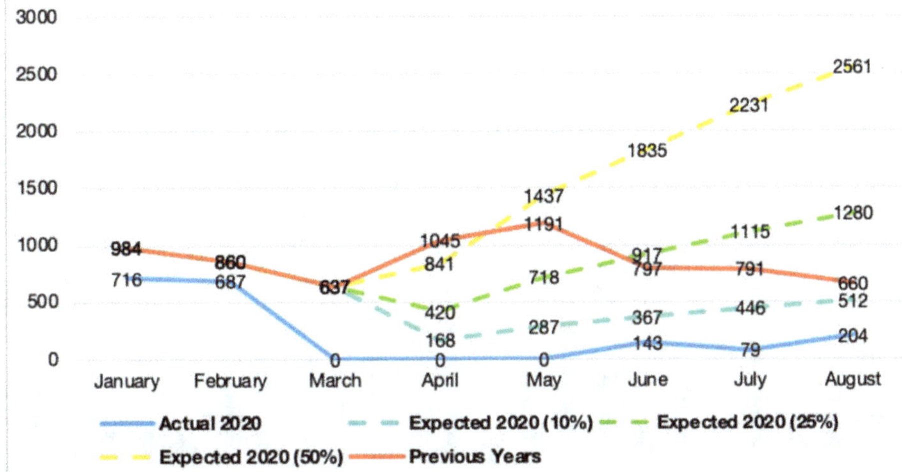

FIGURE 2 | Predicted and actual care seeking rates post the COVID Lockdown. The predicted and actual care-seeking rates as seen as outpatient numbers in the Department of Pediatric and Preventive Dentistry, JSS Dental College and Hospital, Mysuru. Previous year cases are the average values of OP numbers from the years 2017 to 2019. The predicted cases are modeled at 10, 25, and 50% using linear regression analysis. These are compared with the OP numbers of 2020 coming to a halt during the lockdown and inflow during the unlock phase post the lockdown. A statistically significant variation was observed in the number of actual and expected number of out-patients with the p-values 0.021, <0.001, and <0.001 for 10, 25, and 50%, respectively.

Chi square test for trend was performed to compare the actual and expected care-seeking rates (OP numbers) of 10, 25, and 50%. A statistically significant variation was observed in the number of actual and expected number of out-patients seeking dental treatment.

A tabulation of a shift in progression of treatment needs to the next sequela of pulpitis modeled on the predictive progression and accumulation of treatment procedure has been presented in **Table 3** for each procedure. A graph representing the progression and accumulation of treatment procedures for each of the lockdown and unlock stages considered in this study has been prepared (**Figure 3**). The prediction of progression of dental caries as the shift in treatment needs are noted to have increased with every stage of the lockdown, possibly due to the unavailability of treatment during the lockdown (expected 2020 progression) and underutilization of services post the lockdown (expected 2020 due to other treatment needs). Hence, this shift can be attributed to the unavailability (due to restriction of elective procedures by national and international advisories) and underutilization of dental services during the lockdown period.

An increase in the number of temporary restorations, indirect pulp capping, direct pulp capping, pulpectomies, and root canal treatments is seen due to the predictive progression and also the accumulation of newer cases at the end of each month. Whereas, an increase in the treatments requiring glass ionomer cement and light cure composite restorations occurred only due to the accumulation at the end of each month and not due to progression from any other treatment need. Extraction of deciduous and permanent teeth are also noted to have increased in number owing to their progression from pulpectomies and root canal treatments, respectively.

DISCUSSION

This study aims to predict the care-seeking rates, utilization, progression, and accumulation of treatment need in children in a tertiary care hospital during the lockdown and partial lockdown period in a tertiary dental hospital in Mysore city, India.

As per the data processed in this study, there has been a notable underutilization of all dental services in a tertiary care hospital setting post the lockdown due to the coronavirus pandemic. In the Department of Pediatric and Preventive Dentistry, an increase in the utilization of dental manpower was expected post the lockdown. However, the actual care-seeking rates are viewed to have dropped drastically owing primarily to the inherent fear and stigma associated with the virus spread. It was noted in China that despite the large scale transmission of the disease, the urgent dental treatment had decreased by only 38%, indicating the need for urgent dental treatment as an essential service (12).

In the pediatric setting, children are assumed to be potential carriers of the disease until proven otherwise thereby causing further underutilization of services (11). This is despite the lack of evidence that aerosols generated during dental treatment can lead to transmission of the virus (13). The fear of the spread of COVID due to aerosols generated during dental procedures caused several national and international bodies including WHO, CDC, IDA, DCI, and MoHFW to restrict all elective dental procedures. The risk of caries in children has increased compared with previous decades because of high sugar diets, sedentary lifestyles, and chronic health conditions (14). This may impact the pediatric population with a greater number of urgent dental treatments required for advanced dental conditions, including acute irreversible pulpitis and abscesses.

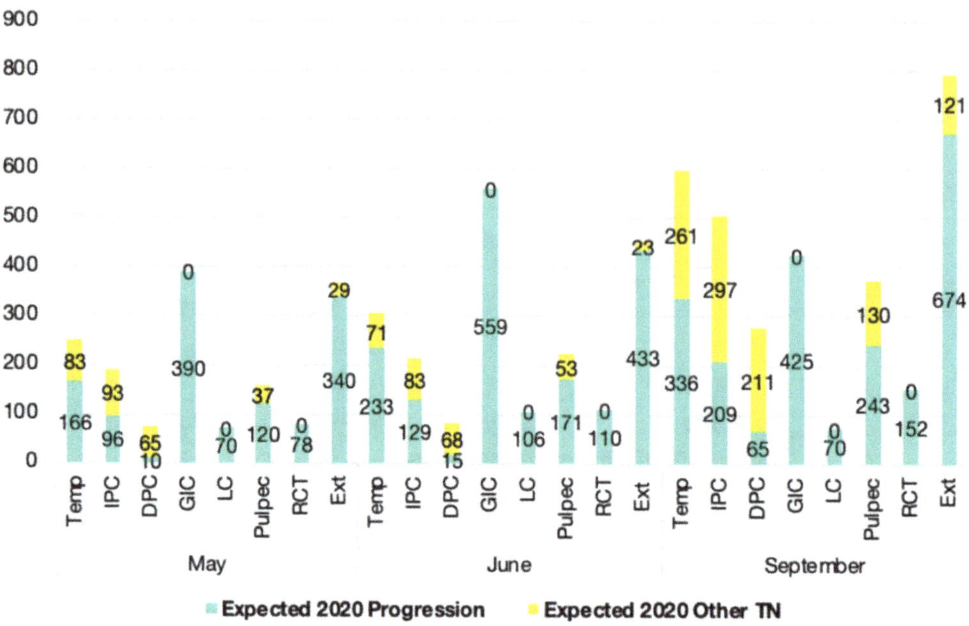

FIGURE 3 | Prediction of shift in progression of treatment needs. The prediction of progress of dental caries as shift in treatment needs are noted to have increased with every stage of the lockdown.

The shift in progression of treatment needs may have increased due to progression, accumulation as well as newer incoming cases owing to the inherent progressive nature of dental caries. However, various problems are associated with such an increase in number of cases advancing to pulpectomies as they require a specialist for the provision of treatment. This would create a load for the limited specialists, including post graduate students and staff. Further referral from local centers or private practitioners hesitant to work during an ongoing pandemic might increase the load.

According to an online survey conducted in the country, the preparedness of Indian dental professionals seemed inadequate during and after the pandemic due to professional as well as medico-legal concerns (15). A survey assessing the knowledge, attitudes, practices of practitioners regarding the current pandemic across various countries, including most Asian ones, found dentists having good knowledge and practice scores. These scores were found to be significantly associated with years of practice and qualifications (16). Another study done in the Indian scenario among dental health professionals to assess the knowledge, awareness, and hygiene practices showed notable deficiencies regarding some vital aspects of COVID-19. The authors recommended an urgent need for health education and training programs for improving the knowledge of dentists (17). A similar cross-sectional study was carried out to evaluate the knowledge, attitude, and practices along with the perceived barriers in practicing dentistry during the pandemic elicited poor median score for "knowledge." However, the "attitude" median score was observed to be good and "practices scores" for participants over 40 years of age were significantly better (18). These surveys indicate that health care professionals treating and not treating COVID-19 positive patients seem unprepared and urge the policymakers for better protocols. A model to assess the impact of lockdown and the disease transmission in India suggested a reduction in the transmission of the COVID-19 virus as well as in the burden on the health care system (19). At the time of writing this paper, we did not come across any study with respect to the accumulation or progression of disease states in pediatric dentistry.

A literature review on the current clinical practices in pediatric dentistry post COVID 19 concluded that behavior management would include a thorough explanation with regard to the professional dressing up in PPEs (20). Treatments avoiding aerosol procedures and those that incorporated minimally invasive procedures were sought to be preferred wherever possible (20). Hence, a change in the way routine pediatric dental treatments are managed may be seen with more focus on minimal interventional dentistry, atraumatic restorative treatments, application of fissure sealants, usage of silver diamine fluoride, and Hall technique (21, 22).

The increased number of cases in the dental operatory warrants a proper disinfection protocol with special personal protective gear for treatments generating aerosols and those not generating aerosols (21). Therefore, a structured pretreatment, treatment and posttreatment protocol need to be followed with proper hand hygiene, oral hygiene, and tele-dentistry practices for future implications (3, 23). An increased emphasis on disinfection and prevention of cross contamination with the use of preprocedural mouth rinses and environmental disinfection is warranted (20, 24). The Hospital was fully geared as per the interim guidance by WHO and other guidelines by MoHFW with PPEs, UV and chemical sterilizations, screening procedures, and triage. The dental hospital was also backed up with the Medical Hospital in case of any emergency. Despite the increased preparedness, a fall in the care-seeking rates was noted in this study.

CONCLUSION

Although there is plenty of literature around the biosafety of dental practices in pediatric dentistry post COVID, none provides a perspective on the increased suffering due to the progression of dental caries and the pain it can cause. This in turn can have a decreased quality of life in children due to perceived pain leading to chewing difficulties. From this study, it can be safely concluded that the care-seeking rates after removal of lockdown were lesser than the assumed 10% values in a tertiary health care hospital in Mysuru, a city in Southern Karnataka. The progression of dental disease as modeled in this study is significantly high with underutilization of services. This adds to the burden on society and the caregivers due to the progression of disease states and the increased cost of treatments. Thus, we urge the medical practitioners to help make patients aware of safe utilization of dental services at the appropriate time before further advancement of the disease occurs, leading to disability in children. The fear of cross infection is also advocated to be limited due to the high standards of infection control followed in the field of dentistry, which have improved further to avoid cross infection of the coronavirus as well.

LIMITATIONS

i. Gender and age distribution of data was missing electronically.
ii. Shift in treatment needs was assumed to be 10%, which may not be accurate due to the absence of direct literature on the same.
iii. Further studies are required to generalize the results to a global population.

AUTHOR CONTRIBUTIONS

All authors listed have made a substantial, direct and intellectual contribution to the work, and approved it for publication.

REFERENCES

1. Featherstone JDB. Dental caries: a dynamic disease process. *Aust Dent J.* (2008) 53:286–91. doi: 10.1111/j.1834-7819.2008.00064.x
2. Chen ZM, Fu JF, Shu Q, Chen YH, Hua CZ, Li FB, et al. Diagnosis and treatment recommendations for pediatric respiratory infection caused by the 2019 novel coronavirus. *World J Pediatr.* (2020) 16:240–6. doi: 10.1007/s12519-020-00345-5
3. Bhanushali P, Katge F, Deshpande S, Chimata VK, Shetty S, Pradhan D. COVID-19: changing trends and its impact on future of dentistry. *Int J Dent.* (2020) 2020:8817424. doi: 10.1155/2020/8817424
4. Paital B, Das K, Parida SK. Inter nation social lockdown versus medical care against COVID-19, a mild environmental insight with special reference to India. *Sci Total Environ.* (2020) 728:138914. doi: 10.1016/j.scitotenv.2020.138914
5. Rammohan A, Rela M. COVID-19: could India still escape?. *J Glob Health.* (2020) 10:1–4. doi: 10.7189/jogh.10.010372
6. The Lancet. *India Under COVID-19 Lockdown.* Lancet. (2020) 395:1315. doi: 10.1016/S0140-6736(20)30938-7
7. WHO. *Coronavirus Disease Case Report - 18 May 2020.* World Health Organization (2020) 2633 p.
8. Sharma N, Hasan Z, Velayudhan A, A EM, Mangal DK, Gupta SD. Personal protective equipment: challenges and strategies to combat COVID-19 in India: a narrative review. *J Health Manag.* (2020) 22:157–68. doi: 10.1177/0972063420935540
9. Mallineni S, Innes PN, Raggio DP, Robertson MD, Jayaraman J. Coronavirus disease (COVID-19): characteristics in children and considerations for dentists providing their care. *Int J Paediatr Dent.* (2020) 30:245–50. doi: 10.1111/ipd.12653
10. Mathur R. Ethics preparedness for infectious disease outbreaks research in India: a case for novel coronavirus disease 2019. *Indian J Med Res.* (2020) 151:124–31. doi: 10.4103/ijmr.IJMR_463_20
11. Al-Halabi M, Salami A, Alnuaimi E, Kowash M, Hussein I. Assessment of paediatric dental guidelines and caries management alternatives in the post COVID-19 period. A critical review and clinical recommendations. *Eur Arch Paediatr Dent.* (2020) 21:543–56. doi: 10.1007/s40368-020-00547-5
12. Guo H, Zhou Y, Liu X, Tan J. The impact of the COVID-19 epidemic on the utilization of emergency dental services. *J Dent Sci.* (2020) 15:564–7. doi: 10.1016/j.jds.2020.02.002
13. Epstein JB, Chow K, Mathias R. Dental procedure aerosols and COVID-19. *Lancet Infect Dis.* (2021) 21:e73. doi: 10.1016/S1473-3099(20)30636-8
14. Lamont RJ, Egland PG. Dental caries. *Mol Med Microbiol.* (2014) 3:945–55. doi: 10.1016/B978-0-12-397169-2.00052-4
15. Kinariwala N, Perera Samaranayake L, Perera I, Patel Z. Concerns and fears of indian dentists on professional practice during the coronavirus disease-2019 (COVID-19) pandemic. *Oral Dis.* (2020). 730–732. doi: 10.1111/odi.13459
16. Kamate SK, Sharma S, Thakar S, Srivastava D, Sengupta K, Hadi AJ, et al. Assessing knowledge, attitudes and practices of dental practitioners regarding the covid-19 pandemic: a multinational study. *Dent Med Probl.* (2020) 57:11–7. doi: 10.17219/dmp/119743
17. Gambhir RS, Dhaliwal JS, Aggarwal A, Anand S. Covid-19: a survey on knowledge, awareness and hygiene practices among dental health professionals in an Indian scenario. *Rocz Państwowego Zakładu Hig.* (2020) 71:223–9. doi: 10.32394/rpzh.2020.0115
18. Singh KT, Mishra G, Shukla AK, Behera S, Tiwari AK, Panigrahi S, et al. Preparedness among dental professionals towards COVID-19 in India. *Pan Afr Med J.* (2020) 36:1–7. doi: 10.11604/pamj.2020.36.108.23694
19. Ambikapathy B, Krishnamurthy K. Mathematical modelling to assess the impact of lockdown on COVID-19 transmission in India: model development and validation. *J Med Internet Res.* (2020) 6:e19368. doi: 10.2196/preprints.19368
20. Sales SC, Meyfarth S, Scarparo A. The clinical practice of Pediatric Dentistry post-COVID-19: the current evidences. *Pediatr Dent J.* (2021) 31:25–32. doi: 10.1016/j.pdj.2021.01.002
21. Cianetti S, Pagano S, Nardone M, Lombardo G. Model for taking care of patients with early childhood caries during the SARS-CoV-2 pandemic. *Int J Environ Res Public Health.* (2020) 17:1–17. doi: 10.3390/ijerph17113751
22. BaniHani A, Gardener C, Raggio DP, Santamaría RM, Albadri S. Could COVID-19 change the way we manage caries in primary teeth? Current implications on Paediatric Dentistry. *Int J Paediatr Dent.* (2020) 30:523–5. doi: 10.1111/ipd.12690
23. World Health Organization. *Considerations for the Provision of Essential Oral Health Services in the Context of COVID-19: Interim Guidance.* (2020). 1–5 p.
24. de Amorim LM, Maske TT, Ferreira SH, Dos Santos RB, Feldens CA, Kramer PF. New post-COVID-19 biosafety protocols in pediatric dentistry. *Pesqui Bras Odontopediatr Clin Integr.* (2020) 20:1–9. doi: 10.1590/pboci.2020.117

27

COVID-19 Impact on Community-Based Participatory Randomized Controlled Trials—Lessons from the Oral Health Disparities in Children Consortium

Francisco J. Ramos-Gomez[1,2†], Molly A. Martin[3†], Suchitra S. Nelson[4†], Belinda Borrelli[5†], Michelle M. Henshaw[6†], Shelley Curtan[4], Helen E. Lindau[1], Nicolle Rueras[5], Anna S. Sandoval[3] and Stuart A. Gansky[2,7†]*

[1] Department of Pediatric Dentistry, University of California, Los Angeles, Los Angeles, CA, United States, [2] Center to Address Disparities in Children's Oral Health (CAN DO), University of California, San Francisco, San Francisco, CA, United States, [3] Institute for Health Research and Policy, University of Illinois Chicago, Chicago, IL, United States, [4] Department of Community Dentistry, Case Western Reserve University, Cleveland, OH, United States, [5] Center for Behavioral Sciences Research, Henry M. Goldman School of Dental Medicine, Boston University, Boston, MA, United States, [6] Global and Population Health, Henry M. Goldman School of Dental Medicine, Boston University, Boston, MA, United States, [7] School of Dentistry, University of California, San Francisco, San Francisco, CA, United States

***Correspondence:**
Stuart A. Gansky
stuart.gansky@ucsf.edu*

† These authors have contributed equally to this work

The COVID-19 pandemic has had a major impact on nearly every sector of science and industry worldwide, including a significant disruption to clinical trials and dentistry. From the beginning of the pandemic, dental care was considered high risk for viral transmission due to frequent aerosol-generating procedures. This resulted in special challenges for dental providers, oral health care workers, patients, and oral health researchers. By describing the effect that the COVID-19 pandemic had on four community-based randomized clinical trials in the Oral Health Disparities in Children (OHDC) Consortium, we highlight major challenges so researchers can anticipate impacts from any future disruptions.

Keywords: COVID-19, pandemic (COVID-19), clinical trials, community-based participatory research, dentistry, behavioral science, health disparities, health inequities

INTRODUCTION

In the beginning of the COVID-19 pandemic, roughly 80% of non–COVID-related trials were interrupted or stopped (1). The nature of COVID-19, a highly contagious respiratory virus spread *via* respiratory droplets, requires handwashing, masking, and social (physical) distancing—even with quarantines—to prevent viral spread. These measures create many complications for clinical trials with in-person visits for intervention delivery and/or data collection (2, 3). From the beginning of the pandemic, dental care was considered high risk for viral transmission due to aerosol-generating procedures that are frequently used. Dental providers and oral health care workers were at high risk for both being infected by, and spreading, COVID-19. This risk carried over into dental research.

TABLE 1 | Overview of challenges by domain for the 4 OHDC Consortium trials.

	BEECON	COOP	iSmile	PACT
Change in timeline	X	X	X	X
Increased retention	X		X	
Challenges to obtaining PPE		X	X	
Change to participant compensation		X	X	
Extended data collection windows	X	X	X	X
Change to data collection protocols	X	X		X
Change to handling missing data and change in analytic plan			X	

The Oral Health Disparities in Children (OHDC) Consortium is composed of four separate trials focused on the oral health of US children. All trials receive support from a single Coordinating Center (CC) that provides data acquisition and quality assurance services. The OHDC Consortium reflects the National Institute for Dental and Craniofacial Research's (NIDCR) efforts to support research using community engagement to answer scientific questions. Each study addresses various health determinants and risk factors at multiple influence levels, such as individual, family, community, organization/institution, health services, and public policy.

The four OHDC Consortium trials include the BEhavioral EConomics for Oral health iNnovation (BEECON) trial (ClinicalTrials.gov registration number NCT03576326), the Coordinated Oral Health Promotion Chicago (CO-OP) trial (NCT03397589), the Interactive Short Messages to Initiate Lasting Education (iSmile) trial (NCT03294590) and the Pediatric Providers Against Cavities in Children's Teeth (PACT) trial (NCT03385629). The BEECON trial tests financial incentives for families to improve oral health behaviors that could prevent early childhood caries. BEECON is conducted jointly by University of California San Francisco (UCSF) and University of California Los Angeles (UCLA), with participants in Los Angeles County, CA (4). The CO-OP trial tests a family-focused community health worker program. CO-OP Chicago is led by the University of Illinois at Chicago (UIC) with participants from Cook County, IL (5). The iSmile trial tests an interactive, automated, and customized parent-targeted text message program to improve oral health among children attending urban pediatric clinics. iSmile is led by Boston University, Henry M. Goldman School of Dental Medicine (BU-GSDM) with participants in Boston, MA (6). The PACT trial tests bundled practice- and provider-level interventions in primary care that include oral health education, referral to dental care, and integrating oral health assessment into electronic health records. PACT is conducted by Case Western Reserve University (CWRU) in Cleveland, OH (7).

While all four OHDC Consortium community-based prevention trials had already completed enrollment before COVID-19 began to spread widely in the USA, the pandemic greatly disrupted in-person follow-up visits that were integral to collecting primary outcome variables (e.g., oral health examinations to assess dental caries, dental plaque assessments). This paper aims to discuss the impact that the COVID-19 pandemic had on conducting the OHDC Consortium trials specifically, and on community-based participatory research, in general. Moreover, this paper provides recommendations for modifying community-based research during future unforeseen disruptions.

MATERIALS AND METHODS

Data Collection and Analysis

In March, the states in which the studies were conducted (California, Illinois, Ohio, and Massachusetts) implemented stay-at-home orders which required the OHDC Consortium trials to pause in-person visits. All projects had to cease in-person research in March due to the shut-down, but each project had very different timelines for restart given the various approvals required at universities and at external sites. From February 2020 through January 2021, the standing monthly OHDC Consortium Steering Committee (SC) meeting of Principal Investigators (PIs) and lead staff from each trial, the CC, and NIDCR project scientists became an important virtual venue to discuss the impacts of COVID-19 on trial operations and shared strategies for how to address pandemic-caused interruptions. Based on information documented during these discussions, COVID-19 specific barriers and strategies were compiled to describe the main issues the OHDC Consortium SC identified. Staff from the CC distributed the notes that were compiled and each study team contributed to the list of barriers and strategies. Then the PIs reviewed these qualitative data and consolidated the information into four domains as shown in **Table 1**: timeline adjustments; data collection, retention, and analysis; logistical challenges; scientific challenges.

RESULTS

Domain 1: Timeline Adjustments (Table 2)

BEECON

All in-person clinical components were halted on March 16, 2020, when UCLA shut down research, following stay-at-home orders in Los Angeles County and remained halted until October 1, 2020, when clinic visits were approved to resume. BEECON text messages regarding the incentive intervention continued without impact during COVID-19. Visits occurred daily from October 1 to October 19 and then were approved to resume twice per week starting November 6. Subsequent holiday related surges in Los Angeles County caused clinic visits to be halted again from January 6, 2021 to February 25, 2021.

The reviewing IRB (UCSF) posted guidance about COVID-19 related study modifications not needing pre-approval in minimal risk studies, which included changes from in-person to remote data collection. No modification was required until the annual

TABLE 2 | Trial timelines and activities before and during COVID-19.

Trial	Area	2017	2018	2019	Q1/2020	Q2/2020	Q3/2020	Q4/2020	Q1/2021	Q2/2021	Q3/2021	Q4/2021	Q1/2022	Q2/2022
CO-OP	Chicago, IL		e+r	e+r	r r r	r r r	r r							
BEECON	Los Angeles, CA		e+r	e+r	r r r	r r r	r r r	r r r	r r r	r r				
PACT	Cleveland, OH	e	e+r	r	r r r	r r r	r r r	r r r	r r r	r r r	r r r	r r r	r r r	r
iSMILE	Boston, MA		e+r	e+r	e+r e+r r*	r r r	r r r	r r r	r r r	r r r	r r r	r r r	r r r	

e Enrollment/randomization.
e+r Enrollment/randomization and retention (follow-up visits).
r Retention (follow-up visits).
r During COVID—remote retention (follow-up visits).
r During COVID—partial remote retention (follow-up visits), some sites and/or some part of the month.
*Enrollment/randomization ended March 6, 2019 (pre-COVID shutdown).

Continuing Review since the changes did not increase participant risk. Therefore, where possible questionnaires that could be administered over the telephone were used so some data collection could continue, only pausing clinical visit portions of data collection (dental caries screening, plaque disclosing, plaque photograph, and fluoride varnish application). Study staff mailed participants supplies (toothbrush heads, tooth paste pumps, brushing calendars, and written materials). In January 2021, the trial submitted an IRB modification to extend the 12-month data collection visit window for an extra 90 days due to clinic closures caused by the winter COVID-19 surge in Los Angeles County.

CO-OP

The CO-OP timeline was delayed a total of 90 days. When UIC shut down on March 16, 2020, CO-OP Chicago had completed all intervention delivery and had follow-up data collection pending on only 38 of enrolled 420 participants. On April 19, 2020, CO-OP Chicago received IRB approval extending data collection visit windows another 90 days. Starting April 21, 2020, the study team resumed data collection *via* phone, reaching 21 participants. One participant did not want any further data collection beyond the phone visit, 20 agreed to attempt the extended window period. When home visits clearly would not be in the best interests of staff and participants for the foreseeable future, CO-OP Chicago obtained IRB approval (on July 6, 2020) for families to complete the objective data collection themselves with trial staff supporting them by applying disclosing solution and using their smartphones to take photographs. The final data collection window then closed and all data collection subsequently ended August 20, 2020.

iSmile

In-person study visits were suspended on March 12, 2020, when the University halted all in-person research. The iSmile intervention is delivered electronically *via* text messages, so there was no disruption in intervention delivery. Because the original protocol included participant completion of online questionnaires remotely, this portion of the study was not affected by the shut-down. The primary outcome variable, however, is collected during in-person visits at four pediatric clinics, which each had a different timeline for resumption of research activities. In all cases, clinics resumed patient care but indicated that they needed to delay resumption of research. Before resuming research activities, iSmile staff had to obtain approval from both the University and from the medical campus of the University because it was clinical research conducted off-campus. The approval process required submission of different forms that detailed the precautions for participants and staff, including personal protective equipment (PPE), social distancing, travel, and scheduling.

Once approved, the team met with leadership from each clinic *via* Zoom to discuss restart guidelines and timelines. iSmile received approval to resume research at its first site on September 10, 2020, and its second on October 1, 2020. Due to the COVID-19 surge that began in late 2020, the January 1, 2021 start date to resume research at the third site was further delayed. During the pandemic, the final site underwent a merger which required new approvals be attained and agreements drafted, reviewed, and executed. Research restart is expected March 2021 in the final two sites. Importantly, different protocols have been required for each clinic regarding staff COVID-19 testing and vaccination, participant scheduling, participant COVID-19 screening, participant arrival, use of waiting rooms, and inter-participant intervals. Study visit windows were extended because of the lengthy suspension of in-person research activities.

PACT

The PACT study conducts in-person visits at the time children are seen for their well-child visits (WCVs). At the WCVs, the pediatricians/nurse practitioners deliver the intervention, and study staff complete questionnaires with parents and conduct the clinical dental screening examination for the child. Between March 20, 2020 and May 25, 2020, all in-person follow-up WCVs were paused in accordance with the CWRU, University Hospitals, and Ohio guidelines. When the shutdown began, 666 (65%) and 349 (6%) of 1,024 participants were seen for their subsequent Well Child Visit (WCV) 2 and 3. During this period, some participants were seen at WCVs that the study staff missed due to COVID-19 restrictions. However, questionnaire data were still collected by mailing paper forms for parents/caregivers to complete and return. US Postal Service delays during the pandemic were slightly more frequent for participants receiving forms and the study receiving completed forms from participants; however, this had a minor impact on data collection. In-person visits resumed on May 26, 2020. Again, due to staff being quarantined from October 5 to 19, 2020 all in-person WCVs were paused. The same protocol was followed to obtain questionnaire data for visits that were missed during this period. In-person visits resumed on October 20, 2020. Visit windows for the PACT study are ±3 months of the follow-up WCVs. In addition, the PACT protocol had specified from the beginning that visits may occur out-of-window and that the duration between visits will be accounted for in the analysis. Therefore, the necessity to extend the windows was not an issue with the PACT study.

Domain 2: Data Collection, Retention, and Analysis

Data Collection Innovations

The BEECON and CO-OP trials before COVID-19 had been collecting images of children's teeth after applying a disclosing solution to assess plaque. Research staff conducted this process in homes (CO-OP) and at the clinic (BEECON). Because in-home data collection could not resume before study follow-up would end, the CO-OP study delivered plaque disclosing solution and asked the parents to apply the solution and collect the images. Of the 20 families eligible, 6 completed the process and submitted adequate images for plaque assessment. The BEECON staff created infographics, educational videos, and other resources that would guide participants how to apply the disclosing solution and take plaque photographs, but did not ultimately use them due to the return to the clinic for in-person visits.

Retention Improvements

Before COVID-19, the BEECON trial relied on participants to come to clinic for data collection. With the COVID-19 modifications, the BEECON study saw a boost in retention as data collection was able to be completed telephonically. The iSmile trial had an increase in the number of 12- and 24-month self-report surveys that were completed during the stay-at-home order. Study staff in both trials had more time to devote to retention activities because in-person oral health assessments were suspended.

Furthermore, participants were more easily reached *via* text message and phone during the stay-at-home orders. In the PACT trial, retention rates were slightly decreased with some participants not returning questionnaires to the study team even with multiple calls to the participants. Also, even with WCVs resuming in June 2020, some parents were hesitant to schedule their children's WCVs or canceled visits. Consequently, this extended study windows for follow-up visits.

Missing Data

Before the COVID-19 pandemic, these trials expected that data would be missing at random (MAR) and the failure to complete the oral health examination would be expected to depend on participant characteristics. Due to the COVID-19 pandemic, the data would be missing completely at random (MCAR) because the clinics were closed and participants could not attend their visits; therefore, missing data are not dependent upon participant characteristics. During analysis, models will have to account for both types of missing data. These assumptions would then drive the choice of analytic model. For example, these trials cannot use inverse probability weighting to account for missing data because the weights are based on the propensity for missing data, and that changes occurred during the trial. Multiple imputation may be a better approach for analysis for these trials which is a departure from the original plan to do Inverse Probability Weighting (IPW).

Analysis Modifications

The BEECON trial modified data collection to allow for fewer data collection visits if more than one planned in-person data collection was missed during COVID-19. Final analyses for the primary endpoint of toothbrushing behavior will use the planned visit times. Final analyses of the secondary endpoints of caries screening and plaque from photo of disclosed F incisor teeth will use actual dates to account for the delays due to COVID-19. Final analyses for the CO-OP trial will be conducted both with and without the 21 participants whose data were collected after COVID-19 started due to concerns their data would not adequately represent their normal experiences. Due to the extended window for data collection, the iSmile trial will need to add a time-to-event analysis. For example, because a large number of participants could not complete their 24-month oral health examination within window, and because this is the primary outcome variable, iSmile expanded the window end date and will control for time since baseline in analyses. Time of the oral examination (months from baseline) will be included as a predictor since caries increases with age; for a logistic regression analysis predicting any caries, this adjusts for the chance of any caries increasing with oral examinations later than planned. For the primary analysis at 24 months, this is just another predictor. In longitudinal analyses assessing oral examination data from baseline, to 12–24 months, this could be a time-dependent covariate, reflecting the timing of the 12-month examination and the timing of the 24-month examination. The PACT study will use Medicaid data for its primary endpoint which will be available for almost all participants regardless of WCV attendance. The PACT study will have missing data for the secondary endpoints using questionnaire data. PACT will use actual time between baseline and follow-up visit to perform longitudinal analysis.

Domain 3: Logistical Challenges

The COVID-19 pandemic presented logistical challenges primarily related to personal protective equipment (PPE), participant compensation, and staffing that required changes to study protocols.

PPE and Risk of Aerosolization

Before COVID-19, BEECON trial PPE requirements for dental providers included surgical masks, safety glasses, disposable gowns, and gloves, while research assistants were not required to wear any PPE. To reduce aerosolization risk after COVID-19, the in-person data collection protocol was revised. Dental providers were instructed not to dip the toothbrush in water before removing the disclosing solution from the participating child's teeth to reduce possible aerosols. Dental providers instead used a dry toothbrush or gauze to remove the disclosing solution from the child's teeth. When in-person data collection resumed in October 2020, PPE requirements included disposable gowns, surgical masks, face shields, safety glasses, and gloves for both the dental providers and research assistants. Dental providers also wore surgical bonnets and had the option to wear N95 masks, which were not required because BEECON dental screenings are not aerosol-generating procedures. There were no issues obtaining necessary PPE for the BEECON Study.

The iSmile data collection protocol includes dry brushing the teeth before the oral health assessment; plus, the participants' young age frequently resulted in crying during the examination; both of these produce aerosols. A decision was made not to change the clinical examination protocol. Therefore, after COVID-19, the PPE required for the clinical examiners changed from surgical masks, disposable gowns, safety glasses, and gloves to also include an N95 mask covered with a surgical mask, face shield, surgical bonnet, and surgical booties.

The research assistants use the same PPE as the clinical examiners since maintaining a 6-foot distance from the participant was challenging when recording data. Parents with children also had to wear a surgical mask.

PPE, especially N95 masks, were not available when research was restarted due to limited global supply. This was one of the limiting factors in approval to resume in-person research visits.

PACT trial data collection was conducted in primary care clinics, but included a dental examination with tooth brushing with a potential risk of aerosolization. Shortly after returning to visits, primary care physicians did not have N95 masks available and therefore study staff had more PPE concerns. To avoid conflict, the study team changed the protocol to stop tooth brushing children and to use gauze to wipe teeth before examination, thereby reducing aerosolization risk. With this change, the hygienists were comfortable using a surgical mask, face shield, gowns, gloves to conduct the brief dental examination. Primary care clinics later changed their requirements with all study hygienists required to wear a N95 mask while examining the child.

The CO-OP trial completed data collection; therefore, it did not have to secure any PPE.

Participant Compensation Reimbursement

Before COVID-19, the BEECON trial provided $30 in grocery store gift cards to participants for attending clinic visits. When BEECON moved to telephonic data collection in March 2020, participants were offered electronic gift cards for payment immediately or participants could receive their grocery store gift cards at a later date when the clinic reopened. Reimbursement did not depend on completing plaque images to be collected at clinic visits later. The delay for clinic reopening became longer than expected, resulting in the BEECON team coordinating contactless delivery of grocery store gift cards to participants who had chosen that option.

In the CO-OP trial, reimbursement changed from cash at data collections to a check for the same amount that was sent *via* mail. Participants were reimbursed immediately after the telephone data collection and reimbursement was not dependent on completing plaque images attempted later.

While the total amount of participant compensation remained constant in the iSmile trial, timing of the compensation changed during COVID-19. Before COVID-19, participants received a $60 gift card after completing both the online questionnaire and the child's oral health assessment. This was adjusted to give a $30 electronic gift card upon completing the online questionnaire and an additional $30 gift card when in-person oral health assessments were completed later after resuming in-person research activities. This change was initiated to motivate remote questionnaire completion while waiting for permission to restart the study in the clinic.

In the PACT trial, participants received cash at WCVs and after completing follow-up questionnaires. The only change made was that the incentive was mailed to the participants instead of distributing in person. After participants signed a mailed receipt, the money was mailed to them. The PACT trial did not have any instances of people reporting not receiving the incentive after mailing.

Staffing Changes

The BEECON trial staff did not change its hours or staffing numbers, although all moved remotely once the stay-at-home was declared. Because in-person visits could not happen, project staff and providers usually responsible for those activities assisted the project manager with designing a drive-thru dental clinic option that was ultimately not implemented.

When the stay-at-home order was initiated in March 2020, some CO-OP staff had to convert computer equipment to allow for effective working at home. This included hooking up computers to TV monitors and purchasing home office supplies like chairs. Before COVID-19, the plan had been for the intervention and research assistant staff positions to end in Spring 2020 as intervention and data collection ended. During the initial months of the pandemic, UIC put a hold on all staffing changes. The extended data window also made it necessary to retain research staff longer. Therefore, employment for five full-time staff continued for many months despite almost no work for them, impacting the study budget.

iSmile had no reduction in its research staff. All study staff and investigators moved to working remotely, in accordance with stay-at-home orders. Research assistants continued working on retention activities and ensuring participants completed questionnaires within their scheduled window. Clinical examiners also helped with retention activities and assisted the project manager with administrative tasks that included activities to increase participant engagement (e.g., creating "activity packets" for children), drafting new clinical procedures to comply with COVID-19 guidelines and assisting with return to research documents. All staff and clinical examiners were necessary for data collection that resumed in September 2020; this delay in timeline and associated staffing costs had significant budget impacts. Reduction in force was avoided due to the lengthy training required to replace research assistants, and that the dental hygienists were already trained and calibrated.

The PACT trial moved all staff to remote and kept them occupied with manuscript writing, checking the electronic health record for missed and upcoming visits, sending questionnaire packages home to participants who were missed at WCVs, and data entry of returned questionnaires. Because in-person data collection resumed at the end of May 2020 staffing was not affected beyond that point.

Other Protocol Changes

BEECON focus groups that were slotted to take place in Fall 2020 were changed to virtual focus groups that had good attendance and participation. iSmile eliminated the option of clinic data collection visits being conducted in the home. The BU IRB also required study staff to read a script about COVID-19 risks to participants.

Domain 4: Scientific Challenges

Challenges With Community-Based Research Ramp-Up

At each of the participating universities, special committees were established early in the pandemic to monitor research safety during COVID-19. All studies had to submit proposals and be approved to resume research operations. These committees prioritized laboratory research. Clinical research was next. Community research was the last group to receive review and approval.

In June, 2020 UCLA approved the ramp up of research operations University wide. The BEECON study was not required to submit a Research Operational Plan to the University because the research activities took place off campus at a community health clinic. The required approval needed to come from the community health clinic, which did not approve resuming clinical visits until October 2020. UCSF created a COVID Community Advisory Board (CCAB) to review community-based research in the San Francisco Bay Area and required the CCAB approve plans to resume research; because BEECON's performance site is in LA, the UCSF CCAB approval was not required.

In June 2020, UIC approved the CO-OP trial for restart with the same safety instructions that applied to clinical and laboratory research. The trial did not resume in-person data collection because the State of Illinois safety orders were clear that everyone should stay at home except for essential activities and the trial leadership determined that study data collection was not essential.

After iSmile submitted to the BU COVID-19 research committee for restart approval, trial leadership was informed that because the study took place in community settings, an additional proposal and protocol also needed to be submitted to the affiliated hospital's research resumption committee. The hospital committee required that the study receive approval from each of the four study sites before granting approval.

However, each site wanted BU approval before granting approval at its site. At GSDM, laboratory and clinical research conducted within the dental school had overarching COVID-19 protocols to customize for its research. iSmile, BU GSDM's only community-based clinical trial, had to develop its own protocols that adhered to protocols from GSDM, the hospital granting the approval and that were tailored to each site's COVID procedures.

For PACT, the State of Ohio and CWRU deemed research as essential and allowed feasible activities to continue. Since the PACT trial was conducted using hospital-based primary care clinics, the study team had to follow hospital system guidelines. When the trial resumed, the study PI had to submit a COVID-19 plan to the CWRU leadership for approval and list study staff who would be going to the community. The hospital IRB also required a COVID-19 plan be submitted before visits could be resumed.

DISCUSSION

The four trials in the ODHC Consortium all experienced challenges in their timelines and staffing due to COVID-19, all of which increased budget expenditures. These pediatric oral health trials were all conducted in community settings. The priority in research restart activities at all the participating institutions was on laboratory restart followed by restart of clinical research. The reasons for this are well-understood. Laboratory research includes substantial investments in animals and specimens with limited lifespans. Also, laboratory research cannot generally be conducted remotely. Clinical research often addresses life-threatening health conditions, necessitating rapid re-opening. While clinical researchers could use the COVID-19 protocols that were developed for the site where the research was operating, community research trials could not easily do the same due to the considerable variation in setting and procedures at each research site. The importance of community research was difficult for the organizations to operationalize and often organizational protocols to guide the return of community research do not exist. The other big difference is the specific risks associated with dental clinical care in the research being conducted by these four trials.

Not all changes caused by COVID-19 were negative. Some studies experienced boosts in retention and remote data collection techniques were implemented. These studies also encountered other unanticipated challenges throughout the pandemic lockdown and return to clinic which would provide helpful lessons learned to other trials navigating the COVID-19 pandemic.

The BEECON study found it difficult to navigate different levels of staff stress and anxiety about returning to clinic. Scheduling fewer participants than usual during the first 2 days at the clinic in an effort to allow the staff to get used to increased cleaning and safety protocols helped to reduce some staff anxiety. Some participants expressed that they were not comfortable returning to clinic due to fear of contracting the virus.

In particular, because many participants lacked their own transportation, they were nervous about taking public transit during the pandemic. BEECON study staff found integrating oral health into overall health was essential, and that Medical/Dental integration was an effective way for children to continue to be able to be screened for caries during routine medical visits that were allowed to occur while clinic research and preventative dental visits were not allowed to occur. The CO-OP study found that while it is feasible for parents to apply disclosing solution to their child's teeth on their own and take adequate images, it was not easy.

The iSmile study were given fewer blocks to schedule participants at clinics. Because of the visit backlog, these blocks filled up quickly which sometimes required that participants were scheduled out-of-window.

Study staff had to be flexible when contacting participants and found that during the lockdown, participants were eager to talk with the research staff, reducing the number of follow up calls that could be made each day.

Both the Research Assistants and clinical examiners had anxiety about returning to the field, however, after the first day in the field, everyone reported feeling better about being able to return to "normal." Return to clinic started slow with a very light participant load. This helped staff gain confidence, and acclimate to cleaning protocols and new clinic protocols. A few participants expressed concern about coming to the clinic, especially when COVID-19 cases began to rise. Some participants were reticent to schedule appointments; however, once an appointment was scheduled, it was more likely to occur than pre-COVID-19. Study staff tried to pair participants' research appointments with their medical appointments, even when out-of-window.

The PACT study experienced several challenges related to staff being sick and having to quarantine for 2 weeks. Some parents delayed WCV visits, but there were no major changes to no-show rates.

Guidance for Future Interruptions in Research

In case of future local/regional emergencies (e.g., blizzards, wild fires), national public health crises (e.g., PPE shortage), or global pandemics, having a plan in place to outline what a halt in research would look like and the steps needed to pivot to virtual/remote research activities would be helpful. Developing specific guidelines and return to research protocols for community research is critical. This could be achieved by having representatives experienced in community-based research involved in the process of intervention development, as some of the trials have done here (6). Having an emergency plan in place would also make IRB modifications easier. In addition, during the developmental stages of a trial, discussing emergency plans with community partners would be helpful so there is a general sense of what research activities will be allowed if the protocols had to change. While this planning would be helpful, there are many variables that could change if another public health crisis or pandemic occurred, such as type of virus, how contagious it is, and how it is transmitted. Having alternative options and scenarios for different situations that might affect trials in the future would be helpful to address these negative conditions. The implementation of telehealth and/or teledentistry in conjunction as a way to continue to be able to carry out clinical research would be a potential aid. Adding these platforms to our set of tools would be very beneficial in an effort to support ongoing and uninterrupted community-based participatory research. Ultimately, being flexible, persistent, and focused on adhering to the science and safety protocols will add consistency and provide alternative options.

Emergency plans need to consider how to best maintain treatment fidelity and internal validity of the study according to NIH guidelines during these crises (8).

AUTHOR CONTRIBUTIONS

All authors listed have made a substantial, direct and intellectual contribution to the work, and approved it for publication.

REFERENCES

1. van Dorn A. COVID-19 and readjusting clinical trials. *Lancet*. (2020) 396:523–4. doi: 10.1016/S0140-6736(20)31787-6
2. Sathian B, Asim M, Banerjee I, Pizarro AB, Roy B, van Teijlingen ER, et al. Impact of COVID-19 on clinical trials and clinical research: a systematic review. *Nepal J Epidemiol.* (2020) 10:878–87. doi: 10.3126/nje.v10i3.31622
3. Tuttle KR. Impact of the COVID-19 pandemic on clinical research. *Nat Rev Nephrol.* (2020) 16:562–4. doi: 10.1038/s41581-020-00336-9
4. Ramos-Gomez F, White JS, Lindau HE, Lin TK, Finlayson TL, Liu JX, et al. Family monetary incentives as a value-based care model for oral hygiene: rationale and design of the behavioral economics for oral health innovation (BEECON) trial. *J Public Health Dent.* (2020) 80:S17–26. doi: 10.1111/jphd.12406
5. Martin MA, Zimmerman LJ, Rosales GF, Lee HH, Songthangtham N, Pugach O, et al. Design and sample characteristics of coordinated oral health promotion (CO-OP) Chicago: a cluster-randomized controlled trial. *Contemp Clin Trials.* (2020) 92:105919. doi: 10.1016/j.cct.2019.105919

6. Borrelli B, Henshaw M, Endrighi R, Adams WG, Heeren T, Rosen RK, et al. An interactive parent-targeted text messaging intervention to improve oral health in children attending urban pediatric clinics: feasibility randomized controlled trial. *JMIR MHealth UHealth.* (2019) 7:e14247. doi: 10.2196/14247
7. Nelson S, Slusar MB, Curtan S, Selvaraj D, Hertz A. Formative and pilot study for an effectiveness-implementation hybrid cluster randomized trial to incorporate oral health activities into pediatric well-child visits. *Dent J.* (2020) 8:101. doi: 10.3390/dj8030101
8. Borrelli B. The assessment, monitoring, and enhancement of treatment fidelity in public health clinical trials. *J Public Health Dent.* (2011) 71:S52–63. doi: 10.1111/j.1752-7325.2011.00233.x

Permissions

All chapters in this book were first published by Frontiers; hereby published with permission under the Creative Commons Attribution License or equivalent. Every chapter published in this book has been scrutinized by our experts. Their significance has been extensively debated. The topics covered herein carry significant findings which will fuel the growth of the discipline. They may even be implemented as practical applications or may be referred to as a beginning point for another development.

The contributors of this book come from diverse backgrounds, making this book a truly international effort. This book will bring forth new frontiers with its revolutionizing research information and detailed analysis of the nascent developments around the world.

We would like to thank all the contributing authors for lending their expertise to make the book truly unique. They have played a crucial role in the development of this book. Without their invaluable contributions this book wouldn't have been possible. They have made vital efforts to compile up to date information on the varied aspects of this subject to make this book a valuable addition to the collection of many professionals and students.

This book was conceptualized with the vision of imparting up-to-date information and advanced data in this field. To ensure the same, a matchless editorial board was set up. Every individual on the board went through rigorous rounds of assessment to prove their worth. After which they invested a large part of their time researching and compiling the most relevant data for our readers.

The editorial board has been involved in producing this book since its inception. They have spent rigorous hours researching and exploring the diverse topics which have resulted in the successful publishing of this book. They have passed on their knowledge of decades through this book. To expedite this challenging task, the publisher supported the team at every step. A small team of assistant editors was also appointed to further simplify the editing procedure and attain best results for the readers.

Apart from the editorial board, the designing team has also invested a significant amount of their time in understanding the subject and creating the most relevant covers. They scrutinized every image to scout for the most suitable representation of the subject and create an appropriate cover for the book.

The publishing team has been an ardent support to the editorial, designing and production team. Their endless efforts to recruit the best for this project, has resulted in the accomplishment of this book. They are a veteran in the field of academics and their pool of knowledge is as vast as their experience in printing. Their expertise and guidance has proved useful at every step. Their uncompromising quality standards have made this book an exceptional effort. Their encouragement from time to time has been an inspiration for everyone.

The publisher and the editorial board hope that this book will prove to be a valuable piece of knowledge for researchers, students, practitioners and scholars across the globe.

List of Contributors

Stefan Serban
School of Dentistry, University of Leeds, Leeds, United Kingdom
Public Health England, North East and Yorkshire Regional Office, Leeds, United Kingdom

Zhain Mustufvi and Gail Douglas
School of Dentistry, University of Leeds, Leeds, United Kingdom

Sally Eapen Simon and Siobhan Grant
Public Health England, North East and Yorkshire Regional Office, Leeds, United Kingdom

Feiyang Guo, Bojun Tang and Tingting Zhao
Department of Orthodontics, Hubei-MOST KLOS & KLOBM, School & Hospital of Stomatology, Wuhan University, Wuhan, China

Eugenio Beltrán-Aguilar
Department Epidemiology and Health Promotion, World Health Organization Collaborating Center Quality Improvement and Evidence-Based Dentistry, College of Dentistry, New York University, New York, United States

Habib Benzian
Department Epidemiology and Health Promotion, World Health Organization Collaborating Center Quality Improvement and Evidence-Based Dentistry, College of Dentistry, New York University, New York, United States
Global Health Center, Geneva Graduate Institute for Policy Studies, Geneva, Switzerland

Li Li, Mianyan Zeng, Xiao Chen, Shuman Cai, Cuixia Xu, Wei Xia, Lijun Jiang, Xiaoyan Zou, Pei Chen and Mingdeng Rong
Department of Periodontology and Oral Implantology, Stomatological Hospital, Southern Medical University, Guangzhou, China

Zhen Li, Yuhong Li, Han Jiang, Chenzheng Zhang and Minquan Du
The State Key Laboratory Breeding Base of Basic Science of Stomatology (Hubei-MOST) & Key Laboratory of Oral Biomedicine Ministry of Education, School and Hospital of Stomatology, Wuhan University, Wuhan, China

Shenuka Singh
Discipline of Dentistry, School of Health Sciences, University of KwaZulu-Natal (UKZN), Durban, South Africa

Danchen Qin, Jiarong Yan and Hong He
Department of Orthodontics, Hubei-MOST KLOS & KLOBM, School & Hospital of Stomatology, Wuhan University, Wuhan, China

Fang Hua
Department of Orthodontics, Hubei-MOST KLOS & KLOBM, School & Hospital of Stomatology, Wuhan University, Wuhan, China
Center for Evidence-Based Stomatology, Hubei-MOST KLOS & KLOBM, School & Hospital of Stomatology, Wuhan University, Wuhan, China
Division of Dentistry, Faculty of Biology, Medicine and Health, Manchester Academic Health Science Centre, School of Medical Sciences, University of Manchester, Manchester, United Kingdom

Mei Zhong, Bingpeng Lin, Xinhong Wang, Kaibin Wu, Mingxiao Liu, Jian-ming Chen and Jiangyong Huang
Guangzhou Key Laboratory of Basic and Applied Research of Oral Regenerative Medicine, Affiliated Stomatology Hospital of Guangzhou Medical University, Guangzhou, China

Janak L. Pathak and Linhu Ge
Guangzhou Key Laboratory of Basic and Applied Research of Oral Regenerative Medicine, Affiliated Stomatology Hospital of Guangzhou Medical University, Guangzhou, China
Institute of Oral Disease, Guangzhou Medical University, Guangzhou, China

Hongbin Gao
Key Laboratory of Guangdong Laboratory Animals, Guangdong Laboratory Animals Monitoring Institute, Guangzhou, China

Andrew J. Young
Columbus Inpatient Care, Grove City, OH, United States

Chang Liu
Stomatology School of Ji'nan University, Guangzhou, China
The State Key Laboratory Breeding Base of Basic Science of Stomatology (Hubei-MOST) & Key Laboratory of Oral Biomedicine Ministry of Education, School and Hospital of Stomatology, Wuhan University, Wuhan, China

Learn-Han Lee
Novel Bacteria and Drug Discovery Research Group (NBDD), Microbiome and Bioresource Research Strength (MBRS), Jeffrey Cheah School of Medicine and Health Sciences, Monash University Malaysia, Bandar Sunway, Malaysia

Cui-ling Qi
School of Life Science and Biopharmaceutics, Vascular Biology Research Institute, Guangdong Pharmaceutical University, Guangzhou, China

Lijing Wang
Guangzhou Key Laboratory of Basic and Applied Research of Oral Regenerative Medicine, Affiliated Stomatology Hospital of Guangzhou Medical University, Guangzhou, China
School of Life Science and Biopharmaceutics, Vascular Biology Research Institute, Guangdong Pharmaceutical University, Guangzhou, China

Devi Sewvandini Atukorallaya and Ravindra K. Ratnayake
Department of Oral Biology, Dr. Gerald Niznick College of Dentistry, Rady Faculty of Health Sciences, University of Manitoba, Winnipeg, MB, Canada

Sami Aldhuwayhi, Saquib Ahmed Shaikh, Amar Ashok Thakare and Mohammed Ziauddeen Mustafa
Department of Prosthodontics, College of Dentistry, Majmaah University, Al-Majmaah, Saudi Arabia

Sreekanth Kumar Mallineni
Department of Preventive Dental Science, College of Dentistry, Majmaah University, Al-Majmaah, Saudi Arabia
Department of Pediatric and Preventive Dentistry, Saveetha Dental College and Hospital, Saveetha Institute of Medical and Technical Science, Saveetha University, Chennai, India

Matthew Wen Jian Lau
National Dental Research Institute Singapore, National Dental Centre Singapore, Singapore

Bee Tin Goh
National Dental Research Institute Singapore, National Dental Centre Singapore, Singapore
Duke-NUS Graduate Medical School, Singapore, Singapore

Chaminda Jayampath Seneviratne
Oral Health Academic Clinical Programme, Duke-NUS Medical School, Singapore
National Dental Research Institute Singapore, National Dental Centre Singapore, Singapore
Duke-NUS Graduate Medical School, Singapore, Singapore

Giusy Rita Maria La Rosa, Rocco De Pasquale, Sebastiano Ferlito and Eugenio Pedullà
Department of General Surgery and Medical-Surgical Specialties, University of Catania, Catania, Italy

Massimo Libra
Department of Biomedical and Biotechnological Sciences, Oncologic, Clinic and General Pathology Section, University of Catania, Catania, Italy

Colman McGrath
Faculty of Dentistry, Universiti Kebangsaan Malaysia (The National University of Malaysia), Kuala Lumpur, Malaysia
Faculty of Dentistry, The University of Hong Kong, Sai Ying Pun, Hong Kong
Applied Oral Sciences & Community Dental Care, Faculty of Dentistry, The University of Hong Kong, Hong Kong, China

Shahida Mohd-Said, Tuti Ningseh Mohd-Dom, Nawal Suhaimi and Haslina Rani
Faculty of Dentistry, Universiti Kebangsaan Malaysia (The National University of Malaysia), Kuala Lumpur, Malaysia

Aneta Olszewska
Department of Developmental Facial Malformation, Poznan University of Medical Sciences, Poznań, Poland

Elzbieta Paszynska
Department of Integrated Dentistry, Community Dentistry Section, Poznan University of Medical Sciences, Poznań, Poland

Magdalena Roszak
Department of Computer Science and Statistics, Poznan University of Medical Sciences, Poznań, Poland

Agata Czajka-Jakubowska
Department of Temporomandibular Joint Disorders, Poznan University of Medical Sciences, Poznań, Poland

John Rong Hao Tay and Ethan Ng
Department of Restorative Dentistry, National Dental Centre Singapore, Singapore

Ken Tan
Oral Health Academic Clinical Programme, Duke-NUS Medical School, Singapore

Marianne Meng Ann Ong
Department of Restorative Dentistry, National Dental Centre Singapore, Singapore
Oral Health Academic Clinical Programme, Duke-NUS Medical School, Singapore, Singapore

Chelsia Sim
Department of Oral and Maxillofacial Surgery, National Dental Centre Singapore, Singapore

Basim Almulhim, Abdullah Alassaf and Sara Alghamdi
Department of Preventive Dental Science, College of Dentistry, Majmaah University, Al-Majmaah, Saudi Arabia

Riyadh Alroomy
Department of Restorative Dental Sciences, College of Dentistry, Majmaah University, Al-Majmaah, Saudi Arabia

Abdullah Aljabr
Department of Medical Education, College of Dentistry, Majmaah University, Al-Majmaah, Saudi Arabia

Fang Yu, Bohao Cheng, Ziqing Zhu, Sheng Liao, Yu Chen and Fang Wang
Department of Endocrinology, The Third Xiangya Hospital of Central South University, Changsha, China

Haojun Yang
Department of Endocrinology, The Third Xiangya Hospital of Central South University, Changsha, China
Department of Neurology, Xiangya Hospital of Central South University, Changsha, China

Yue Zheng
West China School of Medicine, Sichuan University, Chengdu, China

Jianzhen Wu
The Third Xiangya Hospital of Central South University, Changsha, China

Richard Niederman
WHO Collaborating Center Quality Improvement & Evidence-Based Dentistry, Department Epidemiology & Health Promotion, College of Dentistry, New York University, New York, United States

Harriet Larvin
School of Dentistry, University of Leeds, Leeds, United Kingdom

Sheryl Wilmott
Leeds Dental Institute, Leeds Teaching Hospitals Trust, Leeds, United Kingdom

Jianhua Wu
School of Dentistry, University of Leeds, Leeds, United Kingdom
Leeds Institute for Data Analytics, University of Leeds, Leeds, United Kingdom

Jing Kang
Oral Biology, School of Dentistry, University of Leeds, Leeds, United Kingdom

Jingya Jane Pu, Yiu Yan Leung, Wing Shan Choi, Wei-fa Yang, Kar Yan Li and Yu-xiong Su
Division of Oral and Maxillofacial Surgery, Faculty of Dentistry, The University of Hong Kong, Pokfulam, Hong Kong

Colman Patrick McGrath
Division of Applied Oral Sciences and Community Dental Care, Faculty of Dentistry, The University of Hong Kong, Pokfulam, Hong Kong

Anas F. Mahdee
Department of Restorative and Aesthetic Dentistry, College of Dentistry, University of Baghdad, Baghdad, Iraq

Sarhang S. Gul
Department of Periodontics, College of Dentistry, University of Sulaimani, Sulaimani, Iraq

Ali A. Abdulkareem
Department of Periodontics, College of Dentistry, University of Baghdad, Baghdad, Iraq

Syed Saad B. Qasim
Department of Bioclinical Sciences, Faculty of Dentistry, Kuwait University, Safat, Kuwait

Armelia Sari Widyarman
Department of Microbiology, Faculty of Dentistry, Trisakti University, Jakarta, Indonesia

Endang W. Bachtiar, Citra Fragrantia Theodorea and Boy M. Bachtiar
Department of Oral Biology, Faculty of Dentistry, Universitas Indonesia, Depok, Indonesia

M. Ihsan Rizal, M. Orliando Roeslan, Melanie S. Djamil and Didi N. Santosa
Department of Oral Biology, Faculty of Dentistry, Trisakti University, Jakarta, Indonesia

Mohamed G. Hassan
Department of Orthodontics, Faculty of Oral and Dental Medicine, South Valley University, Qena, Egypt
Department of Orthodontics, Faculty of Dentistry, October 6 University, Giza, Egypt

Hala Amer
Department of Pediatric Dentistry and Dental Public Health, Faculty of Dentistry, Alexandria University, Alexandria, Egypt

Syeda Afshan Manzoor
Department of Operative Dentistry & Endodontics, Bakhtawar Amin Medical & Dental College, Multan, Pakistan

Abdul-Hakeem Alomari
Biomedical Engineering Department, College of Engineering, Imam Abdulrahman Bin Faisal University (IAU), Dammam, Saudi Arabia

Mousumi Goswami, Tanu Nangia, Aditya Saxena, Sakshi Chawla, Anam Mushtaq and Palak Jain
I.T.S Dental College, Hospital and Research Centre, Noida, India

Shrey R. Singh
School of Medical Science and Research, Sharda University, Noida, India

Bhojraj Nandlal and Birti Singh
Department of Pediatric and Preventive Dentistry, Jagadguru Sri Shivarathreeshwara Dental College and Hospital, Jagadguru Sri Shivarathreeshwara Academy of Higher Education and Research, Mysuru, India

Arun Gopi
Department of Community Medicine, Jagadguru Sri Shivarathreeshwara Medical College and Hospital, Jagadguru Sri Shivarathreeshwara Academy of Higher Education and Research, Mysuru, India

Helen E. Lindau
Department of Pediatric Dentistry, University of California, Los Angeles, Los Angeles, CA, United States

Francisco J. Ramos-Gomez
Department of Pediatric Dentistry, University of California, Los Angeles, Los Angeles, CA, United States
Center to Address Disparities in Children's Oral Health (CAN DO), University of California, San Francisco, San Francisco, CA, United States

Anna S. Sandoval and Molly A. Martin
Institute for Health Research and Policy, University of Illinois Chicago, Chicago, IL, United States

Suchitra S. Nelson and Shelley Curtan
Department of Community Dentistry, Case Western Reserve University, Cleveland, OH, United States

Belinda Borrelli and Nicolle Rueras
Center for Behavioral Sciences Research, Henry M. Goldman School of Dental Medicine, Boston University, Boston, MA, United States

Michelle M. Henshaw
Global and Population Health, Henry M. Goldman School of Dental Medicine, Boston University, Boston, MA, United States

Stuart A. Gansky
Center to Address Disparities in Children's Oral Health (CAN DO), University of California, San Francisco, San Francisco, CA, United States
School of Dentistry, University of California, San Francisco, San Francisco, CA, United States

Index

www.ingramcontent.com/pod-product-compliance
Lightning Source LLC
LaVergne TN
LVHW060547210926
848485LV00005B/1269
* 9 7 8 1 6 4 6 4 7 5 5 7 5 *